Endodontic Irrigation

Bettina Basrani
Editor

Endodontic Irrigation

Chemical Disinfection of the Root Canal System

Springer

Editor
Bettina Basrani
Department of Dentistry
University of Toronto
Toronto
Canada

ISBN 978-3-319-37126-9 ISBN 978-3-319-16456-4 (eBook)
DOI 10.1007/978-3-319-16456-4

Springer Cham Heidelberg New York Dordrecht London

Softcover reprint of the hardcover 1st edition 2015

Printed on acid-free paper

Springer International Publishing AG Switzerland is part of Springer Science+Business Media (www.springer.com)

This book is dedicated:

To my father, Enrique, for leaving his fingerprints of endodontic passion in my life
To my mother, Clarita, and mother-in-law, Enid, for being my dearest and most unconditional fans
To my husband, Howard, for helping me, every day, in becoming a better person
To my children, Jonathan and Daniel, for teaching me what life is really about
To my coworkers, Shimon, Cal, Anil, Andres, Gevik, and Pavel, for being my second family
Finally, to my students for making me a better teacher

Foreword

Apical periodontitis is an infectious disease related to the presence of microorganisms in the root canal system of teeth. Its treatment therefore must be directed at eliminating or, at the very least, reducing the infecting microbiota, to levels that allow healing to occur. Advances in microbiology have identified the nature and complexity of the infecting microbiota and the ability of some of its members to collectively survive under the harshest of conditions. The treatment of apical periodontitis has historically been based upon two pillars, the mechanical removal of necrotic tissue and microorganisms from the root canal system and the irrigation of the root canal system with chemical agents, to supplement removal of tissue and microorganisms from areas of the system that were mechanically prepared, as well as address the presence of tissue and microorganisms at sites in the system that mechanical preparation could not reach. Research has shown that despite the nature and design of the instruments used in the mechanical preparation of the system, significant reduction in the concentrations of tissue and microorganisms in complex root canal systems can only be achieved when irrigation of the system is an integral part of the treatment undertaken. Over the years, different irrigants have been used in endodontic treatment, but only one, sodium hypochlorite, has proven itself to be consistently effective. Its effectiveness is a product of its concentration and the manner in which it is introduced into the root canal system. Because of the toxic nature of sodium hypochlorite, both of these factors pose a potential risk to the patient if tissues surrounding the tooth are inadvertently exposed to the agent during use.

In this textbook, Dr. Basrani, a noted authority in root canal irrigation, has recruited a panel of prominent authors to discuss the merits, limitations, and safety of the various sodium hypochlorite delivery systems currently being used in endodontic treatment. Some attention is also paid to the influence that mechanical root canal preparation has in impeding or promoting their therapeutic effect. With an eye to the future, Dr. Basrani has also included chapters concerned with evolving technologies in the field of supplemental root canal disinfection, technologies that have shown promise in avoiding the potential risks associated with sodium hypochlorite use, while achieving and, in some instances, exceeding sodium hypochlorite's effectiveness in tissue and microbial reduction.

In view of the importance of irrigation of the root canal system in its broadest form, to the outcome of endodontic treatment, this textbook is a must-read for all clinicians who include endodontics as an integral part of their dental practice.

Toronto, ON, Canada Calvin D. Torneck, DDS, MS, FRCD(C)

Preface

When I was invited by Springer International Publishing to edit a book in irrigation, I felt like a dream came true. I have been working on endodontic irrigation for close to 20 years. While doing my PhD at Maimonides University in Buenos Aires, Argentina, I was invited work with a periodontist, Dr. Piovano, and microbiologist, Dr. Marcantoni, who became my initial mentors. After a couple of meetings together, we recognized how much periodontics and endodontics have in common: (a) similar etiological factor of the diseases (bacterial /biofilm related causes), (b) similar treatments (both disciplines mechanically clean the tooth surface either with curettes or endodontic files), and (c) both chemically disinfect the surface (medicaments and irrigants). However, the big difference is that, as endodontists, we seal the canal as tridimensionally as possible, while in periodontal treatment this step is difficult to achieve.

When we recognized the similarity in the procedure, we started to analyze the medicaments that periodontal therapy applied, and chlorhexidine (CHX) was the "new" topical drug at that time. We wondered: if CHX is used for periodontics, why not for endodontics? This is how my irrigation pathway began in 1995, and that path opened to new amazing and unexpected routes. I was able to complete my PhD and published in vitro papers on the use of CHX as an intracanal medicament and other papers on the mixture of CHX with calcium hydroxide with my new supervisors Dr. Tjadehane and Dr. Canete. Finally, this motivation and interest in irrigation research brought me to Canada to continue this line of investigation with the research group at the University of Toronto, under the wise guidance of Dr. Shimon Friedman and Dr. Calvin Torneck and the inquisitive minds of the residents who went through our program. Today, the disinfection research is reaching for new horizons with the leading research of Dr. Anil Kishen and his lab. I am so proud of being part of such a prestigious group of researchers and remarkable group of human beings.

Chemical disinfection of the root canal system is now the bread and butter of modern endodontic therapy. Even though we have new and sophisticated file systems in the market, the key to endodontic success is based on chemical disinfection. This book is intended to convey the most recent challenges and advances in cleaning the root canal. We start by analyzing the main etiological factors of apical periodontitis in Chapter 1, and Dr. Luis Chaves de Paz explains the importance of the biofilms in causing endodontic diseases. In Chapter 2 Dr. Marco A. Versiani, Jesus D. Pécora, and Manoel D. Sousa-Neto, with distinctive studies on microCT, explain dental anatomy in great detail. In Chapter 3 on irrigation dynamics was written by Dr. Christos Boutsioukis and Lucas W.M. van der Sluis explained in detail why the irrigants do not reach the apical part of the canal and what we can do to improve irrigation dynamics. For the more academic-oriented readers, we have Chapter 4 Drs. Shen Y, Gao Y, Lin J, Ma J, Wang Z, and Haapasalo M described different methods on studying irrigation. In Chapter 5, Dr. Gevik Malkhassian and I put together the most common irrigant solutions used in endodontics along with the pros and cons of their use. Chapter 6 Dr Gary Glassman describes accidents and mishaps during irrigation. We then have Dr Jorge Vera in Chapter 7 describing how patency file may (or may not) affect irrigation efficacy Chapters 8 to 14 are dedicated to each irrigation technique written by experts in each of these fields: Dr. Pierre Matchou for manual dynamic technique, Drs. Gary Glassman and Karine Charara for apical negative pressure, Dr. John Nusstein for sonic and ultrasonics, Drs. Zvi Metzger and Anda Kfir for SAF, Drs. Amir Azarpahazoo and Zahed Mohammadi for ozone, Dr. David Jaramillo for PIPS, and Dr. Anil Kishen and Anie Shersta for photo activation disinfection. Two chapters are dedicated to inter-appointment therapy, with Dr. Zahed Mohammadi and Dr. Paul Abbott (Chap. 15) describing the use of antibiotics in endodontics and Professor José F. Siqueira Jr and Isabela N. Rôças describing the details on intracanal medications (Chap. 16).

Two chapters are dedicated to modern and current points of interest, Chap. 17 on irrigation in the era of re-treatment written by Dr. Rodrigo Sanches Cunha and Dr. Carlos Eduardo da Silveira Bueno and Chap.18 on irrigation in the era of revascularization by Dr. Anibal R. Diogenes and Nikita B. Ruparel.

The vision of this book would never have been possible without the dedication and hard work of this astounding team of scientists with such different backgrounds but with the same enthusiasm for endodontic disinfection. The collaborators of this textbook are bringing their expertise and knowledge from Brazil, Iran, Peru, Mexico, Canada, Australia, USA, Israel, France, Greece, and Holland. To all of them, to my coauthors, thank you!

Toronto, ON, Canada Bettina Basrani

Acknowledgments

I would like to start by thanking Springer International Publishing for giving me the wonderful opportunity of editing a textbook on chemical disinfection of the root canal system. I appreciate the trust, patience, and knowledge they demonstrated throughout the whole process. I also want to thank Dean Haas, Faculty of Dentistry, University of Toronto, for granting me the 6-month sabbatical to focus on this project, and I have a deep appreciation to the whole endodontic department of the faculty of dentistry for their motivation and constant support. Special thanks to Warrena Wilkinson for editing some of the chapters and Dr. Calvin Torneck for the thoughtful writing of the preface.

Gratitude goes to the collaborators of this book. It was a great pleasure to invite you to participate in this project, and your motivated and enthusiastic responses were always encouraging. Thanks for your expertise and dedication.

Finally, I want to recognize my family. I have to start by thanking my father, Professor Emeritus Dr. Enrique Basrani, for showing me what a life of an endodontist looks like. He lived in Buenos Aires, Argentina, and divided his time between academics and clinical practice, while he wrote six textbooks in endodontics, finishing his last one on his death bed. He never stopped working. I should say: he never stopped doing what he loved. Now, as I follow in his steps, dividing my own time between academics and clinical practice, and feel him guiding me in spirit in all that I do. Secondly, I want to thank my mother, Clarita, and mother-in-law, Enid Alter for listening and understanding when sometimes I think that life is overpowering. My brother Dr. Damian Basrani and his family always have a special place in my heart. Howard, my beloved and precious husband, thanks for being there for me, always. Without your presence in my life, I would not be able to be the person that I am today. And to my beautiful children, Jonathan and Daniel, for being as enthusiastic as I am in everything they do.

I want to conclude by thanking all my students, from the undergraduate to graduate program and participants in lectures and workshops. You are the ones who make us better teachers, the ones who challenge us, who inspire us to give our best, and the ones who I also dedicate this book to.

Contents

Contributors

Paul V. Abbott, BDSc, MDS, FRACDS(Endo), FIADT Department of Endodontics, School of Dentistry, The University of Western Australia, Nedlands, WA, Australia

Amir Azarpazhooh, DDS, MSc, PhD, FRCD(C) Division of Endodontics, Department of Dentistry, and Clinician Scientist, Lunenfeld-Tanenbaum Research Institute, Mount Sinai Hospital, Toronto, ON, Canada

Dental Public Health and Endodontics, Faculty of Dentistry, University of Toronto, Toronto, ON, Canada

Bettina Basrani, DDS, MSc, RCDC (F), PhD Associate Professor, Director M.Sc. Endodontics Program, Faculty of Dentistry, University of Toronto, Toronto, ON, Canada

Christos Boutsioukis, DDS, MSc, PhD Department of Endodontology, Academic Centre for Dentistry Amsterdam (ACTA), Amsterdam, The Netherlands

Karine Charara, DMD Adjunct Professor of Dentistry, Université de Montréal, Montréal, QC, Canada

Private Practice, Clinique Endodontique Mont-Royal, Mont-Royal, QC, Canada

Rodrigo Sanches Cunha, DDS, MSc, PhD, FRCD(C) Department Restorative Dentistry, Faculty of Health Sciences, College of Dentistry, University of Manitoba, Winnipeg, MB, Canada

Luis E. Chávez de Paz, DDS, MS, PhD Endodontics, The Swedish Academy for Advanced Clinical Dentistry, Gothenburg, Sweden

Carlos Eduardo da Silveira Bueno, DDS, MSc, PhD Faculty of Dentistry, São Leopoldo Mandic Centre for Dental Research, Campinas, SP, Brazil

Anibal R. Diogenes, DDS, MS, PhD Department of Endodontics, University of Texas Health Center at San Antonio, San Antonio, TX, USA

Yuan Gao, DDS, PhD Department of Endodontics and Operative Dentistry, West China Stomatological College and Hospital Sichuan University, Chengdu, P.R. China

Gary Glassman, DDS, FRCD(C) Associate in Dentistry, Graduate, Department of Endodontics, Faculty of Dentistry, University of Toronto, Toronto, ON, Canada

Adjunct Professor of Dentistry, University of Technology, Kingston, Jamaica

Private Practice, Endodontic Specialists, Toronto, ON, Canada

Markus Haapasalo, DDS, PhD Division of Endodontics, Department of Oral Biological and Medical Sciences, Faculty of Dentistry, University of British Columbia, Vancouver, BC, Canada

David E. Jaramillo, DDS Department of Endodontics, University of Texas Health Science Center at Houston, School of Dentistry, Houston, TX, USA

Anda Kfir, DMD Department of Endodontology, The Goldschlager School of Dental Medicine, Tel Aviv University, Tel Aviv, Israel

Anil Kishen, PhD, MDS, BDS Department of Endodontics, Facility of Dentistry, University of Toronto, Toronto, ON, Canada

James Lin, DDS, MSc, FRCD(C) Division of Endodontics, Department of Oral Biological and Medical Sciences, Faculty of Dentistry, University of British Columbia, Vancouver, BC, Canada

Jingzhi Ma, DDS, PhD Department of Stomatology, Tongji Hospital, Tongji Medical College, Huazhong University of Science and Technology, Wuhan, P.R. China

Pierre Machtou, DDS, MS, PhD Endodontie, UFR d'Odontologie Paris 7-Denis Diderot, Paris Ile de France, France

Gevik Malkhassian, DDS, MSc, FRCD(C) Assistant Professor, Discipline of Endodontics, Faculty of Dentistry, University of Toronto, Toronto, ON, Canada

Zvi Metzger, DMD Department of Endodontology, The Goldschlager School of Dental Medicine, Tel Aviv University, Tel Aviv, Israel

Zahed Mohammadi, DMD, MSD Iranian Center for Endodontic Research (ICER), Research Institute of Dental Sciences, Shahid Beheshti University of Medical Sciences, Tehran, Iran

John M. Nusstein, DDS, MS Division of Endodontics, The Ohio State University College of Dentistry, Columbus, OH, USA

Jesus D. Pécora, DDS, MSc, PhD Department of Restorative Dentistry, Dental School of Ribeirao Preto, University of Sao Paulo, Ribeirao Preto, Brazil

Isabella N. Rôças, DDS, MSc, PhD PostGraduate Program in Endodontics and Molecular Microbiology Laboratory, Faculty of Dentistry, Estácio de Sá University, Rio de Janeiro, RJ, Brazil

Nikita B. Ruparel, MS, DDS, PhD Department of Endodontics, University of Texas Health Center at San Antonio, San Antonio, TX, USA

Ya Shen, DDS, PhD Division of Endodontics, Department of Oral Biological and Medical Sciences, Faculty of Dentistry, University of British Columbia, Vancouver, BC, Canada

Annie Shrestha, PhD, MSc, BDS Faculty of Dentistry, Department of Endodontics, University of Toronto, Toronto, ON, Canada

José F. Siqueira Jr., DDS, MSc, PhD PostGraduate Program in Endodontics, Faculty of Dentistry, Estácio de Sá University, Rio de Janeiro, RJ, Brazil

Lucas W.M. van der Sluis, DDS, PhD Department of Conservative Dentistry, University Medical Center Groningen, Groningen, The Netherlands

Manoel D. Sousa-Neto, DDS, MSc, PhD Department of Restorative Dentistry, Dental School of Ribeirao Preto, University of Sao Paulo, Ribeirao Preto, Brazil

Jorge Vera, DDS Department of Endodontics, University of Tlaxcala Mexico, Puebla, Puebla, Mexico

Marco A. Versiani, DDS, MSc, PhD Department of Restorative Dentistry, Dental School of Ribeirao Preto, University of Sao Paulo, Ribeirao Preto, SP, Brazil

Zhejun Wang, DDS, PhD Division of Endodontics, Department of Oral Biological and Medical Sciences, Faculty of Dentistry, University of British Columbia, Vancouver, BC, Canada

Microbial Biofilms in Endodontics

1

Luis E. Chávez de Paz

Abstract

Microorganisms colonizing different sites in humans have been found to grow predominantly in complex structures known as biofilms. Biofilms are dynamic systems with attributes of both primordial multicellular organisms and represent a protected mode of growth that allows cells to survive. The initial stage of biofilm formation includes the attachment of bacteria to the substratum. Bacterial growth and division then leads to the colonization of the surrounding area and the maturation of the biofilm. The environment in a biofilm is not homogeneous; the bacteria in multispecies biofilms are not randomly distributed, but rather are organized to best meet their requirements. The implications of this mode of microbial growth in the context of endodontic infections are discussed in this chapter. Although there is an initial understanding on the mechanisms of biofilm formation in root canals and its associated resistance to clinical antimicrobial regimens, this topic is still under investigation. A greater understanding of biofilm processes should lead to novel, effective control strategies for endodontic biofilm control and a resulting improvement in patient management.

Introduction

In nature, bacteria are able to live either as independent free-floating cells (planktonic state) or as members of organized surface-attached microbial communities called biofilms. Biofilms are composed of microorganisms that are embedded in a self-produced extracellular matrix which bind cells together [17, 18, 30]. Biofilms have major clinical relevance as they provide bacteria with protective environments against stresses, immune responses, antibacterial agents, and antibiotics [31, 33]. After several decades of intense research, it is now well established that biofilm formation is a developmental process that begins when a cell attaches to a surface and it is strictly regulated in response to environmental conditions [33].

L.E. Chávez de Paz, DDS, MS, PhD
Endodontics, The Swedish Academy for Advanced Clinical Dentistry, Gothenburg, Sweden
e-mail: luis.chavez.de.paz@gmail.com

B. Basrani (ed.), *Endodontic Irrigation: Chemical Disinfection of the Root Canal System*,
DOI 10.1007/978-3-319-16456-4_1

One of the most relevant features of oral bacteria is their intrinsic ability to continuously form complex biofilm communities, also known as dental plaque. Oral biofilm formation serves not only to aid in retention of bacteria in the oral cavity, but also results in their increased survival [34, 35]. In root canals of teeth, biofilms have been confirmed by examinations of extracted teeth with periapical lesions [71]. For example, when sections were viewed by transmission electron microscopy, dense aggregates of cocci and rods embedded in an extracellular matrix were observed along the walls [61], while studies using scanning electron microscopy have shown microcolonies of cocci, rods, and filaments on root canal walls [59, 74, 83]. The biofilm mode of growth contributes to resistance to host defenses, and within the biofilm, there are formed subpopulations of cells that are phenotypically highly resistant to antibiotics and biocides [13, 16, 24, 46]. Although there is no generally agreed upon mechanism to account for this broad resistance to antimicrobials, the extent of the problem in endodontics is considerable.

Formation of Microbial Biofilms

Formation of a bacterial biofilm is a developmental process that begins when a cell attaches to a surface. The formation of microbial biofilms includes several steps that can be divided in two main parts: (a) the initial interactions of cells with the substrate and (b) growth and development of the biofilm (see Figs. 1.1 and 1.2).

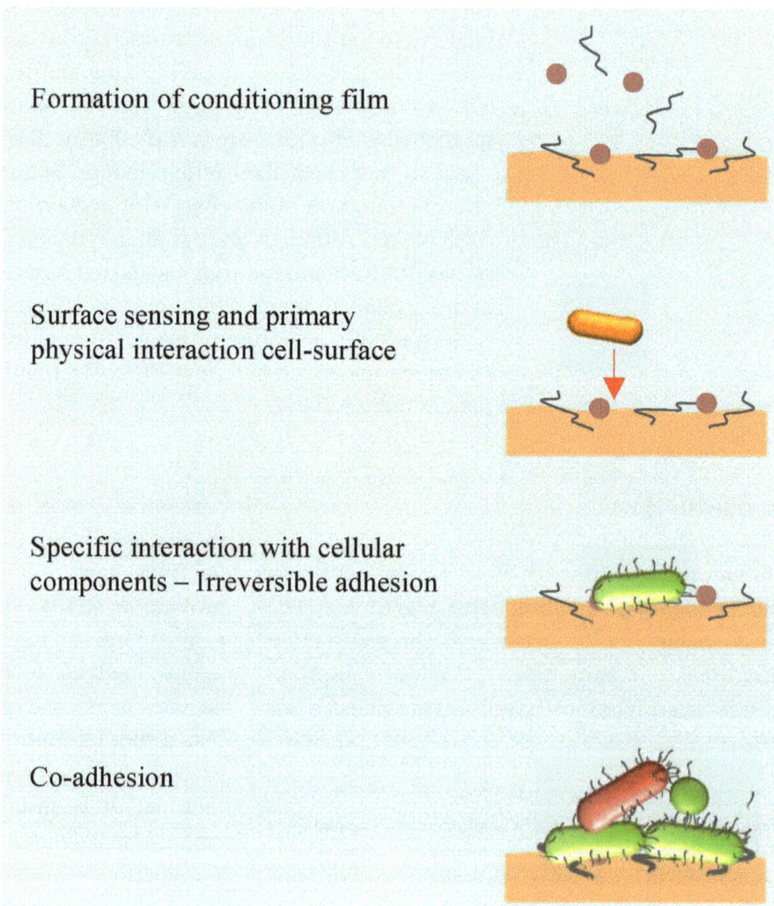

Fig. 1.1 Initial stages of biofilm formation. Schematic outlining the general approaches of initial cellular interaction of planktonic cells with coated substrates. In the initial phase, a "clean" surface is coated with environmental elements. At the second stage, a planktonic cell that approaches the coated surface initiates adhesion by adjusting a number of regulatory mechanisms known as surface sensing. In the following stage, irreversible adhesion occurs by association of specific cell components such as pili, flagella, exopolymers, etc. Lastly, co-adhesion with other organisms is achieved by specific interspecies interactive mechanisms

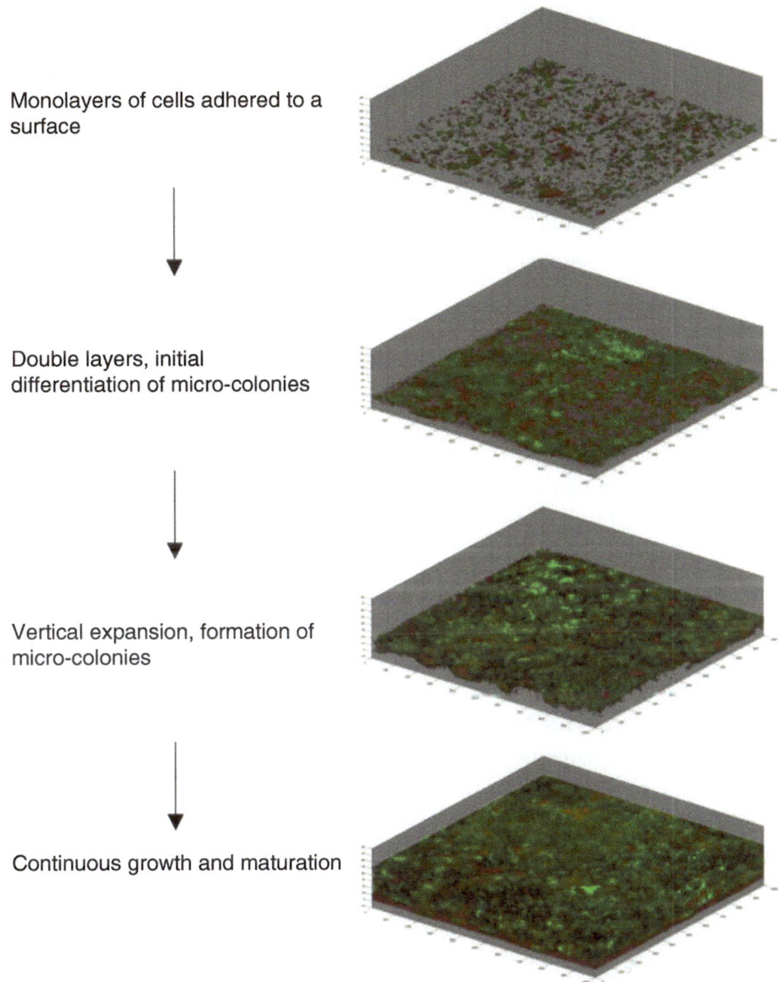

Fig. 1.2 Biofilm growth and maturation. Image sections showing reconstructed three-dimensional biofilm images at a magnification of ×100. Biofilms were stained with LIVE/DEAD stain, resulting in live and dead bacteria appearing as green or red, respectively. 3D images show confocal images of biofilm formation by oral bacteria at 1, 3, 5, and 7 days of growth, respectively. *Upper image* shows the first stage of biofilm growth at day 1; second and third images show subsequent stages of biofilm formation at day 3 and 5, respectively. *Bottom image* shows the fourth stage of biofilm formation at day 7. Damaged organisms appear red and undamaged organisms appear *green*

Biofilms initiate formation when a free-floating cell (cell in planktonic state) is deposited on a substratum coated with an organic conditioning polymeric matrix or "conditioning film" (Fig. 1.1). Conditioning films are composed by constituents of the local environment like water, salt ions, albumin, or fibronectin. When the first bacterial cells arrive, there is a weak and reversible contact between the cell and the conditioning film resulting from physical interactions such as Brownian motion, gravitation, diffusion, or electrostatic interactions [21]. Specific interactions with bacterial surface structures such as flagella and pilus are also important in the initial formation of a biofilm. The next step is when the adhesion of the cell to the substrate becomes irreversible. This is partly due to surface appendages overcoming the repulsive forces between the two surfaces and also helped by the sticky exopolymers secreted by the cells. These hydrophilic exopolymers have a complex and dynamic structure [22].

As depicted in Fig. 1.2, the second part of the formation of a biofilm comprises its growth and development. Development of a biofilm occurs as a result of adherent cells replicating and by additional cells adhering to the biofilm [37]. This is an overall dynamic process where many microorganisms co-adhere to one another and interact in the now active communities. Consequently during growth some cells will be detaching from the biofilm over time [6, 8, 28, 47].

Biofilms Developed in Root Canals

As surface-associated microbial communities are the main form of colonization and retention by oral bacteria in the mouth, it is not unreasonable to assume that biofilms also form in root canals having the same properties as the parent communities colonizing the enamel and cementum surfaces [10]. Microorganisms have been found to colonize by adhering to dentine walls in all the extension of the root canals. These aggregations of microorganisms have been observed adhered to the inner walls of complex apex anatomies and accessory canals [61, 71]. When these biofilm communities are formed on surfaces located beyond the reach of mechanical removal and the effects of antimicrobials, host-derived proteins from remaining necrotic tissues and bacterially produced adhesive substances will provide the proper prerequisites for the survival of microbes.

In 2004, Svensäter and Bergenholtz [83] proposed a hypothesis for biofilm formation in root canals. Biofilm formation in root canals is probably initiated just after the first invasion of the pulp chamber by oral organisms following the pulp tissue inflammatory breakdown. The inflammatory lesion frontage will then move successively towards the apex providing the fluid vehicle for the invading organisms so these can multiply and continue attaching to the root canal walls. Interestingly, bacteria have been observed to detach from inner root canal surfaces and occasionally mass in the inflammatory lesion per se [61, 71]. This observation could explain how the inflammatory lesion front serves as a fluid source for bacterial biofilm detachment and colonization of other remote sites in the root canal.

Resistance to Antimicrobials

Biofilm bacteria usually have an increased resistance to antimicrobial agents, in some cases up to 1,000-fold greater than that of the same microorganisms living in liquid suspension [27, 38]. Biofilms formed by oral bacteria are more resistant to chlorhexidine, amine fluoride, amoxicillin, doxycycline, and metronidazole than planktonic cells [46, 75]. Therefore, it is reasonable to assume that biofilms formed in root canals will also share the same resistant properties as oral bacteria, a fact that will affect the overall prognosis of root canal treatments. The high resistance capacity of biofilm communities from root canal bacteria was shown in a series of experiments that tested the resistance of biofilms formed by bacteria isolated from infected root canals to alkaline stress [12]. In this study, the viability of susceptible root canal strains in planktonic cultures was found to be considerably increased when the same strains were exposed to the same alkaline stress in biofilms.

The reasons for the increased resistance of bacteria when forming a biofilm are believed to be multiple, and currently, there is no generally agreed upon specific mechanism(s). It would seem that resistance is dependent in multiple factors such as the substrate, microenvironment, and age of the biofilm [80, 81]. There are, however, a number of known mechanisms that account for this broad resistance and can be divided in two main groups: (a) physical and (b) acquired. The physical protection is mainly related to the impaired penetration of antibiotics through the biofilm matrix. As it is illustrated in Fig. 1.3, acquired resistance is divided into three subcategories: differentiation of cells with low metabolic activity, differentiation of cells that actively respond to stress, and differentiation of cells with a very high persistent phenotype.

Physical Barrier to the Penetration of Antimicrobials in Biofilms

The main barrier that will hinder the penetration of antibiotics into the biofilm is the extracellular matrix [7, 26]. The extracellular matrix is the backbone of the biofilm and it is very complex in its composition, wide ranging between polysaccharides, proteins, nucleic acids, and lipids. The extracellular polymeric substances (EPS) provide not only physical and adhesive stability to the biofilm, but they also form the scaffold for the three-dimensional architecture that interconnects and organizes cells in biofilms [26].

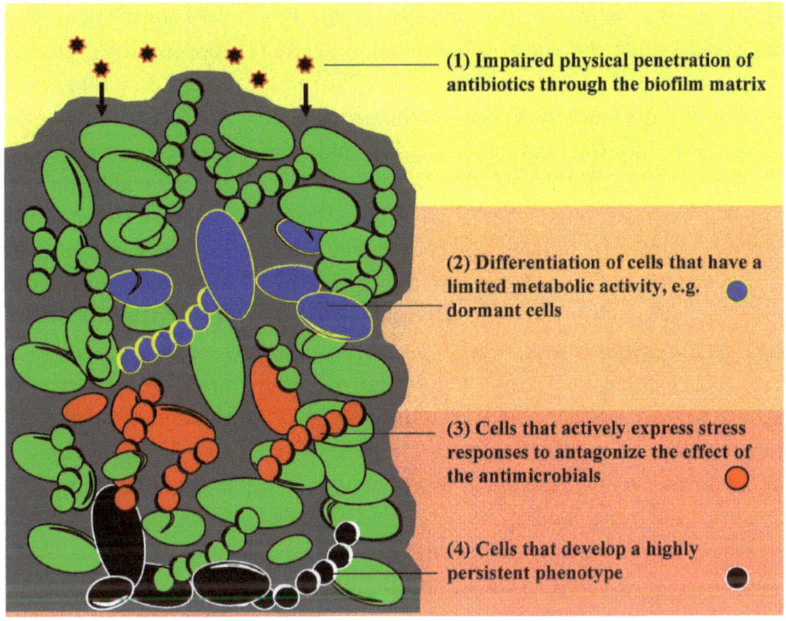

Fig. 1.3 Mechanisms of resistance by biofilm bacteria. The illustration depicts different mechanisms of resistance by biofilm bacteria. Slow or incomplete penetration of antimicrobials through the matrix (*1*). Concentration gradients of metabolites and waste will form zones where subpopulations of bacteria are differentiated. These subpopulations have different antimicrobial resistance capacities depending on their metabolic activity (dormant cells labeled blue) (*2*) or if they develop an active stress response mechanism (*red cells*) (*3*). Finally, a subpopulation of persister cells may also develop (*black cells*) (*4*)

Table 1.1 Novel biofilm matrix components recently found and under current research

Biofilm matrix component	Biofilm-forming species	Reference
Exopolysaccharide	*Bacillus subtilis (NCIB3610)*	[7]
Poly-gamma-DL-glutamic acid	*B. subtilis (RO-FF-1)*	[79]
Poly-N-acetyl glucosamine (PNAG)	*S. aureus*	[66]
Amyloid fibers of the protein TasA	*B. subtilis*	[72]
Protein BapL	*L. monocytogenes*	[39]
BAP proteins	*S. aureus*	[87]
Extracellular protein, MabA	*Lactobacillus rhamnosus*	[88]
Extracellular DNA (eDNA)	*Bacillus cereus, S. aureus, and L. monocytogenes*	[55, 70, 91]

Critical to matrix function is the distribution of the varied molecular-complex components that influences the developmental, homeostatic, and defensive processes in biofilms. Because of the marked diversity of EPS – inclusive of glycoproteins, proteoglycans, and insoluble hydrophobic polymers, among other components depending on the species involved – it is not surprising that this slimy substance delays considerably the diffusion of antimicrobials [81]. For example, it has been directly observed a profound retardation in the delivery of a penicillin antibiotic from penetrating a biofilm formed by a betalactamase-positive bacterium [3].

Due to the physical protection provided by the biofilm matrix, intense research is ongoing that aim to target the identification of novel matrix components. This novel research on matrix components will provide evidence for the identification and application of matrix-degrading enzymes that may prevent formation and/or activate dispersal of biofilms [45]. Some examples of novel biofilm matrix components that are currently studied are listed in Table 1.1.

State of Nutrient Deprivation and Dormancy

It has been observed that throughout the various sections of the biofilm, cells are in different physiological states. Cells at the base of the film, for example, may be dead or lysing, while those near the surface may be actively growing [19, 80].

However, the majority of time cells in biofilms are in a dormant state that is equivalent to cells in the stationary phase of growth [64, 65]. In particular this dormant state is hypothesized to be common in biofilms that are formed in microenvironments where nutrients are scarce, such as treated root canals of teeth [14]. This dormant physiological state related to the general stress response and associated survival responses may offer an explanation for the resistance of biofilm cells to antimicrobials.

Bacteria under the stress of nutrient deprivation have developed efficient adaptive regulatory mechanisms to modify their metabolic balance away from biosynthesis and reproduction [40, 73]. One such mechanism involves the stringent response, a global bacterial response to nutritional stress that is mediated by the accumulation of the alarmones guanosine tetraphosphate and guanosine pentaphosphate, collectively known as (p) ppGpp [25, 68, 85]. For example, (p)ppGpp plays an important role for low-nutrient survival of *E. faecalis*, an organism that is known to withstand prolonged periods of starvation and remain viable in root-filled teeth for at least 12 months [58, 67]. Furthermore, the alarmone system (p)ppGpp has also a profound effect on the ability of *E. faecalis* to form, develop, and maintain stable biofilms [15]. These improved understanding of the alarmone mechanisms underlying biofilm formation and survival by *E. faecalis* may facilitate the identification of pathways that could be targeted to control persistent infections by this organism.

From the perspective of the persisting root canal flora, it is reasonable to assume that such dormant cells might "wake up" at some point in time and resume their metabolic activity to provoke periapical inflammation. Thus, from the metabolic perspective, the reactivation of dormant cells will render biofilm bacteria able to contribute to the persistence of inflammation. For example, a recent case report of a tooth that was adequately treated and showed no signs of disease revealed recurrent disease after 12 years. Histopathologic and histobacteriologic analyses showed a heavy dentinal tubule infection surrounding the area of a lateral canal providing evidence on the persistence of an intraradicular infection caused by bacteria possibly located in dentinal tubules [90].

The above hypothesis on the reactivation of biofilm cells was tested in a recent study [14]. Biofilm cultures of oral isolates of *Streptococcus anginosus* and *Lactobacillus salivarius* were forced to enter a state of dormancy by exposing them to nutrient deprivation for 24 h in buffer. After the starvation period the number of metabolically active cells decreased dramatically to zero and their cell membrane integrity was kept intact. Biofilm cells were then exposed to a "reactivation period" with fresh nutrients, but even after 96 h, the cultures were dominated by undamaged cells that were metabolically inactive. This phenomenon was not observed for cells in a planktonic state that were rapidly reactivated after 2 h. The data produced by this study showed that biofilm cells exhibit a slow physiological response and, unlike cells in planktonic culture, do not reactivate in short time periods even under optimal conditions. This observation highlights the difference in physiology between the biofilm and planktonic cultures and also confirms the slower physiological response of biofilm cells [53, 54], a mechanism that may account as a strategy of biofilm bacteria to resist stressful conditions.

Formation of Phenotypically Different Subpopulations

Bacteria within biofilms differ in their phenotype, depending on the spatial location of the cells within the community [81, 96]. There is now consistent evidence that has proven the presence of subpopulations of cells within biofilms that significantly differ in their antibiotic susceptibility [32, 41]. This phenomenon is correlated with differences in chemical concentration gradients that create unique microenvironments within biofilm communities. Simultaneously, adaptive variability allows the cells to respond to their local environmental conditions [69, 97]. Numerous studies have investigated the creation of these phenotypically different subpopulations and their mechanisms including genetic alterations, mutations, genetic recombination, and stochastic gene expression. For example, Weiser et al. described two distinct phenotypic variants in *S. pneumoniae* that switched between a phenotype with the ability to adhere and coexist among eukaryotic cells and a phenotype that was less capable to adhere but was better adapted to evade the host immune response during inflammation or invasive infection [94]. Of interest is the fact that both phenotypes of *S. pneumoniae* differed in their production of capsular polysaccharide having the inflammation-resistant phenotype an increased production of up to two to six times more capsular polysaccharide. These differences were accentuated by changes in the environmental concentration of oxygen; decreased oxygen levels correlated with an increase in capsular polysaccharide expression.

Interestingly, the formation of subpopulation in biofilms, where physiological differences are in play, has been demonstrated to occur in multispecies biofilms by root canal bacteria [11]. This was shown using four root canal bacterial isolates that, when cocultured, reacted concurrently to the absence of glucose in the culture medium. Although the overall cell viability of the four-species community was not affected by the lack of glucose, there was a significant variation in the 3D structure of the biofilms. In addition, patterns of physiologic adaptation by members of the community to the glucose-deprived medium were observed. The metabolic activity was concentrated in the upper levels of the biofilms, while at lower levels the metabolism of cells was considerably decreased. Subpopulations of species with high glycolytic demands, streptococcus, and lactobacilli were found predominating in the upper levels of the biofilms. This distinct spatial organization in biofilms grown in the lack of glucose shows a clear reorganization of the community in order to satisfy their members' metabolic pathways in order to enable the long-term persistence of the community. This result lends support to the hypothesis that the reorganization of subpopulations of cells in multispecies biofilms is also important for survival to stress factors from the environment [76].

Bacterial Cells That Persist

Groups of cells have been found to persist following exposure to lethal doses of antibiotics and new growing populations appear in the culture [48, 49]. These persister cells (a) may represent cells in some protected part of their cell cycle, (b) are capable of rapid adaptation, (c) are in a dormant state, or (d) are unable to initiate programmed cell death in response to the stimulus [49]. Thus, such persister cells represent a recalcitrant subpopulation that will not die and are capable of initiating a new population with normal susceptibility once the antibacterial effect has been dissipated. To date, these cells have only been reported to occur after the exposure of a bacterial population to high doses of a single antimicrobial agent, which triggered the appearance of persister cells exhibiting multiple drug resistance [51]. The frequency of persister occurrence and the mechanism(s) involved in their appearance are unclear, although one hypothesis with *Escherichia coli* suggests that persister cells are regulated by the expression of chromosomal toxin–antitoxin genes [42]. In this case, the operon HipA seems to be responsible for tolerance to ciprofloxacin and mitomycin C in stationary-phase planktonic cells and *E. coli* biofilms [42]. It has also been proposed that the expression of toxins drives bacteria reversibly into the slow-growing, multiple drug-tolerant phenotypes by "shutting down" antibiotic targets [50]. In the context of root canal bacteria, the formation of such persisting populations that are capable of surviving imposed endodontic treatment measures, as rise of the alkaline levels due to application of calcium hydroxide [12], would explain how organisms are able to survive and remain in the environment until the effects of noxious stimuli have dissipated.

Methods to Study Bacteria in Biofilms

The previous discussion relative to the capacity of biofilm bacteria to resist exposure to antimicrobials indicates the importance of studying the physiological state of bacteria with respect to their potential level of activity in the disease processes. However, the exact description of the status of a microorganism can be complex especially in chronic infections such as apical periodontitis. Currently, a variety of microscopic in situ methods have been developed to identify subpopula-

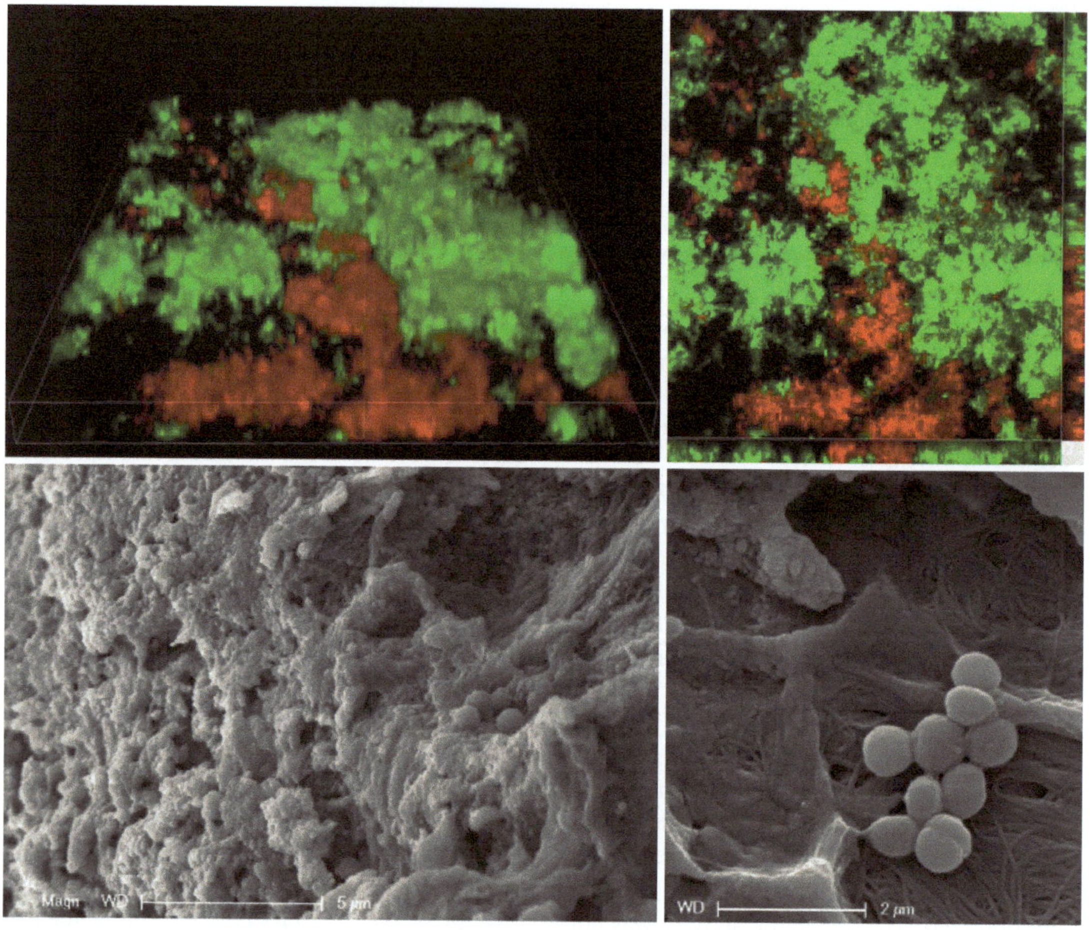

Fig. 1.4 LSM and SEM techniques. Observation of biofilm features by laser scanning microscopy and SEM. The panel above shows 3D reconstruction of biofilm structures labeled with LIVE/DEAD, a fluorescent marker of cell viability; green represents cells with intact cell membranes, while red represents cells with damaged membranes. The panel below shows ultrastructure of biofilms formed on apex of teeth as imaged by SEM. Scale bars: 5 and 2 μm (SEM images are courtesy of Dr. David Jaramillo)

tions and assess the physiological status of bacterial cells in biofilms. Some of these methods include molecular markers to study cell membrane integrity, metabolic activity, or the identification of stress encoding genes.

SEM and LSM

Electron microscopy (EM) in the transmission and scanning mode allows higher magnifications of fixed and dehydrated samples and, in combination with specific detectors, analysis of the elemental composition in specific regions of the sample [92]. EM provides resolution and magnification to offer a more detailed insight into the ultrastructure of the biofilm as well as its environment (Fig. 1.4). One of the main drawbacks of this technique, however, is that it requires the sample to be dehydrated prior to its analysis.

The invention of laser scanning microscopy (LSM) in the 1980s caused a revolution in light microscopy. The LSM technique, usually called confocal laser scanning microscopy (CLSM), is nowadays the most important and indispensable tool for three-dimensional in situ imaging of microbial communities [9]. The LSM technique is mainly used to visualize multiple features in different channels that are spectrally resolved. By means of this imaging procedure, it is possible to analyze the structure, composition, microhabitats, activity, and processes using a variety of specific color probes. Finally, LSM allows the volumetric and structural quantification of multichannel signals in four dimensions [63]. One of the main disadvantages of LSM, however, is that the information captured from detailed ultrastructure of the biofilm is difficult. Very recently, this problem of LSM has been overcome with the advent of super-resolution microscopy (SRM). SRM encompasses a suite of cutting-edge microscopy methods able to surpass the resolution limits of common light microscopy [60]. It is foreseen that the application of SRM in combination with rRNA FISH (see below) would allow the tracking of ribosome-associated changes in activity levels and subcellular localization at the single-cell level [2].

rRNA Fluorescence In Situ Hybridization (FISH)

The combination of FISH with confocal laser scanning microscopy is one of the most powerful tools in modern microbiology as it allows visualization of specific subpopulation of cells while maintaining unaltered the 3D structure of the biofilm [1]. This high-throughput microscopy technique allows the specific detection and enumeration of biofilm subpopulations in situ in their natural environment without the need for cultivation [1]. Up to date a number of studies have demonstrated the direct use of CLSM-FISH on biofilm cultures growing in different surfaces [11, 23]. The most frequent application of FISH is the hybridization of oligonucleotide probes to ribosomal RNA, most often 16S but also 23S rRNA, for identification of single cells in their natural habitat [2]. Since ribosomes are the protein factories of all cells, their numbers are good proxies of general metabolic activity and of the physiological state of cells. Sequences of oligonucleotide probes targeting 16S rRNA have been developed for specific detection of different bacterial species and can be found in online databanks. In endodontics, FISH has been used to visualize and identify bacteria from periapical lesions of asymptomatic root-filled teeth [82]. Furthermore, biofilm models using CLSM-FISH can be of great advantage to investigate distribution of species in multispecies biofilms.

Markers of Cell Viability

Viability of bacteria is conventionally defined as the capacity of cells to perform all cell functions necessary for survival under given conditions [62]. The common method to assess bacterial viability is growth on plates, where the number of viable cells approximates the number of colony-forming units. In root canal infections, culture techniques have been the standard method used to assess bacterial viability. Once the living bacterial cells from root canals were isolated after growth on specific substrate, the metabolic properties of these bacterial isolates were then used to infer the potential roles of these and related microorganisms in a clinical context. Under some circumstances, however, such methods may underrepresent the number of viable bacteria for a variety of reasons, such as cases where slightly damaged organisms are present [4], the laboratory growth media employed are deficient for one or more essential nutrients required for the growth of some bacteria in the sample [93], or viable cells are present that have lost their ability to form colonies [95]. Furthermore, if the bacteria exist in a biofilm, they may assume a status of low metabolic activity similar to stationary-phase planktonic growth for the majority of time [65]. The bacteria in such low active states may be undetectable by regular culture techniques. The extent of this problem is reflected in the indiscriminate use of terms that are used to assess non-viable states, such as dead, moribund, starved, dormant, resting, quiescent, viable but not culturable, injured, sublethally damaged, inhibited, and resuscitable [62]. Many of these terms are used conceptually and do not reflect the actual knowledge of the exact viability state of the organism in question.

A number of viability indicators that can be assessed at the single-cell level without culturing cells have gained increased popularity in the latest years. These indicators are based mostly on fluorescent molecules, which can be detected with epifluorescence microscopy or laser scanning microscopy.

The LIVE/DEAD kit tests the integrity of the cell membrane by applying two nucleic acid stains, SYTO-9 and propidium iodide (PI), which can simultaneously detect dead/injured (fluorescent red by stain with PI) and intact cells (fluorescent green by staining with SYTO-9) [5]. This fluorescent probe has been used to assess the viability of root canal strains ex vivo [10] and to determine the autoaggregation and coaggregation of bacteria isolated from teeth with acute endodontic infections [44].

Alternative fluorescent probes to test bacterial viability are those that target specific cell metabolic functions, such as the tetrazolium salts 2-(4-iodophenyl)-3-(4-nitrophenyl)-5-phenyl tetrazolium chloride (INT) and 5-cyano-2,3-ditolyl tetrazolium chloride (CTC). The tetrazolium salts INT and CTC are often used as markers of bacterial respiratory activity, as well as viability [20]. With these relatively simple methods, a good correlation between the number of INT/CTC-positive cells and the CFU count can be obtained.

In Vivo Models for Biofilm Testing

To better understand the pathogenesis of human polybacterial diseases, such as oral infections including apical periodontitis, there is a great need of experimental models that will closely mimic in vivo features of the disease. However, modeling polybacterial infections presents specific challenges such as establishing a mixed infection and, in some cases, managing the effects of the native microbiota.

Oral infections including periodontitis and endodontic infections have been modeled in the oral cavity of antibiotic-treated rats or in mouse skin wound infections [56, 84, 89]. Although the former model is a closer representation of the disease, the wound infection model is easier to administer and monitor. It is also easier to exclude other bacteria in this model. Both models have been useful in revealing some of the interbacterial interactions that influence oral diseases [43]. Advances in in vivo models will make it possible in the future to observe the events of human infections in detail. It is likely that these in vivo biofilm models will help improve the resolution of our understanding of chronic infections and will bridge the gap from the lab to the clinic.

Antibiofilm Strategies

Along the years, different therapeutic strategies have been developed to prevent biofilm formation and to eliminate established biofilm-related infections. Most of these strategies are summarized in Fig. 1.5. Although the majority of these antibiofilm approaches arise from basic science research, most of them have been developed with the prospective view for them to be applied to fight root canal biofilms. Up until now, the most common and efficient antibiofilm strategy used in root canal therapy is the mechanical removal with instrumentation and irrigation. Biofilm basic research that focuses to test novel antibiofilm strategies allows the characterization and effect of antimicrobials on specific biofilm properties. The validation of these new strategies will likely require efficient translational collaborations between basic research and clinical practice before these strategies can be included in future clinical measures.

Surface Coating

A reasonable approach to prevent or reduce secondary biofilm formation in root canals is to replace the conditioning film with repelling substances that will alter the chemical composition of the substrates [36]. Once a surface has been artificially conditioned, its properties become permanently altered, so that the affinity of an

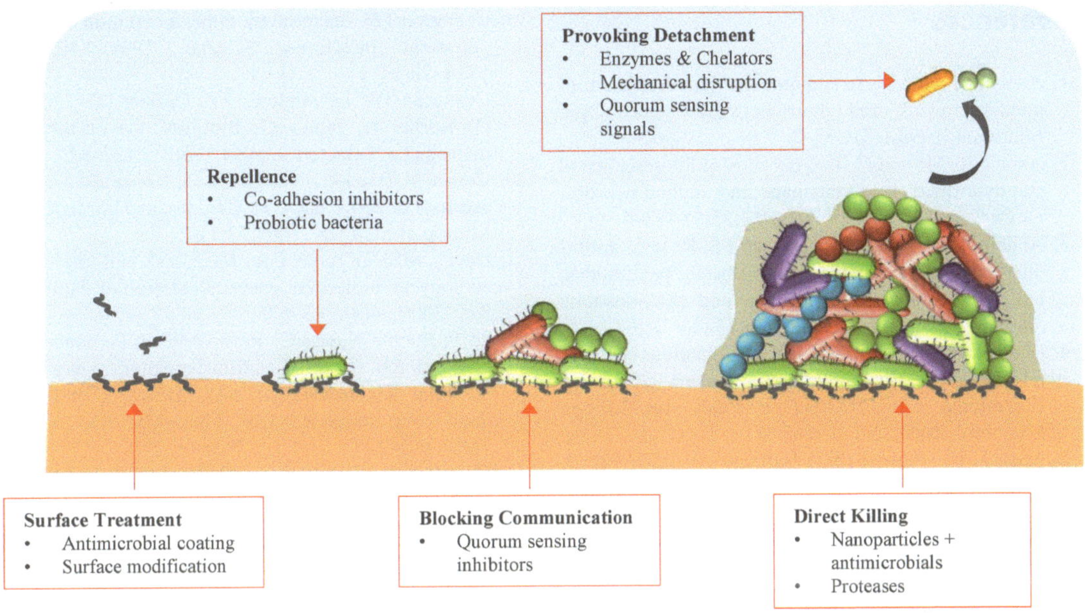

Fig. 1.5 Antibiofilm strategies. Schematic outlining the general approaches for antibiofilm strategies currently used and under research

organism for a native or a conditioned surface can vary greatly depending on the molecules in the new conditioning film [52, 77]. In the biomedical industry, surface modifications have been shown to prevent or reduce bacterial adhesion and biofilm formation by the incorporation of antimicrobial products into surface materials and by modifying the surface's physicochemical properties [29, 86]. Several studies have reported that surface preconditioning with biocides has the potential to prevent bacterial adhesion [57, 78]. For example, it was shown that biocides can increase the cell wall charge of bacteria and therefore reduce their ability to attach and form biofilms [78].

In a recent study it was shown that a surface coating with a solution of benzalkonium chloride diminished biofilm formation by oral bacteria in a dentin disk model and by a consortium of three root canal isolates in an in vitro biofilm model [36]. Benzalkonium chloride was found to exhibit an overall 70-fold reduction in the biofilm biomass accumulation. In parallel, it was also found that NaOCl (1 %) also had good effects in reducing biofilm formation. However, one of the main problems with this method to prevent biofilm formation is that the coating at some point in time may get exhausted; thus, its antibiofilm effect may stop. Hence, the development of a coated surface that prevents bacterial colonization for long periods remains still a challenge.

Concluding Remarks

It is clear that endodontic infections are caused by multispecies biofilms and that the interactions between different organisms can contribute to apical periodontitis progress and clinical outcome. Biofilm research in endodontics is still an open field of research that should greatly contribute into a better understanding of the mechanistic behind the complex interplay between pathogenic agents, commensal organisms, and their eukaryotic hosts. Further research in basic microbiological processes such as the molecular basis and biological effect of these host–bacterial connections may lead to an improvement of treatment regimens and also may identify new objectives and strategies for disease control.

References

1. Amann R, Kuhl M. In situ methods for assessment of microorganisms and their activities. Curr Opin Microbiol. 1998;1(3):352–8.
2. Amann R, Moraru C. Two decades of fluorescence in situ hybridization in systematic and applied microbiology. Syst Appl Microbiol. 2012;35(8):483–4.
3. Anderl JN, Franklin MJ, Stewart PS. Role of antibiotic penetration limitation in Klebsiella pneumoniae biofilm resistance to ampicillin and ciprofloxacin. Antimicrob Agents Chemother. 2000;44(7):1818–24.
4. Blackburn CW, McCarthy JD. Modifications to methods for the enumeration and detection of injured Escherichia coli O157:H7 in foods. Int J Food Microbiol. 2000;55(1–3):285–90.
5. Boulos L, Prevost M, Barbeau B, Coallier J, Desjardins R. LIVE/DEAD BacLight: application of a new rapid staining method for direct enumeration of viable and total bacteria in drinking water. J Microbiol Methods. 1999;37(1):77–86.
6. Bowden GH, Hamilton IR. Survival of oral bacteria. Crit Rev Oral Biol Med. 1998;9(1):54–85.
7. Branda SS, Vik S, Friedman L, Kolter R. Biofilms: the matrix revisited. Trends Microbiol. 2005;13(1):20–6.
8. Brecx M, Theilade J, Attstrom R. An ultrastructural quantitative study of the significance of microbial multiplication during early dental plaque growth. J Periodontal Res. 1983;18(2):177–86.
9. Bridier A, Briandet R. Contribution of confocal laser scanning microscopy in deciphering biofilm tridimensional structure and reactivity. Methods Mol Biol. 2014;1147:255–66.
10. Chavez de Paz LE. Redefining the persistent infection in root canals: possible role of biofilm communities. J Endod. 2007;33(6):652–62.
11. Chavez de Paz LE. Development of a multispecies biofilm community by four root canal bacteria. J Endod. 2012;38(3):318–23.
12. Chavez de Paz LE, Bergenholtz G, Dahlen G, Svensater G. Response to alkaline stress by root canal bacteria in biofilms. Int Endod J. 2007;40(5):344–55.
13. Chavez de Paz LE, Bergenholtz G, Svensater G. The effects of antimicrobials on endodontic biofilm bacteria. J Endod. 2010;36(1):70–7.
14. Chavez de Paz LE, Hamilton IR, Svensater G. Oral bacteria in biofilms exhibit slow reactivation from nutrient deprivation. Microbiology. 2008;154(Pt 7):1927–38.
15. Chavez de Paz LE, Lemos JA, Wickstrom C, Sedgley CM. Role of (p)ppGpp in biofilm formation by Enterococcus faecalis. Appl Environ Microbiol. 2012;78(5):1627–30.
16. Clegg MS, Vertucci FJ, Walker C, Belanger M, Britto LR. The effect of exposure to irrigant solutions on apical dentin biofilms in vitro. J Endod. 2006;32(5):434–7.
17. Costeron JW, Lewandowski Z, Caldwell DE, Korber DR, Lappin-Scott HM. Microbial biofilms. Annu Rev Microbiol. 1995;49:711–45.
18. Costerton JW. Bacterial biofilms: a common cause of persistent infections. Science. 1999;284(5418):1318–22.
19. Costerton JW, Lewandowski Z, DeBeer D, Caldwell D, Korber D, James G. Biofilms, the customized microniche. J Bacteriol. 1994;176(8):2137–42.
20. Creach V, Baudoux AC, Bertru G, Rouzic BL. Direct estimate of active bacteria: CTC use and limitations. J Microbiol Methods. 2003;52(1):19–28.
21. Davey ME, O'Toole GA. Microbial biofilms: from ecology to molecular genetics. Microbiol Mol Biol Rev. 2000;64(4):847–67.
22. de la Fuente-Nunez C, Reffuveille F, Fernandez L, Hancock RE. Bacterial biofilm development as a multicellular adaptation: antibiotic resistance and new therapeutic strategies. Curr Opin Microbiol. 2013;16(5):580–9.
23. Delatolla R, Tufenkji N, Comeau Y, Lamarre D, Gadbois A, Berk D. In situ characterization of nitrifying biofilm: minimizing biomass loss and preserving perspective. Water Res. 2009;43(6):1775–87.
24. Dunavant TR, Regan JD, Glickman GN, Solomon ES, Honeyman AL. Comparative evaluation of endodontic irrigants against Enterococcus faecalis biofilms. J Endod. 2006;32(6):527–31.
25. Ezequiel W, Jehoshua K, Gad G, Roee V. ppGpp analogues as antibacterial compounds. Nucleic Acids Symp Ser (Oxf). 2008;52:633–4.
26. Flemming HC. The perfect slime. Colloids Surf B Biointerfaces. 2011;86(2):251–9.
27. Gilbert P, Das J, Foley I. Biofilm susceptibility to antimicrobials. Adv Dent Res. 1997;11(1):160–7.
28. Gilbert P, Evans DJ, Brown MR. Formation and dispersal of bacterial biofilms in vivo and in situ. J Appl Bacteriol. 1993;74(Suppl):67S–78.
29. Gottenbos B, Grijpma DW, van der Mei HC, Feijen J, Busscher HJ. Antimicrobial effects of positively charged surfaces on adhering Gram-positive and Gram-negative bacteria. J Antimicrob Chemother. 2001;48(1):7–13.
30. Hall-Stoodley L, Costerton JW, Stoodley P. Bacterial biofilms: from the natural environment to infectious diseases. Nat Rev Microbiol. 2004;2(2):95–108.
31. Hall-Stoodley L, Stoodley P. Evolving concepts in biofilm infections. Cell Microbiol. 2009;11(7):1034–43.
32. Hallet B. Playing Dr Jekyll and Mr Hyde: combined mechanisms of phase variation in bacteria. Curr Opin Microbiol. 2001;4(5):570–81.
33. Hoiby N, Bjarnsholt T, Givskov M, Molin S, Ciofu O. Antibiotic resistance of bacterial biofilms. Int J Antimicrob Agents. 2010;35(4):322–32.
34. Hope CK, Wilson M. Biofilm structure and cell vitality in a laboratory model of subgingival plaque. J Microbiol Methods. 2006;66(3):390–8.
35. Huang R, Li M, Gregory RL. Bacterial interactions in dental biofilm. Virulence. 2011;2(5):435–44.
36. Jaramillo DE, Arriola A, Safavi K, Chavez de Paz LE. Decreased bacterial adherence and biofilm growth on surfaces coated with a solution of benzalkonium chloride. J Endod. 2012;38(6):821–5.

37. Jenkinson HF, Lappin-Scott HM. Biofilms adhere to stay. Trends Microbiol. 2001;9(1):9–10.
38. Johnson SA, Goddard PA, Iliffe C, Timmins B, Rickard AH, Robson G, Handley PS. Comparative susceptibility of resident and transient hand bacteria to para-chloro-meta-xylenol and triclosan. J Appl Microbiol. 2002;93(2):336–44.
39. Jordan SJ, Perni S, Glenn S, Fernandes I, Barbosa M, Sol M, Tenreiro RP, Chambel L, Barata B, Zilhao I, Aldsworth TG, Adriao A, Faleiro ML, Shama G, Andrew PW. Listeria monocytogenes biofilm-associated protein (BapL) may contribute to surface attachment of L. monocytogenes but is absent from many field isolates. Appl Environ Microbiol. 2008;74(17):5451–6.
40. Kaprelyants AS, Gottschal JC, Kell DB. Dormancy in non-sporulating bacteria. FEMS Microbiol Rev. 1993;10(3–4):271–85.
41. Kaufmann SH, Schaible UE. 100th anniversary of Robert Koch's Nobel Prize for the discovery of the tubercle bacillus. Trends Microbiol. 2005;13(10): 469–75.
42. Keren I, Kaldalu N, Spoering A, Wang Y, Lewis K. Persister cells and tolerance to antimicrobials. FEMS Microbiol Lett. 2004;230(1):13–8.
43. Kesavalu L, Sathishkumar S, Bakthavatchalu V, Matthews C, Dawson D, Steffen M, Ebersole JL. Rat model of polymicrobial infection, immunity, and alveolar bone resorption in periodontal disease. Infect Immun. 2007;75(4):1704–12.
44. Khemaleelakul S, Baumgartner JC, Pruksakom S. Autoaggregation and coaggregation of bacteria associated with acute endodontic infections. J Endod. 2006;32(4):312–8.
45. Landini P, Antoniani D, Burgess JG, Nijland R. Molecular mechanisms of compounds affecting bacterial biofilm formation and dispersal. Appl Microbiol Biotechnol. 2010;86(3):813–23.
46. Larsen T. Susceptibility of Porphyromonas gingivalis in biofilms to amoxicillin, doxycycline and metronidazole. Oral Microbiol Immunol. 2002;17(5): 267–71.
47. Lee SF, Li YH, Bowden GH. Detachment of Streptococcus mutans biofilm cells by an endogenous enzymatic activity. Infect Immun. 1996;64(3): 1035–8.
48. Lewis K. Riddle of biofilm resistance. Antimicrob Agents Chemother. 2001;45(4):999–1007.
49. Lewis K. Persister cells and the riddle of biofilm survival. Biochemistry (Mosc). 2005;70(2):267–74.
50. Lewis K. Persister cells, dormancy and infectious disease. Nat Rev Microbiol. 2007;5(1):48–56.
51. Lewis K. Persister cells. Annu Rev Microbiol. 2010;64:357–72.
52. Lorite GS, Rodrigues CM, de Souza AA, Kranz C, Mizaikoff B, Cotta MA. The role of conditioning film formation and surface chemical changes on Xylella fastidiosa adhesion and biofilm evolution. J Colloid Interface Sci. 2011;359(1):289–95.
53. Mah TF. Biofilm-specific antibiotic resistance. Future Microbiol. 2012;7(9):1061–72.
54. Mah TF, O'Toole GA. Mechanisms of biofilm resistance to antimicrobial agents. Trends Microbiol. 2001;9(1):34–9.
55. Mann EE, Rice KC, Boles BR, Endres JL, Ranjit D, Chandramohan L, Tsang LH, Smeltzer MS, Horswill AR, Bayles KW. Modulation of eDNA release and degradation affects Staphylococcus aureus biofilm maturation. PLoS One. 2009;4(6), e5822.
56. Meka A, Bakthavatchalu V, Sathishkumar S, Lopez MC, Verma RK, Wallet SM, Bhattacharyya I, Boyce BF, Handfield M, Lamont RJ, Baker HV, Ebersole JL, Kesavalu L. Porphyromonas gingivalis infection-induced tissue and bone transcriptional profiles. Mol Oral Microbiol. 2010;25(1):61–74.
57. Meylheuc T, Methivier C, Renault M, Herry JM, Pradier CM, Bellon-Fontaine MN. Adsorption on stainless steel surfaces of biosurfactants produced by gram-negative and gram-positive bacteria: consequence on the bioadhesive behavior of Listeria monocytogenes. Colloids Surf B Biointerfaces. 2006;52(2):128–37.
58. Molander A, Reit C, Dahlen G, Kvist T. Microbiological status of root-filled teeth with apical periodontitis. Int Endod J. 1998;31(1):1–7.
59. Molven O, Olsen I, Kerekes K. Scanning electron microscopy of bacteria in the apical part of root canals in permanent teeth with periapical lesions. Endod Dent Traumatol. 1991;7(5):226–9.
60. Moraru C, Amann R. Crystal ball: fluorescence in situ hybridization in the age of super-resolution microscopy. Syst Appl Microbiol. 2012;35(8):549–52.
61. Nair P. Light and electron microscopic studies on root canal flora and periapical lesions. J Endod. 1987;13: 29–39.
62. Netuschil L, Auschill TM, Sculean A, Arweiler NB. Confusion over live/dead stainings for the detection of vital microorganisms in oral biofilms–which stain is suitable? BMC Oral Health. 2014;14:2.
63. Neu TR, Manz B, Volke F, Dynes JJ, Hitchcock AP, Lawrence JR. Advanced imaging techniques for assessment of structure, composition and function in biofilm systems. FEMS Microbiol Ecol. 2010;72(1): 1–21.
64. Nystrom T. Not quite dead enough: on bacterial life, culturability, senescence, and death. Arch Microbiol. 2001;176(3):159–64.
65. Nystrom T. Conditional senescence in bacteria: death of the immortals. Mol Microbiol. 2003;48(1):17–23.
66. O'Gara JP. ica and beyond: biofilm mechanisms and regulation in Staphylococcus epidermidis and Staphylococcus aureus. FEMS Microbiol Lett. 2007; 270(2):179–88.
67. Portenier I, Waltimo T, Orstavik D, Haapasalo M. The susceptibility of starved, stationary phase, and growing cells of Enterococcus faecalis to endodontic medicaments. J Endod. 2005;31(5):380–6.
68. Potrykus K, Cashel M. (p)ppGpp: still magical? Annu Rev Microbiol. 2008;62:35–51.
69. Qi X, Gao J, Sun D, Liang W, Wan Y, Li C, Xu X, Gao T. Biofilm formation of the pathogens of fatal bacterial granuloma after trauma: potential mechanism

underlying the failure of traditional antibiotic treatments. Scand J Infect Dis. 2008;40(3):221–8.
70. Rice KC, Mann EE, Endres JL, Weiss EC, Cassat JE, Smeltzer MS, Bayles KW. The cidA murein hydrolase regulator contributes to DNA release and biofilm development in Staphylococcus aureus. Proc Natl Acad Sci U S A. 2007;104(19):8113–8.
71. Ricucci D, Siqueira Jr JF. Biofilms and apical periodontitis: study of prevalence and association with clinical and histopathologic findings. J Endod. 2010;36(8):1277–88.
72. Romero D, Aguilar C, Losick R, Kolter R. Amyloid fibers provide structural integrity to Bacillus subtilis biofilms. Proc Natl Acad Sci U S A. 2010;107(5):2230–4.
73. Sachidanandham R, Yew-Hoong Gin K. A dormancy state in nonspore-forming bacteria. Appl Microbiol Biotechnol. 2009;81(5):927–41.
74. Sen BH, Piskin B, Demirci T. Observation of bacteria and fungi in infected root canals and dentinal tubules by SEM. Endod Dent Traumatol. 1995;11(1):6–9.
75. Shani S, Friedman M, Steinberg D. The anticariogenic effect of amine fluorides on Streptococcus sobrinus and glucosyltransferase in biofilms. Caries Res. 2000;34(3):260–7.
76. Shapiro JA. Bacteria are small but not stupid: cognition, natural genetic engineering and sociobacteriology. Stud Hist Philos Biol Biomed Sci. 2007;38(4):807–19.
77. Siboni N, Martinez S, Abelson A, Sivan A, Kushmaro A. Conditioning film and initial biofilm formation on electrochemical CaCO3 deposition on a metallic net in the marine environment. Biofouling. 2009;25(7):675–83.
78. Splendiani A, Livingston AG, Nicolella C. Control of membrane-attached biofilms using surfactants. Biotechnol Bioeng. 2006;94(1):15–23.
79. Stanley NR, Lazazzera BA. Defining the genetic differences between wild and domestic strains of Bacillus subtilis that affect poly-gamma-dl-glutamic acid production and biofilm formation. Mol Microbiol. 2005;57(4):1143–58.
80. Stewart PS. Mechanisms of antibiotic resistance in bacterial biofilms. Int J Med Microbiol. 2002;292(2):107–13.
81. Stewart PS. Biophysics of biofilm infection. Pathog Dis. 2014;70(3):212–8.
82. Sunde PT, Olsen I, Gobel UB, Theegarten D, Winter S, Debelian GJ, Tronstad L, Moter A. Fluorescence in situ hybridization (FISH) for direct visualization of bacteria in periapical lesions of asymptomatic root-filled teeth. Microbiology. 2003;149(Pt 5):1095–102.
83. Svensäter G, Bergenholtz G. Biofilms in endodontic infections. Endodontic Topics. 2004;9:27–36.
84. Tobias Duarte PC, Gomes-Filho JE, Ervolino E, Marcal Mazza Sundefeld ML, Tadahirowayama M, Lodi CS, Dezan-Junior E, Angelo Cintra LT. Histopathological condition of the remaining tissues after endodontic infection of rat immature teeth. J Endod. 2014;40(4):538–42.
85. Traxler MF, Summers SM, Nguyen HT, Zacharia VM, Hightower GA, Smith JT, Conway T. The global, ppGpp-mediated stringent response to amino acid starvation in Escherichia coli. Mol Microbiol. 2008;68(5):1128–48.
86. Tsibouklis J, Stone M, Thorpe AA, Graham P, Peters V, Heerlien R, Smith JR, Green KL, Nevell TG. Preventing bacterial adhesion onto surfaces: the low-surface-energy approach. Biomaterials. 1999;20(13):1229–35.
87. Valle J, Latasa C, Gil C, Toledo-Arana A, Solano C, Penades JR, Lasa I. Bap, a biofilm matrix protein of Staphylococcus aureus prevents cellular internalization through binding to GP96 host receptor. PLoS Pathog. 2012;8(8), e1002843.
88. Velez MP, Petrova MI, Lebeer S, Verhoeven TL, Claes I, Lambrichts I, Tynkkynen S, Vanderleyden J, De Keersmaecker SC. Characterization of MabA, a modulator of Lactobacillus rhamnosus GG adhesion and biofilm formation. FEMS Immunol Med Microbiol. 2010;59(3):386–98.
89. Verma RK, Rajapakse S, Meka A, Hamrick C, Pola S, Bhattacharyya I, Nair M, Wallet SM, Aukhil I, Kesavalu L. Porphyromonas gingivalis and Treponema denticola mixed microbial infection in a rat model of periodontal disease. Interdiscip Perspect Infect Dis. 2010;2010:605125.
90. Vieira AR, Siqueira Jr JF, Ricucci D, Lopes WS. Dentinal tubule infection as the cause of recurrent disease and late endodontic treatment failure: a case report. J Endod. 2012;38(2):250–4.
91. Vilain S, Pretorius JM, Theron J, Brozel VS. DNA as an adhesin: Bacillus cereus requires extracellular DNA to form biofilms. Appl Environ Microbiol. 2009;75(9):2861–8.
92. Wang J, Chen W, Jiang Y, Liang J. Imaging of extraradicular biofilm using combined scanning electron microscopy and stereomicroscopy. Microsc Res Tech. 2013;76(9):979–83.
93. Ward DM, Weller R, Bateson MM. 16S rRNA sequences reveal uncultured inhabitants of a well-studied thermal community. FEMS Microbiol Rev. 1990;6(2–3):105–15.
94. Weiser JN, Austrian R, Sreenivasan PK, Masure HR. Phase variation in pneumococcal opacity: relationship between colonial morphology and nasopharyngeal colonization. Infect Immun. 1994;62(6):2582–9.
95. Xu HS, Roberts N, Singleton FL, Attwell RW, Grimes DJ, Colwell RR. Survival and viability of nonculturable *Escherichia coli* and *Vibrio cholerae* in the estuarine and marine environment. Microbial Ecol. 1982;8:313–23.
96. Xu KD, McFeters GA, Stewart PS. Biofilm resistance to antimicrobial agents. Microbiology. 2000;146(Pt 3):547–9.
97. Xu KD, Stewart PS, Xia F, Huang CT, McFeters GA. Spatial physiological heterogeneity in Pseudomonas aeruginosa biofilm is determined by oxygen availability. Appl Environ Microbiol. 1998;64(10):4035–9.

Update in Root Canal Anatomy of Permanent Teeth Using Microcomputed Tomography

2

Marco A. Versiani, Jesus D. Pécora, and Manoel D. Sousa-Neto

Abstract

The primary goals of endodontic treatment are to debride and disinfect the root canal space to the greatest possible extent and to seal the root canal system as effectively as possible, aiming to establish or maintain healthy periapical tissues. Treating complex and anomalous anatomy requires knowledge of the internal anatomy of all types of teeth before undertaking endodontic therapy. Recently, three-dimensional imaging of teeth using microcomputed tomography has been used to reveal the internal anatomy of the teeth to the clinician. This chapter is focused on the complexity of root canal anatomy and discusses its relationship on the understanding of the principles and problems of shaping and cleaning procedures.

A Brief History of the First Studies on Root Canal Anatomy

Since the first attempts of using contemporary advanced imaging systems, such as X-ray computerized tomography [1–5], a lot of research work has been done in relation to the root canal anatomy and its remarkable influence on the endodontic procedures. However, to understand the contemporary approaches regarding this issue, it would be appropriate to take a brief look to the past. Authors that preceded this new image-processing technological era, to whom endodontics is greatly indebted, should be always revisited.

Although the Hungarian dentist and professor György Carabelli, from the University of Vienna, was eternized in the dental literature by his description of an additional cusp on the palatal surface of the mesiopalatal maxillary molar cusp [6], the so-called Carabelli's cusp, he was also the first author to provide a comprehensive description of the number and location of root canals. In his textbook, *Anatomie des Mundes* [6], he reproduced some illustrations of sectioned

M.A. Versiani, DDS, MSc, PhD (✉)
Department of Restorative Dentistry,
Dental School of Ribeirao Preto,
University of Sao Paulo,
Avenida do Café, s/n Bairro Monte Alegre,
Ribeirao Preto 14049-904, SP, Brazil
e-mail: marcoversiani@yahoo.com

J.D. Pécora, DDS, MSc, PhD
M.D. Sousa-Neto, DDS, MSc, PhD
Department of Restorative Dentistry, Dental School of Ribeirao Preto, University of Sao Paulo,
Ribeirao Preto, Brazil

B. Basrani (ed.), *Endodontic Irrigation: Chemical Disinfection of the Root Canal System*,
DOI 10.1007/978-3-319-16456-4_2

teeth detailing the root canal system and the external morphology of all groups of teeth. Thirty years later, Mühlreiter [7] published the first systematic study on the root canal anatomy in which teeth was sectioned in all planes and the internal anatomy described in details. After a few decades, Greene Vardiman Black published the first edition of his classic book [8] in which he systematized the dental terminology and detailed the internal and external anatomy of the teeth. According to him, "anatomy is not to be learned from books alone, but also by bringing the parts to be studied into view, and closely examining them in connection with the descriptions given." In 1894, Professor Alfred Gysi, from the University of Zürich, published a collection of photomicrographs in which impressive pictures of histological sections of human teeth demonstrated the complexity of the root canal system [9]. Nevertheless, at this point, the methodological approaches for studying the root canal anatomy were predominantly based on sectioning techniques.

At the beginning of the twentieth century, Preiswerk introduced the "modeling technique" for the study of the root canal anatomy [10]. His method consisted in the injection of molten metal (70 °C) into the canal space in which, after complete tooth decalcification, it was possible to obtain a metal model of its internal anatomy. The main limitation of this method was that it led to tooth overheating and the replicas were obviously incomplete as the metal could not penetrate the finer branches of the root canal system. Despite these methodological drawbacks, Preiswerk was one of the first researchers who stated that "a canal-anastomosis system can be found in some roots and is not rare" [10]. In 1908, Fischer [11] obtained better results filling approximately 700 teeth with a collodion solution, made up of 1 part small-piece collodion to 8 parts of pure acetone. The collodion solution was able to penetrate all the branches of the root canal system and harden in 2 or 3 weeks, providing a full replica of the root canal system. Fisher deeply studied ramifications and little lateral canal branches, especially those near the apical foramen. However, the hardened collodion solution was fragile, and replicas of the more subtle ramifications fractured easily. In later years, improved techniques for injecting different materials, such as paraffin [12], were also used to obtain a model of the root canal space.

In 1914, the German anatomist Werner Spalteholz developed a process in which organs could be made translucent and stained using different colors [13]. This process was based on dehydration of the removed organs and the use of anoptically transparent embedding material that had the same refractive index as the tissue of the organ itself. Some researchers in the endodontic field modified and simplified the Spalteholz's method employing this "clearing technique" (diaphanization) for the study of the root canal anatomy. Basically, this method renders the surrounding hard tissues transparent through demineralization after injecting fluid materials, such as molten Wood's metal [14], gelatin-containing cinnabar [15], and China ink [16], into the root canal system.

After considering that the available research methods did not fit for the study of a large number of teeth, Professor Walter Hess developed his own technique and studied the root canal morphology of approximately 3,000 teeth [17, 18]. Basically, he used the demineralizing method, packing and pressing softened natural rubber, which was vulcanized later into teeth. Then, specimens were washed in running water and placed in 50 % hydrochloric acid. After decalcification, the teeth were washed again, organic debris removed, and vulcanite samples mounted on blocks of chalk. Hess corroborated his results performing some histological preparations by carrying out serial sections. He established a correlation between the presence of ramifications and the patient's age and published details about the percentage number of root canals in all groups of teeth [17]. A few years later, Okumura specified the percentage values concerning the number and divisions of the main root canal in 1,339 teeth using dye injection and diaphanization technique [19].

In the following decades, the morphology of the root canal system was described by several in vivo and ex vivo methods such as three-dimensional wax models [20], conventional radiography [21–32], digital radiography [33–35], resin injection [36–38], macroscopic evaluation [27, 39, 40], tooth sectioning on different planes [39, 41–46], microscopy evaluation [43–45, 47, 48], clearing techniques [49–59], radiographic methods with radiopaque contrast media [60], and scanning electron microscopy [61].

Without doubt, these techniques have shown potential for endodontic research and have been used successfully over many years [62]; however, some of them may provide questionable data. The accuracy of radiographic methods, longitudinal and transverse cross sectioning, and microscopic approaches in assessing the morphology of the root canal system is reduced because they provide only a two-dimensional image of a three-dimensional structure [63]. It may be pointed out that in the process of making the sections, the specimens are also destroyed, and an accurate image of the root canal as a whole cannot be obtained because of the large thickness of the sections [64]. Modeling techniques with the removal of all surrounding tissues from casts of root canals with wood metal, celluloid, resin, or wax, as well as, decalcification and clearing techniques, produce irreversible changes in the specimens [65] and many artifacts [66] which, therefore, cannot accurately reflect the canal morphology [67, 68]. Furthermore, these techniques do not allow for the three-dimensional analysis of the external and internal anatomy of the teeth at the same time [64]. These inherent limitations have repeatedly been discussed, encouraging the search for new methods with improved possibilities [62].

Computational Methods for the Study of Root Canal Anatomy

In 1986, Mayo et al. [69] introduced computer-assisted imaging in the field of endodontic research. According to these authors, endodontics needed "a model for studying canal morphology before, during, or after endodontic therapy on actual teeth." They adapted a technique that allowed three-dimensional imaging of objects [70] for the evaluation of the root canals of single-rooted premolars. Briefly, after the injection of a contrast medium into the root canal, six radiographs of each tooth were taken from known angles. By combining all six views, a mathematically determined three-dimensional (3D) representation of the canals was obtained. From this data, the volume and diameters of the root canals were estimated using a computerized video image-processing program. Despite a significant discrepancy in the results, essentially caused by technological computer-processing limitations, authors stated that "applications of this technique in the fields of research and education are very promising." This radiographic volume interpolation method from two-dimensional radiographs taken in different angles was also used in further studies to evaluate the root canal anatomy [71–73]. Some years later, a new computerized method for 3D visualization of the root canal before and after instrumentation was introduced [74]. Five cross-sectional images of the mesial root of mandibular first molars before and after canal preparation, at intervals of 1 mm, were obtained. Then, micrographs of these sections were transferred to a graphics computer, which rebuilt, superimposed, and elaborated the sections, providing a 3D model of the root with the image of the canal system. Subsequently, this computer-based method was improved by decreasing the cross-sectional thickness of the root [75–79].

These computerized methods allowed the development of 3D models of the root as well as the measurements of parameters such as distance, contour, diameter, perimeter, area, surface, and volume of the canal. Despite the improvements achieved with this newer approach, it was still a destructive technique, and the thickness of sections and material loss were found to influence the obtained results [79]. The invention of X-ray computed tomography (CT) brought a significant step forward in diagnostic medicine [70]. CT produces a two-dimensional map of X-ray absorption into a two-dimensional slice of the subject. This is achieved by taking a series of X-ray projections through the slice at various angles around an axis perpendicular to the slice. From this set of projections, the X-ray absorption map is computed. By taking a number of slices, a three-dimensional map is produced [5]. To maximize their effectiveness in differentiating tissues while minimizing patient exposure, medical CT systems need to use a limited dose of relatively low-energy X-rays (≤125 keV). Besides, they must also acquire their data rapidly because the patient should not move during scanning. Then, to obtain as much data as possible given these requirements, they use relatively large scale in mm and high-efficiency detectors [80].

In 1990, Tachibana and Matsumoto [1] were the first authors to suggest and evaluate the feasibility of CT imaging in endodontics. Because of high costs, inadequate software, and a low spatial resolution (0.6 mm), they concluded that CT had only a limited usefulness in endodontics as achieved images were not detailed enough to allow a proper analysis. Further improvements in digital image systems have been used to evaluate the root canal anatomy in either ex vivo or in vivo conditions using nondestructive tools such as conventional medical CT [81–86], magnetic resonance microscopy [87–93], tuned-aperture computed tomography (TACT) [94, 95], optical coherence tomography [96], and volumetric or cone beam CT (CBCT) [97–114]. However, these digital image systems were hampered mainly by insufficient spatial resolution and slice thickness for the study of root canal anatomy [3, 4].

A decade after the CT scanner was created, Elliott and Dover [2] developed the first high-resolution X-ray microcomputed tomographic device, and using a resolution of 12 μm, the image of the shell of a *Biomphalaria glabrata* snail was produced. The term "micro" in this new device was used to indicate that the pixel sizes of the cross sections were in the micrometer range. This also meant that the machine was smaller in design compared to the human version and was indicated to model smaller objects [115]. X-ray microcomputed tomography (micro-CT) has also been denominated as microcomputed tomography, microcomputer tomography, high-resolution X-ray tomography, X-ray microtomography, and similar terminologies. Nowadays, despite the impossibility of employing micro-CT for in vivo human imaging, it has been considered the most important and accurate research tool for the study of root canal anatomy [63, 67, 68, 116].

The Micro-CT Technology in Endodontics

Like conventional medical tomography, micro-CT also uses X-rays to create cross sections of a 3D object that later can be used to recreate a virtual model without destroying the original model [115]. Therefore, whereas a typical digital image is composed of pixels (picture elements), a CT slice image is composed of voxels (volume elements) [80, 115] (Fig. 2.1).

Because micro-CT is mostly used in nonliving objects, the scanners were designed to take advantage of the fact that the items being studied do not move and are not harmed by X-rays. Basically, micro-CT technology employs four optimizations in comparison to conventional CT [80]:

(a) It uses high-energy X-rays which are more effective at penetrating dense materials.
(b) X-ray focal spots are smaller providing increased resolution at a cost in X-ray output.
(c) X-ray detectors are finer and more densely packed which increases resolution at a cost in detection efficiency.
(d) It uses longer exposure times increasing the signal-to-noise ratio to compensate for the loss in signal from the diminished output and efficiency of the source and detectors.

Application of micro-CT technology to endodontic research was recognized only 13 years after its development and described in a paper entitled *Microcomputed Tomography: An Advanced System for Detailed Endodontic Research* [3]. In this article, Nielsen et al. [3] evaluated the reliability of micro-CT in the reconstruction of the external and internal anatomy of four maxillary first molars, assessing the morphological changes in the root canal after instrumentation and obturation, using an isotropic resolution of 127 μm. Authors concluded that micro-CT had "potential as an advanced system for research, but also provides the foundation as an exciting interactive educational tool." In this study, three-dimensional images of the internal

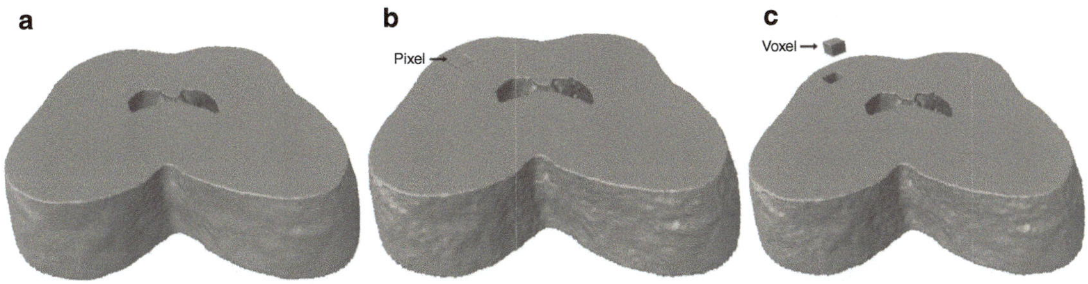

Fig. 2.1 Three-dimensional cross section of the coronal third of a mandibular second molar root (**a**) illustrating the difference between pixel (**b**) and voxel (**c**). The word pixel stands for picture element. Every digital image is made up of pixels. They are the smallest unit of information arranged in a two-dimensional grid that makes up a picture. Voxel stands for volumetric element, and it is the three-dimensional equivalent of a pixel and the tiniest distinguishable element of a 3D object

and external structures of the teeth were also presented in a format previously unattainable [3].

With further developments of the micro-CT scanners, improvements in the speed of data collection, resolution, and image quality yielded greater accuracy compared with the first studies using computational methods, with voxel sizes decreasing to less than 40 μm [4, 117]. Dowker et al. [4] demonstrated the feasibility of this technology using a resolution of 38.7 μm to evaluate the morphological characteristics of the root canal before and after different steps of root canal treatment. Authors concluded that micro-CT technology would offer the possibility of learning tooth morphology by interactive study of surface-rendered images and slices, contributing to the development of virtual reality techniques for endodontic teaching. Later, the reliability of micro-CT as a methodological tool was also demonstrated in the quantitative assessment of the root canal preparation [62, 116–119], obturation [120], and retreatment [121], using innovative image software that allowed the alignment of pre- and post-image volumes.

Therefore, micro-CT has gained increasing significance in the detailed study of canal anatomy in endodontics because it offered a nondestructive reproducible technique that could be applied quantitatively as well as qualitatively for two- and three-dimensional accurate assessment of the root canal system [116]. Conversely, given that scanning and reconstruction procedures take considerable time, the technique is not suitable for clinical use, the equipment is expensive, and the complexity of the technical procedures requires a high learning curve and an in-depth knowledge of dedicated software. The technical procedures related to the micro-CT methodology with the aim to evaluate aspects related to the morphological analysis of the root canal anatomy are a complicated subject, and a thorough discussion is beyond the scope of this text. However, an understanding of basic principles is desirable to ensure a better comprehension of its potential as a tool for endodontic teaching and researching.

A typical micro-CT scanner consists of a microfocus X-ray source, a motorized high-precision sample rotation stage, a detection array, a system control mechanism, and computing software resources for reconstruction, visualization, and analysis of the root canal anatomy [122]. The source sends X-ray radiation through the tooth attached to the sample stage (Fig. 2.2a), and a detector array – coupled to a digital charge-couple device camera – records attenuated intensities of the X-ray beam, while the object rotates on its own axis (Fig. 2.2b); i.e., micro-CT involves gathering projection data of the tooth from multiple directions. If many projections are recorded from different viewing angles of the same tooth, each projection image will contain different information about its internal structure. At this stage, the only preparation that is absolutely necessary for scanning is to ensure that the previously cleaned tooth fits inside the field of

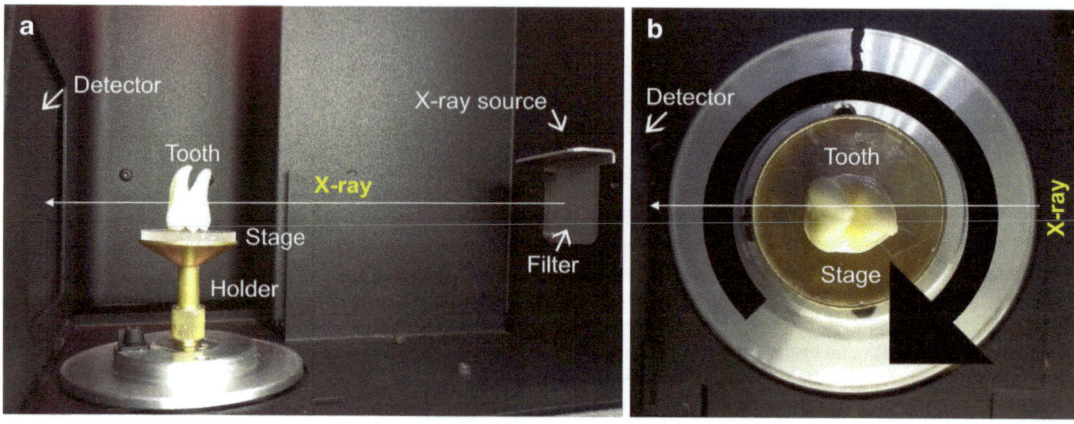

Fig. 2.2 Inside view of the chamber of a SkyScan 1174 v2 (Bruker-microCT, Kontich, Belgium) micro-CT device. Common elements of micro-CT: (**a**) X-ray source, an object attached to the sample stage to be imaged through which the X-rays pass, and a detector(s) that measures the extent to which the X-ray signal has been attenuated by the object. The source sends X-ray radiation through the tooth, and a detector array records attenuated intensities of the X-ray beam, while the object rotates on its own axis (**b**)

view and does not move during the scan [80]. The entire operation of the scanner, including X-ray exposure, type of filter, flat-field correction, resolution, rotation step, rotation angle, number of frames, data collection, etc., is controlled by a software – the system control mechanism – which allows setting up these parameters in order to improve the further 3D reconstruction of the tooth.

After recording the X-ray images, the projection data of the tooth from multiple directions (Fig. 2.3a) is then used as input for a reconstruction algorithm. This algorithm computes a three-dimensional image of the internal anatomy of the tooth, based on the two-dimensional projection images (Fig. 2.3b) [123]. The resulting volumetric images are then subjected to image segmentation using dedicated software. Image segmentation is a manual or automatic procedure that can remove the unwanted structures from the image based on the object density. The goal of segmentation is to simplify the representation of an image into something that is more meaningful and easier to analyze. More precisely, image segmentation is the process of assigning a label to every pixel in an image as such that pixels with the same label share certain visual characteristics [124]. Concerning the tooth, the different radiographic densities of the enamel, dentin, and root canal facilitate the segmentation procedures (Fig. 2.3c). The result of image segmentation is a set of segments that collectively cover the entire image. When applied to a stack of images, as in the study of the internal anatomy of the teeth, the resulting contours after image segmentation can be used to create 3D models with the help of interpolation algorithms, which can be visualized (Fig. 2.3d) or analyzed using different software.

Evaluation of Root Canal Anatomy Using Micro-CT

The first attempt to use micro-CT as a quantitative tool for the analysis of the root canal anatomy was done by Bjørndal et al. [125]. Authors correlated the shape of the root canals to the corresponding roots of five maxillary molars scanned at a resolution of 33 μm. However, the real potential for the analysis of several quantitative parameters using micro-CT was reported in the following year [116]. Peters et al. [116] evaluated the potential and accuracy of micro-CT for detailing the root canal geometry of 12 maxillary molars regarding volume, surface area, diameter, and structured model index. Then, micro-CT was used by different groups to evaluate geometrical changes in root canals after preparation with different instruments and techniques [62, 119, 126–129], as well as, for educa-

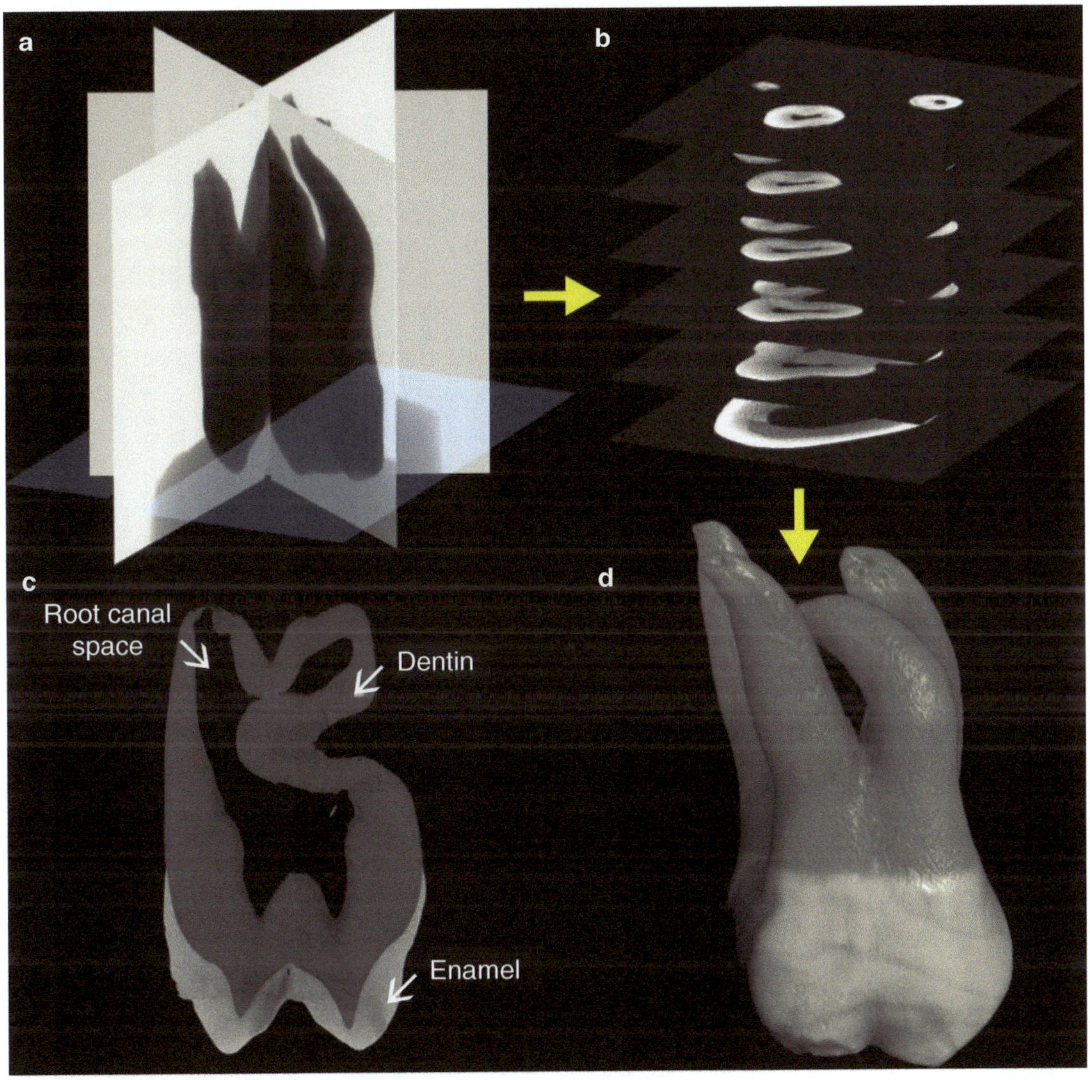

Fig. 2.3 The projection data of the tooth from multiple directions (**a**) is used as input for a reconstruction algorithm which computes a 3D image of the internal anatomy of the tooth, based on the 2D projection images (**b**). The different radiographic densities of the tooth tissues (**c**) facilitate its segmentation which can be used to create 3D models (**d**)

tional purposes [64, 130, 131]. Though, it took over 18 years for the micro-CT scanners gain accessibility [3] and the first in-depth studies evaluating the root canal anatomy started to be published. The main results of the studies published in indexed journals in English language are summarized in Tables 2.1, 2.2, 2.3, and 2.4.

Most of the micro-CT studies on root canal anatomy evaluated anatomical variations present in specific groups of teeth, such as the second canal in the mesiobuccal root of maxillary first molars [161–165, 167–170], three-rooted mandibular premolars [135, 143, 144] and molars [154–156], four-rooted maxillary second molar [67], two-rooted mandibular canines [68] and premolars [141], C-shaped canals in mandibular premolars [136–138] and molars [145, 146, 148–152, 159], radicular grooves [134, 136, 139, 140, 144], and isthmuses [147, 153, 157, 158, 160]. Other authors evaluated the anatomical configuration of conventional mandibular incisors [132, 133], mandibular canines [63], mandibular first

Table 2.1 Micro-CT studies on the root and root canal morphology of incisors and canines

Authors	Aim	Scanner specifications	Main conclusions
Almeida et al. 2013 (Brazil) [132]	To investigate the root canal anatomy of mandibular incisors ($n = 340$)	SkyScan 1174 v2 (50 kV, 80 μA, voxel size: 19.6 μm)	Vertucci's type III configuration represented 92 % of the samples. Oval-shaped canals in the apical third were not uncommon and were more prevalent in the type III anatomy. The incidence of 2 or more root canals at the apical third was 3.2 %
Leoni et al. 2014 (Brazil) [133]	To investigate the root canal anatomy of mandibular central ($n = 100$) and lateral ($n = 100$) incisors	SkyScan 1174 v2 (50 kV, 80 μA, voxel size: 22.9 μm)	Vertucci's types I and III were the most prevalent canal configurations; however, 8 new types were described. Accessory canals were observed only at the apical third; however, most of the incisors had no accessory canals. No difference was observed in the comparison of the morphometric parameter analyzed between central and lateral incisors. The area of the root canal in both teeth increased gradually in the coronal direction. The average roundness represented a flat- or oval-shaped configuration of the canal in the apical third of both groups of teeth
Gu 2011 (China) [134]	To investigate the anatomical features of radicular grooves (RG) in maxillary lateral incisors ($n = 11$)	Siemens Inveon (n.r., voxel size: 15 μm)	RG were classified into type I ($n = 3$), short RG at the coronal third; type II ($n = 5$), long and shallow RG extended beyond the coronal third of the root (in one specimen, a cross-sectional teardrop-like canal was observed); and type III ($n = 3$), long and deep RG associated with a complex root canal system (C shaped, invagination, and additional root/canal). RG were located at mesial ($n = 3$), distal ($n = 6$), and in both ($n = 1$) aspects of the root
Versiani et al. 2011 (Brazil) [68]	To investigate the root canal anatomy of mandibular canines ($n = 14$) with two roots and two distinct canals	SkyScan 1174 v2 (50 kVp, 80 μA, voxel size: 16.7 μm)	Bifurcation was located in both apical (44 %) and middle (58 %) thirds of the root. From a buccal view, no curvature toward the lingual or buccal direction occurred in either roots. From a proximal view, no straight lingual root occurred. In both views, S-shaped roots were found in 21 % of the specimens. Location of the apical foramen tended to the mesiobuccal aspect of both roots. Lateral and furcation canals were observed mostly in the cervical third. SMI ranged from 1.87 to 3.86. Mean volume and area of the canals were 11.52 ± 3.44 mm^3 and 71.16 ± 11.83 mm^2, respectively
Versiani et al. 2013 (Brazil) [63]	To investigate the root canal anatomy of single-rooted mandibular canines ($n = 100$)	SkyScan 1174 v2 (50 kVp, 80 μA, voxel size: 19.6 μm)	31 % of the samples had no accessory canals. The location of the apical foramen varied considerably and its major diameter ranged from 0.16 to 0.72 mm. The mean distance from the root apex to the major apical foramen was 0.27 ± 0.25 mm. Mean major and minor diameters of the canal 1 mm short of the foramen were 0.43 and 0.31 mm, respectively. The mean area, perimeter, form factor, roundness, major and minor diameters, volume, surface area, and SMI were 0.85 ± 0.31 mm^2, 3.69 ± 0.88 mm, 0.70 ± 0.09, 0.59 ± 0.11, 1.36 ± 0.36 mm and 0.72 ± 0.14 mm, 13.33 ± 4.98 mm^3, 63.5 ± 16.4 mm^2, and 3.35 ± 0.64, respectively

n.r. not reported

Table 2.2 Micro-CT studies on the root and root canal morphology of premolars

Authors	Aim	Scanner specifications	Main conclusions
Cleghorn et al. 2008 (Canada) [135]	To investigate unusual variations in the root and canal morphology of mandibular first ($n=1$) and second ($n=1$) premolars	Feinfocus 160 (n.r., voxel size: 30 μm)	Mandibular first premolar exhibited three distinct, separate roots. Corresponding canals divided in the middle to apical third of the root. A prominent furcation canal was present. The mandibular second premolar exhibited a single root, a single apical foramen, and a prominent vertical root groove on buccal surface. Canal system had a C-shaped morphology through the majority of the mid-canal system, which terminated in a single apical foramen
Fan et al. 2008 (China) [136]	To investigate the root and canal morphology of C-shaped mandibular first premolars with ($n=86$) and without ($n=54$) radicular groove (RG) by accessing the morphology of canal orifices	Scanco μCT-80 (n.r., voxel size: 37 μm)	Two canals and bifurcations were dominant at the middle and apical third. It was not possible to define the canal configurations in the middle and apical canal third by just assessing the morphology of coronal canal. Detection and instrumentation of a second canal of a bifurcation located further apically may be a difficult task
Fan et al. 2012 (China) [137]	To investigate the root and canal morphology of C-shaped mandibular first premolars with ($n=146$) and without ($n=181$) radicular groove (RG)	Scanco μCT-20 and μCT-80 (n.r., voxel size: 38 and 30 μm)	No C-shaped canals were found in teeth without RG. C-shaped canals were identified in 66.2 % of premolars with RG. C-shaped mandibular first premolars had a groove on the external root surface. The morphology of C-shaped canals was classified as continuous, semilunar, continuous combined with semilunar, and interrupted by non-C-shaped canal. Seventy furcation canals were observed and 57 were located in C-shaped premolars
Gu et al. 2013 (China) [138]	To investigate the wall thickness and groove configuration in C-shaped mandibular first premolars ($n=148$) with radicular groove (RG)	Siemens Inveon (n.r., voxel size: 15 μm)	C-shaped canals was observed in 29 teeth (19.6 %) and 107 cross sections. 102 sections exhibited a mesial groove. The root length ranged from 9.7 to 14.9 mm. The wall thickness decreased at increasing distances from the CEJ. Buccal and lingual walls were thicker than the distal and mesial walls. Overall, the minimum thickness occurred at the lingual aspect of the mesial (67.3 %) and distal (69.2 %) root walls
Gu et al. 2013 (China) [139]	To investigate the relation between the root canal and the groove in C-shaped mandibular first premolars ($n=148$) with radicular groove (RG)	Siemens Inveon (80 kVp, 500 μA, voxel size: 15 μm)	Mean root length was 12.98 ± 1.36 mm. Shallow and deep RGs were found on 37.5 % and 18.5 % of the specimens, respectively. 155 RGs were observed in 140 premolars. If one RG was present ($n=125$), the location was mostly on the mesiolingual side of the root; if two RGs were present ($n=15$), another groove was located on the distobuccal side. C-shaped canals were found in 29 specimens (19.6 %) and 107 cross sections. The complexity of canal systems in mandibular premolars may be determined by the severity of the RGs
Li et al. 2013 (China) [140]	To investigate the furcation grooves in the buccal root of bifurcated maxillary first premolars ($n=42$)	Scanco μCT-80 (n.r., voxel size: 36 μm)	The prevalence of furcation grooves was 85.7 %. Most of them (69.4 %) were located in the coronal and middle thirds of the buccal roots. The mean groove length was 3.94 mm. The wall thickness of the buccal roots was buccopalatally asymmetric
Li et al. 2012 (China) [141]	To evaluate the anatomical aspects of the lingual canal in mandibular first premolars with Vertucci's type V canal configuration ($n=26$)	Siemens Inveon (80 kVp, 500 μA, voxel size: 14.97 μm)	The lingual canal orifice was located at the middle-apical third with severe angle. 69 % of lingual canals began at the middle third and the remainder at the apical third. The greatest angles "a" [curvature at the beginning of the lingual canal] and "b" [lingual canal curvature] were 65.24° and 43.39°, respectively

(continued)

Table 2.2 (continued)

Authors	Aim	Scanner specifications	Main conclusions
Liu et al. 2013 (China) [142]	To investigate the canal morphology of mandibular first premolars ($n=115$)	Siemens Inveon (80 kVp, 500 µA, voxel size: 14.97 µm)	The shape of the canal orifice was classified as oval (84.3 %), flattened ribbon shaped (7.0 %), eight shaped (7.0 %), and triangular (1.7 %). Root canal configuration was identified as types I (65.2 %), V (22.6 %), III (2.6 %), and VII (0.9 %). Ten specimens did not fit Vertucci's classification. Accessory canals were present in 35.7 % of the teeth and most of them (92.7 %) located in the apical third. The presence of one (50.4 %), two (28.7 %), three (14.8 %), or four (6.1 %) apical foramens was observed mostly laterally (77.4 %). Apical delta and intercanal communications were present in 6.1 % and 3.5 % of the samples, respectively. Mesial invagination of the root was observed in 27.8 % of teeth
Marca et al. 2013 (Brazil) [143]	To evaluate the applicability of micro-CT and iCat CBCT system to study the anatomy of three-rooted maxillary premolars ($n=16$)	SkyScan 1072 (50 kVp, voxel size: 34×34×42 µm)	Mesiobuccal (MB) canal area was greater than distobuccal (DB) canal. Micro-CT images revealed more details than CBCT including the presence of 3 and 2 canals in the middle third of the MB and DB root of one specimen, lateral canals, canal trifurcation in the apical third, and differences in cross-sectional canal shapes in different levels of the root
Ordinola-Zapata et al. 2013 (Brazil) [144]	To describe the morphometric aspects of the external and internal anatomy of mandibular premolars with Vertucci's type IX canal configuration ($n=16$)	SkyScan 1174 v2 (50 kVp, 80 µA, voxel size: 18 µm)	Type IX configuration was found in 15.2 % of mandibular premolars with radicular grooves. Most of them had a triangle-shaped pulp chamber in which the distance between the MB and L canals was the largest. Complexities of the root canal systems such as the presence of furcation canals, fusion of canals, oval-shaped canals at the apical level, small orifices at the pulp chamber level, and apical delta were observed

n.r. not reported

Table 2.3 Micro-CT studies on the root and root canal morphology of mandibular molars

Authors	Aim	Scanner specifications	Main conclusions
Cheung et al. 2007 (China) [145]	To investigate the apical canal morphology of C-shaped mandibular second molars ($n=44$)	Scanco μCT-20 (n.r., voxel size: 30 μm)	Most of the samples had 2 (i.e., type II, IV, V, or VI) or 3 (i.e., type VIII) root canals. 1/5 of specimens showed 4 or more canals. Prevalence of accessory and lateral canals ranged from 11 to 41 %. A total of 115 main and 41 accessory foramina were observed. The diameters of the main and accessory foramina ranged from 0.19 to 0.32 mm and from 0.07 to 0.10 mm, with a mean form factor of 0.73 and 0.82, respectively
Fan et al. 2009 (China) [146]	To investigate effective ways to negotiate the root canal system of C-shaped mandibular second molars ($n=44$)	Scanco μCT-20 (n.r., voxel size: n.r.)	8 teeth had a continuous C-shaped orifice (type I), 16 had a type II configuration, 14 a type III configuration, and 6 a type IV configuration. The total number of the orifices was 83 including 8 continuous C-shaped, 14 mesiobuccal-distal, 14 flat, 41 oval, and 6 round orifices
Fan et al. 2010 (China) [147]	To investigate the morphology of the isthmuses in the mesial root of mandibular first ($n=70$) and second ($n=56$) molars	Scanco μCT-80 (n.r., voxel size: 37 μm)	107 molars (85 %) had isthmuses in the apical 5 mm of mesial roots. The total number of isthmuses was 120, in which 94 samples had only 1 isthmus, and 13 samples had 2. Mandibular first molars had more isthmuses with separate and mixed morphological types, while second molars had more isthmuses with sheet connections
Fan et al. 2004 (China) [148]	To investigate the canal morphology of C-shaped mandibular second molars ($n=54$)	Scanco μCT-20 (n.r., voxel size: n.r.)	C-shaped canals varied in shape at different levels. None of the orifices was found at the level of the CEJ. 1/4 of the orifices were found 1 mm below CEJ, while 98.1 % were located within 3 mm below the CEJ. Canal bifurcation was observed in the apical 4 mm of 17 teeth, with most of them occurring within 2 mm from the apex
Fan et al. 2004 (China) [149]	To investigate the predictability of the radiography in detecting C-shaped canals in mandibular second molars ($n=54$)	Scanco μCT-20 (n.r., voxel size: n.r.)	C1 (uninterrupted "C") and C2 (shape resembled a semicolon) configurations always have narrow isthmuses closed to the groove. C1 and C2 configurations were prevalent in types I (mesial and distal canals merge into one before exiting) and III (separated canals) teeth, suggesting that the debridement of these canals would be more demanding than type II (canals continue on their own pathway to the apex). C-shaped canal system in mandibular molars might be predicted according to the radiographic appearance
Fan et al. 2007 (China) [150]	To investigate the predictability of the radiography in detecting C-shaped canals in mandibular second molars ($n=30$), using a contrast medium	Scanco μCT-20 (n.r., voxel size: n.r.)	The contrast medium helped to discern the C-shaped canal anatomy in mandibular second molars. The development of a device for contrast medium introduction into anatomically complex root canal systems might lead to a useful clinical diagnostic tool

(continued)

Table 2.3 (continued)

Authors	Aim	Scanner specifications	Main conclusions
Fan et al. 2008 (China) [151]	To investigate the predictability of the digital subtraction radiography (DSR) in detecting C-shaped canals in mandibular second molars ($n=30$), using a contrast medium	Scanco μCT-20 (n.r., voxel size: n.r.)	It was observed that some factors, such as the X-ray-projecting angulation and the degree to which the contrast medium is distributed within the canal system, could change the shape and size of canal images, affecting the classification of the canal anatomy. This discrepancy could be the result of incomplete cleaning in the apical canal merging area, which would prevent contrast media from entering this area
Gao et al. 2006 (China) [152]	To investigate the morphology and canal wall thickness at different levels of C-shaped mandibular second molars ($n=98$)	Scanco μCT-20 (n.r., voxel size: 11×11×500 μm/30×30×100 μm)	C-shaped canals were assigned as follows: in type I ($n=32$), canals merged into one major canal before exiting at the apical foramen. In type II ($n=38$), separated mesial and distal canals were located at the mesial part and distal part of the root, respectively. Symmetry of the mesial canal and distal canal was present along the root. In type III ($n=28$), separate mesial and distal canals were evident. The distal canal may have a large isthmus across the furcation area, which commonly made the mesial and distal canals asymmetrical. Differences in the minimum canal wall thickness were observed in the apical and middle portion, but not in the coronal portion
Gu et al. 2009 (China) [153]	To investigate the isthmuses in mesial roots of mandibular first molars ($n=36$)	GE Explore Locus SP (n.r., voxel size: 15 μm)	The morphology of the isthmuses includes the presence of fin, web, or ribbon connecting the individual canals. In the apical third, 32 teeth had isthmus somewhere along its length. Seven out of 32 roots had a continuous isthmus from coronal to apical end, while 25 roots showed a pattern of sections with and without isthmus. The prevalence of an isthmus was higher at the apical 4- to 6-mm level in the 20- to 39-year-old age group (up to 81 %)
Gu et al. 2010 (China) [154]	To investigate the root canal configuration in three- ($n=20$) and two-rooted ($n=25$) mandibular first molars	GE Explore Locus SP (n.r., voxel size: 21 μm)	Pulp floors with two mesial and two distal orifices were frequent ($n=16$). The third root usually curved severely in the proximal view. The lingual edge of the orifice might form a dentinal shelf, which blocks the view of the canal. Grooves could be observed between adjacent orifices. In 65 % of the 3-rooted teeth, mesial root contained a type 2-2 root canal configuration. Type 1-1 canal occurred more frequently in the DL and DB roots. In mesial and distal roots of three-rooted molars, the incidences of lateral canals were 65 % and 40 %, respectively. Furcation canals were not observed

Gu et al. 2010 (China) [155]	To investigate the root canal curvature in three- ($n=20$) and two-rooted ($n=25$) mandibular first molars	GE Explore Locus SP (n.r., voxel size: 21 μm)	In the 3-rooted molars, the mean degrees of curvature in the MB and ML canals were 24.34° and 22.39°, respectively (Schneider method). Secondary curvature was rare in the mesial root. The frequency of S-shaped canals was 60 % of the DB canals. The mean angle of the second curvature was approximately twice that of the primary one. In proximal view, the DL canal exhibited the greatest degree of curvature (32.06°). Using Pruett method, the mean angle and radius of the DL canals were 59.04° and 6.17 mm in proximal view and 26.17° and 20.99 mm in central view, respectively. The curvature in the DL canals had a more severe angle and smaller radius in the proximal view
Gu et al. 2011 (China) [156]	To investigate the root canal morphology in three- ($n=20$) and two-rooted ($n=25$) mandibular first molars	GE Explore Locus SP (n.r., voxel size: 21 μm)	The length of DL roots was shorter than the DB and mesial roots. The buccal and lingual canal walls were thicker than the distal and mesial for MB, ML, and DB canals. The distal wall of the MB/ML canal and the mesial wall of the DB and DL canals were the thinnest zones. It was suggested that the initial apical file for a DL canal should be 2 sizes smaller than that for a DB canal; DB, DL, and MB/ML canals should be instrumented to a mean size of #55, #40, and #45, respectively. The MB, ML, and DB canals were mostly oval, while the DL canals were relatively rounder
Harris et al. 2013 (USA) [157]	To investigate the canal morphology of the mandibular first molars ($n=22$)	n.r. (n.r., voxel size: 11.41 × 12.21 × 17.53 μm)	Mean distance from the mesial to distal orifices at the pulpal floor was 4.35 mm. In the apical third of the distal root, the mean thickness of dentin on the furcation side ranged from 0.25 to 1.47 mm. Types V and I were the most common configurations of the canal in the mesial and distal roots, respectively. Isthmuses were found along the length of all of the mesial roots (100 %) and within 9.1 % of the distal roots. In the mesial and distal roots, an average of 3.73 and 3.36 portals of exit was observed in the apical 0.5 mm of the roots
Mannocci et al. 2005 (U.K.) [158]	To investigate the isthmus at the apical third of the mesial root of mandibular first molars ($n=20$)	GE Testing Lab (100 kVp, voxel size: 12.5 × 12.5 × 25.0 μm)	17 roots had isthmuses in one or more sections of the apical third. Only 4 out of 17 roots with isthmuses had a continuous isthmus from coronal to the apical end. The other 3 roots showed sections with and without isthmuses. The percentage of sections showing isthmuses ranged from 17.25 to 50.25 % in the apical 5 mm of the root canals. The morphology of the isthmuses varied between teeth and within the same tooth

(continued)

Table 2.3 (continued)

Authors	Aim	Scanner specifications	Main conclusions
Min et al. 2006 (China) [159]	To investigate the morphology of the pulp chamber floor of C-shaped mandibular second molars ($n=44$)	Scanco μCT-20 (n.r. voxel size: n.r.)	90.91 % of the pulp chamber floors were within 3 mm below the CEJ. The location of grooves was usually 4 mm below the CEJ. Eight teeth had a continuous C-shaped orifice and type I canal configuration. Types II and III were observed in 16 and 14 teeth, respectively. Six teeth with a C-shaped canal system showed non-C-shaped chamber floors. In type II teeth, the canal configuration was similar to those present in conventional mandibular molars with separated roots. In type III teeth, there was a large MB-D orifice and a small ML orifice
Villas-Boas et al. 2011 (Brazil) [160]	To evaluate the morphology of the canal and the presence of isthmus at the apical third of the mesial root of mandibular first and second molars ($n=60$)	SkyScan 1076 (n.r., voxel size: 18 μm)	The median mesiodistal diameter (in mm) at the 1-, 2-, 3-, and 4-mm levels were 0.22, 0.23, 0.27, and 0.27 in the MB canal and 0.3, 0.3, 0.36, and 0.35 in the ML canal, respectively; while the buccolingual diameters were 0.37, 0.55, 0.54, and 0.54 in the MB canal and 0.35, 0.41, 0.49, and 0.6 in the ML canal, respectively. The presence of isthmuses was more prevalent at the 3- to 4-mm level. 27 teeth presented complete or incomplete isthmuses at the 1-mm apical level. The volume of the apical third ranged from 0.02 to 2.4 mm^3

n.r. not reported

Table 2.4 Micro-CT studies on the root and root canal morphology of maxillary molars

Authors	Aim	Scanner specifications	Main conclusions
Bjørndal et al. 1999 (Denmark) [125]	To analyze the correlation between the shapes of the outer surface of the root and the canal in maxillary molars ($n=5$)	THX1430 GKV (n.r., voxel size: 33 μm)	There was a strong correlation between the shape of the canals and the root components. Authors suggested that 3D volumes generated by micro-CT technology would constitute a platform for preclinical training in fundamental endodontic procedures
Domark et al. 2013 (USA) [161]	To evaluate the reliability of radiography, CBCT, and micro-CT in determining the number of canals in the MB root of maxillary first ($n=13$) and second ($n=14$) molars	Scanco VivaCT 40 (70 kVp, 114 μA, voxel size: 20 μm)	Using human cadavers, it was verified that the number of canals determined with micro-CT was different compared to digital radiography, but similar from those acquired using CBCT system (Kodak 9000). In all maxillary first molars, MB roots had 2 canals, of which 69 % (9 out of 13) exited as 2 or more foramina. Fifty-seven percent (8 out of 14) of maxillary second molar MB root had 2 canals exiting as 2 or more foramina
Gu et al. 2011 (South Korea) [162]	To evaluate the use of minimum-intensity projection technique as an adjunct to evaluate the morphology of the MB root of maxillary first molars ($n=110$)	SkyScan 1172 (n.r., voxel size: 31.8 μm)	24 roots had a single canal. Multiple canals were observed in 76.2 % of the MB roots. 15 MB roots had a completely independent second canal, while 9 had 3 canals. 53 roots had 2 canals that joined into 1 or had 1 canal that divided into 2. Eleven roots showed 6 new configuration types. 82.2 % of roots had multiple apical foramina. Intercanal communications were found in all roots having multiple canals. The incidences of intercanal communication in the coronal, middle, and apical thirds were 40.6 %, 49.5 %, and 44.6 %, respectively
Hosoya et al. 2012 (Japan) [163]	To evaluate the reliability of different methods in detecting a second canal in the MB root of maxillary first molars ($n=86$)	Hitachi MCT100-MFZ (65 kVp, 100 μA, voxel size: n.r.)	A second canal in the MB root was observed in 60.5 % of the samples. Types I, II, III, and IV (Weine's configuration) were observed in 39.5, 15.1, 27.9, and 17.5 % of the samples, respectively. Detection of the second canal was higher for micro-CT and dental CT than the other diagnostic tools
Kim et al. 2013 (South Korea) [164]	To investigate the canal configuration in the MB roots of maxillary first molars ($n=154$)	SkyScan 1172 (100 kVp, 100 μA, voxel size: 15.9 μm)	73.4 % roots presented additional canals. 94 roots had two canals and 19 roots had three or more canals. The most prevalent configurations were Weine's types III (32.8 %), II (23 %), and IV (15 %). Using Vertucci's classification, the most common configurations were types II (23 %), IV (19.5 %), VI (13.3 %), III (10.6 %), V (9.7 %), VII (5.3 %), and VIII (0.9 %). Twenty (17.7 %) roots had 12 new configuration types
Lee et al. 2006 (South Korea) [165]	To evaluate the root canal curvature in maxillary first molars ($n=46$)	SkyScan 1072 (n.r., voxel size: 19.5×19.5×39.0 μm)	Curvatures were most pronounced in the MB canals, moderate in the DB canals, and least in the P canals. Accessory canals within the apical third were present in almost half of the MB canals and nearly a quarter of the DB canals. The curvatures increased in the apical third when accessory canals are present, particularly in MB and DB canals

(continued)

Table 2.4 (continued)

Authors	Aim	Scanner specifications	Main conclusions
Meder-Cowherd et al. 2011 (USA) [166]	To evaluate the apical morphology of the palatal canal of maxillary first and second molars ($n=40$)	Siemens Micro-CAT II (n.r. voxel size: n.r.)	65 % of the specimens had no constriction in the apical 1–3 mm, while the 35 % had a constriction. The morphology frequencies of apical constrictions were parallel (35 %), single (19 %), flaring (18 %), tapered (15 %), and delta (12 %)
Park et al. 2009 (South Korea) [167]	To investigate the canal configuration of the MB root of maxillary first molars ($n=46$)	SkyScan 1072 (n.r., voxel size: 19.5 × 19.5 × 39 μm)	65.2 % of the roots had 2 canals, 28.3 % had 1 canal, and 6.5 % had 3 canals. The most common configuration was type III (2 distinct MB canals; 37 %) followed by types I (single canal; 28.3 %), II (2 MB canals that joined; 17.4 %), IV (1 MB canal that split into 2; 10.9 %), and V (3 canals; 6.5 %)
Somma et al. 2009 (Italy) [168]	To investigate the canal configuration of the MB root of maxillary first molars ($n=30$)	SkyScan 1072 (100 kVp, 98 μA, voxel size: 19.1 × 19.1 × 38 μm)	80 % of the roots had 2 canals. An independent canal was observed in 42 % of roots. Communications between canals were found mainly in the coronal and middle thirds, while accessory canals and loops were mainly found in apical third. In 5 teeth (21 %), a second canal had its origin some distance down the orifice. Isthmus and intercanal connections were observed in different regions of the same root. A single apical foramen was found in 37 % of the samples, while 2 foramina were present in 23 % of the samples. Three separated apical foramina and apical delta were present in 20 % of the samples
Verma and Love 2011 (New Zealand) [169]	To investigate the canal configuration of the MB root of maxillary first molars ($n=20$)	SkyScan 1172 (80 kVp, 85 μA, voxel size: 11.6 μm)	Multiple foramina and accessory canals were found in 17 roots. Types II and III (Weine's classification) were the most prevalent configuration; however, 40 and 30 % of the roots had configurations that could not be classified by Weine's or Vertucci's classification systems, respectively. Intercanal communications were found in 55 % of the roots located in all areas of the roots. In 18 roots with multiple canals, two had completely independent MB canals. Two roots had three canals with separate orifices, while 14 roots had two canals that either joined into one canal, or one canal divided into two or multiple canals, or showed multiple intercanal communications
Versiani et al. 2012 (Brazil) [67]	To investigate the canal morphology of four-rooted maxillary second molars ($n=25$)	SkyScan 1174 v2 (50 kVp, 80 μA, voxel size: 22.6 μm)	Most of the roots presented straight with 1 main canal, except the MB root, which presented 2 canals in 24 % of the sample. No furcation canals were observed. Accessory canals were located mostly in the apical third of the roots, and apical delta was observed in 12 % of the roots. 56 % of the sample presented an irregular quadrilateral-shaped orifice configuration. The mean distance from the pulp chamber floor to the furcation was 2.15 ± 0.57 mm. No difference was observed between roots by considering their length, the configuration of the root canal in the apical third, the SMI, the volume, and the surface area of the root canals
Yamada et al. 2011 (Japan) [170]	To investigate the canal anatomy of the MB root of maxillary first molars ($n=90$)	HMX225 ACTIS4 (100 kVp, 75 μA, voxel size: n.r.)	Single root canals were observed in 44.5 % of the samples, incomplete separation of root canals in 22.3 %, and completely separated canals in 33.3 %. Accessory canals were observed in 76.6 % of the samples

n.r. not reported

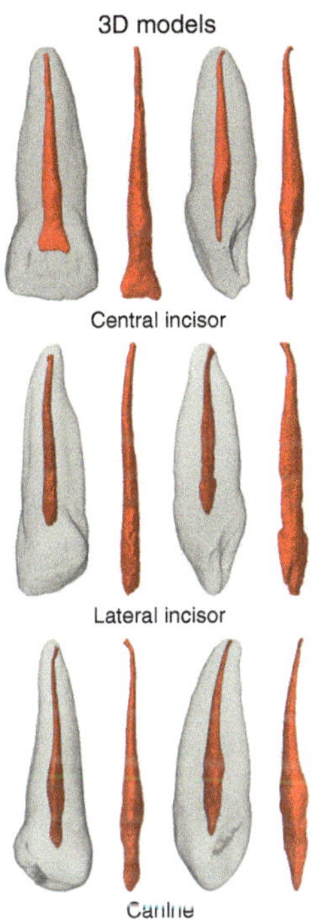

3D models	Normal anatomy[a]	Variations	Anomalies	Clinical remarks[u]
Central incisor	1 canal	2 canals[b] 3 canals[c] 4 canals[d]	Two-rooted[i] Radicular groove[j] Fusion/gemination[k]	- A total of 79.7 % of all foramina were located approximately 0.5 mm or less from the apex and 94.9 % were approximately 1.0 mm or less away - 56.4 % of the lateral canals has a mean diameter less than an size 10 K-file - Average length: 22.5 mm
Lateral incisor	1 canal	2 canals[e] 3 canals[f] 4 canals[g]	Two-rooted[l] Radicular groove[m] Fusion/gemination[n] *Dens invaginatus*[o] *Dens evaginatus*[p] C-shaped[p] Talon cusp[r] Apical curvature[s]	- High frequency of apical root curvature to the disto-buccal direction - Average length: 22 mm
Canine	1 canal	2 canals[h]	*Dens invaginatus*[t]	- Root canal cross-section is usually oval-shaped - Large midroot canal diameter - Average length: 26.5 mm

Fig. 2.4 Morphology of the permanent maxillary anterior teeth. References: (*a*) [171]; (*b*) [172–174]; (*c*) [175]; (*d*) [176]; (*e*) [177–179]; (*f*) [180, 181]; (*g*) [182]; (*h*) [183–185]; (*i*) [172–174]; (*j*) [186]; (*k*) [187]; (*l*) [188]; (*m*) [186]; (*n*) [189]; (*o*) [32]; (*p*) [190]; (*q*) [191]; (*r*) [192]; (*s*) [193]; (*t*) [194]; (*u*) [50, 171, 195]

premolars [142], and maxillary molars [166]. Summarized data for canal numbers and its variations, extracted from selected references, are presented in Figs. 2.4, 2.5, 2.6, and 2.7.

The quantitative morphological data of the first studies [41, 61] on root canal anatomy using conventional methods were taken from measuring some parameters such as area, diameter, and perimeter, acquired from a few cross sections of the root. In contrast, these same parameters can be easily measured by means of micro-CT technology using automatic computer tools in hundreds of slices at once. Based on cross sections of the root, the canal shape has been also qualitatively classified as round, flat, oval, or irregular shaped [242]. Despite its applicability, a qualitative evaluation is always subjective, which may lead to inaccurate results. Algorithms used in micro-CT evaluation allow a mathematical description of these cross-sectional appearances using two morphometric parameters: form factor and roundness. Roundness is defined as 4.A/(p.[dmax]^2), where "A" is the area and "dmax" is the major diameter. The value of roundness ranges from 0 to 1, with 1 signifying a circle. The form factor is calculated by the equation (4.p.A)/P^2, where "A" and "P" are object area and perimeter, respectively. Elongation of individual objects results in smaller values of form factor. Previous results using these parameters in single-rooted canines have demonstrated different cross-sectional forms throughout the root canal [63]. This is an important data as different canal shapes in the same root may have impact on the selected chemomechanical protocol on root canal treatment. Form factor was also used to describe that the shape of the accessory foramen was more round than that of the main foramen in C-shaped canals of mandibular second molars [145] (Fig. 2.8a).

In the earlier studies, 3D analysis was applied qualitatively to evaluate the number and configuration of the main canal, as well as, the presence and location of accessory, lateral, and furcation

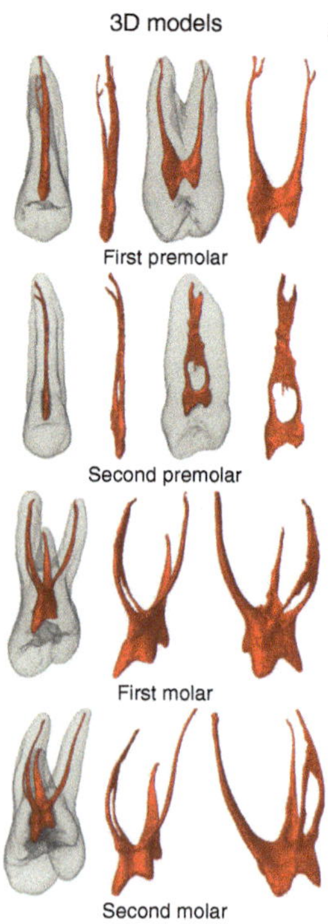

Tooth	Normal anatomy[a]	Second most frequent[a]	Variations	Anomalies	Clinical remarks[v]
First premolar	2 canals	1 canal	3 canals[b]	Furcation groove[l] Gemination/fusion[m] *Dens evaginatus*[n]	- In cross-section at the CEJ, the palatal orifice is wider buccolingually and kidney-shaped because of the mesial concavity of the root - The palatel canal usually is slightly larger than the buccal canal - Incidence of furcation groove on the palatal aspect of the buccal root has been reported as between 62 % and 100 % - Average length: 20.6 mm
Second premolar	1 canal	2 canals	3 canals[c]	*Dens invaginatus*[o]	- The root canal system is wider buccolingually than mesiodistally - 2 or 3 canals can occur in a single root - Average length: 21.5 mm
First molar	4 canals	3 canals	1 canal[d] 5 canals[e] 6 canals[f] 7 canals[g] 8 canals[h]	C-shaped[p] Four-rooted[q] Hypertaurodontism[r]	- There are 2 MB canals in majority of cases - Location of the MB2 canal varies greatly - The palatal root often curves buccally at the apical third - Palatal and MB roots contain 1 (most commom), 2 or 3 root canals, while DB have 1 or 2 canals - A concavity exists on the distal aspect of the MB root, which makes this wall thin - Average length: 20.8 mm
Second molar	3 canals	4 canals	1 canal[i] 2 canals[j] 5 canals[k]	Gemination/fusion[s] Four-rooted[t] Hypertaurodontism[u]	- Generally, the 3 roots are grouped closer together and are sometimes fused - The 2nd molar usually has one canal in each root; however, it may have 2 or 3 MB canals, 1 or 2 DB canals, or 2 palatal canals - Teeth with fused roots occasionally have only 2 canals (buccal and palatal) of equal length and diameter - Average length: 20 mm

Fig. 2.5 Morphology of the permanent maxillary posterior teeth. References: (*a*) [171]; (*b*, *c*) [196]; (*d*) [197]; (*e*) [198]; (*f*) [199]; (*g*) [200]; (*h*) [201]; (*i*, *j*) [202]; (*k*) [203]; (*l*) [204]; (*m*) [205]; (*n*) [206]; (*o*) [207]; (*p*) [208]; (*q*) [209]; (*r*) [210]; (*s*) [211]; (*t*) [67]; (*u*) [212]; (*v*) [50, 171, 195]

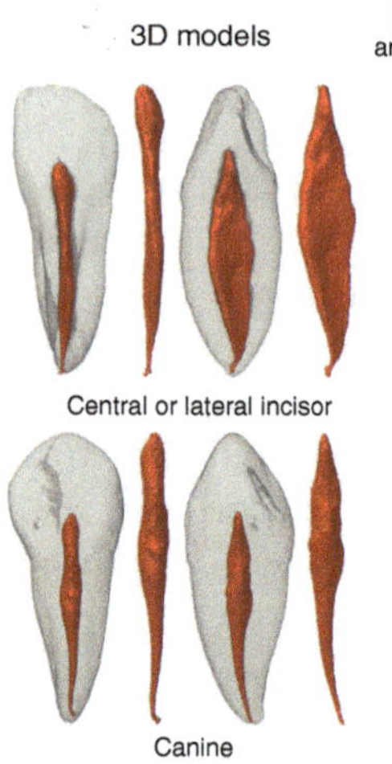

Tooth	Normal anatomy[a]	Second most frequent[a]	Variations	Anomalies	Clinical remarks[i]
Central or lateral incisor	1 canal	2 canals	3 canals[c]	Gemination/fusion[e] *Dens invaginatus*[f] Two-rooted[g]	- Most incisors have a single root - Often a dentinal bridge is present in the pulp chamber that divides the root into 2 canals - The 2 canals usually join and exit through a single apical foramen; but, they may persist as 2 separate canals - Removal of the lingual shoulder is critical, because this tooth often has 2 canals - Canal cross-section is oval-shaped, wider buccolingually than mesiodistally - Average length: 20.7 mm
Canine	1 canal	2 canals[b]	3 canals[d]	Two-rooted[h]	- The root canal is narrow mesiodistally but usually very broad buccolingually - In two-rooted canines, a lingual shoulder must be removed to gain access to the entrance of a second canal - The lingual wall is almost slit-like compared with the larger buccal wall, which makes the canal. - Average length: 25.6 mm

Fig. 2.6 Morphology of the permanent mandibular anterior teeth. References: (*a*) [171]; (*b*) [68]; (*c*) [133]; (*d*) [213]; (*e*) [214]; (*f*) [215]; (*g*) [216]; (*h*) [68]; (*i*) [50, 171, 195]

canals, and apical deltas. Nowadays, 3D analysis using micro-CT algorithms allows also for the calculation of volume and surface area [116]. The clinical significance of such parameters has been emphasized by studies demonstrating that variations in canal geometry before cleaning and shaping had a greater effect on the changes that occurred during preparation than did the instrumentation techniques [119]. Besides, considering that the main role of laboratory-based studies is to develop well-controlled condition, these morphological data should be taken into account in

3D models	Normal anatomy[(a)]	Second most frequent[(a)]	Variations	Anomalies	Clinical remarks[(ak)]
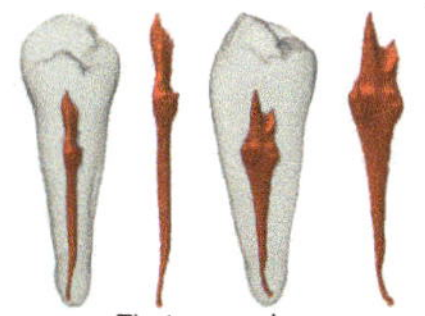 First premolar	1 canal	2 canals	3 canals[(b)] 4 canals[(c)]	Radicular groove[(m)] C-shaped[(n)] *Dens evaginatus*[(o)] *Dens invaginatus*[(p)] Gemination/fusion[(q)]	- The root canal system is extremely variated. - The root canal system is wider buccolingually than mesiodistally - At the cervical third is oval-shaped and tends to become round at the middle and apical thirds - The lingual canal, when present, tends to diverge from the main canal at a sharp angle - Average length: 21.6 mm
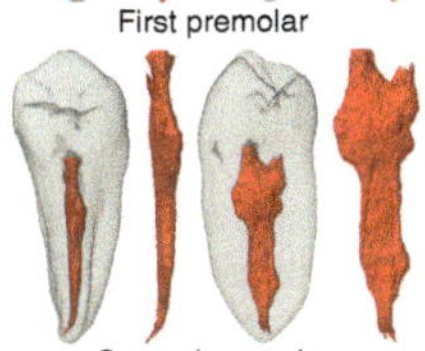 Second premolar	1 canal	2 canals	3 canals[(d)] 4 canals[(e)] 5 canals[(f)]	Two rooted[(r)] C-shaped[(s)] *Dens evaginatus*[(t)] Taurodontism[(u)] Gemination/fusion[(v)]	- The root canal is more often oval than round - The lingual canal, when present, tends to diverge from the main canal at a sharp angle - The canal morphology may present many variation - Average length: 22.3 mm
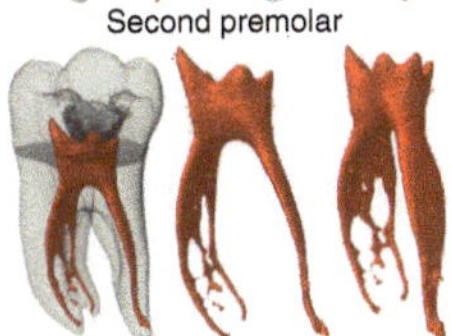 First molar	4 canals	3 canals	5 canals[(g)] 6 canals[(h)] 7 canals[(i)]	Radix[(w)] Taurodontism[(x)] Apical curvature[(y)] Gemination/fusion[(z)] Isthmuses[(aa)] Three-rooted[(ab)] C-shaped[(ac)] Middle mesial[(ad)] Middle distal[(ae)]	- It usually has 2 roots, but occasionally it has 3, with 2 or 3 canals in the mesial root and 1,2, or 3 canals in the distal root - The distal surface of the mesial root and the mesial surface of the distal root have a concavity, which makes the dentin wall very thin - The presence of root canal isthmuses averages 55% in the mesial root and 20 % in the distal root - Multiple accessory foramina may be present in the furcation area. - Average length: 21 mm
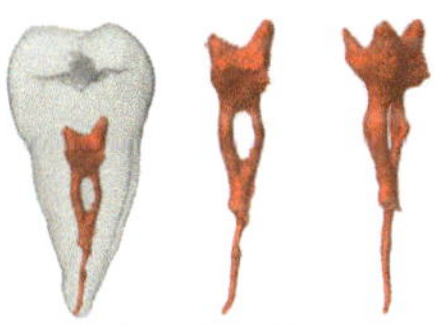 Second molar	3 canals	4 canals	1 canal[(j)] 2 canals[(k)] 5 canals[(l)]	Apical curvature[(af)] Gemination/fusion[(ag)] Isthmuses[(ah)] C-shaped[(ai)] Middle mesial[(aj)]	- It may have 1 to 5 canals, although the most prevalent configurations are 3 and 4 canals - The 2 mesial orifices are located closer together - A variation in root morphology is the presence of C-shaped canal - The apices of this tooth often are close to the mandibular canal - Average length: 19.8 mm

Fig. 2.7 Morphology of the permanent mandibular posterior teeth. References: (*a*) [171]; (*b*) [144]; (*c*) [217]; (*d*) [218]; (*e*) [219]; (*f*) [220]; (*g*) [221]; (*h*) [222]; (*i*) [223]; (*j*) [224]; (*k*) [225]; (*l*) [226]; (*m*) [139]; (*n*) [136]; (*o*) [227]; (*p*) [228]; (*q*) [229]; (*r*) [230]; (*s*) [135]; (*t*) [231]; (*u*) [220]; (*v*) [232]; (*w*) [233]; (*x*) [234]; (*y*) [35]; (*z*) [235]; (*aa*) [147]; (*ab*) [236]; (*ac*) [237]; (*ad*) [238]; (*ae*) [239]; (*af*) [35]; (*ag*) [240]; (*ah*) [147]; (*ai*) [148, 149]; (*aj*) [241]; (*ak*) [50, 171, 195]

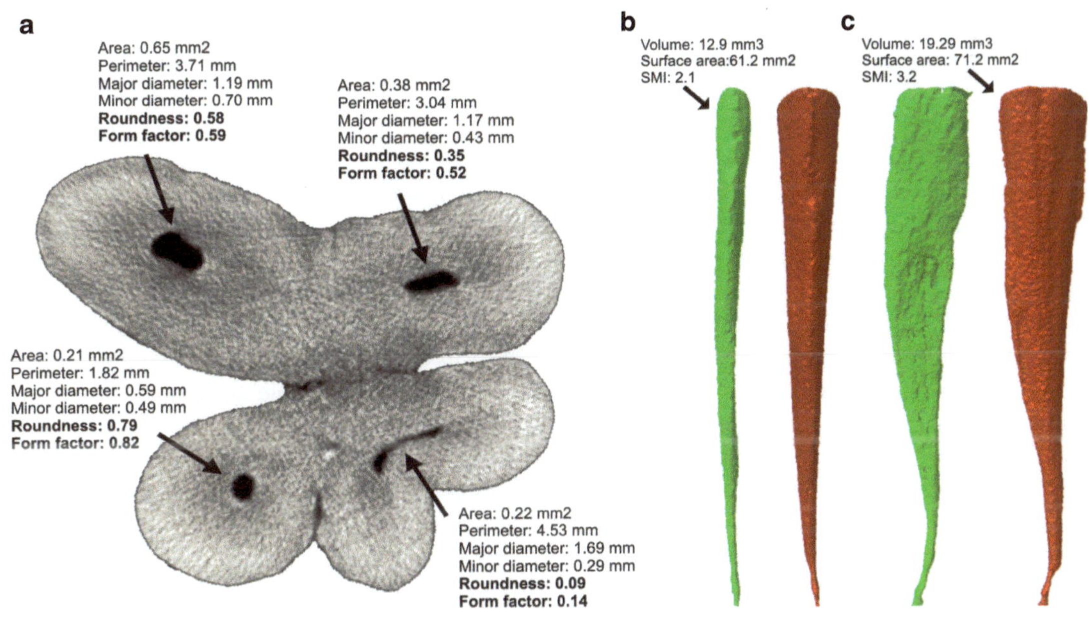

Fig. 2.8 (**a**) Two-dimensional micro-CT cross section of the cervical third of a maxillary first molar root showing the 2D parameter measurements of the four root canals. (**b**) Frontal and (**c**) lateral views of 3D models of a mandibular canine root canal before (*green*) and after (*red*) preparation with a conventional multiple-file rotary system, demonstrating the qualitative and quantitative changes in the canal geometry

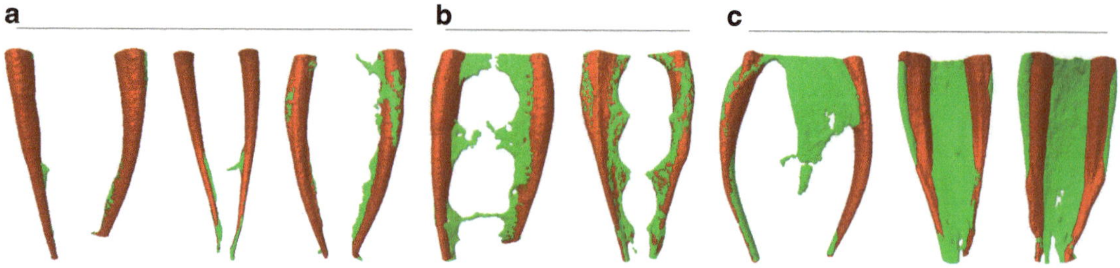

Fig. 2.9 Three-dimensional micro-CT models of the mesial root system of 8 mandibular molars presenting regular (**a**) and irregular (**b**) tapered root canals, as well as, canals connected by isthmus (**c**), after preparation (in *red*) with single-file reciprocating systems. From *left* to *right*, it is possible to observe that with the increase of the complexity of the root canal system, the amount of non-prepared canal surface areas (in *green*) also increases

the sample selection, as the results of such studies might demonstrate the effect of canal anatomy rather than the variable of interest [63, 68, 119, 243, 244].

Another interesting 3D parameter that can be evaluated using micro-CT is the so-called structure model index (SMI). SMI is derived as 6. ((S'.V)/S2), where S is the object surface area before dilation and S' is the change in surface area caused by dilation. V is the initial, undilated object volume. An ideal plate, cylinder, and sphere have SMI values of 0, 3, and 4, respectively. SMI is impossible to achieve using conventional techniques such as radiographs or grinding, and describes the plate- or cylinder-like geometry of an object. The SMI is determined by an infinitesimal enlargement of the surface, while the change in volume is related to changes of surface area, that is, to the convexity of the structure. This parameter has been used to assess root canal geometry three-dimensionally in anatomical studies of different groups of teeth [63, 67, 68, 116] (Fig. 2.8b, c). A recent study has shown a large discrepancy between the minimum and maximum values of SMI in the comparison of the root canal thirds in a same tooth [63]. These dissimilarities should be taken into consideration during the root canal preparation as it might compromise the treatment outcome.

The Influence of Root Canal Anatomy on Irrigation Procedures

Advances with micro-CT analysis brought new perspectives on the overall mechanical preparation quality, confirming the inability of shaping tools in acting within the anatomical complexity of the root canal [81, 118, 126–129, 243, 245, 246]. Preparation of oval-, flattened-, or irregular-shaped cross-sectional root canals using different instruments has shown to leave unprepared extensions or recesses which can harbor remnants of necrotic pulp tissue and biofilms [242, 243]. The disinfecting effects of instruments and irrigants may be additionally hampered in the presence of complex anatomy such as accessory canals, ramifications, intercanal connections, fins, isthmuses, and apical deltas, which cannot be properly accessed and cleaned by conventional techniques [147, 153, 158, 168, 243]. These hard-to-reach areas may also be packed with dentin debris generated and pushed therein by endodontic instruments, interfering with disinfection by both preventing the irrigant flow into them as well as by neutralizing its efficacy [247, 248] (Fig. 2.9).

Based on the aforementioned assumptions, spreading and flushing the irrigant throughout the canal space assumes a pivotal role in treatment because it acts mechanically and chemically on remnants of necrotic pulp tissue and bacterial communities colonizing the main canal [243]. In order to circumvent limitations generated by the unpredictable anatomical configurations of the root canal, making cleaning and disinfection procedures more predictable, several instruments and techniques have been developed and are properly detailed in this book. Ideally, efficient irrigation solutions and protocols are required to provide fluid penetrability to such an extent as to accomplishing a microcirculation flow throughout the intricate root canal anatomy and to counterbalance the suboptimal debridement quality obtained by currently available

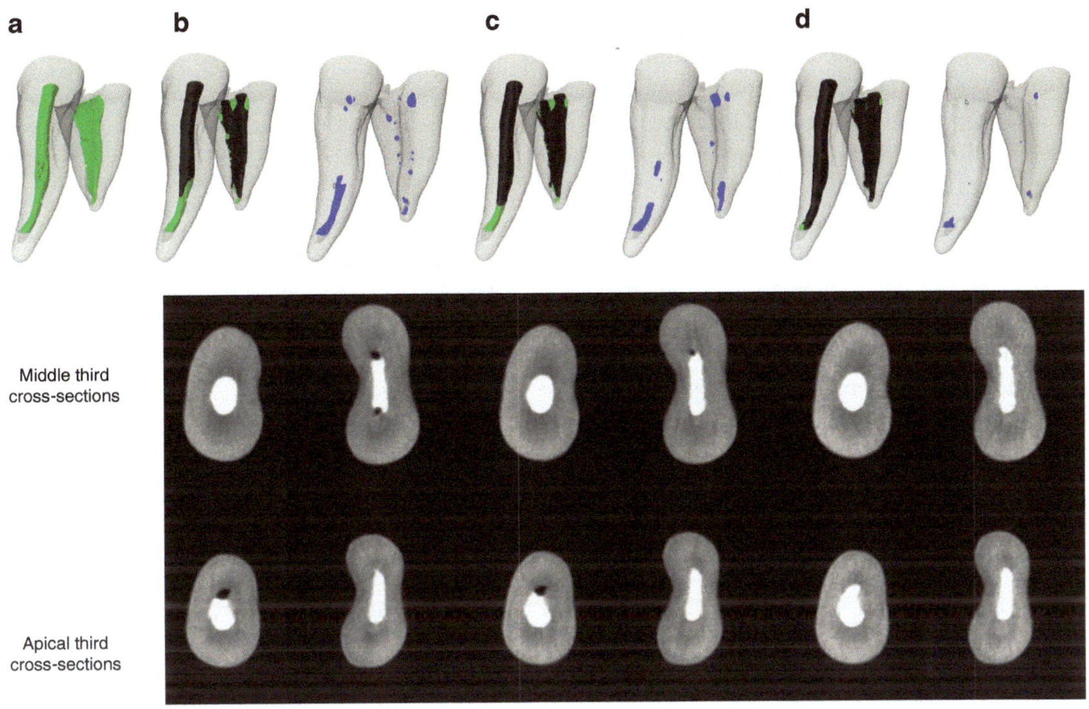

Fig. 2.10 Three-dimensional micro-CT models of a type I root canal configuration molar. Original root canal anatomy (in *green*) prior to treatment (**a**) and after glide path (**b**), root canal preparation (**c**), and ultrasonic passive irrigation technique (**d**), subsequently to the injection of a contrast solution (in *black*). Irrigant-free areas are shown in *blue* after each preparation step. *Below*: same cross sections of the root in different levels showing the root canal space (in *black*) before preparation and the contrast solution (in *white*) and irrigant-free areas (in *black*) after glide path, canal preparation, and ultrasonic irrigation

technology in the mechanical enlargement of the root canal space [246].

In laboratory-based studies, several experimental models have been used to understand the intracanal effect of irrigants by different irrigation protocols. It includes artificially created grooves [249], histological cross sections [250], computational fluid dynamics (CFD) [251–253], and in vivo use of radiopaque solutions [254–256]. These methodological approaches provide valuable information about the quality of cleaning and shaping procedures which cannot otherwise be obtained, but they are unable to show some critical factors, such as the volume of the solution or the root canal areas effectively touched by the irrigant [257]. Besides, the destructive approach of these methods stands for its major drawback, since the preoperative condition of the root canal is unknown.

An ideal experimental model should allow a reliable in situ volumetric quantitative evaluation of the root canal space, offering a deeper and comprehensive understanding on capabilities and limitations of different irrigation protocols. Recently, micro-CT has gained increasing significance in endodontics as it offers a reproducible technique for the three-dimensional assessment of the root canal system [63, 67, 68, 119, 244, 245, 248] in different groups of teeth (Tables 2.1, 2.2, 2.3, and 2.4). Micro-CT technology may also overcome several limitations displayed by the conventional methods on the study of root canal irrigation, as it provides three-dimensional quantitative volumetric and two-dimensional mapping of the irrigant within the root canal space (Fig. 2.10).

Using micro-CT, the volume of irrigant can be correlated to the full root canal volume and with the presence of some anatomical irregularity or the presence of dentin debris that may avoid the spreadability of the irrigant. A comprehensive quantification of irrigant-free areas can also be calculated and correlated, for example, to the irrigant delivery method, fluid activation system, irrigation needle penetration and design, root canal configuration, amount of hard tissue debris, or shaping protocols. Besides, three-dimensional visualization of the hard-to-reach areas can provide useful information related to irrigation efficiency. Data can be further subjected to inferential statistical models to assess the relevance of different irrigation protocols following the established parameters. Recently, a nondestructive experimental model that allows a two- and three-dimensional in situ quantification of several outcome parameters related to irrigation in the complex root canal space was proposed [257]. These interesting aspects definitely open a new methodological appraisal to study irrigation efficiency, bringing the possibility to a better understanding of the irrigant behavior in the near future.

References

1. Tachibana H, Matsumoto K. Applicability of X-ray computerized tomography in endodontics. Endod Dent Traumatol. 1990;6:16–20.
2. Elliott JC, Dover SD. X-ray microtomography. J Microsc. 1982;126:211–3.
3. Nielsen RB, Alyassin AM, Peters DD, Carnes DL, Lancaster J. Microcomputed tomography: an advanced system for detailed endodontic research. J Endod. 1995;21:561–8.
4. Dowker SE, Davis GR, Elliott JC. X-ray microtomography: nondestructive three-dimensional imaging for in vitro endodontic studies. Oral Surg Oral Med Oral Pathol Oral Radiol Endod. 1997;83:510–6.
5. Davis GR, Wong FS. X-ray microtomography of bones and teeth. Physiol Meas. 1996;17:121–46.
6. Carabelli G. Systematisches Handbuch der Zahnheilkunde. II. Anatomic des Mundes. Vienna: Braumuller and Siedel; 1842.
7. Mühlreiter E. Anatomie des menschlichen Gebisses von med. Th. E. de Jonge Cohen. Leipzig: Arthur Felix; 1870.
8. Black GV. Descriptive anatomy of the human teeth. Philadelphia: The Wilmington Dental Manufacturing co.; 1890.
9. Gysi A, Röse C. Sammlung von Mikrophotographien zur Veranschaulichung der mikroscopischen Struktur der Zähne des Menschen. Zürich: Mikrophotographien der Zahnhistologie; 1894.
10. Preiswerk G. Leherbuch und Atlas der Zahnheilkunde mit Einschluβ der Mund-Krankheiten. Munich: J. F Lehmann; 1903.
11. Fisher G. Beitrage zur behandlung enkrankter zahne mit besonderer beucksichtigung der anatomie und pathologie der wurzelkanale. Leipzig: Georg Thiéme; 1908.
12. Dewey M. Dental anatomy. St. Louis: C.V. Mosby Company; 1916.
13. Spalteholz W. Über das durchsichtigmachen von menschlichen und tierischen präparaten und seine theoretischen bedigungen. Leipzig: F. Hirzel; 1914.
14. Adloff P. Das Durchsichtigmachen von Zähnen und unsere Wurzelfüllungsmethoden. Dtsch Monatsschr Zahnheifkd. 1913;31:445.
15. Fasoli G. Sull'anatomia dei canali radicolari dei denti umani. Stomatologia 1913;11:409–15.
16. Moral H. Uber das vorkommen eines vierten kanals in oberen molaren. Österr.-Ungar Vjschr Zahnheilk 1915;31:313–25.
17. Hess W, Zurcher E. The anatomy of the root canals of the teeth of the permanent and deciduous dentitions. London: John Bale, Sons & Danielsson, Ltd.; 1925.
18. Hess W. Die pulpaamputation als selbstandige wurzelbehandlungsmethod. Leipzig: Georg Thiéme; 1917.
19. Okumura T. Anatomy of the root canals. J Am Dent Assoc. 1927;14:632–6.
20. Meyer W, Scheele E. Die Anatomie der Wurzelkanäle der oberen Frontzähne. Dtsch Zahnärztl. 1955;10: 1041–5.
21. Mueller AH. Anatomy of the root canals of the incisors, cuspids and bicuspids of the permanent teeth. J Am Dent Assoc. 1933;20:1361–86.
22. Barker BC, Lockett BC, Parsons KC. The demonstration of root canal anatomy. Aust Dent J. 1969;14: 37–41.
23. Sykaras SN. Endodontic treatment of teeth with variations of the root canals. J Br Endod Soc. 1971;5: 28–31.
24. Pineda F, Kuttler Y. Mesiodistal and buccolingual roentgenographic investigation of 7,275 root canals. Oral Surg Oral Med Oral Pathol. 1972;33:101–10.
25. Kaffe I, Kaufman A, Littner MM, Lazarson A. Radiographic study of the root canal system of mandibular anterior teeth. Int Endod J. 1985;18:253–9.
26. Fabra-Campos H. Three canals in the mesial root of mandibular first permanent molars: a clinical study. Int Endod J. 1989;22:39–43.
27. Baratto-Filho F, Fariniuk LF, Ferreira EL, Pécora JD, Cruz-Filho AM, Sousa-Neto MD. Clinical and macroscopic study of maxillary molars with two palatal roots. Int Endod J. 2002;35:796–801.
28. Ferraz JA, de Carvalho Junior JR, Saquy PC, Pécora JD, Sousa-Neto MD. Dental anomaly: dens evaginatus (talon cusp). Braz Dent J. 2001;12:132–4.
29. Sousa Neto MD, Paiva EP, Saquy PC, Pécora JD. Treatment of dens invaginatus in supernumerary teeth. Aust Endod J. 1998;24:85–7.
30. Estrela C, Pereira HL, Pécora JD. Radicular grooves in maxillary lateral incisor: case report. Braz Dent J. 1995;6:143–6.
31. Pécora JD, Conrado CA, Zuccolotto WG, Sousa-Neto MD, Saquy PC. Root canal therapy of an anomalous

maxillary central incisor: a case report. Endod Dent Traumatol. 1993;9:260–2.
32. Pécora JD, Saquy PC, de Souza JE, Sousa-Neto MD. Endodontic treatment of a maxillary lateral incisor presenting dens invaginatus and transposition to the region of the canine–case report. Braz Dent J. 1991;2:5–8.
33. Nattress BR, Martin DM. Predictability of radiographic diagnosis of variations in root canal anatomy in mandibular incisor and premolar teeth. Int Endod J. 1991;24:58–62.
34. Burger CL, Mork TO, Hutter JW, Nicoll B. Direct digital radiography versus conventional radiography for estimation of canal length in curved canals. J Endod. 1999;25:260–3.
35. Schäfer E, Diez C, Hoppe W, Tepel J. Roentgenographic investigation of frequency and degree of canal curvatures in human permanent teeth. J Endod. 2002;28:211–6.
36. Barker BC, Parsons KC, Mills PR, Williams GL. Anatomy of root canals. I. Permanent incisors, canines and premolars. Aust Dent J. 1973;18:320–7.
37. Barker BC, Parsons KC, Mills PR, Williams GL. Anatomy of root canals. III. Permanent mandibular molars. Aust Dent J. 1974;19:408–13.
38. Barker BC, Parsons KC, Mills PR, Williams GL. Anatomy of root canals. II. Permanent maxillary molars. Aust Dent J. 1974;19:46–50.
39. Green D. Morphology of pulp cavity of the permanent teeth. Oral Surg Oral Med Oral Pathol. 1955;8:743–59.
40. Green D. Double canals in single roots. Oral Surg Oral Med Oral Pathol. 1973;35:689–96.
41. Green EN. Microscopic investigation of root canal diameters. J Am Dent Assoc. 1958;57:636–44.
42. Weine FS, Healey HJ, Gerstein H, Evanson L. Canal configuration in the mesiobuccal root of the maxillary first molar and its endodontic significance. Oral Surg Oral Med Oral Pathol. 1969;28:419–25.
43. Kerekes K, Tronstad L. Morphometric observations on the root canals of human molars. J Endod. 1977;3:114–8.
44. Kerekes K, Tronstad L. Morphometric observations on root canals of human anterior teeth. J Endod. 1977;3:24–9.
45. Kerekes K, Tronstad L. Morphometric observations on root canals of human premolars. J Endod. 1977;3:74–9.
46. Mauger MJ, Schindler WG, Walker 3rd WA. An evaluation of canal morphology at different levels of root resection in mandibular incisors. J Endod. 1998;24:607–9.
47. Green D. A stereomicroscopic study of the root apices of 400 maxillary and mandibular anterior teeth. Oral Surg Oral Med Oral Pathol. 1956;9:1224–32.
48. Burch JG, Hulen S. The relationship of the apical foramen to the anatomic apex of the tooth root. Oral Surg Oral Med Oral Pathol. 1972;34:262–8.
49. Robertson D, Leeb IJ, McKee M, Brewer E. A clearing technique for the study of root canal systems. J Endod. 1980;6:421–4.
50. Vertucci FJ. Root canal anatomy of the human permanent teeth. Oral Surg Oral Med Oral Pathol. 1984;58:589–99.
51. Venturi M, Prati C, Capelli G, Falconi M, Breschi L. A preliminary analysis of the morphology of lateral canals after root canal filling using a tooth-clearing technique. Int Endod J. 2003;36:54–63.
52. Weng XL, Yu SB, Zhao SL, Wang HG, Mu T, Tang RY, Zhou XD. Root canal morphology of permanent maxillary teeth in the Han nationality in Chinese Guanzhong area: a new modified root canal staining technique. J Endod. 2009;35:651–6. doi:10.1016/j.joen.2009.02.010.
53. Guerisoli DM, de Souza RA, de Sousa Neto MD, Silva RG, Pécora JD. External and internal anatomy of third molars. Braz Dent J. 1998;9:91–4.
54. Sharma R, Pécora JD, Lumley PJ, Walmsley AD. The external and internal anatomy of human mandibular canine teeth with two roots. Endod Dent Traumatol. 1998;14:88–92.
55. Rocha LF, Sousa Neto MD, Fidel SR, da Costa WF, Pécora JD. External and internal anatomy of mandibular molars. Braz Dent J. 1996;7:33–40.
56. Pécora JD, Sousa Neto MD, Saquy PC. Internal anatomy, direction and number of roots and size of human mandibular canines. Braz Dent J. 1993;4:53–7.
57. Pécora JD, Sousa Neto MD, Saquy PC, Woelfel JB. In vitro study of root canal anatomy of maxillary second premolars. Braz Dent J. 1993;3:81–5.
58. Pécora JD, Saquy PC, Sousa-Neto MD, Woelfel JB. Root form and canal anatomy of maxillary first premolars. Braz Dent J. 1992;2:87–94.
59. Pécora JD, Woelfel JB, Sousa Neto MD, Issa EP. Morphologic study of the maxillary molars. Part II: internal anatomy. Braz Dent J. 1992;3:53–7.
60. Naoum HJ, Love RM, Chandler NP, Herbison P. Effect of X-ray beam angulation and intraradicular contrast medium on radiographic interpretation of lower first molar root canal anatomy. Int Endod J. 2003;36:12–9.
61. Gilles J, Reader A. An SEM investigation of the mesiolingual canal in human maxillary first and second molars. Oral Surg Oral Med Oral Pathol. 1990;70:638–43.
62. Bergmans L, Van Cleynenbreugel J, Wevers M, Lambrechts P. A methodology for quantitative evaluation of root canal instrumentation using microcomputed tomography. Int Endod J. 2001;34:390–8.
63. Versiani MA, Pécora JD, Sousa-Neto MD. Microcomputed tomography analysis of the root canal morphology of single-rooted mandibular canines. Int Endod J. 2013;46:800–7. doi:10.1111/iej.12061.
64. Grande NM, Plotino G, Gambarini G, Testarelli L, D'Ambrosio F, Pecci R, Bedini R. Present and future in the use of micro-CT scanner 3D analysis for the study of dental and root canal morphology. Ann Ist Super Sanita. 2012;48:26–34. doi:10.4415/ANN_12_01_05.
65. Grover C, Shetty N. Methods to study root canal morphology: a review. Quintessence Int. 2012;6:171–82.

66. Perrini N, Castagnola L. W Hess & O. Keller's anatomical plates: studies on the anatomical structure of root canals in human dentition by a method of making the tooth substance transparent (1928). Milan: Altini Communicazioni Grafiche; 1998.
67. Versiani MA, Pécora JD, Sousa-Neto MD. Root and root canal morphology of four-rooted maxillary second molars: a micro-computed tomography study. J Endod. 2012;38:977–82. doi:10.1016/j.joen.2012.03.026.
68. Versiani MA, Pécora JD, Sousa-Neto MD. The anatomy of two-rooted mandibular canines determined using micro-computed tomography. Int Endod J. 2011;44:682–7. doi:10.1111/j.1365-2591.2011.01879.x.
69. Mayo CV, Montgomery S, de Rio C. A computerized method for evaluating root canal morphology. J Endod. 1986;12:2–7.
70. Hounsfield GN. Computerized transverse axial scanning (tomography). 1. Description of system. Br J Radiol. 1973;46:1016–22.
71. Pao YC, Reinhardt RA, Krejci RF, Taylor DT. Computer-graphics aided instruction of three-dimensional dental anatomy. J Dent Educ. 1984;48:315–7.
72. Gullickson DC, Montgomery S. The study of root canal morphology using a digital image processing technique. J Endod. 1987;13:158–63. doi:10.1016/S0099-2399(87)80133-4.
73. Dobó-Nagy C, Keszthelyi G, Szabó J, Sulyok P, Ledeczky G, Szabó J. A computerized method for mathematical description of three-dimensional root canal axis. J Endod. 2000;26:639–43.
74. Berutti E. Computerized analysis of the instrumentation of the root canal system. J Endod. 1993;19:236–8.
75. Blašković-Šubat V, Smojver B, Marićić B, Sutalo J. A computerized method for the evaluation of root canal morphology. Int Endod J. 1995;28:290–6.
76. Lyroudia K, Mikrogeorgis G, Nikopoulos N, Samakovitis G, Molyvdas I, Pitas I. Computerized 3-D reconstruction of two "double teeth". Endod Dent Traumatol. 1997;13:218–22.
77. Lyroudia K, Samakovitis G, Pitas I, Lambrianidis T, Molyvdas I, Mikrogeorgis G. 3D reconstruction of two C-shape mandibular molars. J Endod. 1997;23:101–4.
78. Lyroudia K, Mikrogeorgis G, Bakaloudi P, Kechagias E, Nikolaidis N, Pitas I. Virtual endodontics: three-dimensional tooth volume representations and their pulp cavity access. J Endod. 2002;28:599–602.
79. Hegedus C, Flora-Nagy E, Martos R, Juhasz A, Fulop I, Pomahazi S, Nagy IP, Toth Z, Marton I, Keszthelyi G. 3D reconstruction based on hard tissue microtome cross-section pictures in dentistry. Comput Methods Programs Biomed. 2000;63:77–84. doi:S0169-2607(00)00059-6 [pii].
80. Ketcham RA, Carlson WD. Acquisition, optimization and interpretation of X-ray computed tomographic imagery: applications to the geosciences. Comput Geosci. 2001;27:381–4000.
81. Gambill JM, Alder M, del Rio CE. Comparison of nickel-titanium and stainless steel hand-file instrumentation using computed tomography. J Endod. 1996;22:369–75.
82. Robinson S, Czerny C, Gahleitner A, Bernhart T, Kainberger FM. Dental CT evaluation of mandibular first premolar root configurations and canal variations. Oral Surg Oral Med Oral Pathol Oral Radiol Endod. 2002;93:328–32.
83. Garg AK, Tewari RK, Agrawal N. Prevalence of three-rooted mandibular first molars among Indians using SCT. Int J Dent. 2013;2013:183869. doi:10.1155/2013/183869.
84. Nayak BG, Singh I. Using spiral computed tomography for endodontic management of a mandibular first molar with a middle mesial canal: a case report. Gen Dent. 2013;61:43–6.
85. Reuben J, Velmurugan N, Kandaswamy D. The evaluation of root canal morphology of the mandibular first molar in an Indian population using spiral computed tomography scan: an in vitro study. J Endod. 2008;34:212–5. doi:10.1016/j.joen.2007.11.018.
86. Cimilli H, Cimilli T, Mumcu G, Kartal N, Wesselink P. Spiral computed tomographic demonstration of C-shaped canals in mandibular second molars. Dentomaxillofac Radiol. 2005;34:164–7.
87. Appel TR, Baumann MA. Solid-state nuclear magnetic resonance microscopy demonstrating human dental anatomy. Oral Surg Oral Med Oral Pathol Oral Radiol Endod. 2002;94:256–61.
88. Baumann MA. A new approach to demonstration of root canal anatomy. J Dent Educ. 1994;58:704–8.
89. Baumann MA, Doll GM. Spatial reproduction of the root canal system by magnetic resonance microscopy. J Endod. 1997;23:49–51.
90. Baumann MA, Schwebel T, Kriete A. Dental anatomy portrayed with microscopic volume investigations. Comput Med Imaging Graph. 1993;17:221–8.
91. Sustercic D, Sersa I. Human tooth pulp anatomy visualization by 3D magnetic resonance microscopy. Radiol Oncol. 2012;46:1–7. doi:10.2478/v10019-012-0018-y.
92. Idiyatullin D, Corum C, Moeller S, Prasad HS, Garwood M, Nixdorf DR. Dental magnetic resonance imaging: making the invisible visible. J Endod. 2011;37:745–52. doi:10.1016/j.joen.2011.02.022.
93. Tanasiewicz M. Magnetic resonance imaging in human teeth internal space requirements for visualization of dental prosthetics. J Exp Clin Dent. 2010;2:19–24.
94. Barton DJ, Clark SJ, Eleazer PD, Scheetz JP, Farman AG. Tuned-aperture computed tomography versus parallax analog and digital radiographic images in detecting second mesiobuccal canals in maxillary first molars. Oral Surg Oral Med Oral Pathol Oral Radiol Endod. 2003;96:223–8.
95. Nance R, Tyndall D, Levin LG, Trope M. Identification of root canals in molars by tuned-aperture computed tomography. Int Endod J. 2000;33:392–6.

96. Shemesh H, van Soest G, Wu MK, van der Sluis LW, Wesselink PR. The ability of optical coherence tomography to characterize the root canal walls. J Endod. 2007;33:1369–73. doi:10.1016/j.joen.2007.06.022.
97. Huang CC, Chang YC, Chuang MC, Lai TM, Lai JY, Lee BS, Lin CP. Evaluation of root and canal systems of mandibular first molars in Taiwanese individuals using cone-beam computed tomography. J Formos Med Assoc. 2010;109:303–8. doi:10.1016/S0929-6646(10)60056-3.
98. Lee JH, Kim KD, Lee JK, Park W, Jeong JS, Lee Y, Gu Y, Chang SW, Son WJ, Lee WC, Baek SH, Bae KS, Kum KY. Mesiobuccal root canal anatomy of Korean maxillary first and second molars by cone-beam computed tomography. Oral Surg Oral Med Oral Pathol Oral Radiol Endod. 2011;111:785–91. doi:10.1016/j.tripleo.2010.11.026.
99. Matherne RP, Angelopoulos C, Kulild JC, Tira D. Use of cone-beam computed tomography to identify root canal systems in vitro. J Endod. 2008;34:87–9. doi:10.1016/j.joen.2007.10.016.
100. Michetti J, Maret D, Mallet JP, Diemer F. Validation of cone beam computed tomography as a tool to explore root canal anatomy. J Endod. 2010;36:1187–90. doi:10.1016/j.joen.2010.03.029.
101. Neelakantan P, Subbarao C, Ahuja R, Subbarao CV, Gutmann JL. Cone-beam computed tomography study of root and canal morphology of maxillary first and second molars in an Indian population. J Endod. 2011;36:1622–7. doi:10.1016/j.joen.2010.07.006.
102. Tian YY, Guo B, Zhang R, Yu X, Wang H, Hu T, Dummer PM. Root and canal morphology of maxillary first premolars in a Chinese subpopulation evaluated using cone-beam computed tomography. Int Endod J. 2012;45:996–1003. doi:10.1111/j.1365-2591.2012.02059.x.
103. Yu X, Guo B, Li KZ, Zhang R, Tian YY, Wang H, Tao Hu DDS. Cone-beam computed tomography study of root and canal morphology of mandibular premolars in a western Chinese population. BMC Med Imaging. 2012;12:18. doi:10.1186/1471-2342-12-18.
104. Zhang R, Yang H, Yu X, Wang H, Hu T, Dummer PM. Use of CBCT to identify the morphology of maxillary permanent molar teeth in a Chinese subpopulation. Int Endod J. 2011;44:162–9. doi:10.1111/j.1365-2591.2010.01826.x.
105. Shenoi RP, Ghule HM. CBVT analysis of canal configuration of the mesio-buccal root of maxillary first permanent molar teeth: an in vitro study. Contemp Clin Dent. 2012;3:277–81. doi:10.4103/0976-237X.103618.
106. Hassan BA, Payam J, Juyanda B, van der Stelt P, Wesselink PR. Influence of scan setting selections on root canal visibility with cone beam CT. Dentomaxillofac Radiol. 2012;41:645–8. doi:10.1259/dmfr/27670911.
107. Han X, Yang H, Li G, Yang L, Tian C, Wang Y. A study of the distobuccal root canal orifice of the maxillary second molars in Chinese individuals evaluated by cone-beam computed tomography. J Appl Oral Sci. 2012;20:563–7. doi:S1678-7757 2012000500012 [pii].
108. Kim Y, Lee SJ, Woo J. Morphology of maxillary first and second molars analyzed by cone-beam computed tomography in a korean population: variations in the number of roots and canals and the incidence of fusion. J Endod. 2012;38:1063–8. doi:10.1016/j.joen.2012.04.025.
109. Szabo BT, Pataky L, Mikusi R, Fejerdy P, Dobo-Nagy C. Comparative evaluation of cone-beam CT equipment with micro-CT in the visualization of root canal system. Ann Ist Super Sanita. 2012;48:49–52. doi:10.4415/ANN_12_01_08.
110. Seo DG, Gu Y, Yi YA, Lee SJ, Jeong JS, Lee Y, Chang SW, Lee JK, Park W, Kim KD, Kum KY. A biometric study of C-shaped root canal systems in mandibular second molars using cone-beam computed tomography. Int Endod J. 2012;45:807–14. doi:10.1111/j.1365-2591.2012.02037.x.
111. Zhang R, Wang H, Tian YY, Yu X, Hu T, Dummer PM. Use of cone-beam computed tomography to evaluate root and canal morphology of mandibular molars in Chinese individuals. Int Endod J. 2011;44:990–9. doi:10.1111/j.1365-2591.2011.01904.x.
112. Zheng Q, Zhang L, Zhou X, Wang Q, Wang Y, Tang L, Song F, Huang D. C-shaped root canal system in mandibular second molars in a Chinese population evaluated by cone-beam computed tomography. Int Endod J. 2011;44:857–62. doi:10.1111/j.1365-2591.2011.01896.x.
113. Bauman R, Scarfe W, Clark S, Morelli J, Scheetz J, Farman A. Ex vivo detection of mesiobuccal canals in maxillary molars using CBCT at four different isotropic voxel dimensions. Int Endod J. 2011;44:752–8. doi:10.1111/j.1365-2591.2011.01882.x.
114. Wang Y, Zheng QH, Zhou XD, Tang L, Wang Q, Zheng GN, Huang DM. Evaluation of the root and canal morphology of mandibular first permanent molars in a western Chinese population by cone-beam computed tomography. J Endod. 2010;36:1786–9. doi:10.1016/j.joen.2010.08.016.
115. Stock SR. Microcomputed tomography: methodology and applications. Boca Raton: CRC Press; 2009.
116. Peters OA, Laib A, Ruegsegger P, Barbakow F. Three-dimensional analysis of root canal geometry by high-resolution computed tomography. J Dent Res. 2000;79:1405–9. doi:10.1177/00220345000790060901.
117. Rhodes JS, Ford TR, Lynch JA, Liepins PJ, Curtis RV. Micro-computed tomography: a new tool for experimental endodontology. Int Endod J. 1999;32:165–70.
118. Rhodes JS, Pitt Ford TR, Lynch JA, Liepins PJ, Curtis RV. A comparison of two nickel-titanium instrumentation techniques in teeth using microcomputed tomography. Int Endod J. 2000;33:279–85.

119. Peters OA, Laib A, Gohring TN, Barbakow F. Changes in root canal geometry after preparation assessed by high-resolution computed tomography. J Endod. 2001;27:1–6.
120. Jung M, Lommel D, Klimek J. The imaging of root canal obturation using micro-CT. Int Endod J. 2005;38:617–26.
121. Hammad M, Qualtrough A, Silikas N. Three-dimensional evaluation of effectiveness of hand and rotary instrumentation for retreatment of canals filled with different materials. J Endod. 2008;34: 1370–3. doi:10.1016/j.joen.2008.07.024.
122. Wang G, Vannier MW. Overview on micro-CT scanners for biomedical applications. Adv Imaging. 2001;16:22–7.
123. Feldkamp LA, Davis LC, Kress JW. Practical cone-beam algorithm. J Opt Soc Am. 1984;1:612–9.
124. Pham DL, Xu C, Prince JL. Current methods in medical image segmentation. Annu Rev Biomed Eng. 2000;2:315–37. doi:10.1146/annurev.bioeng.2.1.315.
125. Bjørndal L, Carlsen O, Thuesen G, Darvann T, Kreiborg S. External and internal macromorphology in 3D-reconstructed maxillary molars using computerized X-ray microtomography. Int Endod J. 1999;32:3–9.
126. Peters OA, Schönenberger K, Laib A. Effects of four Ni-Ti preparation techniques on root canal geometry assessed by micro computed tomography. Int Endod J. 2001;34:221–30.
127. Hübscher W, Barbakow F, Peters OA. Root-canal preparation with FlexMaster: canal shapes analysed by micro-computed tomography. Int Endod J. 2003;36:740–7.
128. Bergmans L, Van Cleynenbreugel J, Beullens M, Wevers M, Van Meerbeek B, Lambrechts P. Smooth flexible versus active tapered shaft design using NiTi rotary instruments. Int Endod J. 2002;35:820–8.
129. Bergmans L, Van Cleynenbreugel J, Beullens M, Wevers M, Van Meerbeek B, Lambrechts P. Progressive versus constant tapered shaft design using NiTi rotary instruments. Int Endod J. 2003;36: 288–95.
130. Rao AK. The computerized, three-dimensional reconstruction of human teeth for pedagogical purposes. Stanford Undergrad Res J. 2002;1:55–9.
131. Suebnukarn S, Hataidechadusadee R, Suwannasri N, Suprasert N, Rhienmora P, Haddawy P. Access cavity preparation training using haptic virtual reality and microcomputed tomography tooth models. Int Endod J. 2011;44:983–9. doi:10.1111/j.1365-2591.2011.01899.x.
132. Almeida MM, Bernardineli N, Ordinola-Zapata R, Villas-Boas MH, Amoroso-Silva PA, Brandão CG, Guimaraes BM, Moraes IG, Hungaro Duarte MA. Micro–computed tomography analysis of the root canal anatomy and prevalence of oval canals in mandibular incisors. J Endod. 2013;39:1529–33. doi:10.1016/j.joen.2013.08.033.
133. Leoni GB, Versiani MA, Pécora JD, Sousa-Neto MD. Micro–computed tomographic analysis of the root canal morphology of mandibular incisors. J Endod. 2014;40:710–6. doi:10.1016/j.joen.2013.09.003.
134. Gu YC. A micro-computed tomographic analysis of maxillary lateral incisors with radicular grooves. J Endod. 2011;37:789–92. doi:10.1016/j.joen.2011.03.002.
135. Cleghorn BM, Christie WH, Dong CC. Anomalous mandibular premolars: a mandibular first premolar with three roots and a mandibular second premolar with a C-shaped canal system. Int Endod J. 2008;41:1005–14. doi:10.1111/j.1365-2591.2008.01451.x.
136. Fan B, Yang J, Gutmann JL, Fan M. Root canal systems in mandibular first premolars with C-shaped root configurations. Part I: microcomputed tomography mapping of the radicular groove and associated root canal cross-sections. J Endod. 2008;34: 1337–41. doi:10.1016/j.joen.2008.08.006.
137. Fan B, Ye W, Xie E, Wu H, Gutmann JL. Three-dimensional morphological analysis of C-shaped canals in mandibular first premolars in a Chinese population. Int Endod J. 2012;45:1035–41. doi:10.1111/j.1365-2591.2012.02070.x.
138. Gu YC, Zhang YP, Liao ZG, Fei XD. A micro-computed tomographic analysis of wall thickness of C-shaped canals in mandibular first premolars. J Endod. 2013;39:973–6. doi:10.1016/j.joen.2013.04.039.
139. Gu Y, Zhang Y, Liao Z. Root and canal morphology of mandibular first premolars with radicular grooves. Arch Oral Biol. 2013;58:1609–17. doi:10.1016/j.archoralbio.2013.07.014.
140. Li J, Li L, Pan Y. Anatomic study of the buccal root with furcation groove and associated root canal shape in maxillary first premolars by using micro-computed tomography. J Endod. 2013;39:265–8. doi:10.1016/j.joen.2012.10.003.
141. Li X, Liu N, Ye L, Nie X, Zhou X, Wen X, Liu R, Liu L, Deng M. A micro-computed tomography study of the location and curvature of the lingual canal in the mandibular first premolar with two canals originating from a single canal. J Endod. 2012;38:309–12. doi:10.1016/j.joen.2011.12.038.
142. Liu N, Li X, Ye L, An J, Nie X, Liu L, Deng M. A micro-computed tomography study of the root canal morphology of the mandibular first premolar in a population from southwestern China. Clin Oral Investig.2013;17:999–1007.doi:10.1007/s00784-012-0778-1.
143. Marca C, Dummer PM, Bryant S, Vier-Pelisser FV, So MV, Fontanella V, Dutra VD, de Figueiredo JA. Three-rooted premolar analyzed by high-resolution and cone beam CT. Clin Oral Investig. 2013;17:1535–40. doi:10.1007/s00784-012-0839-5.
144. Ordinola-Zapata R, Bramante CM, Villas-Boas MH, Cavenago BC, Duarte MH, Versiani MA. Morphologic micro-computed tomography analysis

of mandibular premolars with three root canals. J Endod. 2013;39:1130–5. doi:10.1016/j.joen.2013.02.007.

145. Cheung GS, Yang J, Fan B. Morphometric study of the apical anatomy of C-shaped root canal systems in mandibular second molars. Int Endod J. 2007;40:239–46. doi:10.1111/j.1365-2591.2007.01193.x.

146. Fan B, Min Y, Lu G, Yang J, Cheung GS, Gutmann JL. Negotiation of C-shaped canal systems in mandibular second molars. J Endod. 2009;35:1003–8. doi:10.1016/j.joen.2009.04.011.

147. Fan B, Pan Y, Gao Y, Fang F, Wu Q, Gutmann JL. Three-dimensional morphologic analysis of isthmuses in the mesial roots of mandibular molars. J Endod. 2010;36:1866–9. doi:10.1016/j.joen.2010.08.030.

148. Fan B, Cheung GS, Fan M, Gutmann JL, Bian Z. C-shaped canal system in mandibular second molars: part I–anatomical features. J Endod. 2004;30:899–903.

149. Fan B, Cheung GS, Fan M, Gutmann JL, Fan W. C-shaped canal system in mandibular second molars: part II–radiographic features. J Endod. 2004;30:904–8.

150. Fan W, Fan B, Gutmann JL, Cheung GS. Identification of C-shaped canal in mandibular second molars. Part I: radiographic and anatomical features revealed by intraradicular contrast medium. J Endod. 2007;33:806–10. doi:10.1016/j.joen.2007.04.007.

151. Fan W, Fan B, Gutmann JL, Fan M. Identification of a C-shaped canal system in mandibular second molars. Part III. Anatomic features revealed by digital subtraction radiography. J Endod. 2008;34:1187–90. doi:10.1016/j.joen.2008.06.013.

152. Gao Y, Fan B, Cheung GS, Gutmann JL, Fan M. C-shaped canal system in mandibular second molars part IV: 3-D morphological analysis and transverse measurement. J Endod. 2006;32:1062–5.

153. Gu L, Wei X, Ling J, Huang X. A microcomputed tomographic study of canal isthmuses in the mesial root of mandibular first molars in a Chinese population. J Endod. 2009;35:353–6. doi:10.1016/j.joen.2008.11.029.

154. Gu Y, Lu Q, Wang H, Ding Y, Wang P, Ni L. Root canal morphology of permanent three-rooted mandibular first molars – part I: pulp floor and root canal system. J Endod. 2010;36:990–4. doi:10.1016/j.joen.2010.02.030.

155. Gu Y, Lu Q, Wang P, Ni L. Root canal morphology of permanent three-rooted mandibular first molars: part II-measurement of root canal curvatures. J Endod. 2010;36:1341–6. doi:10.1016/j.joen.2010.04.025.

156. Gu Y, Zhou P, Ding Y, Wang P, Ni L. Root canal morphology of permanent three-rooted mandibular first molars: part III–an odontometric analysis. J Endod. 2011;37:485–90. doi:10.1016/j.joen.2011.01.013.

157. Harris SP, Bowles WR, Fok A, McClanahan SB. An anatomic investigation of the mandibular first molar using micro-computed tomography. J Endod. 2013;39:1374–8. doi:10.1016/j.joen.2013.06.034.

158. Mannocci F, Peru M, Sherriff M, Cook R, Pitt Ford TR. The isthmuses of the mesial root of mandibular molars: a micro-computed tomographic study. Int Endod J. 2005;38:558–63.

159. Min Y, Fan B, Cheung GS, Gutmann JL, Fan M. C-shaped canal system in mandibular second molars. Part III: the morphology of the pulp chamber floor. J Endod. 2006;32:1155–9. doi:10.1016/j.joen.2006.07.004.

160. Villas-Boas MH, Bernardineli N, Cavenago BC, Marciano M, Del Carpio-Perochena A, de Moraes IG, Duarte MH, Bramante CM, Ordinola-Zapata R. Micro-computed tomography study of the internal anatomy of mesial root canals of mandibular molars. J Endod. 2011;37:1682–6. doi:10.1016/j.joen.2011.08.001.

161. Domark JD, Hatton JF, Benison RP, Hildebolt CF. An ex vivo comparison of digital radiography and cone-beam and micro computed tomography in the detection of the number of canals in the mesiobuccal roots of maxillary molars. J Endod. 2013;39:901–5. doi:10.1016/j.joen.2013.01.010.

162. Gu Y, Lee JK, Spangberg LS, Lee Y, Park CM, Seo DG, Chang SW, Hur MS, Hong ST, Kum KY. Minimum-intensity projection for in-depth morphology study of mesiobuccal root. Oral Surg Oral Med Oral Pathol Oral Radiol Endod. 2011;112:671–7. doi:10.1016/j.tripleo.2011.04.036.

163. Hosoya N, Yoshida T, Iino F, Arai T, Mishima A, Kobayashi K. Detection of a secondary mesiobuccal canal in maxillary first molar: a comparative study. J Conserv Dent. 2012;15:127–31. doi:10.4103/0972-0707.94579.

164. Kim Y, Chang SW, Lee JK, Chen IP, Kaufman B, Jiang J, Cha BY, Zhu Q, Safavi KE, Kum KY. A micro-computed tomography study of canal configuration of multiple-canalled mesiobuccal root of maxillary first molar. Clin Oral Investig. 2013;17:1541–6. doi:10.1007/s00784-012-0852-8.

165. Lee JK, Ha BH, Choi JH, Heo SM, Perinpanayagam H. Quantitative three-dimensional analysis of root canal curvature in maxillary first molars using micro-computed tomography. J Endod. 2006;32:941–5.

166. Meder-Cowherd L, Williamson AE, Johnson WT, Vasilescu D, Walton R, Qian F. Apical morphology of the palatal roots of maxillary molars by using micro-computed tomography. J Endod. 2011;37:1162–5. doi:10.1016/j.joen.2011.05.012.

167. Park JW, Lee JK, Ha BH, Choi JH, Perinpanayagam H. Three-dimensional analysis of maxillary first molar mesiobuccal root canal configuration and curvature using micro-computed tomography. Oral Surg Oral Med Oral Pathol Oral Radiol Endod. 2009;108:437–42. doi:10.1016/j.tripleo.2009.01.022.

168. Somma F, Leoni D, Plotino G, Grande NM, Plasschaert A. Root canal morphology of the mesiobuccal root of maxillary first molars: a micro-computed tomographic analysis. Int Endod J. 2009;42:165–74. doi:10.1111/j.1365-2591.2008.01472.x.
169. Verma P, Love RM. A micro CT study of the mesiobuccal root canal morphology of the maxillary first molar tooth. Int Endod J. 2011;44:210–7. doi:10.1111/j.1365-2591.2010.01800.x.
170. Yamada M, Ide Y, Matsunaga S, Kato H, Nakagawa K. Three-dimensional analysis of mesiobuccal root canal of Japanese maxillary first molar using micro-CT. Bull Tokyo Dent Coll. 2011;52:77–84. doi:JST.JSTAGE/tdcpublication/52.77 [pii].
171. Vertucci FJ. Root canal morphology and its relationship to endodontic procedures. Endod Top. 2005;10:3–29. doi:10.1111/j.1601-1546.2005.00129.x.
172. Gonzalez-Plata RR, Gonzalez-Plata EW. Conventional and surgical treatment of a two-rooted maxillary central incisor. J Endod. 2003;29:422–4.
173. Lambruschini GM, Camps J. A two-rooted maxillary central incisor with a normal clinical crown. J Endod. 1993;19:95–6.
174. Lin WC, Yang SF, Pai SF. Nonsurgical endodontic treatment of a two-rooted maxillary central incisor. J Endod. 2006;32:478–81.
175. Gondim Jr E, Setzer F, Zingg P, Karabucak B. A maxillary central incisor with three root canals: a case report. J Endod. 2009;35:1445–7. doi:10.1016/j.joen.2009.05.028.
176. Mangani F, Ruddle CJ. Endodontic treatment of a "very particular" maxillary central incisor. J Endod. 1994;20:560–1.
177. Ghoddusi J, Javidi M, Vatanpour M. Treatment of a two-canal maxillary lateral incisor. N Y State Dent J. 2010;76:40–1.
178. Pécora JD, Santana SV. Maxillary lateral incisor with two roots–case report. Braz Dent J. 1992;2:151–3.
179. Thompson BH, Portell FR, Hartwell GR. Two root canals in a maxillary lateral incisor. J Endod. 1985;11:353–5.
180. Peix-Sanchez M, Minana-Laliga R. A case of unusual anatomy: a maxillary lateral incisor with three canals. Int Endod J. 1999;32:236–40.
181. Walvekar SV, Behbehani JM. Three root canals and dens formation in a maxillary lateral incisor: a case report. J Endod. 1997;23:185–6.
182. Kottoor J, Murugesan R, Albuquerque DV. A maxillary lateral incisor with four root canals. Int Endod J. 2012;45:393–7. doi:10.1111/j.1365-2591.2011.01984.x.
183. Alapati S, Zaatar EI, Shyama M, Al-Zuhair N. Maxillary canine with two root canals. Med Princ Pract. 2006;15:74–6.
184. Barkhordar RA, Nguyen NT. Maxillary canine with two roots. J Endod. 1985;11:224–7.
185. Bolla N, Kavuri SR. Maxillary canine with two root canals. J Conserv Dent. 2011;14:80–2. doi:10.4103/0972-0707.80726.
186. Pécora JD, da Cruz Filho AM. Study of the incidence of radicular grooves in maxillary incisors. Braz Dent J. 1992;3:11–6.
187. Libfeld H, Stabholz A, Friedman S. Endodontic therapy of bilaterally geminated permanent maxillary central incisors. J Endod. 1986;12:214–6.
188. Fried IL, Winter AA. Diagnosis and treatment of a two-rooted maxillary lateral incisor. Periodontal Case Rep. 1984;6:40–4.
189. Wong M. Treatment considerations in a geminated maxillary lateral incisor. J Endod. 1991;17:179–81.
190. Mupparapu M, Singer SR, Goodchild JH. Dens evaginatus and dens invaginatus in a maxillary lateral incisor: report of a rare occurrence and review of literature. Aust Dent J. 2004;49:201–3.
191. Boveda C, Fajardo M, Millan B. Root canal treatment of an invaginated maxillary lateral incisor with a C-shaped canal. Quintessence Int. 1999;30:707–11.
192. Ozcelik B, Atila B. Bilateral palatal talon cusps on permanent maxillary lateral incisors: a case report. Eur J Dent. 2011;5:113–6.
193. Park PS, Kim KD, Perinpanayagam H, Lee JK, Chang SW, Chung SH, Kaufman B, Zhu Q, Safavi KE, Kum KY. Three-dimensional analysis of root canal curvature and direction of maxillary lateral incisors by using cone-beam computed tomography. J Endod. 2013;39:1124–9. doi:10.1016/j.joen.2013.06.001.
194. Sousa Neto MD, Zuccolotto WG, Saquy PC, Grandini SA, Pécora JD. Treatment of dens invaginatus in a maxillary canine case report. Braz Dent J. 1992;2:147–50.
195. Hargreaves KM, Cohen S. Cohen's pathways of the pulp. 10th ed. St. Louis: Mosby; 2011.
196. Soares JA, Leonardo RT. Root canal treatment of three-rooted maxillary first and second premolars–a case report. Int Endod J. 2003;36:705–10.
197. Gopikrishna V, Bhargavi N, Kandaswamy D. Endodontic management of a maxillary first molar with a single root and a single canal diagnosed with the aid of spiral CT: a case report. J Endod. 2006;32:687–91.
198. Beatty RG. A five-canal maxillary first molar. J Endod. 1984;10:156–7.
199. Albuquerque DV, Kottoor J, Dham S, Velmurugan N, Abarajithan M, Sudha R. Endodontic management of maxillary permanent first molar with 6 root canals: 3 case reports. Oral Surg Oral Med Oral Pathol Oral Radiol Endod. 2010;110:e79–83. doi:10.1016/j.tripleo.2010.04.017.
200. Kottoor J, Velmurugan N, Sudha R, Hemamalathi S. Maxillary first molar with seven root canals diagnosed with cone-beam computed tomography scanning: a case report. J Endod. 2010;36:915–21. doi:10.1016/j.joen.2009.12.015.
201. Kottoor J, Velmurugan N, Surendran S. Endodontic management of a maxillary first molar with eight root canal systems evaluated using cone-beam computed

tomography scanning: a case report. J Endod. 2011;37:715–9. doi:10.1016/j.joen.2011.01.008.
202. Peikoff MD, Christie WH, Fogel HM. The maxillary second molar: variations in the number of roots and canals. Int Endod J. 1996;29:365–9.
203. Kottoor J, Hemamalathi S, Sudha R, Velmurugan N. Maxillary second molar with 5 roots and 5 canals evaluated using cone beam computerized tomography: a case report. Oral Surg Oral Med Oral Pathol Oral Radiol Endod. 2010;109:e162–5. doi:10.1016/j.tripleo.2009.09.032.
204. Lammertyn PA, Rodrigo SB, Brunotto M, Crosa M. Furcation groove of maxillary first premolar, thickness, and dentin structures. J Endod. 2009;35:814–7. doi:10.1016/j.joen.2009.03.012.
205. Nahmias Y, Rampado ME. Root-canal treatment of a trifid crown premolar. Int Endod J. 2002;35:390–4.
206. Colak H, Aylikci BU, Keklik H. Dens evaginatus on maxillary first premolar: report of a rare clinical case. J Nat Sci Biol Med. 2012;3:192–4. doi:10.4103/0976-9668.101915.
207. Rotstein I, Stabholz A, Friedman S. Endodontic therapy for dens invaginatus in a maxillary second premolar. Oral Surg Oral Med Oral Pathol. 1987;63:237–40.
208. De Moor RJ. C-shaped root canal configuration in maxillary first molars. Int Endod J. 2002;35:200–8.
209. Di Fiore PM. A four-rooted quadrangular maxillary molar. J Endod. 1999;25:695–7.
210. Sert S, Bayrl G. Taurodontism in six molars: a case report. J Endod. 2004;30:601–2.
211. Koenen DJ, Pahncke D. Gemination or fusion: use of a CT scan to assist in diagnosis and endodontic treatment of a maxillary second molar – a case report. ENDO. 2008;2:145–51.
212. Radwan A, Kim SG. Treatment of a hypertaurodontic maxillary second molar in a patient with 10 taurodonts: a case report. J Endod. 2014;40:140–4. doi:10.1016/j.joen.2013.08.017.
213. Orguneser A, Kartal N. Three canals and two foramina in a mandibular canine. J Endod. 1998;24:444–5.
214. Sachdeva GS, Malhotra D, Sachdeva LT, Sharma N, Negi A. Endodontic management of mandibular central incisor fused to a supernumerary tooth associated with a talon cusp: a case report. Int Endod J. 2012;45:590–6. doi:10.1111/j.1365-2591.2012.02029.x.
215. Khabbaz MG, Konstantaki MN, Sykaras SN. Dens invaginatus in a mandibular lateral incisor. Int Endod J. 1995;28:303–5.
216. Loushine RJ, Jurcak JJ, Jeffalone DM. A two-rooted mandibular incisor. J Endod. 1993;19:250–1.
217. Vaghela DJ, Sinha AA. Endodontic management of four rooted mandibular first premolar. J Conserv Dent. 2013;16:87–9. doi:10.4103/0972-0707.105307.
218. De Moor RJ, Calberson FL. Root canal treatment in a mandibular second premolar with three root canals. J Endod. 2005;31:310–3.
219. Farmakis ET. Four-rooted mandibular second premolar. Aust Endod J. 2008;34:126–8. doi:10.1111/j.1747-4477.2007.00092.x.
220. Demiryürek EO, Gönülol N, Bulucu B. Endodontic treatment of a taurodontic premolar with five canals. Aust Endod J. 2013;39:81–4. doi:10.1111/j.1747-4477.2010.00250.x.
221. Friedman S, Moshonov J, Stabholz A. Five root canals in a mandibular first molar. Endod Dent Traumatol. 1986;2:226–8.
222. Ryan JL, Bowles WR, Baisden MK, McClanahan SB. Mandibular first molar with six separate canals. J Endod. 2011;37:878–80. doi:10.1016/j.joen.2011.03.005.
223. Reeh ES. Seven canals in a lower first molar. J Endod. 1998;24:497–9.
224. Fava LR, Weinfeld I, Fabri FP, Pais CR. Four second molars with single roots and single canals in the same patient. Int Endod J. 2000;33:138–42.
225. Chokshi S, Mehta J, Chokshi P, Vaidya R. Morphological variations in the root canal system of mandibular second molar: a case series. Endodontology. 2013;25:135–8.
226. Beatty RG, Krell K. Mandibular molars with five canals: report of two cases. J Am Dent Assoc. 1987;114:802–4.
227. Stecker S, DiAngelis AJ. Dens evaginatus: a diagnostic and treatment challenge. J Am Dent Assoc. 2002;133:190–3.
228. Tavano SM, de Sousa SM, Bramante CM. Dens invaginatus in first mandibular premolar. Endod Dent Traumatol. 1994;10:27–9.
229. Aryanpour S, Bercy P, Van Nieuwenhuysen JP. Endodontic and periodontal treatments of a geminated mandibular first premolar. Int Endod J. 2002;35:209–14.
230. Goswami M, Chandra S, Chandra S, Singh S. Mandibular premolar with two roots. J Endod. 1997;23:187.
231. Koh ET, Ford TR, Kariyawasam SP, Chen NN, Torabinejad M. Prophylactic treatment of dens evaginatus using mineral trioxide aggregate. J Endod. 2001;27:540–2.
232. Muthukumar RS, Arunkumar S, Sadasiva K. Bilateral fusion of mandibular second premolar and supernumerary tooth: a rare case report. J Oral Maxillofac Pathol. 2012;16:128–30. doi:10.4103/0973-029X.92990.
233. De Moor RJ, Deroose CA, Calberson FL. The radix entomolaris in mandibular first molars: an endodontic challenge. Int Endod J. 2004;37:789–99.
234. Ashwin R, Arathi R. Taurodontism of deciduous and permanent molars: report of two cases. J Indian Soc Pedod Prev Dent. 2006;24:42–4.
235. Tsesis I, Steinbock N, Rosenberg E, Kaufman AY. Endodontic treatment of developmental anomalies in posterior teeth: treatment of geminated/fused teeth-report of two cases. Int Endod J. 2003;36:372–9.
236. Schäfer E, Breuer D, Janzen S. The prevalence of three-rooted mandibular permanent first molars in a

German population. J Endod. 2009;35:202–5. doi:10.1016/j.joen.2008.11.010.
237. Bolger WL, Schindler WG. A mandibular first molar with a C-shaped root configuration. J Endod. 1988;14:515–9.
238. Baugh D, Wallace J. Middle mesial canal of the mandibular first molar: a case report and literature review. J Endod. 2004;30:185–6.
239. Kottoor J, Sudha R, Velmurugan N. Middle distal canal of the mandibular first molar: a case report and literature review. Int Endod J. 2010;43:714–22. doi:10.1111/j.1365-2591.2010.01737.x.
240. Ballal S, Sachdeva G, Kandaswamy D. Endodontic management of a fused mandibular second molar and paramolar with the aid of spiral computed tomography: a case report. J Endod. 2007;33: 1247–51. doi:10.1016/j.joen.2007.06.021.
241. Pomeranz HH, Eidelman DL, Goldberg MG. Treatment considerations of the middle mesial canal of mandibular first and second molars. J Endod. 1981;7:565–8.
242. Wu MK, R'Oris A, Barkis D, Wesselink PR. Prevalence and extent of long oval canals in the apical third. Oral Surg Oral Med Oral Pathol Oral Radiol Endod. 2000;89:739–43.
243. Siqueira Jr JF, Alves FRF, Versiani MA, Rocas IN, Almeida BM, Neves MAS, Sousa Neto MD. Correlative bacteriologic and micro–computed tomographic analysis of mandibular molar mesial canals prepared by Self-Adjusting File, Reciproc, and Twisted File systems. J Endod. 2013;39: 1044–50. doi:10.1016/j.joen.2013.04.034.
244. Versiani MA, Steier L, De-Deus G, Tassani S, Pécora JD, Sousa-Neto MD. Micro–computed tomography study of oval-shaped canals prepared with the Self-adjusting File, Reciproc, WaveOne, and Protaper Universal systems. J Endod. 2013;39: 1060–6. doi:10.1016/j.joen.2013.04.009.
245. Versiani MA, Pécora JD, Sousa-Neto MD. Flat-oval root canal preparation with self-adjusting file instrument: a micro-computed tomography study. J Endod. 2011;37:1002–7. doi:10.1016/j.joen.2011.03.017.
246. Gulabivala K, Patel B, Evans G, Ng YL. Effects of mechanical and chemical procedures on root canal surfaces. Endod Top. 2006;10:103–22.
247. Paqué F, Al-Jadaa A, Kfir A. Hard-tissue debris accumulation created by conventional rotary versus self-adjusting file instrumentation in mesial root canal systems of mandibular molars. Int Endod J. 2012. doi:10.1111/j.1365-2591.2011.01991.x.
248. Paqué F, Laib A, Gautschi H, Zehnder M. Hard-tissue debris accumulation analysis by high-resolution computed tomography scans. J Endod. 2009;35:1044–7. doi:10.1016/j.joen.2009.04.026.
249. van der Sluis LW, Gambarini G, Wu MK, Wesselink PR. The influence of volume, type of irrigant and flushing method on removing artificially placed dentine debris from the apical root canal during passive ultrasonic irrigation. Int Endod J. 2006;39:472–6.
250. Ribeiro MVM, Silva-Sousa YT, Versiani MA, Lamira A, Steier L, Pécora JD, Sousa Neto MD. Comparison of the cleaning efficacy of self-adjusting file and rotary systems in the apical third of oval-shaped canals. J Endod. 2013;39:398–410. doi:10.1016/j.joen.2012.11.016.
251. Boutsioukis C, Lambrianidis T, Kastrinakis E. Irrigant flow within a prepared root canal using various flow rates: a Computational Fluid Dynamics study. Int Endod J. 2009;42:144–55. doi:10.1111/j.1365-2591.2008.01503.x.
252. Boutsioukis C, Verhaagen B, Versluis M, Kastrinakis E, van der Sluis LW. Irrigant flow in the root canal: experimental validation of an unsteady Computational Fluid Dynamics model using high-speed imaging. Int Endod J. 2010;43:393–403. doi:10.1111/j.1365-2591.2010.01692.x.
253. Gao Y, Haapasalo M, Shen Y, Wu H, Li B, Ruse ND, Zhou X. Development and validation of a three-dimensional computational fluid dynamics model of root canal irrigation. J Endod. 2009;35:1282–7. doi:10.1016/j.joen.2009.06.018.
254. Vera J, Arias A, Romero M. Effect of maintaining apical patency on irrigant penetration into the apical third of root canals when using passive ultrasonic irrigation: an in vivo study. J Endod. 2011;37:1276–8. doi:10.1016/j.joen.2011.05.042.
255. Vera J, Arias A, Romero M. Dynamic movement of intracanal gas bubbles during cleaning and shaping procedures: the effect of maintaining apical patency on their presence in the middle and cervical thirds of human root canals-an in vivo study. J Endod. 2012;38:200–3. doi:10.1016/j.joen.2011.10.026.
256. Vera J, Hernandez EM, Romero M, Arias A, van der Sluis LW. Effect of maintaining apical patency on irrigant penetration into the apical two millimeters of large root canals: an in vivo study. J Endod. 2012;38:1340–3. doi:10.1016/j.joen.2012.06.005.
257. Versiani MA, De-Deus G, Vera J, Souza E, Steier L, Pécora JD, Sousa Neto MD. 3D mapping of the irrigated areas of the root canal space using micro-computed tomography. Clin Oral Investig. 2015; 19:859–66. doi:10.1007/s00784-014-1311-5.

Syringe Irrigation: Blending Endodontics and Fluid Dynamics

3

Christos Boutsioukis and Lucas W.M. van der Sluis

Abstract

Syringe irrigation remains a widely used irrigant delivery method during root canal treatment. An interdisciplinary approach involving well-established methods from the field of fluid dynamics can provide new insights into the mechanisms involved in cleaning and disinfection of the root canal system by this method. In addition to the equipment used clinically (syringes and needles), this chapter will also discuss the physical properties of commonly used irrigants, the flow developed inside the root canal system, irrigant refreshment, forces applied on the root canal wall, entrapment and removal of air bubbles, and the anatomical challenges faced by syringe irrigation. Essential background knowledge on fluid dynamics will also be provided.

Introduction

Irrigant delivery by a syringe and a needle during root canal treatment dates back more than a century [91]. Despite its long history and the development of newer and more sophisticated irrigation systems, it is still recommended for use [51, 76]. In fact, a recent survey indicated that approximately half of the responding AAE members only used conventional syringe irrigation in their practices [31].

Over the years, the interest to investigate and optimize the various parameters related to this technique has diminished. Nowadays, most publications primarily aim to evaluate new irrigation techniques, so syringe irrigation is frequently used just as a control regarded *a priori* not effective and unnecessary bias is introduced. It seems rather unlikely that syringe irrigation will be totally replaced by other delivery techniques any time soon. Therefore, this chapter will focus on the specific aspects of syringe irrigation that need to be optimized and will also highlight its advantages and limitations. An interdisciplinary approach combining endodontics and fluid

C. Boutsioukis, DDS, MSc, PhD (✉)
Department of Endodontology, Academic Centre for Dentistry Amsterdam (ACTA), Gustav Mahlerlaan 3004, Amsterdam 1081 LA, The Netherlands
e-mail: c.boutsioukis@acta.nl

L.W.M. van der Sluis, DDS, PhD
Department of Conservative Dentistry, University Medical Center Groningen, Groningen, The Netherlands

B. Basrani (ed.), *Endodontic Irrigation: Chemical Disinfection of the Root Canal System*,
DOI 10.1007/978-3-319-16456-4_3

dynamics will be employed, and essential background knowledge on fluid dynamics will also be provided to facilitate comprehension.

Redefining the Aims

The traditional long list of aims of root canal irrigation can be found in every endodontic textbook and also elsewhere in this book. This list has been refined several times in the past but has always reflected the clinician's and microbiologist's point of view, undoubtedly because of the decisive role of microorganisms in the development of apical periodontitis [57, 64, 99]. However, most of the aims and objectives mentioned in this list can be grouped together since they are actually realized by two simultaneous but distinct effects:

- The *chemical effect*, i.e., chemical disruption or inactivation of biofilms, killing of microorganisms and inactivation of endotoxin, dissolution of pulp tissue remnants, dentin debris and of the smear layer by the active chemical component(s) of the irrigant. Clearly, the chemical effect can only be exerted by chemically active solutions (e.g., sodium hypochlorite).
- The *mechanical effect*, i.e., mechanical disruption, detachment and removal of microorganisms/biofilms, pulp tissue remnants, and dentin debris from the root canal system via forces applied by the flowing irrigant. Mechanical effects can be exerted by both chemically active and inert irrigants (e.g., water, saline) [42, 45, 88, 117].

Evidently, both effects cannot take place unless the irrigant comes into close contact with the targeted microorganisms and tissue remnants [45, 90]. The chemical effect strongly depends upon the concentration of the active component(s) of the irrigant, the area of contact, and the duration of interaction with the targeted material. During the interaction, most commonly used irrigants are rapidly consumed, so the concentration decreases [44, 65, 78, 79]. Thus, apart from the initial delivery and penetration, frequent refreshment of the irrigant in all areas of the root canal system is also of utmost importance for an optimum chemical effect.

Irrigants can reach the sites of interest preferably by the flow developed during delivery (or during agitation). This way, chemically active particles (molecules/ions) are transported quickly and efficiently by the fluid motion, a process termed *convection*. In addition, while flowing, the irrigant applies forces on the targeted material, thus exerting the mechanical effect. In areas of the root canal where a flow cannot be created, irrigant transport may still take place by *diffusion,* the random movement of particles in a fluid, but this process is markedly slower than convection, and its rate is further affected by the size of the particles, temperature, and concentration gradients [104]. Moreover, no mechanical effect is exerted by diffusion.

At the moment, there is no consensus on the relative importance of each one of these effects (chemical and mechanical) for the overall success of root canal treatment. Both effects are primarily produced by the flow of a chemically active irrigant and require its penetration to the full extent of the root canal system. Thus, efforts to obtain additional insight and optimize irrigant flow seem justified, and this can be achieved by understanding the fluid dynamics of root canal irrigation.

Fluid dynamics is the study of fluids in motion and the subsequent effects of the fluids upon the boundaries, either solid surfaces or interfaces with other fluids. Fluids are substances that cannot withstand any attempt to change their shape when at rest; they include both liquids and gases, as both have the ability to flow [113]. A flow is caused by the action of externally applied forces, like pressure difference, gravity, or buoyancy [4, 7, 34]. Applications of fluid dynamics in the biomedical field are anything but uncommon. An increasing number of challenging problems have been investigated by interdisciplinary approaches involving fluid dynamics. Notable examples include blood flow in the cardiovascular system and air flow in the respiratory system [23, 30, 54, 59, 71, 75, 114].

Root canal irrigation can be viewed as the microscale flow of a liquid (irrigant) inside an irregularly shaped domain of very small dimensions (root canal system). Consequently, it falls clearly within the scope of fluid dynamics and especially microfluidics. The need to investigate in detail the flow of the irrigants inside the root canal has been stressed repeatedly [2, 24, 29, 42, 82, 93, 117]; however, speculations have dominated this aspect of root canal irrigation for decades. For example, the limited performance of syringe irrigation has been attributed to its inability to deliver the irrigant into all the parts of the complicated root canal system, but without strong experimental evidence [29, 82, 84]. This lack of scientific data may still be reflected on the way this procedure is described in endodontic textbooks as well as taught in dental schools. Wide variations have been found among endodontists in the way they perform syringe irrigation *ex vivo* [8]. Only recently have the abundant data from experiments on the removal of microorganisms, tissue remnants, and dentin debris been coupled with detailed numerical and experimental evaluation of the irrigant flow to provide new insights into root canal cleaning and disinfection.

Based on such an interdisciplinary approach, the basic aims of root canal irrigation can be restated briefly as follows:

- Flow of the irrigant to the full extent of the root canal system and subsequently to the canal orifice, in order to come in close contact with microorganisms/biofilm, debris, and tissue remnants, carry them away and provide lubrication for the instruments. (*Flow*)
- Frequent refreshment of the irrigant, in order to retain a high concentration of its active component(s) at the sites of interest and compensate for their rapid consumption (applicable only to chemically active irrigants). (*Chemical effect*)
- Application of force on the root canal wall (wall shear stress), in order to detach/disrupt microorganisms/biofilm, debris, and tissue remnants. (*Mechanical effect*)
- Restriction of the flow within the constraints of the root canal system and prevention of irrigant extrusion towards the periapical tissues. (*Safety*) [11]

The remainder of this chapter will focus on the first three aims; safety aspects will be discussed in more detail in a separate chapter.

Syringes

In order to perform irrigation, syringes of variable capacity ranging from 1 to 20 mL have been suggested for use (Fig. 3.1) [2, 24, 46, 56, 66, 86, 93, 94]. Although little attention has been put on the size of the syringe used, this can affect the tactile force needed to irrigate at a certain flow rate [8]. Elementary fluid dynamics can provide an explanation for this effect.

During syringe irrigation, a clinician applies tactile force to the syringe plunger. This force is transmitted to the irrigant into the syringe, where pressure is built up (Text Box 3.1). A clinician will need to apply different amounts of force and will feel different levels of difficulty to push the plunger when syringes of a different size are used, even if the actually developed pressure inside the syringe is identical; this results from the definition of pressure. Larger syringes are more difficult to depress and control. For the same reason, the clinician cannot draw reliable conclusions about the pressure.

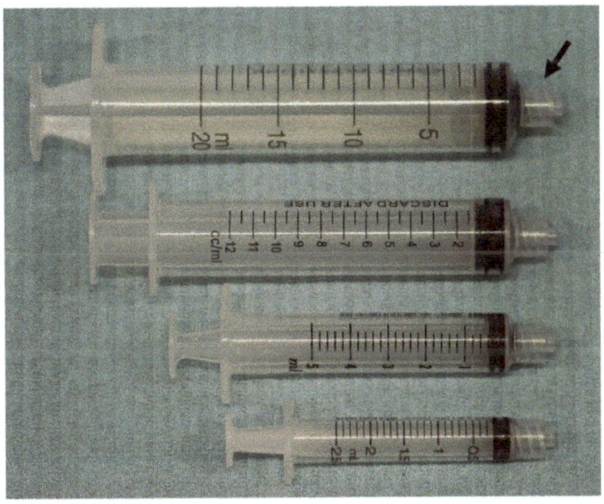

Fig. 3.1 Syringes of variable capacity (from *top* to *bottom*: 20, 12, 5 and 2.5 mL) used for root canal irrigation. All syringes have a Luer Lock threaded fitting (*arrow*)

Text Box 3.1

Pressure

The *pressure* (P) developed inside the syringe barrel is defined as:

$$P = \frac{F}{A}$$

where F is the tactile force applied to the syringe plunger and A is the cross-sectional area of the plunger. Pressure acts uniformly in all directions. In an irrigant confined by solid boundaries (e.g., the wall of the syringe or the root canal), pressure acts perpendicular to the boundary [67].

Flow rate

The *flow rate* (Q) of an irrigant is defined as:

$$Q = \frac{\Delta V}{\Delta t}$$

where ΔV is the volume of the irrigant delivered in the root canal within a time period Δt [67]. The irrigant flow rate is frequently expressed in mL/s or mL/min (1 mL/s = 60 mL/min); in most cases, mL/s is more relevant to clinical practice, since irrigation rarely continues for a whole minute.

Assuming a laminar flow (see Text Box 3.3), the flow rate through a needle is described by the equation:

$$Q = \frac{\pi D^4 \Delta P}{128 \mu L}$$

where D is the internal diameter of the needle, ΔP is the pressure difference along the needle, μ is the viscosity of the irrigant (see Text Box 3.5), and L the length of the needle [103]. Evidently, the needle diameter influences the flow rate much more than the other parameters.

While depressing the plunger, the pressure inside the syringe barrel remains considerably higher than the ambient pressure around the tip of the needle (which is nearly atmospheric). This pressure difference drives the irrigant through the needle and into the root canal, and that is why syringe irrigation is categorized as a *positive-pressure* technique [21]. The irrigant flow rate is proportional to this difference, but is also affected by the size of the needle and several other parameters (Text Box 3.1). So, for the same pressure difference, the flow rate through a smaller needle will be much less than through a larger needle. In other words, a larger pressure difference is required to achieve the same flow rate through a smaller needle.

A common mistake among clinicians which is also reproduced in several publications is that delivery of the irrigant at high flow rate is erroneously termed *forceful delivery* or *delivery under pressure.* Using a very large syringe combined with a fine-diameter needle would require a large tactile force, but the flow rate would still be low. In addition, it must be emphasized that the pressure of the irrigant delivered inside the root canal is always much lower than the pressure inside the syringe, because a significant pressure drop occurs along the needle. Thus, neither "force" nor "pressure" is an appropriate term to describe how fast the irrigant is delivered. Such information can only be provided by the flow rate [8, 10], which can also be estimated clinically.

A 5-mL syringe has been recommended as a reasonable compromise between less-frequent refilling and ease of use. This syringe can be used to reach flow rates at least up to 0.20–0.25 mL/s even when combined with fine irrigation needles [8]. Because of the very high pressures developed inside the syringe, a Luer Lock threaded fitting (Fig. 3.1) is always necessary to avoid accidental detachment of the needle during irrigation [8].

Needles

Over the years, several types of needles have been used to deliver irrigants into the root canals [13, 37, 38, 50, 56, 66, 95, 112, 115]. These needles mainly differ in the presence of an open or closed tip and one or more outlets (Fig. 3.2).

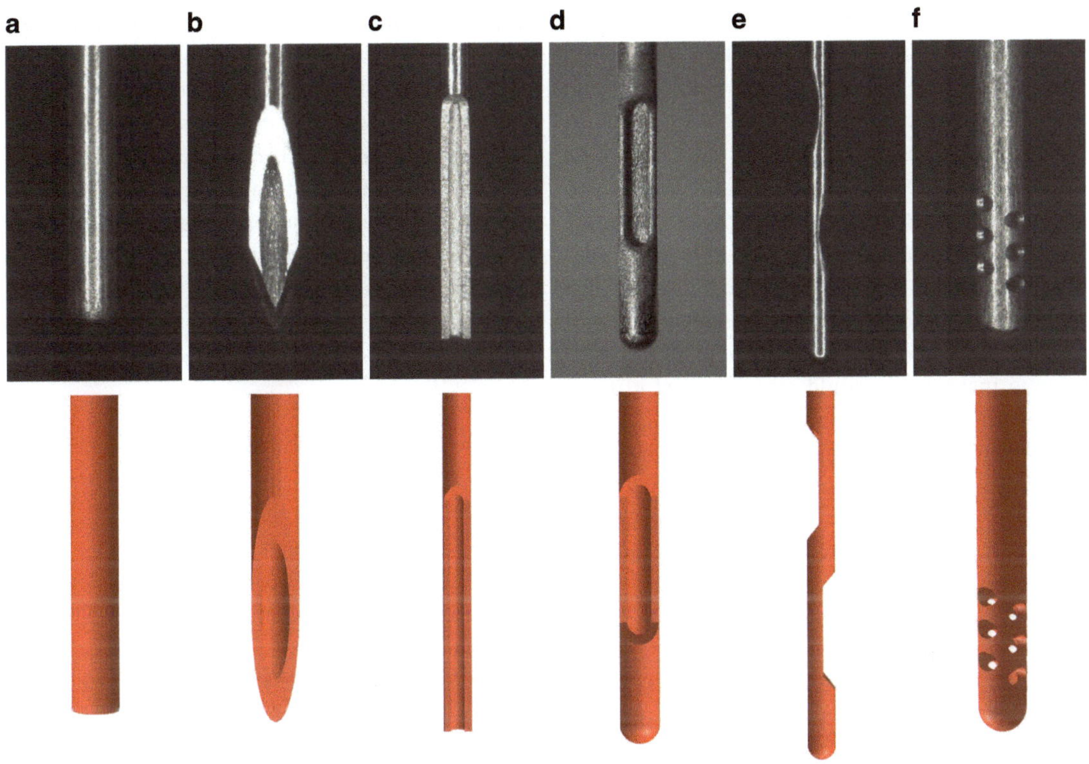

Fig. 3.2 Various types of 30G needles used for root canal irrigation [open-ended needles: flat (**a**), beveled (**b**), and notched (**c**); closed-ended needles: side-vented (**d**), double-side-vented (**e**), and multi-vented (**f**)]. Variable views and magnifications were used to highlight differences in tip design. The multi-vented needle is not commercially available at the moment for use with a syringe. Reprinted with permission from Elsevier (Ref. [13])

Table 3.1 Medical needle specifications according to ISO 9626:1991/Amd.1:2001 and corresponding size of endodontic instruments

ISO 9626:1991/Amd.1:2001 (Medical needles)					Instrument size
Gauge size	Metric size (mm)	External diameter (mm) Min	External diameter (mm) Max	Int. diameter (mm) Min	
21	0.80	0.800	0.830	0.490	80
23	0.60	0.600	0.673	0.317	60
25	0.50	0.500	0.530	0.232	50
27	0.40	0.400	0.420	0.184	40
28	0.36	0.349	0.370	0.133	40
29	0.33	0.324	0.351	0.133	35
30	0.30	0.298	0.320	0.133	30
31	0.25	0.254	0.267	0.114	25

Nonexisting instrument sizes were rounded up to the next available size. Even if the nominal size of an instrument and a needle are the same, the actual sizes may be different to some extent due to inevitable variations during the machining procedures (tolerances)

Similarly to all other medical needles, the sizes of irrigation needles are most frequently described by the "gauge" system (Table 3.1) and seem to conform well to the relevant ISO specification [9]. However, the "gauge" units cannot be directly compared to the size of instruments and obturation materials. The adoption of the millimeter as the standard metric unit to express needle size already recommended by the ISO for more than a decade [52], and the development of a color code corresponding to that of the endodontic instruments could greatly assist clinical procedures [9].

In the past, large needles (21–25G) were commonly employed for irrigant delivery [20, 24, 82, 87, 102]. Such needles could hardly penetrate beyond the coronal third of the root canal, even in wide root canals. More recently, the use of finer-diameter needles (28G, 30G or 31G) has been advocated, mainly because they can reach farther into the canal, even to working length (WL) [6, 14, 19, 49, 69, 92, 117]. The effect of needle type and size on root canal irrigation will be discussed in more detail further on.

Physical Properties of Irrigants

Apart from the equipment (syringe and needle), the flow of irrigants is also affected by their physical properties, mainly density and viscosity (Text Box 3.2) [67, 103, 113]. For commonly used endodontic irrigants, these properties are very similar to those of distilled water [41, 105] because most irrigants are sparse aqueous solutions. The surface tension of endodontic irrigants (Text Box 3.2) and its decrease by wetting agents (surfactants) have also been studied extensively, under the assumption that they may have a significant effect on irrigant penetration in dentinal tubules and accessory root canals [1, 36, 100] and on dissolution of pulp tissue [97]. However, while density and viscosity affect the flow in all cases, the effect of surface tension is important only at the interface between two immiscible fluids [58, 113]. Such an interface is formed between the irrigant and an air bubble, but not between the irrigant and the dentinal fluid, because these two liquids are miscible. Recent studies have confirmed that surfactants do not enhance the ability of NaOCl to dissolve pulp tissue [25, 27, 55] or the ability of common chelators to remove calcium from dentin [116] or to remove the smear layer [26, 62]. In addition, bubble entrapment in the apical part of root canals is an unlikely event provided that certain guidelines are followed, as it will be discussed further on.

Text Box 3.2

Density

Density (ρ) is defined as:

$$\rho = \frac{m}{V}$$

where m is the mass of a certain quantity of the irrigant and V is its volume [67, 113].

Viscosity

Viscosity describes the resistance of the irrigant to motion [67, 103, 113]. A more elaborate definition will be given in Text Box 3.5, together with the definition of *wall shear stress*.

Surface tension

The interface between two immiscible fluids in contact (e.g., irrigant and air) is found to behave as if it were under tension, like a stretched membrane. The origin of such tension at an interface is due to the intermolecular attractive forces within each fluid. The net effect of these forces is for the interface to contract and it is called *surface tension*. It depends on the pair of fluids in contact and other factors, such as the temperature and the presence of wetting agents or surfactants [58, 113].

Irrigant Flow During Syringe Irrigation

Evaluating irrigant flow even in a simple straight and uniformly tapered root canal can be a very demanding task. It has been underlined that during irrigation, the root canal behaves mostly like a closed-ended system, so in *ex vivo* and *in vitro* experiments the apical foramen should be sealed [10, 18, 47, 73, 101]. This seemingly minor detail has been overlooked in many experimental studies in the past, giving rise to doubt about the validity of their results, as pointed out by Tay et al. [101]. In fact, a closed apical foramen results in a significantly more complicated flow pattern and adds considerable obstacles for irrigant penetration compared to a root canal open from both sides, even if no air bubbles are entrapped apically [12, 109, 113].

Fluid flows are broadly categorized into *laminar* and *turbulent* ones (Text Box 3.3). In the case of root canal irrigation, turbulence would greatly assist irrigant penetration and refreshment due to the far more effective mixing [34]. However, the development of turbulence inside root canals during syringe irrigation has not been verified experimentally yet. When the irrigant is delivered at very low flow rates (~0.01 mL/s) through a 30G needle, a steady laminar flow is developed within the root canal. At higher flow rates (up to at least 0.26 mL/s), the flow becomes unsteady, but it remains laminar [10, 12, 109], contrary to previous reports [56]. An unsteady flow changes smoothly over time, but it is not necessarily turbulent. It is likely that the formation of vortices (Text Box 3.4) and the unsteady flow during syringe irrigation could have been mistaken for turbulence in the past due to limitations of the visual assessment in real time. According to computer simulations, a higher, yet clinically unrealistic, flow rate (0.53–0.79 mL/s) may lead to the development of turbulence mostly close to the tip of the needle [10]; however, these results have not been verified in experiments.

Text Box 3.3

Laminar and turbulent flow

The type of flow occurring within the root canal depends primarily on the balance between the *inertia* (driving) *forces* and *viscous* (frictional) *forces* affecting the irrigant. This balance is expressed by the *Reynolds number* (*Re*), which combines four parameters influencing the flow: fluid density (ρ) and viscosity (μ), characteristic velocity scale (v), and characteristic length scale (D).

$$\mathrm{Re} = \frac{\rho v D}{\mu}$$

At low Reynolds numbers, viscous forces are dominant over inertia forces, and the flow remains *laminar*, characterized by a smooth variation of the velocity with position and/or time. If the Reynolds number increases further than a critical value (usually taken to be around 2200–3000 for flows in pipes), a complicated series of events leads to a radical change of the flow, which becomes *turbulent*. In such a case, inertia forces are dominant over viscous forces, except adjacent to solid surfaces [39, 58, 63, 77, 80].

Turbulent flows possess a number of characteristic properties that distinguish them from laminar flows. They are *random*, *unpredictable*, and *chaotic*. Moreover, they are highly *unsteady* and generally vary along the three spatial directions. Visualizations of turbulent flows reveal rotational flow structures of various sizes, called *turbulent eddies* (not to be confused with the more stable *vortices* – see Text Box 3.4). The kinetic energy is continuously transferred from large eddies to progressively smaller eddies until it is dissipated and converted into thermal energy. This dissipation results in *increased energy losses* associated with turbulent flows [39, 60, 77, 111]. Turbulent flows are also characterized by substantially *more effective mixing* than laminar flows because of the eddying motions. As a consequence, heat, mass, and momentum are very effectively exchanged [39, 60, 77, 96, 111], and this can be an important advantage for certain chemical or biological applications [34].

Text Box 3.4

Jet

A *jet* is a high-velocity fluid stream forced out of a small-diameter opening or nozzle [103, 113].

Vortex

A *vortex* is a relatively stable rotating flow structure [103, 113]. It should be distinguished from the *eddies* formed in turbulent flows.

The type of the needle has also a substantial effect on the basic flow pattern developed in the root canal during syringe irrigation (Fig. 3.3), while other parameters such as needle insertion depth, root canal size, and taper have only a limited influence [12–16, 109]. Based on the needle design and the resulting flow, the available types of needles can be categorized into two main groups, namely, the *open-ended* and the *closed-ended* [13]. All needles create a jet (Text Box 3.4) at their outlet, but the exact position and shape of the outlet determines the orientation and, to some extent, the intensity of the jet.

In the case of the open-ended needles (flat, beveled, notched), the jet is very intense and extends along the root canal, apically to their tip (Fig. 3.3a–c). Within a certain distance, which depends on the geometry of the root canal, the insertion depth of the needle, and the flow rate, the jet appears to break up gradually. Reverse flow towards the canal orifice occurs near the canal wall. The jet formed by the flat and beveled needle is slightly more intense and extends further apically than that of the notched needle [13, 109].

When closed-ended needles are used (side-vented, double-side-vented), the jet is formed near the apical side of the outlet (the one proximal to the tip for the double-side-vented needle), and it is directed apically with a slight divergence (Fig. 3.3d–e). The irrigant mainly follows a curved path around the tip and then towards the coronal orifice. A series of counterrotating vortices are formed apically to the tip, extending almost to the WL. Their size, position, and

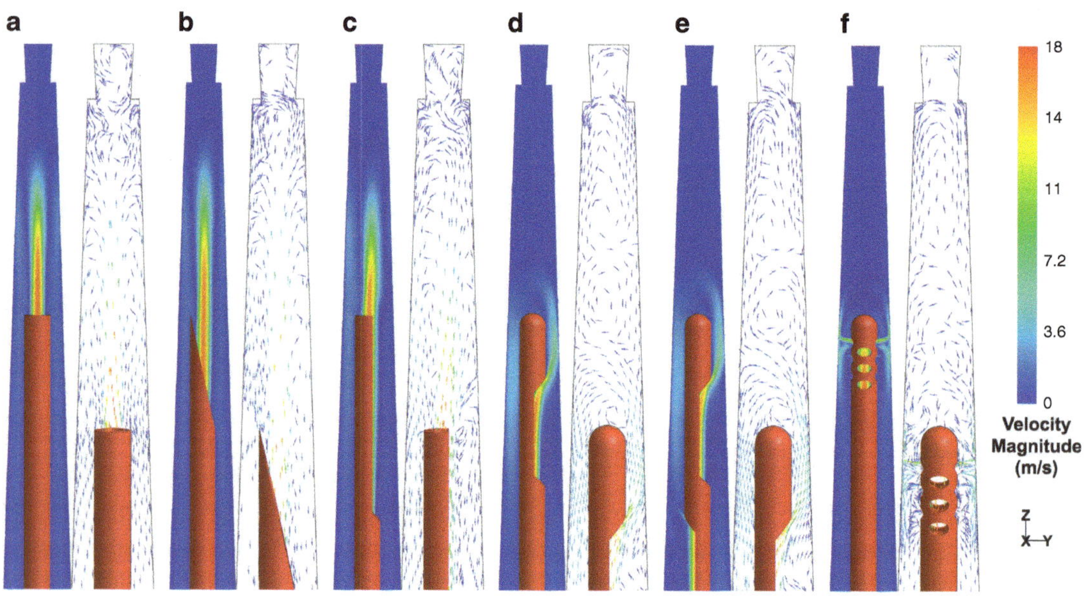

Fig. 3.3 Time-averaged contours (*left*) and vectors (*right*) of irrigant velocity in the apical part of a size 45, 0.06 tapered root canal during syringe irrigation by different types of needles, according to computer simulations [open-ended needles: flat (**a**), beveled (**b**), and notched (**c**); closed-ended needles: side-vented (**d**), double-side-vented (**e**), and multi-vented (**f**)]. All needles are positioned at 3 mm short of WL and are colored in *red*. Reprinted with permission from Elsevier (Ref. [13])

number may differ according to needle insertion depth, root canal shape, and flow rate. Despite the fact that irrigant can flow from one vortex to the next, the velocity decreases significantly towards the apex, so irrigant penetration becomes slower. The distal outlet of the double-side-vented needle has only a minor influence on the overall flow pattern because most of the irrigant (93.5 %) flows out through the proximal outlet; thus, it doesn't provide any important advantage [13, 109].

A special case of closed-ended needle is the multi-vented needle, suggested for root canal irrigation many years ago [37, 38, 66]. Although this needle is not commercially available at the moment, it appears to develop a distinct flow pattern (Fig. 3.3f); several small jets are formed by the irrigant exiting the needle from the outlets proximal to the tip and they are directed perpendicularly to the canal wall. The most intense jets (73 % of the total flow) are formed through the pair of outlets most proximal to the tip. Most of the flowing irrigant is directed towards the canal orifice, while very low velocities are noted apically to the tip [13].

Irrigant Refreshment

As already mentioned, irrigant exchange in the various parts of the root canal system is a crucial requirement for an adequate chemical effect [29, 45, 65]. The type of needle also appears to have a significant effect on the extent of apical irrigant exchange. Earlier reports argued that closed-ended needles are more efficient than open-ended ones [56, 112]. However, recent studies have clarified the limitations in the irrigant refreshment apically to closed-ended needles and clearly proven their inferiority [10, 13–16, 109, 117]. Under the same conditions, closed-ended needles are always less effective in exchanging the irrigant apically than open-ended needles. Very limited differences have been detected between various types of closed-ended or between various types of open-ended needles [13, 112].

A general trend has been well-documented in the literature that needle placement closer to WL results in more efficient irrigant exchange, irrespective of other parameters (Fig. 3.4) [14, 19, 24, 48, 93]. Furthermore, an increase in the preparation size or taper also improves irrigant refreshment [15, 16, 18, 24, 33, 48, 49], in addition to allowing needle placement closer to WL [2]. Increasing the flow rate also seems to have a similar effect. It has been found that hardly any irrigant refreshment is achieved apically to a closed-ended needle when irrigating at a very low flow rate (~0.01 mL/s), but an optimal flow rate (0.26 mL/s) can provide refreshment up to 1 mm apically to the needle [10]. A similar effect has been noted for the open-ended needles, although in this case, refreshment always extends farther compared to the closed-ended ones [109].

Even when an optimal flow rate is attained, it seems that root canal preparation to apical size 25, 0.06 taper does not allow adequate irrigant flow and apical refreshment (Fig. 3.5) [15, 48]. Apical enlargement to size 30 leads to effective exchange 2 mm apically to an open-ended needle when combined at least with 0.06 taper [16], while size 35 combined with 0.05–0.06 taper results into significant irrigant refreshment almost 3 mm apically to the needle [15, 48]. Regarding the closed-ended needles, it appears that irrigant exchange occurs almost 1 mm apically to their tip in a root canal of size 30 and at least 0.06 taper, while further increase of the size or taper has only a minimal additional effect [15, 16, 47]. Therefore, these needles need to be placed within 1 mm from WL, and in order for a 30G needle to reach this position, a minimum apical size 30 or 35 is required. If a multi-vented needle were to be used for syringe irrigation, it would also have to be placed almost at WL, since irrigant exchange apically to its tip is very limited [13]. Interestingly, a minimally tapered root canal preparation (size 60, 0.02 taper) may present an advantage over the usual tapered ones in terms of irrigant refreshment [16]. However, the resistance to root fracture, the possibility of iatrogenic errors, and the requirements of the obturation technique should also be taken into account when deciding the instrumentation strategy.

It has been reported that a *dead-water* or *stagnation* zone may exist apically to the tip of

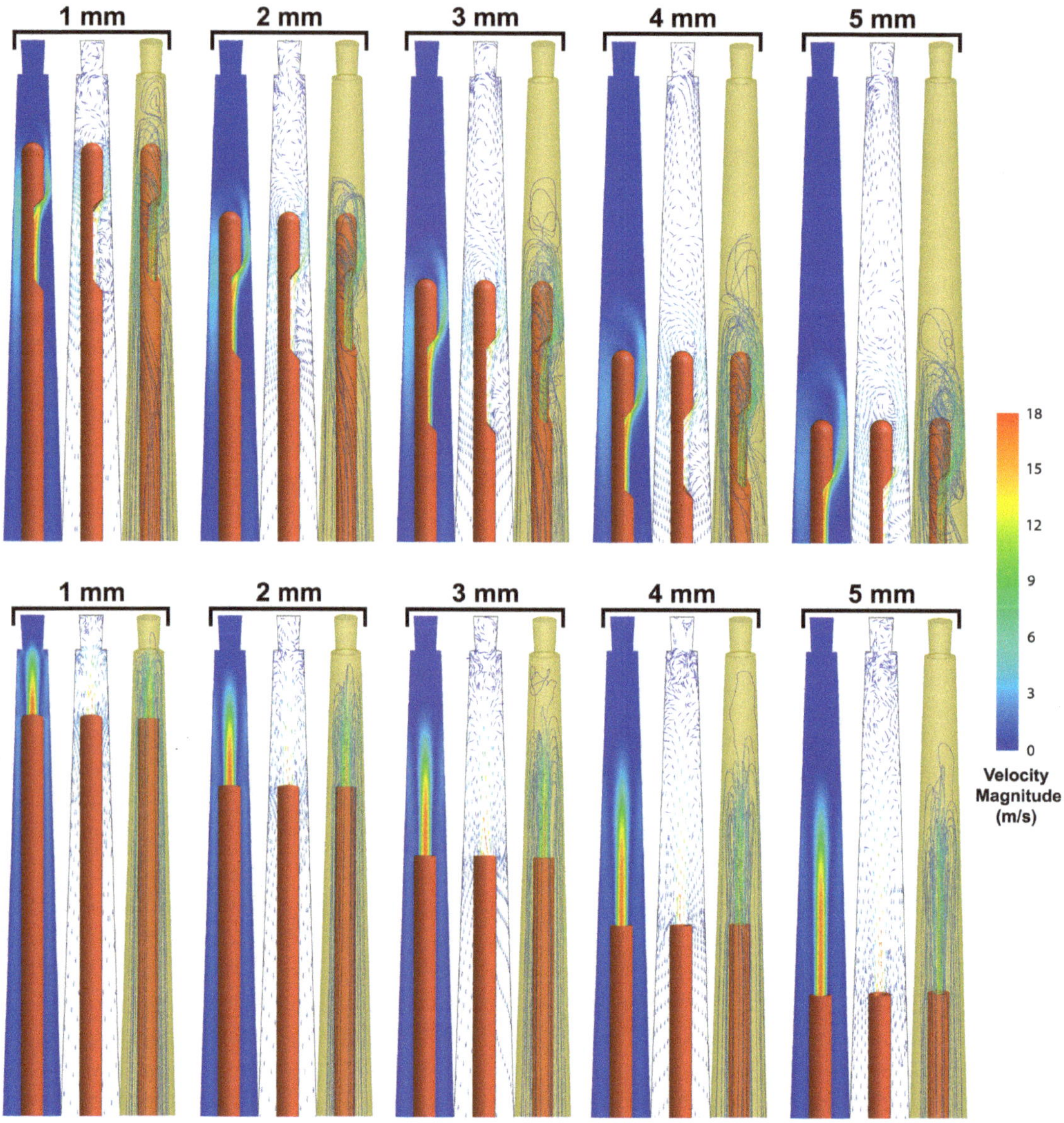

Fig. 3.4 Triads of time-averaged velocity contours (*left*) and vectors (*middle*), and streamlines (*right*) in the apical part of a size 45, 0.06 tapered root canal for a closed-ended (*top*) and an open-ended needle (*bottom*) positioned at 1–5 mm short of WL, according to computer simulations. Needles are colored in *red*. Reprinted and modified with permission from Elsevier (Ref. [14])

closed-ended needles, where no irrigant refreshment takes place [35, 74, 95]. This zone has been observed while irrigating at a medium flow rate (~0.1 mL/s) through closed-ended needles positioned 3–5 mm short of WL. Given the limited irrigant exchange apically to closed-ended needles and the flow rate used, it is possible that a zone of inadequate refreshment may indeed exist near WL in these cases. However, the real-time visual evaluation of dye clearance that was employed has only a very limited ability to detect irrigant flow and true exchange. More detailed studies using high-speed imaging combined with computer simulations have shown that there are no areas in the main root canal where the irrigant is completely stagnant during syringe irrigation at an optimal flow rate (0.26 mL/s), even if closed-ended needles are positioned at 3 mm

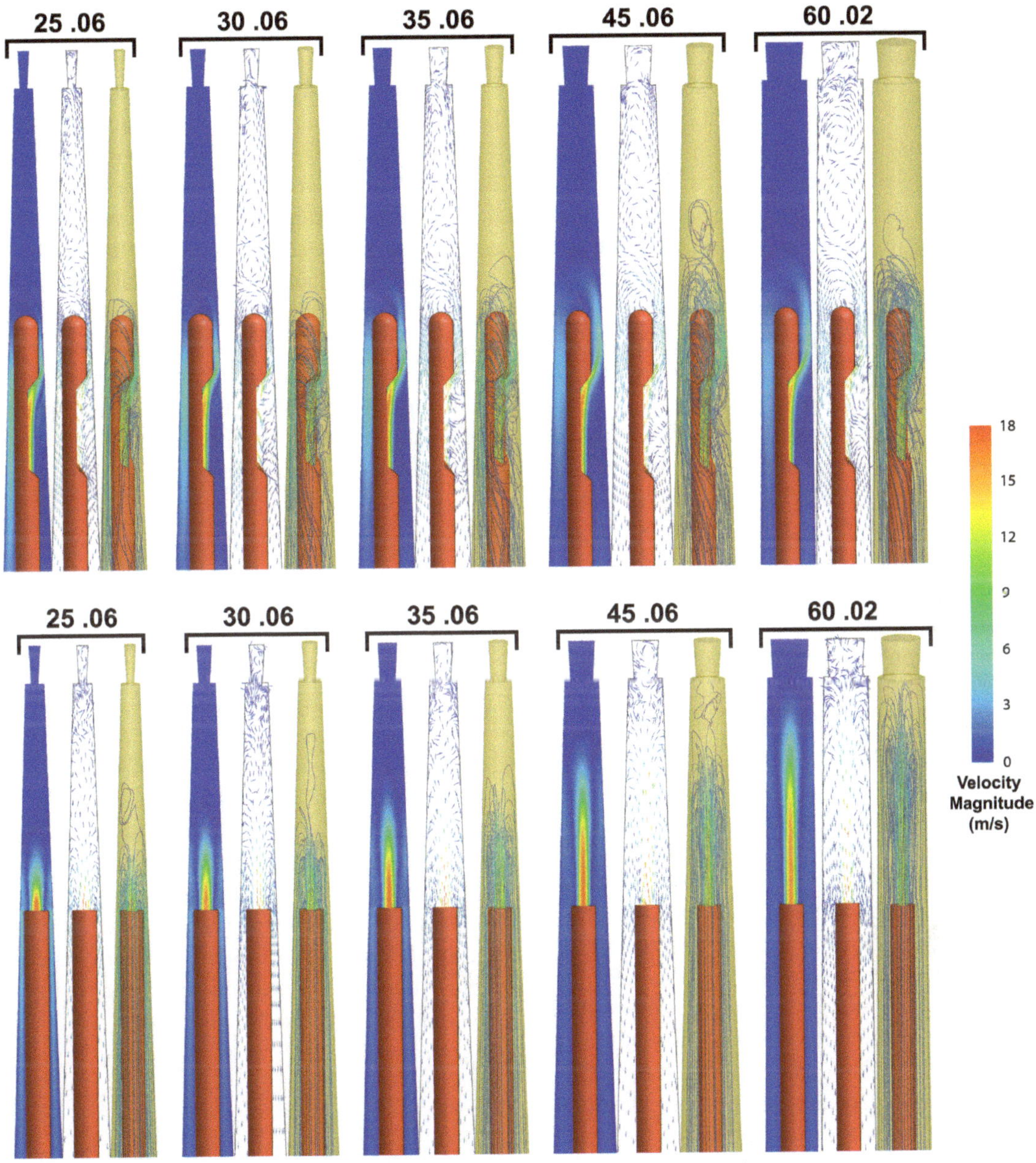

Fig. 3.5 Triads of time-averaged velocity contours (*left*) and vectors (*middle*) and streamlines (*right*) for a closed-ended (*top*) and an open-ended needle (*bottom*) positioned at 3 mm short of WL in the apical part of root canals of various sizes and tapers, according to computer simulations. Needles are colored in *red*. Reprinted and modified with permission from Wiley (Refs. [15, 16])

short of WL. However, the flow may be very slow near WL, not being able to ensure adequate irrigant exchange within the time limitations of a root canal treatment; such areas exist when the needle is placed too far away from WL [12–16, 109]. Increasing the flow rate, delivering additional volume of irrigant or inserting the needle closer to WL could help to improve refreshment in these cases [14, 19, 92, 93].

Most of the data on irrigant flow and refreshment have been obtained from experiments and computer simulations of simple straight root canal. Nonetheless, many root canals are curved in reality. The effect of root canal curvature on irrigant exchange has been studied indirectly by Nguy and Sedgley [69], who evaluated the removal of bioluminescent planktonic bacteria. Based on their results, a curvature up to 24°–28° according to Schneider's method [89] doesn't seem to create additional obstacles for irrigant flow even when a low flow rate is used, provided that a closed-ended needle is placed at 1 mm short of WL [69]. It can be assumed that if needles are positioned within 1–3 mm short of WL in a curved root canal, in many cases they have already bypassed most of the curvature and the remaining curvature apically to their tip is limited. Small size (30G or 31G) flexible irrigation needles widely available nowadays can facilitate placement near WL in many cases, even in severely curved canals.

In addition to improving irrigant exchange in severely curved root canals, fine-diameter needles can reach further and earlier even into straight root canals without the need of excessive enlargement; this way they satisfy better the requirements for irrigant refreshment [14]. Indeed, it has been verified in *ex vivo* studies that finer needles result into improved irrigant exchange and cleaning [24, 29, 82], but this is true even when positioned at the same insertion depth as larger needles [19, 24]. The latter finding probably relates to the space available around the needle for the reverse flow of the irrigant towards the canal orifice. Evidently, a larger needle occupies more space inside the root canal and leaves less space for the reverse flow compared to a finer needle. The development of an effective reverse flow improves irrigant refreshment in the apical part of the root canal and is also necessary for refreshment coronally to the needle tip. Moreover, the reverse flow carries away microorganisms, tissue remnants, and dentin debris detached from the walls by the shear stress [15, 16]. Larger needles also increase the risk of wedging and irrigant extrusion [81]. On the other hand, finer-diameter needles require more effort by the clinician during irrigation [8].

Wall Shear Stress

During irrigant flow, frictional forces occur between the flowing irrigant and root canal walls. These forces give rise to *wall shear stress* (Text Box 3.5), which is of particular interest to irrigation because it can detach material from the root canal wall, so it determines the mechanical effect. At the moment, there are no quantitative data on the minimum shear stress required for the removal of dentin debris, tissue remnants, isolated microorganisms, or biofilm from root canal walls; thus, the overall distribution of wall shear stress can be useful mainly for comparisons of the relative mechanical effect.

Text Box 3.5

Wall shear stress and viscosity

Frictional forces occurring within a flowing irrigant and between flowing irrigant and root canal walls tend to resist its motion. In order to explain this phenomenon, the irrigant is considered to consist of individual layers of infinitely small thickness, which can slide over each other. As the irrigant moves, the layers farther away from the wall tend to move faster than the ones closer to the wall and a shear stress is developed. *Shear stress* (τ) is defined as the force (F) required to slide one layer of the fluid over another divided by the area of contact between the two layers (A):

$$\vec{\tau} = \frac{\vec{F}}{A}$$

For most irrigants, the wall shear stress is proportional to the difference of the velocity (u) between the adjacent irrigant layers close to the wall, also called as the *velocity gradient* (du/dy, where y is the distance from the wall), according to the equation:

$$\tau = \mu \frac{du}{dy}$$

The viscosity of the irrigant (μ) describes its resistance to motion and could be regarded as a measure of its internal friction. It is a property of the irrigant, depending mainly on temperature [67, 103, 113] Obviously, irrigants with higher viscosity will develop a higher wall shear stress, but they will also resist flow and require more effort to deliver

Similarly to the developed irrigant flow, two basic wall shear stress patterns can be distinguished during syringe irrigation (Fig. 3.6) [13]. Regarding the open-ended needles, an area of increased shear stress is developed apically to the needle tip, in the region of jet breakup. This area is approximately symmetrical around the needle and is slightly smaller for the beveled and notched needles, which develop local maxima on the side of the root canal wall not facing the outlet. On the other hand, the closed-ended needles (side-vented and double-side-vented) lead to almost twice as high maximum shear stress, but limited near their tip, on the wall facing the needle outlet (the proximal outlet for the double-side-vented needle) [13]. An area of slightly increased shear stress is also identified opposite to the distal outlet of the double-side-vented needle, but has only a minimum influence on the overall stress pattern [13]. The unidirectional performance of the side-vented and double-side-vented needles has also been reported in *ex vivo* studies that investigated the influence of needle orientation in the debridement of the root canal [49, 115]. Being a special case of closed-ended needles, the multi-vented needles show a slightly

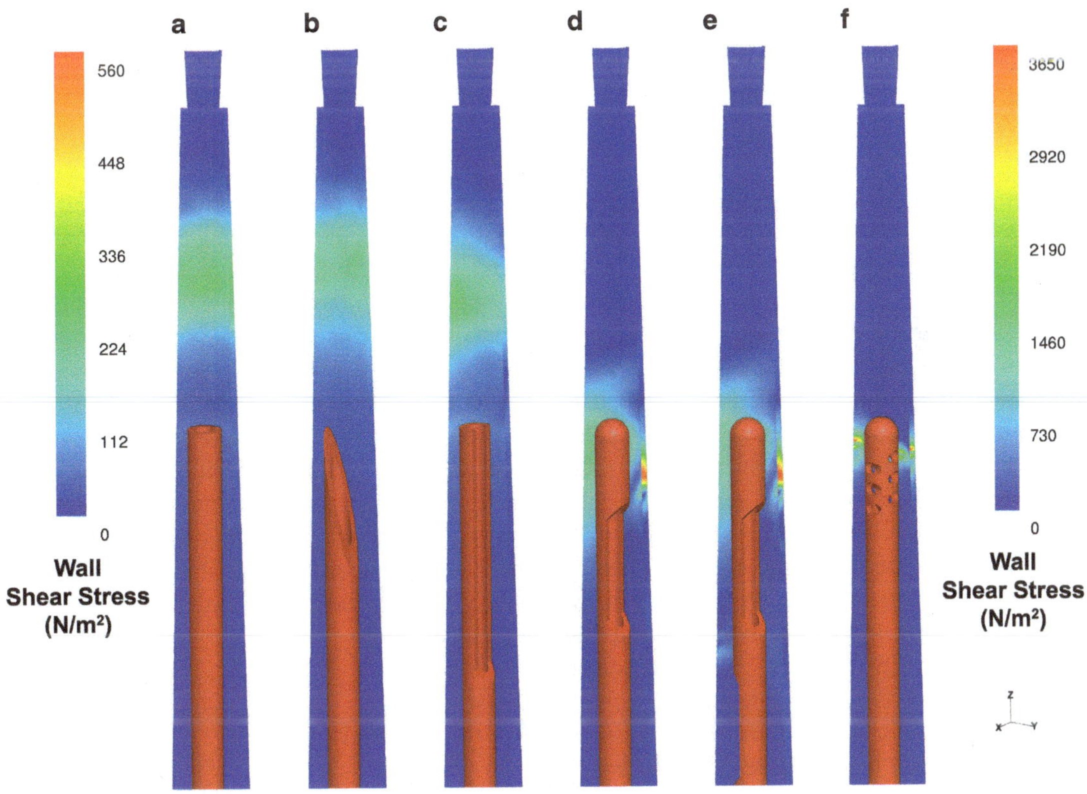

Fig. 3.6 Time-averaged distribution of shear stress on the root canal wall in the apical part of a size 45, 0.06 tapered root canal during syringe irrigation using various types of needles [open-ended needles: flat (**a**), beveled (**b**), and notched (**c**); closed-ended needles: side-vented (**d**), double-side-vented (**e**), and multi-vented (**f**)], according to computer simulation. Only half of the root canal wall is shown to allow simultaneous evaluation of the needle position. Needles are colored in *red*. Reprinted with permission from Elsevier (Ref. [13])

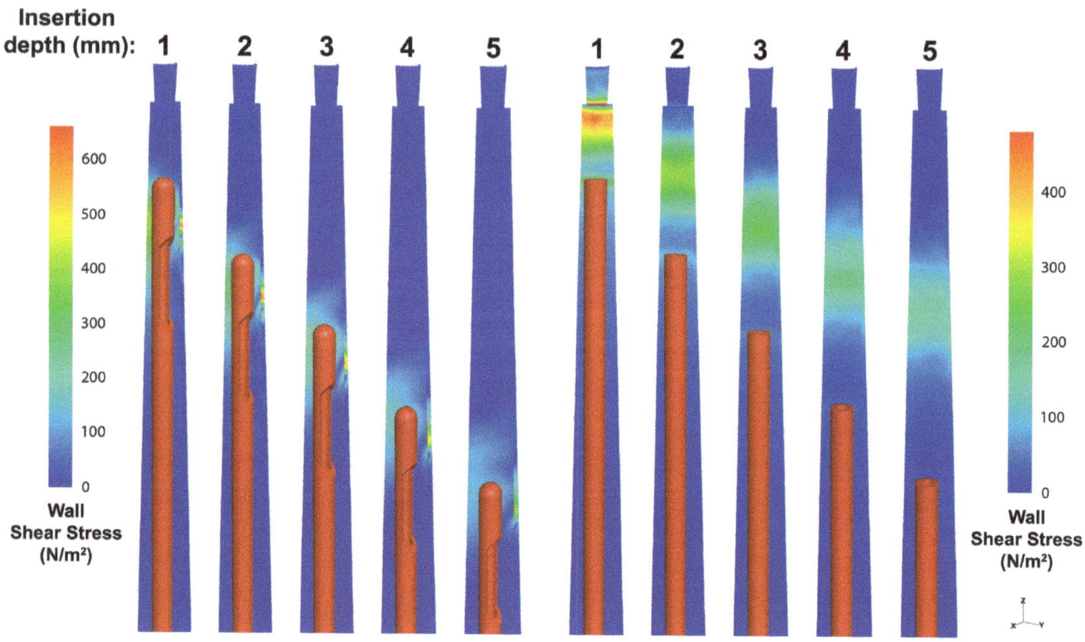

Fig. 3.7 Time-averaged distribution of shear stress on the root canal wall for the a closed-ended (*left*) and an open-ended needle (*right*) positioned at 1–5 mm short of the WL in a size 45, 0.06 tapered root canal, according to computer simulation. Only half of the root canal wall is shown to allow simultaneous evaluation of the needle position. Needles are colored in *red*. Reprinted and modified with permission from Elsevier (Ref. [14])

different pattern. Maximum wall shear stress can be up to seven times more than the other types of needles, but the stress is mainly concentrated on a very limited area opposite to the many needle outlets [13].

Needle insertion depth, root canal size, and taper do not seem to affect the distribution of wall shear stress to a large extent [14–16]. The maximum shear stress decreases as needles move away from WL or with increasing size or taper, because more space is available for the reverse flow of the irrigant, so the irrigant velocity decreases; at the same time, the area affected by maximum shear stress becomes larger. Based on these findings, it could be hypothesized that overenthusiastic enlargement of the root canal further than a certain size or taper may in fact reduce the mechanical effect of irrigation. Currently, no data are available on the effect of irrigant flow rate on wall shear stress. Based on the definition of wall shear stress (Text Box 3.5) and the relation of the flow rate to the velocity distribution in the root canal [10], it is very likely that an increase in the flow rate results in a direct increase in wall shear stress.

Optimum debridement seems to be achieved only in a limited part of the root canal wall near the tip of the needle, irrespective of other parameters [13–16, 49]. Consequently, it appears advantageous to move the needle inside the root canal during syringe irrigation, so that the limited area of high wall shear stress affects as much of the root canal wall as possible (Fig. 3.7). It must also be emphasized that wall shear stress may lead to the detachment of biofilm, tissue remnants, or dentin debris from the root canal wall, but it is not enough to ensure their removal from the root canal space; a favorable reverse flow is needed to carry them towards the canal orifice, as mentioned above.

Apical Vapor Lock

Most of the experiments and simulations already described in this chapter have assumed that the root canal is completely filled with a liquid (*single-phase system*). Recently, it has been demonstrated that air bubbles may be entrapped in the apical part of the root canal during syringe irriga-

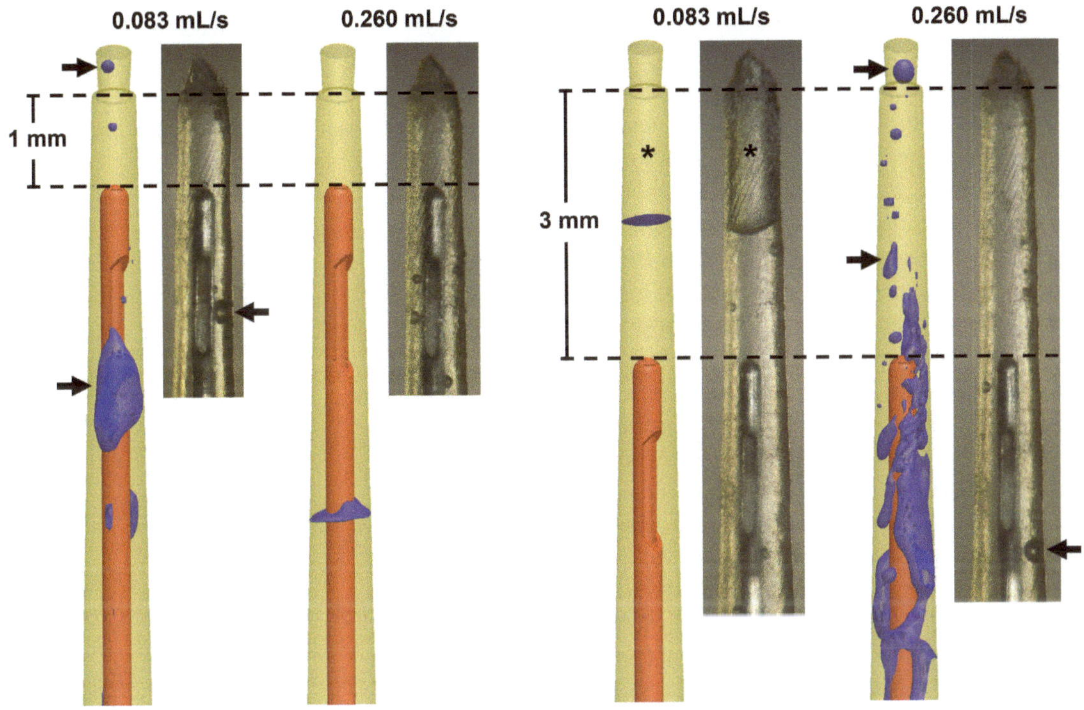

Fig. 3.8 Bubble entrapment (vapor lock) in the apical part of size 50, 0.04 tapered root canals, according to computer simulations and *in vitro* experiments. The irrigant was delivered through a 30G closed-ended needle at a flow rate of 0.083 or 0.260 mL/s. The blue surface depicts the air-irrigant interface in the computer simulations. Only large bubbles occupying completely a part of the apical root canal should be considered a vapor lock (*stars*). Smaller bubbles floating in the irrigant or moving with the irrigant towards the coronal orifice (*arrows*) are of minor importance because they cannot block irrigant penetration to any part of the root canal. Reprinted and modified with permission from Wiley (Ref. [17])

tion and totally block irrigant penetration in that area (Fig. 3.8), a phenomenon also termed *apical vapor lock* [17, 28, 101, 107, 108]. The presence of an air bubble results in the formation of a *two-phase system* (irrigant – air) (Text Box 3.6).

Despite earlier claims [28, 40, 101], bubble entrapment doesn't seem to be a major issue during syringe irrigation. The formation and extent of apical vapor lock is dependent on the same parameters that affect irrigant penetration in general: an increase in the flow rate, use of an open-ended needle, insertion of the needle closer to WL, and enlargement of the root canal all seem to result into a smaller apical vapor lock. In addition, an entrapped bubble can be easily removed during syringe irrigation either by brief insertion of a closed-ended needle to WL or by increasing the flow rate to 0.26 mL/s. So, there seems to be no need for the use of negative pressure systems or agitation techniques to reach this goal [17]. Earlier studies probably overestimated the frequency and importance of apical vapor lock by positioning the needles too far away from WL and irrigating only at a very low flow rate.

In view of these recent findings, it appears that the poorer performance of syringe irrigation in closed-ended root canals (sealed apical foramen) as compared to open-ended ones [28, 40, 73, 98, 101] should not be directly attributed to the presumed apical vapor lock without demonstrating its presence. A more likely explanation is the large differences in irrigant flow between these two cases [12, 109, 113], as explained above.

Anatomical Challenges

Overall, it appears that the *ex vivo* cleaning efficiency of syringe irrigation in the main root canal may be similar even to that of ultrasonic activation, provided that an optimum technique is used [3]. Such technique includes adequate canal enlargement, placement of a fine needle very close to WL, and a relatively high flow rate. However, anatomic irregularities may pose additional challenges for the debridement and disinfection of the root canal system. Syringe irrigation seems unable to remove hard tissue debris or soft tissue remnants from the isthmus between the mesial root canals of mandibular molars *ex vivo* [3, 32, 72] or from artificial grooves and cavities in the apical part of the canal [85]. Clinical studies have corroborated these limitations [22, 68, 83]. Currently, the irrigant flow developed by syringe irrigation in such complicated geometries has not been studied. It could be speculated that flow into narrow spaces connected to the main root canal is very much dependent on adequate agitation, which could force the irrigant laterally into the grooves, cavities, and isthmuses [53]. However, a recently published randomized controlled clinical trial showed that an optimized syringe irrigation protocol still resulted in the same radiographic success rate as the combination of the same protocol with ultrasonic activation [61]. This indicates that a more effective lateral cleaning may not be directly translated to a better treatment outcome, so further research is warranted to clarify the factors influencing the healing of apical periodontitis and especially the role of the biofilm structure.

Irrigant penetration inside dentinal tubules also seems to be a challenge [43, 70]. Recent studies have shown that irrigant flow created by syringe irrigation cannot penetrate farther than a few micrometers from the tubule entrance [110] and diffusion is very slow even under ideal conditions [110, 118]. Nevertheless, the importance of irrigant penetration into dentinal tubules in the apical part of the root canal remains unclear because of the inevitable dentinal sclerosis that blocks most patent tubules as early as the third decade of life [106].

A tooth may have a maxillary, mandibular, or even horizontal orientation, if the usual patient positions during treatment are taken into account. In most cases of syringe irrigation, tooth orientation has no significant effect in the resulting flow [11–13]. The presence of an air bubble in the canal is a noteworthy exception to this statement, because of buoyancy (Text Box 3.6). A maxillary-oriented root canal is the most challenging case for the removal of an entrapped air bubble, but even in such a case, this can still be achieved easily during syringe irrigation [17].

Text Box 3.6
Single- and two-phase systems

If a root canal is assumed to be completely filled with a liquid (irrigant), a *single-phase system* is studied. In a single-phase system, *gravity* affects the irrigant flow through hydrostatic pressure, which is negligible compared to the dynamic pressure developed due to the flow itself. In addition, surface tension has no effect on the irrigant flow [58, 113].

To the contrary, when an air bubble occupies part of the root canal during irrigation, a *two-phase system* is formed (irrigant – air). In such case, gravity also gives rise to *buoyancy*, which always forces the bubble upwards [5, 104]. Moreover, surface tension effects become significant, since irrigant and air are immiscible and form an interface [5, 58, 104, 113].

Summary: Clinical Tips

- Syringe irrigation using 5-mL syringes and fine needles (at least 30G) presents several advantages.
- Closed-ended needles need to be placed at 0–1 mm short of WL.
- Open-ended needles can be placed at 2–3 mm short of WL.
- During irrigation, the needle should be moved longitudinally inside the root canal up to the abovementioned point of maximum insertion.
- Root canals need to be enlarged to size 30 or 35 combined with increased taper, to allow irrigant penetration to WL.
- A relatively high flow rate (~0.25 mL/s) seems to augment both the chemical and the mechanical effects of irrigation.

Acknowledgment The authors would like to thank Dr. Anil Kishen for revising an earlier version of this text.

References

1. Abou-Rass M, Patonai Jr FJ. The effects of decreasing surface tension on the flow of irrigating solutions in narrow root canals. Oral Surg Oral Med Oral Pathol. 1982;53:524–6.
2. Abou-Rass M, Piccinino MV. The effectiveness of four clinical irrigation methods on the removal of root canal debris. Oral Surg Oral Med Oral Pathol. 1982;54:323–8.
3. Adcock JM, Sidow SJ, Looney SW, Liu Y, McNally K, Lindsey K, Tay FR. Histologic evaluation of canal and isthmus debridement efficacies of two different irrigant delivery techniques in a closed system. J Endod. 2011;37:544–8.
4. Batchelor GK. An introduction to fluid dynamics. Cambridge: Cambridge University Press; 2000. p. 92–9.
5. Berthier J, Silberzan P. Microfluidics for biotechnology. 2nd ed. Boston: Artech House; 2010. p. 17–199.
6. Beus C, Safavi K, Stratton J, Kaufman B. Comparison of the effect of two endodontic irrigation protocols on the elimination of bacteria from root canal system: a prospective, randomized clinical trial. J Endod. 2012;38:1479–83.
7. Blazek J. Computational fluid dynamics: principles and applications. Oxford: Elsevier Science; 2001. p. 1–57.
8. Boutsioukis C, Lambrianidis T, Kastrinakis E, Bekiaroglou P. Measurement of pressure and flow rates during irrigation of a root canal *ex vivo* with three endodontic needles. Int Endod J. 2007;40:504–13.
9. Boutsioukis C, Lambrianidis T, Vasiliadis L. Clinical relevance of standardization of endodontic irrigation needle dimensions according to the ISO 9626:1991 & 9626:1991/Amd 1:2001 specification. Int Endod J. 2007;40:700–6.
10. Boutsioukis C, Lambrianidis T, Kastrinakis E. Irrigant flow within a prepared root canal using different flow rates: a computational fluid dynamics study. Int Endod J. 2009;42:144–55.
11. Boutsioukis C. Application of a computational fluid dynamics model to the study of root canal irrigation. Doctoral Thesis. Thessaloniki: Aristotle University of Thessaloniki; 2010. p. 1–530.
12. Boutsioukis C, Verhaagen B, Versluis M, Kastrinakis E, van der Sluis LWM. Irrigant flow in the root canal: experimental validation of an unsteady computational fluid dynamics model using high-speed imaging. Int Endod J. 2010;43:393–403.
13. Boutsioukis C, Verhaagen B, Versluis M, Kastrinakis E, Wesselink P, van der Sluis LWM. Evaluation of irrigant flow in the root canal using different needle types by an unsteady computational fluid dynamics model. J Endod. 2010;36:875–9.
14. Boutsioukis C, Lambrianidis T, Verhaagen B, Versluis M, Kastrinakis E, Wesselink P, van der Sluis LWM. The effect of needle insertion depth on the irrigant flow in the root canal: evaluation using an unsteady computational fluid dynamics model. J Endod. 2010;36:1664–8.
15. Boutsioukis C, Gogos C, Verhaagen B, Versluis M, Kastrinakis E, van der Sluis LWM. The effect of apical preparation size on irrigant flow in root canals evaluated using an unsteady computational fluid dynamics model. Int Endod J. 2010;43:874–81.
16. Boutsioukis C, Gogos C, Verhaagen B, Versluis M, Kastrinakis E, van der Sluis LWM. The effect of root canal taper on the irrigant flow: evaluation using an unsteady computational fluid dynamics model. Int Endod J. 2010;43:909–16.
17. Boutsioukis C, Kastrinakis E, Lambrianidis T, Verhaagen B, Versluis M, van der Sluis LWM. Formation and removal of apical vapor lock during syringe irrigation: a combined experimental and computational fluid dynamics approach. Int Endod J. 2014;47:191–201.
18. Bronnec F, Bouillaguet S, Machtou P. *Ex vivo* assessment of irrigant penetration and renewal during the cleaning and shaping of root canals: a digital subtraction radiographic study. Int Endod J. 2010;43:275–82.
19. Bronnec F, Bouillaguet S, Machtou P. *Ex vivo* assessment of irrigant penetration and renewal during the final irrigation regimen. Int Endod J. 2010;43:663–72.
20. Brown JI, Doran JE. An *in vitro* evaluation of the particle flotation capability of various irrigating solutions. J Calif Dent Assoc. 1975;3:60–3.
21. Brunson M, Heilborn C, Johnson JD, Cohenca N. Effect of apical preparation size and preparation taper on irrigant volume delivered by using negative pressure irrigation system. J Endod. 2010;36:721–4.
22. Burleson A, Nusstein J, Reader A, Beck M. The *in vivo* evaluation of hand/rotary/ultrasound instrumentation in necrotic, human mandibular molars. J Endod. 2007;33:782–7.
23. Calarza M, Giménez A, Valero J, Pellicer OP, Amigó JM. Computational fluid dynamics of ventricular catheters used for the treatment of hydrocephalus: a 3D analysis. Childs Nerv Syst. 2014;30:105–16.
24. Chow TW. Mechanical effectiveness of root canal irrigation. J Endod. 1983;9:475–9.
25. Clarkson RM, Kidd B, Evans GE, Moule AJ. The effect of surfactant on the dissolution of porcine pulpal tissue by sodium hypochlorite solutions. J Endod. 2012;38:1257–60.
26. De-Deus G, Reis C, Fidel S, Fidel R, Paciornik S. Dentine demineralization when subjected to EDTA with or without various wetting agents: a co-site digital optical microscopy study. Int Endod J. 2008;41:279–87.
27. De-Deus G, de Berredo Pinho MA, Reis C, Fidel S, Souza E, Zehnder M. Sodium hypochlorite with reduced surface tension does not improve *in situ* pulp tissue dissolution. J Endod. 2013;39:1039–43.

28. de Gregorio C, Estevez R, Cisneros R, Heilborn C, Cohenca N. Effect of EDTA, sonic, and ultrasonic activation on the penetration of sodium hypochlorite into simulated lateral canals: an *in vitro* study. J Endod. 2009;35:891–5.
29. Druttman ACS, Stock CJR. An *in vitro* comparison of ultrasonic and conventional methods of irrigant replacement. Int Endod J. 1989;22:174–8.
30. Dumont K, Stijnen JM, Vierendeels J, van de Vosse FN, Verdonck PR. Validation of a fluid–structure interaction model of a heart valve using the dynamic mesh method in fluent. Comput Methods Biomech Biomed Engin. 2004;7:139–46.
31. Dutner J, Mines P, Anderson A. Irrigation trends among American Association of Endodontists members: a web-based survey. J Endod. 2012;38:37–40.
32. Endal U, Shen Y, Knut A, Gao Y, Haapasalo M. A high-resolution computed tomographic study of changes in root canal isthmus area by instrumentation and root filling. J Endod. 2011;37:223–7.
33. Falk KW, Sedgley CM. The influence of preparation size on the mechanical efficacy of root canal irrigation *in vitro*. J Endod. 2005;31:742–5.
34. Ferziger JH, Perić M. Computational methods for fluid dynamics. 3rd ed. Berlin: Springer; 2002. p. 1–36, 265–7, 329–64.
35. Gao Y, Haapasalo M, Shen Y, Wu H, Li B, Ruse ND, Zhou X. Development and validation of a three-dimensional computational fluid dynamics model of root canal irrigation. J Endod. 2009;35:1282–7.
36. Giardino L, Ambu E, Becce C, Rimondini L, Morra M. Surface tension comparison of four common root canal irrigants and two new irrigants containing antibiotic. J Endod. 2006;32:1091–3.
37. Goldman M, Kronman JH, Goldman LB, Clausen H, Grady J. New method of irrigation during endodontic treatment. J Endod. 1976;2:257–60.
38. Goldman LB, Goldman M, Kronman JH, Lin PS. Scanning electron microscope study of a new irrigation method in endodontic treatment. Oral Surg Oral Med Oral Pathol. 1979;48:79–83.
39. Griebel M, Dornseifer T, Neunhoeffer T. Numerical simulation in fluid dynamics. A practical introduction. Philadelphia: Society for Industrial and Applied Mathematics; 1998. p. 1–48, 109–20, 153–69.
40. Gu LS, Kim JR, Ling J, Choi KK, Pashley DH, Tay FR. Review of contemporary irrigant agitation techniques and devices. J Endod. 2009;35:791–804.
41. Guerisoli DMZ, Silva RS, Pecora JD. Evaluation of some physico-chemical properties of different concentrations of sodium hypochlorite solutions. Braz Endod J. 1998;3:21–3.
42. Gulabivala K, Patel B, Evans G, Ng YL. Effects of mechanical and chemical procedures on root canal surfaces. Endod Topics. 2005;10:103–22.
43. Haapasalo M, Ørstavik D. In vitro infection and disinfection of dentinal tubules. J Dent Res. 1987;66:1375–9.
44. Haapasalo HK, Sirén EK, Waltimo TM, Ørstavik D, Haapasalo MP. Inactivation of local root canal medicaments by dentine: an *in vitro* study. Int Endod J. 2000;33:126–31.
45. Haapasalo M, Endal U, Zandi H, Coil JM. Eradication of endodontic infection by instrumentation and irrigation solutions. Endod Topics. 2005;10:77–102.
46. Haapasalo M, Shen Y, Qian W, Gao Y. Irrigation in endodontics. Dent Clin N Am. 2010;54:291–312.
47. Hockett JL, Dommisch JK, Johnson JD, Cohenca N. Antimicrobial efficacy of two irrigation techniques in tapered and nontapered canal preparations: an *in vitro* study. J Endod. 2008;34:1374–7.
48. Hsieh YD, Gau CH, Kung Wu SF, Shen EC, Hsu PW, Fu E. Dynamic recording of irrigating fluid distribution in root canals using thermal image analysis. Int Endod J. 2007;40:11–7.
49. Huang TY, Gulabivala K, Ng YL. A bio-molecular film ex-vivo model to evaluate the influence of canal dimensions and irrigation variables on the efficacy of irrigation. Int Endod J. 2008;41:60–71.
50. Hülsmann M, Rödig T, Nordmeyer S. Complications during root canal irrigation. Endod Topics. 2009;16:27–63.
51. Ingle JI, Himel VT, Hawrish CE, Glickman GN, Serene T, Rosenberg PA, Buchanan LS, West JD, Ruddle CJ, Camp JH, Roane JB, Cecchini SCM. Endodontic cavity preparation. In: Ingle JI, Bakland LK, editors. Endodontics. 5th ed. Ontario: BC Decker; 2002. p. 502.
52. ISO 9626. Stainless steel needle tubing for manufacture of medical devices. Amendment 1. Geneva: International Organization for Standardization; 2001. p. 1–5.
53. Jiang LM, Verhaagen B, Versluis M, van der Sluis LW. Influence of the oscillation direction of an ultrasonic file on the cleaning efficacy of passive ultrasonic irrigation. J Endod. 2010;36:1372–6.
54. Jung J, Lyczkowskib RW, Panchal C, Hassaneina A. Multiphase hemodynamic simulation of pulsatile flow in a coronary artery. J Biomech. 2006;39:2064–73.
55. Jungbluth H, Peters C, Peters O, Sener B, Zehnder M. Physicochemical and pulp tissue dissolution properties of some household bleach brands compared with a dental sodium hypochlorite solution. J Endod. 2012;38:372–5.
56. Kahn FH, Rosenberg PA, Gliksberg J. An *in vitro* evaluation of the irrigating characteristics of ultrasonic and subsonic handpieces and irrigating needles and probes. J Endod. 1995;21:277–80.
57. Kakehashi S, Stanley HR, Fitzgerald RJ. The effects of surgical exposure of dental pulps in germ-free and conventional rats. Oral Surg Oral Med Oral Pathol. 1965;20:340–9.
58. Kundu PK, Cohen IM. Fluid mechanics. 3rd ed. San Diego: Elsevier Academic Press; 2004. p. 1–23, 271–377.
59. Lau KD, Diaz V, Scambler P, Burriesci G. Mitral valve dynamics in structural and fluid–structure interaction models. Med Eng Phys. 2010;32:1057–64.
60. Lesieur M. Turbulence in fluids. 4th ed. Dordrecht: Springer; 2008. p. 1–23.

61. Liang YH, Jiang LM, Jiang L, Chen XB, Liu YY, Tian FC, Bao XD, Gao XJ, Versluis M, Wu MK, van der Sluis L. Radiographic healing after a root canal treatment performed in single-rooted teeth with and without ultrasonic activation of the irrigant: a randomized controlled trial. J Endod. 2013;39:1218–25.
62. Lui JN, Kuah HG, Chen NN. Effect of EDTA with and without surfactants or ultrasonics on removal of smear layer. J Endod. 2007;33:472–5.
63. McComb WD. The physics of fluid turbulence. Oxford: Clarendon Press; 1990. p. 1–34.
64. Möller AJR. Microbiological examination of root canals and periapical tissues of human teeth. Methodological studies. Odontol Tidskr. 1966;74(Suppl):1–360.
65. Moorer WR, Wesselink PR. Factors promoting the tissue dissolving capability of sodium hypochlorite. Int Endod J. 1982;15:187–96.
66. Moser JB, Heuer MA. Forces and efficacy in endodontic irrigation systems. Oral Surg Oral Med Oral Pathol. 1982;53:425–8.
67. Mott RL. Applied fluid mechanics. 5th ed. Upper Saddle River: Prentice Hall; 1999. p. 1–188, 221–38.
68. Nair PN, Henry S, Cano V, Vera J. Microbial status of apical root canal system of human mandibular first molars with primary apical periodontitis after "one-visit" endodontic treatment. Oral Surg Oral Med Oral Pathol Oral Radiol Endod. 2005;99:231–52.
69. Nguy D, Sedgley C. The influence of canal curvature in the mechanical efficacy of root canal irrigation *in vitro* using real-time imaging of bioluminescent bacteria. J Endod. 2006;32:1077–80.
70. Ørstavik D, Haapasalo M. Disinfection by endodontic irrigants and dressings of experimentally infected dentinal tubules. Endod Dent Traumatol. 1990;6:142–9.
71. Owida AA, Do H, Morsi YS. Numerical analysis of coronary artery bypass grafts: an over view. Comput Methods Programs Biomed. 2012;108:689–705.
72. Paqué F, Boessler C, Zehnder M. Accumulated hard tissue debris levels in mesial roots of mandibular molars after sequential irrigation steps. Int Endod J. 2011;44:148–53.
73. Parente JM, Loushine RJ, Susin L, Gu L, Looney SW, Weller RN, Pashley DH, Tay FR. Root canal debridement using manual dynamic agitation or the EndoVac for final irrigation in a closed system and an open system. Int Endod J. 2010;43:1001–12.
74. Park E, Shen Y, Khakpour M, Haapasalo M. Apical pressure and extent of irrigant flow beyond the needle tip during positive-pressure irrigation in an *in vitro* root canal model. J Endod. 2013;39:511–5.
75. Pekkan K, De Zélicourt D, Ge L, Sotiropoulos F, Frakes D, Fogel MA, Yoganathan AP. Physics-driven CFD modeling of complex anatomical cardiovascular flows – a TCPC case study. Ann Biomed Eng. 2005;33:284–300.
76. Peters OA. Current challenges and concepts in the preparation of root canal systems: a review. J Endod. 2004;30:559–67.
77. Pope SB. Turbulent flows. Cambridge: Cambridge University Press; 2000. p. 3–9.
78. Portenier I, Haapasalo H, Ørstavik D, Yamauchi M, Haapasalo M. Inactivation of the antibacterial activity of iodine potassium iodide and chlorhexidine digluconate against Enterococcus faecalis by dentin, dentin matrix, type-I collagen, and heat-killed microbial whole cells. J Endod. 2002;28:634–7.
79. Portenier I, Waltimo T, Ørstavik D, Haapasalo M. Killing of Enterococcus faecalis by MTAD and chlorhexidine digluconate with or without cetrimide in the presence or absence of dentine powder or BSA. J Endod. 2006;32:138–41.
80. Potter MC, Wiggert DC. Schaum's outline of fluid mechanics. New York: McGraw-Hill; 2008. p. 47.
81. Psimma Z, Boutsioukis C, Kastrinakis E, Vasiliadis L. The effect of needle insertion depth and root canal curvature on irrigant extrusion *ex vivo*. J Endod. 2013;39:521–4.
82. Ram Z. Effectiveness of root canal irrigation. Oral Surg Oral Med Oral Pathol. 1977;44:306–12.
83. Ricucci D, Siqueira Jr JF. Fate of the tissue in lateral canals and apical ramifications in response to pathologic conditions and treatment procedures. J Endod. 2010;36:1–15.
84. Rosenfeld EF, James GA, Burch BS. Vital pulp tissue response to sodium hypochlorite. J Endod. 1978;4:140–6.
85. Rödig T, Sedghi M, Konietschke F, Lange K, Ziebolz D, Hülsmann M. Efficacy of syringe irrigation, RinsEndo and passive ultrasonic irrigation in removing debris from irregularities in root canals with different apical sizes. Int Endod J. 2010;43:581–9.
86. Sabins RA, Johnson JD, Hellstein JW. A comparison of the cleaning efficacy of short term sonic and ultrasonic passive irrigation after hand instrumentation in molar root canals. J Endod. 2003;29:674–8.
87. Salzgeber RM, Brilliant JD. An *in vivo* evaluation of the penetration of an irrigating solution in root canals. J Endod. 1977;3:394–8.
88. Schäfer E. Irrigation of the root canal. ENDO (Long Engl). 2007;1:11–27.
89. Schneider SW. A comparison of canal preparations in straight and curved root canals. Oral Surg Oral Med Oral Pathol. 1971;32:271–5.
90. Seal GJ, Ng YL, Spratt D, Bhatti M, Gulabivala K. An *in vitro* comparison of the bactericidal efficacy of lethal photosensitization or sodium hypochlorite irrigation on *Streptococcus intermedius* biofilms in root canals. Int Endod J. 2002;35:268–74.
91. Sedgley C. Root canal irrigation–a historical perspective. J Hist Dent. 2004;52:61–5.
92. Sedgley C, Applegate B, Nagel A, Hall D. Real-time imaging and quantification of bioluminescent bacteria in root canals *in vitro*. J Endod. 2004;30:893–8.
93. Sedgley CM, Nagel AC, Hall D, Applegate B. Influence of irrigant needle depth in removing bacteria inoculated into instrumented root canals using real-time imaging *in vitro*. Int Endod J. 2005;38:97–104.

94. Senia ES, Marshall JF, Rosen S. The solvent action of sodium hypochlorite on pulp tissue of extracted teeth. Oral Surg Oral Med Oral Pathol. 1971;31:96–103.
95. Shen Y, Gao Y, Qian W, Ruse ND, Zhou X, Wu H, Haapasalo M. Three-dimensional numeric simulation of root canal irrigant flow with different irrigation needles. J Endod. 2010;36:884–9.
96. Sideridis GA, Kastrinakis EG, Nychas SG. Scalar transport in a quasi two-dimensional turbulent wake interacting with a boundary layer. Int J Heat Mass Trans. 2002;45:1965–82.
97. Stojicic S, Zivkovic S, Qian W, Zhang H, Haapasalo M. Tissue dissolution by sodium hypochlorite: effect of concentration, temperature, agitation, and surfactant. J Endod. 2010;36:1558–62.
98. Susin L, Liu Y, Yoon JC, Parente JM, Loushine RJ, Ricucci D, Bryan T, Weller RN, Pashley DH, Tay FR. Canal and isthmus debridement efficacies of two irrigant agitation techniques in a closed system. Int Endod J. 2010;43:1077–90.
99. Sundqvist G. Bacteriological studies of necrotic dental pulps. PhD thesis. Umeå: Department of Oral Microbiology, Umeå University. Odontological Dissertations No. 7, 1976. p. 1–94.
100. Taşman F, Cehreli ZC, Oğan C, Etikan I. Surface tension of root canal irrigants. J Endod. 2000;26:586–7.
101. Tay FR, Gu LS, Schoeffel GJ, Wimmer C, Susin L, Zhang K, Arun SN, Kim J, Looney SW, Pashley DH. Effect of vapor lock on root canal debridement by using a side-vented needle for positive-pressure irrigant delivery. J Endod. 2010;36:745–50.
102. Teplitsky PE, Chenail BL, Mack B, Machnee CH. Endodontic irrigation–a comparison of endosonic and syringe delivery systems. Int Endod J. 1987;20:233–41.
103. Tilton JN. Fluid and particle dynamics. In: Perry RH, Green DW, Maloney JO, editors. Perry's chemical engineer's handbook. 7th ed. New York: McGraw-Hill; 1999. p. 6.1–6.50.
104. Truskey GA, Yuan F, Katz DF. Transport phenomena in biological systems. 2nd ed. London: Pearson Education; 2009. p. 1–11, 55–110, 261–336.
105. van der Sluis LWM, Voogels MPJM, Verhaagen B, Macedo R, Wesselink PR. Study on the influence of refreshment/activation cycles and irrigants on mechanical cleaning efficiency during ultrasonic activation of the irrigant. J Endod. 2010;36:737–40.
106. Vasiliadis L, Darling AI, Levers BG. The amount and distribution of sclerotic human root dentine. Arch Oral Biol. 1983;28:645–9.
107. Vera J, Arias A, Romero M. Effect of maintaining apical patency on irrigant penetration into the apical third of root canals when using passive ultrasonic irrigation: an *in vivo* study. J Endod. 2011;37:1276–8.
108. Vera J, Arias A, Romero M. Dynamic movement of intracanal gas bubbles during cleaning and shaping procedures: the effect of maintaining apical patency on their presence in the middle and cervical thirds of human root canals-an *in vivo* study. J Endod. 2012;38:200–3.
109. Verhaagen B, Boutsioukis C, Heijnen GL, van der Sluis LWM, Versluis M. Role of the confinement of a root canal on jet impingement during endodontic irrigation. Exp Fluids. 2012;53:1841–53.
110. Verhaagen B, Boutsioukis C, Sleutel CP, Kastrinakis E, van der Sluis L, Versluis M. Irrigant transport into dental microchannels. Microfluid Nanofluidics. 2014;16:1165–77.
111. Versteeg HK, Malalasekera W. An introduction to computational fluid dynamics: the finite volume method. Essex: Longman Group; 1995. p. 1–83, 156–90.
112. Vinothkumar TS, Kavitha S, Lakshminarayanan L, Gomathi NS, Kumar V. Influence of irrigating needle-tip designs in removing bacteria inoculated into instrumented root canals measured using single-tube luminometer. J Endod. 2007;33:746–8.
113. White FM. Fluid mechanics. 4th ed. Boston: McGraw-Hill; 1999. p. 1–56, 129–214, 541.
114. Xu C, Sin SH, McDonough JM, Udupa JK, Guez A, Arens R, Wootton DM. Computational fluid dynamics modeling of the upper airway of children with obstructive sleep apnea syndrome in steady flow. J Biomech. 2006;39:2043–54.
115. Yamamoto A, Otogoto J, Kuroiwa A, Maeda M, Yamaguchi H, Yamada H, Anzai M, Kasahara E. The effect of irrigation using trial-manufactured washing needle. Jpn J Conserv Dent. 2006;49:64–70.
116. Zehnder M, Schicht O, Sener B, Schmidlin P. Reducing surface tension in endodontic chelator solutions has no effect on their ability to remove calcium from instrumented root canals. J Endod. 2005;31:590–2.
117. Zehnder M. Root canal irrigants. J Endod. 2006;32:389–98.
118. Zou L, Shen Y, Li W, Haapasalo M. Penetration of sodium hypochlorite into dentin. J Endod. 2010;36:793–6.

Research on Irrigation: Methods and Models

4

Ya Shen, Yuan Gao, James Lin, Jingzhi Ma, Zhejun Wang, and Markus Haapasalo

Abstract

Irrigation is regarded by many as being the most important part of root canal treatment. It has several different functions and goals depending on the type of the irrigant used: irrigation reduces friction between the instrument and dentin, improves the cutting effectiveness of the files, and dissolves organic and inorganic matter. It also cools the tooth and the file; it has a washing effect and removes loose debris and bacteria from the canal. Last but not least, irrigation acts against root canal biofilms. Irrigation is also the only way to impact those areas of the root canal wall not touched by mechanical instrumentation. The factors that remain a challenge in the irrigation and disinfection of the root canal include biofilm resistance, poor penetration of the irrigant, and exchange of irrigants in the highly complex root canal anatomy. Progress in the search for better irrigants and irrigant delivery is necessary. A variety of different study models have been used in endodontic research on irrigation. One of the issues is how to make a rational choice for a study model that is relevant for the question at hand. This article presents an overview of the methods and models that have been used in endodontic literature to study irrigation.

Y. Shen, DDS, PhD • J. Lin, DDS, MSc, FRCD(C)
Z. Wang, DDS, PhD
Division of Endodontics, Department of Oral Biological and Medical Sciences, Faculty of Dentistry, University of British Columbia, Vancouver, BC, Canada

Y. Gao, DDS, PhD
Department of Endodontics and Operative Dentistry, West China Stomatological College and Hospital Sichuan University, No. 14, 3rd section, Ren Min Nan Road, Chengdu, 610041, P.R. China

J. Ma, DDS, PhD
Department of Stomatology, Tongji Hospital, Tongji Medical College, Huazhong University of Science and Technology, 1095 Jiefang Avenue Wuhan, 430030, P.R. China

M. Haapasalo, DDS, PhD (✉)
Division of Endodontics, Department of Oral Biological and Medical Sciences, Faculty of Dentistry, University of British Columbia, 2199 Wesbrook Mall, Vancouver, BC V6T 1Z3, Canada
e-mail: markush@dentistry.ubc.ca

B. Basrani (ed.), *Endodontic Irrigation: Chemical Disinfection of the Root Canal System*, DOI 10.1007/978-3-319-16456-4_4

Introduction

Safe and effective irrigation is of central importance to successful root canal treatment. It fulfills several important mechanical, chemical, and (micro)biological functions. Instrumentation of the root canal system must always be supported by irrigation to remove pulp tissue remnants and dentin debris. Without irrigation, accumulation of this debris causes instruments to rapidly become ineffective. Several irrigating solutions also have antimicrobial activity against bacteria and yeasts. A bigger challenge for irrigation may be the areas untouched by the files, such as fins, isthmuses, and large lateral canals. Also large areas in oval and flat canals may remain untouched despite careful instrumentation. These areas contain tissue remnants and biofilms which only can be removed by chemical means using irrigation. In order to simulate this in vivo situation, a variety of in vitro biofilm models are currently used in endodontic research, for example, to study how irrigation and instrumentation can kill biofilm bacteria and remove these biofilms. Factors that remain a challenge with irrigants include poor penetration, limited tissue-dissolving ability, and exchange in the highly complex root canal anatomy. Optimal irrigation is based on research using reliable, reproducible, and standardized irrigation models that closely replicate in vivo scenarios in order to predict safe and effective irrigation. New developments such as computational fluid dynamic models help to interpret and better explain the outcomes of ex vivo, microbiological, and clinical studies and help with the design of new strategies. This article presents an overview of the various factors that need to be considered when developing models to study the effect of irrigation on endodontic biofilms, tissue remnants, and debris removal. We attempt to explain how differences in experimental methods may affect the reported behavior, as well as to provide cutting-edge information on recent developments.

Challenges of Root Canal Irrigation

The goal of endodontic therapy is the removal of all vital or necrotic tissue, microorganisms, and microbial by-products from the root canal system. Although this could be accomplished by optimal chemomechanical instrumentation [1], it is difficult to predictably reach this goal [2–4] because of the complex structure of the root canal system and the resistance of biofilms [5–7]. Instrumentation of the root canal system must always be supported by effective irrigation. The efficacy of an irrigation system is dependent on its ability to deliver the irrigant to the apical and uninstrumented regions of the canal space, to clear the debris from the canals [8–12], to dissolve necrotic tissue and biofilm, and to kill planktonic and biofilm microorganisms. Although many new developments have taken place with introduction of new irrigating solutions and equipment, there is currently no solution or method that predictably results in completely cleaned root canals [13–24].

In 1981, Byström and Sundqvist [25] reported that mechanical instrumentation and saline irrigation greatly reduced bacterial numbers in the infected root canal. However, in ca. 50 % of the cases, bacteria could still be detected in the canals after four appointments. Nevertheless, mechanical instrumentation has been considered one of the most important phases in endodontic treatment. In a study by Dalton et al. [26], the root canals were prepared, irrigated with saline solution, and sampled for microbial growth from the canals before, during, and after instrumentation. The results showed that while progressive filing by both rotary and stainless steel hand instrumentation reduced the number of bacteria, none of the techniques resulted in germ-free canals. Similar results were reported also by Siqueira et al. [27] who reported a 90 % reduction in bacteria counts by instrumentation combined with saline irrigation. In another study the authors reported that 1–5 % sodium hypochlorite (NaOCl) solutions were significantly more effective than saline in reducing bacterial counts in the root canal [28].

Models Employing Teeth and Dentin Blocks

Traditionally, CFU counts of bacteria have been used as the gold standard method for evaluating the effectiveness of disinfection. Different experimental designs have been employed, including (1) direct contact tests in vitro, (2) ex vivo studies using contaminated root canals in extracted teeth, and (3) in vivo studies.

In Vitro: Direct Contact Tests

A traditional way of measuring the antimicrobial effectiveness of endodontic irrigants and disinfecting solutions has been with direct contact tests in test tubes. Bacteria in known concentrations (CFU/mL) are incubated for different time periods in disinfecting solutions such as NaOCl and chlorhexidine (CHX) of various concentrations, sampled, diluted, and cultured on solid media, for example, which allows for counting the CFUs after a period of growth [29–31]. Despite the seemingly simple design, the results from different studies have shown considerable variation. There are several reasons for the differences in different studies. The two main reasons are non-standardized exposure conditions and the use of microbial cultures which are at different, often unidentified growth phases. In several studies, bacteria were exposed to the disinfectants while still in their growth medium [29, 30]. This invites several confounding factors, which can greatly impact the results. The culture medium contains a variety of compounds that may inhibit the activity of the antibacterial substances [32–34]. In addition, if the microbes have been grown in a liquid culture for some time, the pH of the broth drops, often even several pH steps. The activity of many disinfecting agents such as calcium hydroxide and NaOCl is dependent on the pH. When the experimental conditions are properly standardized and reported, the results can be expected to be more constant. Nevertheless, direct contact tests with planktonic bacteria cannot replicate the in vivo conditions and the results must be interpreted with great caution. However, a study comparing the effectiveness of disinfecting agents against bacteria in simple in vitro killing studies with planktonic bacteria to results obtained using killing in biofilms indicated that the planktonic killing tests can predict the ranking of the effectiveness of the same agents in biofilms [35]. However, planktonic studies give much too optimistic picture of the sensitivity of root canal bacteria to these agents. Therefore, biofilms are today recommended instead of planktonic bacteria for direct contact tests [35].

The agar diffusion test and CFU counting method have traditionally been used to measure the effectiveness of endodontic disinfecting solutions [28–31]. Unfortunately, both of these methods have considerable shortcomings. The use of the agar diffusion method to test the antimicrobial activity of endodontic materials is not based on accepted standardization of the methods. Chemical interactions between the media and the disinfecting agents are not known. Furthermore, there are no studies that would assist in drawing conclusions from the size of the zones of inhibition to the effect of the same agent in vivo in the root canal. Therefore, the information obtained from agar diffusion studies does not reliably reflect the in vitro or in vivo antimicrobial activity of endodontic antimicrobial agents and should not be used anymore [36]. However, this should not be confused with agar diffusion tests that are used to determine the effectiveness of systemic antibiotics against specific bacteria, which is still a valid method for that purpose.

In Vitro/Ex Vivo: Use of Extracted Teeth

The use of teeth or dentin blocks in in vitro and ex vivo studies of endodontic disinfection is an effort to bring the experimental conditions closer to the in vivo reality of the root canal than direct contact tests with planktonic bacteria. Often a single species, such as *E. faecalis*, or a mixed bacterial flora obtained from an endodontic infection or from the oral cavity is incubated in the root canal space for 1 day to several weeks [37–44]. After the incubation period, different kinds of treatment procedures are completed, and microbiological samples are taken for culture and CFU counting [37, 38, 40, 43]. Although useful information has been obtained from these studies, the dentin block/extracted tooth model has also weaknesses. In several studies, the extent of bacterial growth on the root canal wall and in the dentin canals was not verified, which leaves some room for error. In addition, the time of incubation with the bacteria and frequency of nutrient exchange show great variation [40, 43, 45, 46]. Within the first hours, the bacteria are likely to be mostly planktonic and in either the exponential or stationary growth phase; biofilm formation is in its early stages. Portenier et al. [47] showed that planktonic bacteria in the starvation phase can be 1,000 times more resistant to disinfecting agents than the same bacteria in the exponential or stationary phase. Another key factor affecting bacterial sensitivity is biofilm formation and biofilm maturity, which again is dependent on time of growth, type and frequency of nutrient addition, and the substrate (surface to attach to). Recent studies with young and old biofilms grown from oral bacteria have shown that the biofilm bacteria were sensitive to NaOCl, chlorhexidine, and iodine for the first 2 weeks of growth [41, 44]. After 3 weeks, the biofilms became very resistant to these same agents, in the same concentrations. Furthermore, biofilms grown from different sources showed the same pattern of resistance; biofilms from six different donors all became resistant to the three disinfecting agents between 2 and 3 weeks of growth [44]. These results make it easy to understand the wide variation of the results in many of the earlier studies with dentin blocks and extracted teeth.

In Vivo Models

Studies done in vivo have the great advantage that real environmental factors are present. These include anatomy, temperature, nutrients, chemistry of the tooth and the periapical area, tissue exudate, host defense, and "natural" biofilm. However, many of these factors show great variation from one tooth to another. By selecting only certain teeth, such as the maxillary central incisors, the impact of some factors such as anatomy is reduced. To balance the differences between study groups, a large sample size is usually required, which makes these studies difficult to do because of increasing costs and the time required to collect a large enough group of patients. In vivo studies also have ethical limitations which in vitro studies often do not have. In patients, for example, it is not possible to have standardized infections. This could be possible to some extent in animal studies, but animal studies nowadays face strict ethical considerations and high cost. Another important aspect in animal experiments is that the anatomy of the root canal system is different from human teeth [48–52].

Although there are many challenges facing in vivo studies on endodontic irrigation and disinfection, this should be the ultimate type of study in the search for optimal treatment protocols. It is clear, however, that when new irrigating solutions or irrigation technologies are introduced, they cannot readily be tested by an extensive in vivo study. Instead, relevant in vitro and ex vivo models with strict control of confounding factors should be used in screening for the best candidates for the in vivo studies.

Sampling Methods

Comparison of the antimicrobial effect of different irrigating solutions and other disinfecting agents has often been done by culturing the bacteria at various stages of the experiment or antimicrobial treatment [53–55]. Sampling of the microbes has been done by paper points, endodontic files, or by aspirating the sample fluid from the root canal. The CFU measurement provides information on the amount of viable bacteria one is able to collect in the sample. However, commonly used sampling methods are best suited for planktonic bacteria and bacteria that are only loosely attached to biofilm. Sampling with paper points is unlikely to effectively collect bacteria from a biofilm. In addition, paper points and files only go where files used for instrumentation have created the path and space. Untouched areas are likely left untouched by the sample collecting instrument. To increase the possibility of also obtaining some of the "hidden" microbes, agitation of sample fluid by sonic or ultrasonic energy has been used [56–58], but their effect on biofilm bacteria is questionable. In some in vitro studies, the whole dentin block has been frozen, pulverized, and cultured in an effort to capture all microbes in the specimen [59, 60].

Results obtained by culturing from direct contact tests using planktonic cultures often show great differences with statistical significance between different groups [29, 31, 35, 61]. The reason for this may be that the dynamics (speed) of killing planktonic bacteria by different agents typically results in differences in CFUs of even several logarithmic steps [29, 31, 62, 63]. However, culturing from the root canal (in vivo biofilms) is a very different situation and is complicated by a number of confounding factors. If the differences in killing root canal bacteria are not great, inherent variations due to the method make it difficult or impossible to obtain statistically significant differences. Recently, confocal laser scanning microscopy together with viability staining has been employed to quantitate the killing of bacteria in the biofilm, root canal, and infected dentin [39, 41, 44, 64]. This approach brings promising advantages for the study of the antimicrobial effectiveness of irrigating solutions against microbes in endodontic biofilms.

Culturing method only detects those bacteria that are able to grow and form colonies on solid laboratory media and whose growth requirements are supported by the culture medium and growth atmosphere selected. In vitro studies have demonstrated the ability of multiple bacteria to form a biofilm architecture on root canal walls [65–67]. Biofilm microbes show much greater resistance to antimicrobial agents than planktonic, "free-floating" microbes [68, 69]. This raises concerns about the validity of laboratory studies based on cultures.

Uninstrumented Parts of the Root Canal System

The irrigating solutions must be in direct contact with the root canal wall to be effective. This is particularly important in the apical part of narrow root canals. It is well documented that in many teeth 35–53 % of the canal wall area, especially in the apical third but also in ribbon-shaped and oval canals, are not touched by the instruments [70–74] (Fig. 4.1). Therefore, microbes in these locations have a better chance of surviving. Residual bacteria are commonly found in such hard-to-reach spaces and in lateral canals and dentin canals. In the main root canal, the biofilm which is touched by the instruments is likely to be removed, although some of the bacterial cells may become embedded within the smear of tissue [75]. Contrary to this, biofilms on the uninstrumented areas remain undisturbed by the mechanical action. The uninstrumented surfaces should therefore always be regarded as

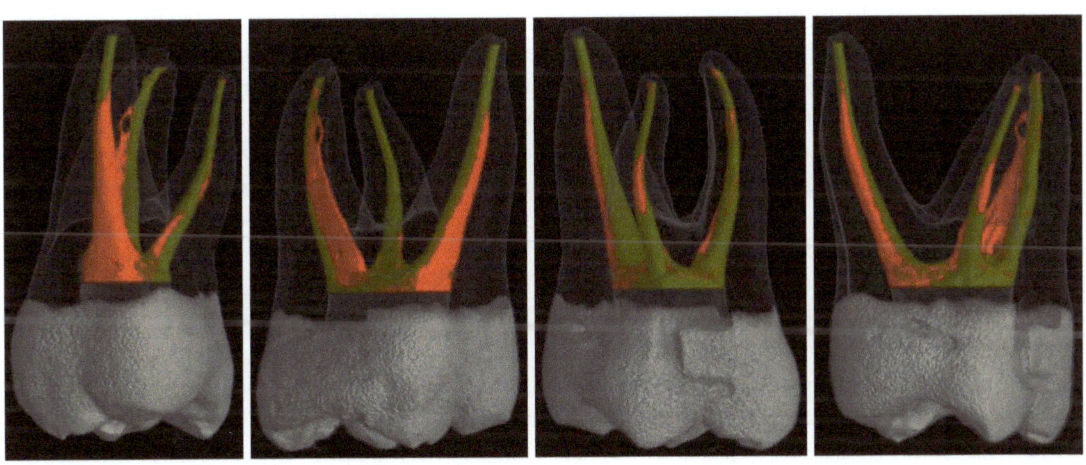

Fig. 4.1 Root canal anatomy of maxillary first molar and the effects of instrumentation as revealed by micro-computed tomography. The preoperative canal system is shown in *red*; the post-instrumentation shape of the canal is indicated by *green* (Courtesy "Visual Endodontics/ Artendo Enterprises Inc.")

contaminated. Removing necrotic tissue, debris, and biofilms from the untouched areas can only be done on chemical means. Sodium hypochlorite is the only irrigant that can dissolve organic matter and (in high concentration) detach biofilms. Therefore, sufficient use of sodium hypochlorite is important in order to obtain maximal cleaning effect in the whole canal.

Models to Study Cleaning of Isthmus Areas

Modern instruments and instrumentation techniques are able of reaching all irregularities of the root canal system. Therefore, dentists must irrigate the uninstrumented areas to remove debris and biofilms. Isthmus areas (connections between two root canals in the same root) in posterior teeth are challenging to irrigate, which may result in survival of microorganisms and only partial removal of dentin debris and tissue remnants. The incidence of canal isthmi varies depending on the type of tooth [76], root level [6], and age [77]. In one study the prevalence of isthmi ranged from 17 to 50 % in the apical 5 mm of the mesial root of mandibular first molars, with the highest prevalence at the 3-mm level [78]. Another study [77] showed that the highest prevalence of isthmus in mandibular first molars is 4–6 mm from the apex.

Use of micro-CT in endodontic research has made it easier to study the effects of instrumentation and irrigation in the root canal system. Recently, a method was presented to quantitatively assess accumulation and removal of inorganic debris in molar teeth instrumentation and irrigation [79, 80]. However, limitations of the micro-CT include that it only can be used on extracted teeth and that it can detect inorganic but not organic matter. Consequently, the chemical effects on soft tissues by NaOCl cannot be measured. A study evaluated the packing of hard tissue debris into isthmus areas of mesial roots of mandibular molars using rotary ProTaper instruments without any irrigation [79]. It showed that ca. 30 % of the original canal system was filled with hard tissue debris after preparation. The study emphasized that debris accumulation can be an undesired consequence of instrumentation. Such packed debris may have a negative impact on the sealability of root canals and reduce the effectiveness of disinfection. Even copious irrigation during and after instrumentation was not able to prevent or remove the debris packed into the isthmus area between the main root canals [80]. Thus, despite rigorous irrigation, the accumulation of dentin debris seems to occur and restrict cleaning and disinfecting the areas blocked by the debris (Fig. 4.2).

In an in vivo situation, the canal is like a closed-end channel, which often results in gas entrapment and a vapor lock effect at its apical end [84–86] during irrigation [12, 81–89]. Studies designed to simulate a closed root canal system have demonstrated incomplete debridement from the apical part of the canal walls with the use of a syringe delivery technique [90–92]. Johnson et al. [93] compared debridement efficacies of a sonic irrigation technique (Vibringe; Cavex Holland BV, Haarlem, the Netherlands) with side-vented needle irrigation (SNI) in the mesiobuccal root of maxillary first molars using a closed canal model. The tooth selection in this study was that the mesiodistal isthmus width of completely patent isthmi or partially obliterated isthmi had to be less than one-quarter of the diameter of the unshaped canals along the canal levels (i.e., 1–2.8 mm from the anatomical apex) from which histological sections would eventually be prepared after completed chemomechanical preparation. Histological sections showed that neither technique could completely remove the debris from the canal or isthmi. A significant difference between the two methods was only identified between the canals and the isthmi. Both instrumented canal spaces and uninstrumented isthmus regions are cleared of soft tissue debris to the same extent using the sonic irrigation device or the conventional SNI technique.

The presence of a complex, variable, multispecies biofilm was recently demonstrated in the entire length of the isthmus of a tooth, which had initially been treated 10 years earlier and then retreated 2 years later [94]. Gram-positive and Gram-negative organisms were both detected. In light of the well-documented challenges in

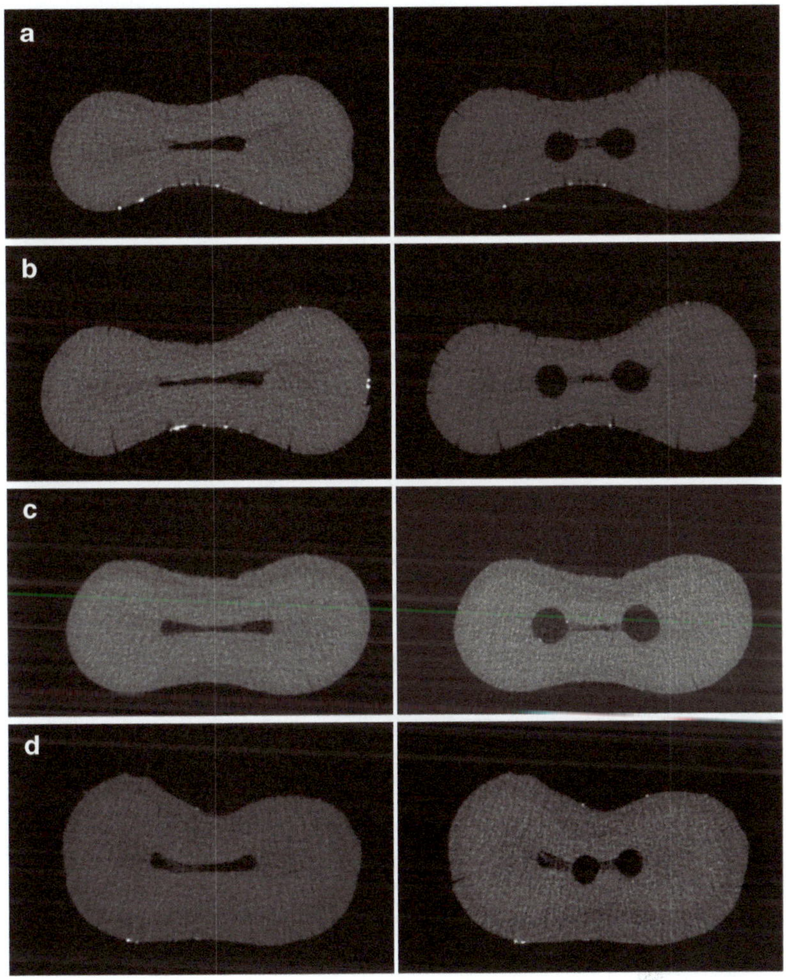

Fig. 4.2 Micro-computed tomographic cross sections of mesial root canals of four mandibular molars treated with rotary NiTi instruments (**a–d**). The cross sections are shown before instrumentation (*left*) and after instrumentation (*right*). Note the presence of accumulated hard tissue debris in the ribbon-shaped isthmus area after instrumentation (the four cross sections on the *right*)

obtaining the desired cleanliness, this area can have a negative impact on the long-term prognosis of non-surgical endodontic treatment.

Dentin Canals

The bulk of root dentin is traversed by the dentin canal (dentinal tubules). Bacteria have been shown to be present in dentinal tubules in most teeth with apical periodontitis [95–97]. Several different approaches have been used to study the effect of irrigation on microbes inside the dentin canals. Ørstavik and Haapasalo [98] investigated the effect of endodontic irrigants and locally used antibacterial agents in standardized bovine dentin blocks infected with test bacteria. The authors reported that bacteria colonized the main root canal lumen and dentin canals. *E. faecalis* infected the entire length of the tubules, whereas *Escherichia coli* penetrated approximately 600 μm. Some other studies have shown that bacteria can penetrate dentinal tubules to depths of 200 μm or more [99, 100] (Fig. 4.3). Mechanical cleaning/disinfection means the removal of some of the infected root canal wall dentin. However, complete uniform enlargement of a root canal by 200 μm is not achieved with any of the contemporary instruments [101, 102]. Berutti et al. [103], using bacterial culture from dentin samples, showed that irrigating the canal with sodium hypochlorite (after removing the smear layer) rendered the dentinal tubules bacteria-free only to a depth of 130 μm from the canal lumen.

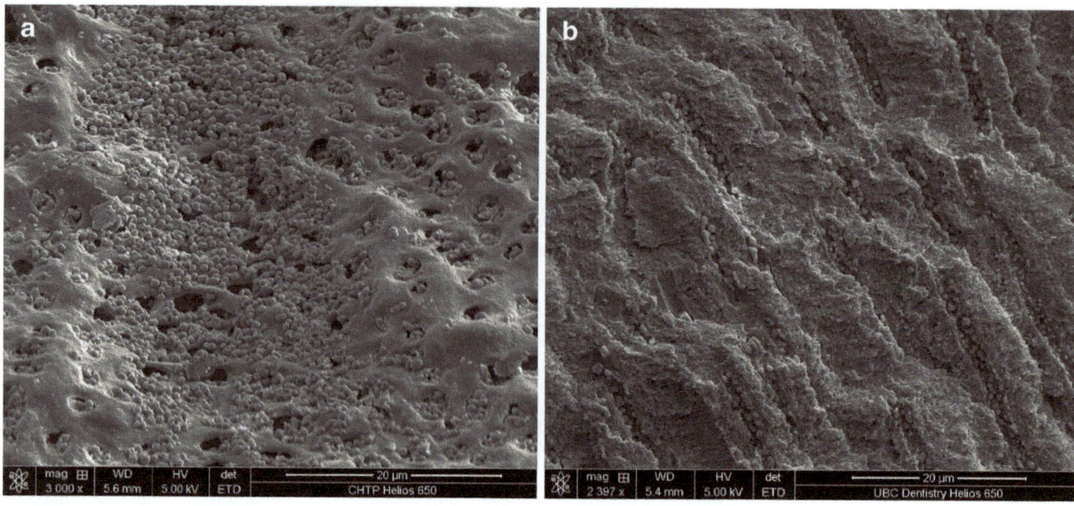

Fig. 4.3 A scanning electron microscope (SEM) image of *Enterococcus faecalis* in dentinal tubules in cross-sectional (**a**) and longitudinal (**b**) view (Courtesy "Visual Endodontics/Artendo Enterprises Inc.")

Berber et al. [54] investigated the efficacy of 0.5, 2.5, and 5.25 % sodium hypochlorite as intracanal irrigants associated with hand and rotary instrumentation techniques against *E. faecalis* within root canals and dentinal tubules. The samples collected from the root canals with paper points were obtained just after biomechanical preparation in order to evaluate the chemicomechanical action immediately after the instrumentation. The dentin samples were obtained using burs of different diameters in order to evaluate the presence of bacterial cells inside the dentinal tubules following the biomechanical procedures. The samples obtained with each bur were placed into brain–heart infusion (BHI) broth, incubated at 37 °C, and plated onto BHI agar. The results indicated that instrumentation and irrigation with saline only removed more than 95 % of the bacterial cells from the root canal. At all depths of the root canals and for all techniques used, 5.25 % NaOCl was shown to be the most effective irrigant solution tested when dentinal tubules were analyzed, followed by 2.5 % NaOCl. No differences between the different hypochlorite concentrations in cleaning the main root canals were found. Although dentin in most teeth with apical periodontitis is infected by bacteria invading from the main root canal, histological sections stained with the Brown and Brenn method and SEM studies have both shown that bacteria are found only in a few dentinal tubules even after a prolonged period of incubation [98, 104]. Such a low level of dentin infection makes it difficult to reliably measure the effects of disinfecting agents by culture or by confocal laser scanning microscopy (CLSM). Therefore, a dentin model that allows predictable, dense, and deep penetration of bacteria would be most useful for the study of endodontic disinfection [100, 105]. Recently, a standardized three-dimensional in vitro model for quantitative assessment of bacterial viability in dentin by CLSM after infection and disinfection of the dentinal tubules was developed [64].

The effect of concentration, time of exposure, and temperature on the penetration of NaOCl into dentinal tubules was recently studied [106]. The depth of penetration of NaOCl was determined by the bleaching of the stain and measured by light microscopy. The results showed that the ability of sodium hypochlorite to penetrate dentinal tubules was dependent on time, concentration, and temperature, but the relative effect of the three factors was much smaller than expected. For instance, penetration after 20-min exposure was only twice (not ten times) as much as after 2-min exposure, and the differences between penetration by 1 and 6 % NaOCl were rather small (Fig. 4.4). Maximum penetration of

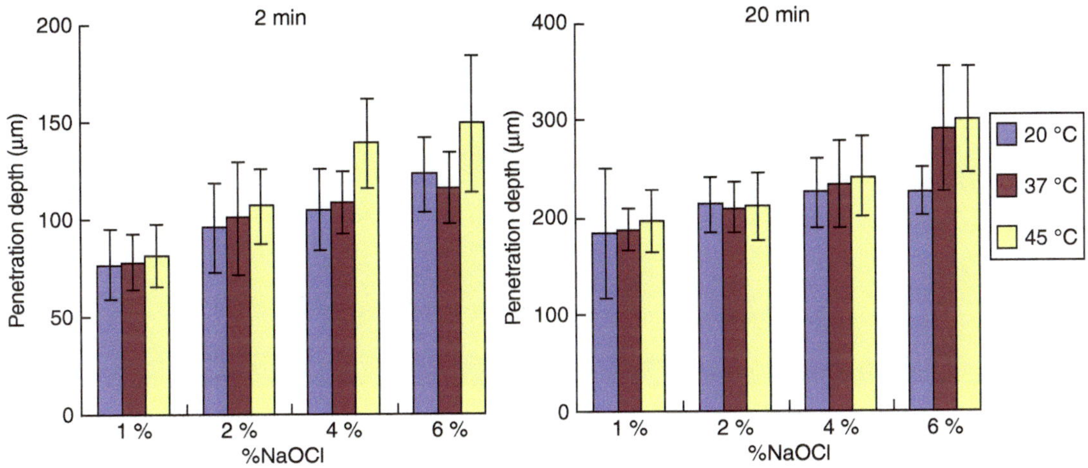

Fig. 4.4 Depth of penetration (in vitro) of sodium hypochlorite in various concentrations and at different temperatures into dentin canals in 2 min (*left*) and 20 min (*right*)

300 µm was seen when 6 % sodium hypochlorite was used for 20 min at 45 °C in coronal and mid-root dentin.

Several studies have reported that dentin weakens the antibacterial effectiveness of calcium hydroxide, iodine potassium iodide, and sodium hypochlorite [32, 33]. The survival of the bacteria could therefore also be attributed to their invasion into the dentinal tubules where they are better protected from endodontic medicaments than in the main canal. This may be caused by the difficulty of the solutions to penetrate into the tubules, inactivation of the medicaments by dentin, or the microbial biomass in the tubules [33]. During chemomechanical preparation of the root canal, use of chelating agents and acids results in selective removal of inorganic dentin components, exposing collagen fibers. Portenier et al. [34] studied the potential inhibitory effect of bovine dentin matrix (collagen), demineralized dentin powder (treated with EDTA or citric acid), and skin collagen on the antibacterial activity of 0.02 % CHX and 0.1/0.2 % iodine potassium iodide (IPI) solution. Dentin matrix (3 % w/v), which mostly consists of purified dentin collagen, was a potent inhibitor of both CHX and IPI, with most *E. faecalis* cells surviving after 24 h of incubation with the medicaments in the given concentrations. Dentin matrix was a slightly less effective inhibitor of IPI than dentin, but on CHX its effect was stronger than that of dentin. This is in accordance with earlier reports which have shown that IPI was more susceptible to dentin than to organic compounds, whereas the opposite was true for CHX [32, 33]. When EDTA or citric acid was first used to dissolve the apatite, dentin inhibited the activity of CHX more than untreated dentin powder but less than purified dentin matrix. No difference was detected between EDTA and citric acid treatment [34]. When IPI was tested, demineralized dentin (pretreated with EDTA or citric acid) showed no inhibitory activity. It can be speculated that rinsing with EDTA or citric acid before irrigation with disinfecting agents might weaken the effect of CHX but strengthen the effect of IPI. Comparative experiments have indicated that skin collagen is a weaker inhibitor of IPI and CHX than dentin matrix [34]. Together with the observation that dentin treated with EDTA or citric acid caused inhibition that was stronger than with skin collagen but weaker than with dentin matrix, this indicates that there are important differences between type I collagen products obtained from different sources and through different production and purification methods. In summary, dentin is a complex chemical and anatomical environment that needs to be carefully considered when designing studies looking at the effects of irrigation.

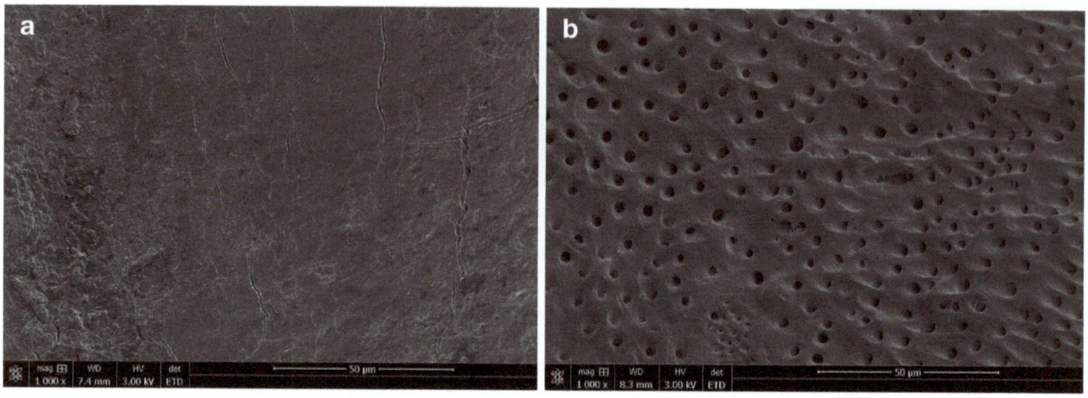

Fig. 4.5 Instrumented canal wall (**a**) with smear layer and (**b**) after removal of the smear layer by NaOCl and EDTA

Lateral Canals

Accessory (lateral) canals branch from the main root canal, with diameters ranging from over 100 μm to a common minimum of 10 μm [107]. Such narrow orifices create a surface tension barrier that does not allow adequate mixing between the irrigant and the liquid within the canal. The narrowing of the root canal apically (toward the root) poses a similar barrier. Any fluid flowing down the accessory canals from the root canal will be laminar flow; turbulent flow will be not be achievable due to the very low Reynolds numbers inherent at such small "pipe" diameters, where edge effects and viscosity become the major factors affecting fluid dynamics [76, 108]. The lateral canals may contain bacteria/bacterial biofilm which may cause lateral, periradicular bone lesions. Histological sections of extracted teeth have indicated that the lateral canals are not completely cleaned and, after root filling, they often still contained vital or necrotic pulp tissue and bacteria [109]. As long as there is no method to completely and predictably clean and disinfect lateral canals, microbes in the lateral canals remain one possible reason for posttreatment endodontic disease.

The small number of studies on irrigant action in lateral or accessory canals is probably due to the difficulty of such studies, as the accessory canal position and status before treatment are difficult to determine. Consequently, there is a need for standardized models that simulate accessory canals. Models of artificially created lateral canals in cleared teeth or an epoxy resin have recently been developed to evaluate efficacy of irrigant penetration [88, 110].

Smear Layer

Use of any kind of metallic instrument in the root canal results in a smear layer wherever the instrument comes into contact with the root canal wall [111, 112] (Fig. 4.5). Smear layer is a 1–2-μm-thick, amorphous, irregular, and granular layer with a deeper part that can penetrate up to 40 μm into the dentinal tubules. The penetration is hypothesized to be the result of capillary action and adhesive forces between the dentinal tubules and the smear layer [113, 114]. Others have estimated the layer to be up to 5 μm thick with inorganic particles of 0.05–0.15 μm diameter [115–117]. Essentially, the smear layer is a complex mixture of inorganic and organic particles, proteins, pulp tissue, blood cells, and, in infected canals, bacteria and fungi [118, 119]. As the irrigation needle is likely to follow the path created by the endodontic instruments, delivery of irrigants to areas covered by the smear layer is usually unproblematic except perhaps in the most apical canal. Irrigation with the needle introduced only to the coronal or middle parts of the root canal (needle too big in size or apical canal not sufficiently enlarged) will result in incomplete removal of the smear layer in the apical root canal.

Various methods have been used to evaluate the smear layer removal in vitro. These include score-based conventional SEM examination or optical microscopy techniques [120, 121]. However, the results obtained from score-based conventional SEM studies are not always reproducible. Therefore, further efforts must be directed to the development of, e.g., computational routines able to automatically extract quantitative data of dentin morphology, thus minimizing human bias. Calcium ions chelated from the root canal have been quantified by atomic absorption spectrophotometry [122, 123].

Therefore, the factors that remain a challenge in the irrigation and disinfection of the root canal include biofilm resistance [124, 125], irrigant penetration [39] and concentration [27], exposure time often very short [38, 39], small overall volume [126], and poor exchange of irrigants in the highly complex root canal system [107, 108]. Progress in the search for safe and more effective irrigant delivery and agitation systems for root canal irrigation is therefore necessary. Newer studies of irrigation have closely examined the same variables associated with irrigation efficiency, but unlike in the previous decades, these studies are increasingly utilizing novel experimental models. An improved understanding of the challenges by microbial biofilms by new research models and designs is likely to help us to better eliminate biofilm infections in the future.

New Models to Study Irrigation

Measuring Antibacterial Activity

Irrigation is complementary to instrumentation in facilitating the removal of pulp tissue and/or microorganisms. However, the available irrigants face great challenges in their effort to eliminate the biofilm from the root canal. Studying endodontic microorganisms adhered to surfaces for their response to antimicrobial agents, e.g., irrigating solutions, calls for relevant in vitro models. Therefore, many in vitro biofilm models have been developed for the testing of the antimicrobial effectiveness and strategies of irrigation. However, the testing of antimicrobial agents against bacteria in biofilms has not been standardized. Not surprisingly, activity of the same disinfectants shows considerable differences between studies and experiments, which may be attributed to the diversity of the microbial growth phase, biofilm models, and procedures utilized for the analysis. Therefore, a number of parameters need to be considered in the design of a representative biofilm model for application in irrigation studies.

Biofilm Substrate, the Surface to Attach to

The structure and susceptibility of biofilms to antimicrobials are affected by a number of factors such as the available nutrients and the substratum where the biofilm has attached to [41, 42]. The majority of endodontic studies on biofilm have been conducted by allowing cells to grow on membranes, glass, or plastic. This allows the film to be first grown on a substrate (e.g., membrane) and then removed and placed in a defined amount of the antimicrobial agent. It has been established that the development and structural organization of a biofilm are influenced by the chemical nature of the substrate [127]. Dentin is a composite material made up of an organic fraction (around 20 wt%), which is mainly collagen, and an interpenetrant inorganic fraction (around 70 wt%). The latter is composed primarily of hydroxyapatite (HA), which exists both within the collagen fibrils (intrafibrillarly mineralized) and between fibers (interfibrillarly mineralized) on a nanometric scale [128]. Type I collagen is the major organic component (90 %) of dentin, although small amounts of several non-collagenous proteins are also present in dentin. Certain bacteria can attach to type I collagen in dentin [97] through the expression of surface adhesins and form biofilms [129, 130]. Biofilm experiments on polycarbonate or glass, due to the different chemistry of the substrate, may not represent a true indication of the bacteria–substrate interaction. It has been reported that HA coated with type I collagen provided an excellent substrate for multi-species

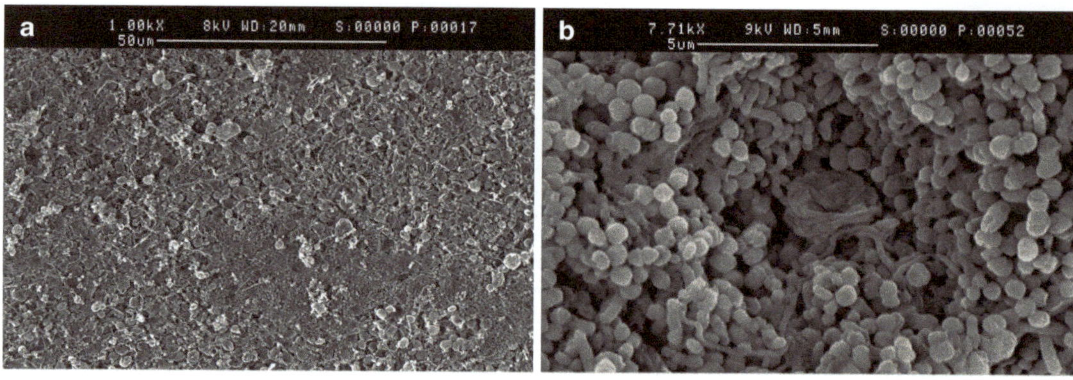

Fig. 4.6 (**a**) Scanning electron micrograph of a 3-week-old biofilm with mixed bacterial flora. (**b**) Several tightly coiled spiral forms which probably represent *Treponema* ssp. can be seen in the biofilm (Courtesy "Visual Endodontics/Artendo Enterprises Inc.")

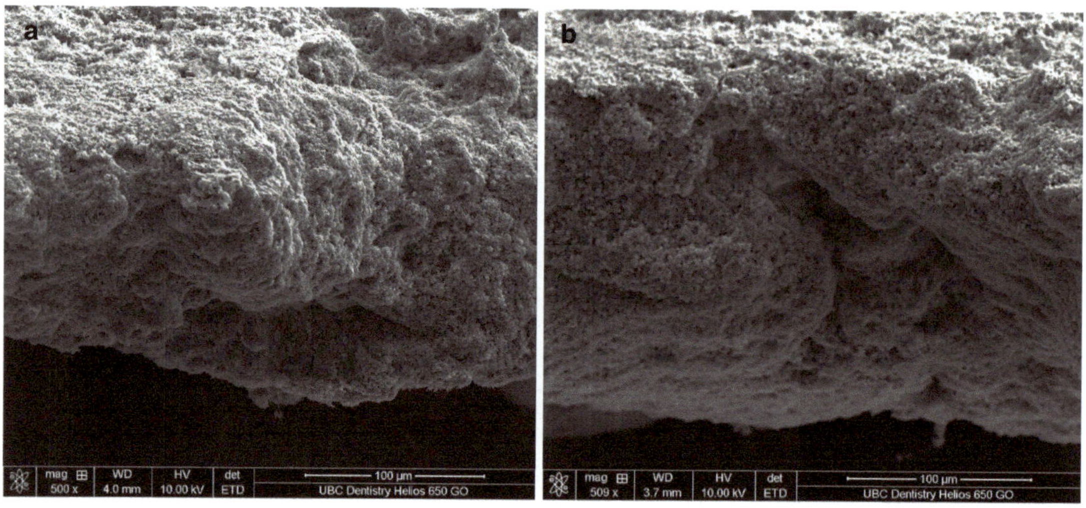

Fig. 4.7 Scanning electron micrograph of a cross section of 3-week-old biofilms. (**a**) Biofilm grown on the hydroxyapatite disc without collagen coating. (**b**) Biofilm grown on a hydroxyapatite disc coated with collagen

biofilm growth (Fig. 4.6) [39]. Chemical similarity with the teeth/dentin and the excellent growth of the multi-species biofilm indicate that this model has the potential to serve as a standard biofilm model for studies of in vitro endodontic biofilms. The abundant growth of oral spiral forms (Fig. 4.6) in this multi-species in vitro biofilm has not been described previously. More bacteria survived in the collagen-treated HA biofilm than in the HA model in the medicament groups and a thicker biofilm was observed (Fig. 4.7) [39, 42]. However, this or any other model does not simulate dentin microanatomy. On the other hand, the standard shape of the discs makes it possible to grow biofilms with consistent characteristics, which has proven difficult when using dentin as the biofilm substrate. However, it is important to keep in mind that several additional local factors in the root canal environment may affect the function of the various irrigating solutions. Therefore, conclusions from in vitro biofilm models must be drawn with caution.

The biofilm substratum (surface where it is attached to) influences both the initial adhesion of the colonizing cells and the production of signaling molecules that control cell physiology and virulence. Chávez de Paz et al. [42] reported that biofilms formed on surfaces preconditioned with collagen showed a more patchy structure than those formed on clean polystyrene surfaces. These differences can be explained by a selection of cells that adhere exclusively to the weakly hydrophobic tracks created by surface oxidation on the collagen–substratum interface [131]. It is possible that such phenomena occurring at the collagen–substratum interface level may influence the stress response in biofilm bacteria when exposed to antimicrobials. In this study, *Streptococcus gordonii*, *E. faecalis*, and *Lactobacillus paracasei* showed a much higher number of viable cells after exposure to 1 % NaOCl on a collagen-coated surface than on an uncoated surface, although the proportion of removed cells was still high. The mechanisms behind these changes are not fully understood. The levels of dehydrogenase and esterase enzyme activities of biofilm cells on collagen-coated surfaces were much lower than on uncoated surfaces [42]. Such documented metabolic downregulation represents one possibility how the substrate surface condition may influence bacterial physiology.

Various hard tissues such as bovine teeth have been used in an attempt to find a replacement for human teeth in scientific research [132]. Lundström et al. [133] developed a "bovine tooth biofilm" model system and used this model to compare the bactericidal activity of concentrated stabilized chlorine dioxide with various concentrations of irrigants commonly used in endodontic treatment protocols. The teeth were coated with mucin; inoculated with standardized suspensions of *Streptococcus sanguinis*, *Actinomyces viscosus*, *Fusobacterium nucleatum*, *Peptostreptococcus micros*, and *Prevotella nigrescens*; and incubated anaerobically. Bovine dentin has a higher mean value of tubules per millimeter but the difference in the diameter of individual tubules is not significant [134]. Several studies have focused on dentin permeability [135–137] and effects of the therapeutic agents applied directly on the exposed dentin which may be dependent on the number and diameter of the dentin tubules [138, 139].

The "infected extracted tooth biofilm" model often uses a single-species biofilm on the root canal walls of extracted single-rooted teeth [45]. Bhuva et al. [46] grew *E. faecalis* biofilms on prepared root canal walls (for 72 h) of longitudinally sectioned, standardized root halves. Scanning electron microscopy was used to measure the effects of different irrigation protocols on the *E. faecalis* biofilms. However, as the length of incubation was only 2 days, the biofilms grown in this study are not as resistant as the true in vivo polymicrobial biofilms. Biofilms found in teeth with apical periodontitis are typically much older, with greater substrate adhesion and dentinal tubule penetration, and therefore much more resistant to the effects of chemomechanical treatment.

Surface modifications are known to prevent or reduce bacterial adhesion and biofilm formation by the incorporation of antimicrobial products into surface materials and by modifying the physicochemical properties of the surface [140–142]. Biofilm formation by oral bacteria after breakdown of temporary or permanent restorations is an unfortunately common challenge to the outcome of root canal treatment. Antibiofilm coatings can alter root canal surface properties and thus interfere with bacterial adhesion. Benzalkonium chloride (BAK) is a cationic detergent expressing a high affinity to membrane proteins. Its antibacterial potential relies on the changes provoked on the ionic resistance of the cell membranes [143]. It was recently reported [144] that a surface coating with a solution of BAK greatly reduced biofilm formation by oral bacteria in a dentin disc model and in an in vitro biofilm model.

Mono- and Multi-species Biofilms

Single-species biofilm models have been the most prevalent in endodontic and microbiologic research [145]. Spratt et al. [146] tested a variety of irrigants against five different facultative and obligate anaerobic single-species biofilms grown on membrane filter discs. Single-species biofilms of *Prevotella intermedia*, *Peptostreptococcus micros*, *Streptococcus intermedius*, *Fusobacterium nucleatum*, and *E. faecalis* were generated on membrane filter discs (incubated for 48 h in an anaerobic cabinet) and subjected to 15-min or 1-h incubation with colloidal silver, 2.25 % sodium hypochlorite, 0.2 % chlorhexidine, or 10 % iodine [146]. The results showed that the effectiveness of a particular agent was dependent on the type of organism and on the contact time. This model has the advantage of at least some level of standardization; it is easily reproducible and allows large quantities of test assays to be performed at one time. The limitations include lack of substrate similar to dentin and the limited number of different bacterial species. Short-term incubation for only 2 days is also a weakness of this model. In a similar study the effect of NaOCl and chlorhexidine on single-species biofilms grown for 10 days on nitrocellulose membranes was examined [147]. The organisms tested were facultative and anaerobic bacteria. The effect of mechanical agitation was also tested. The results indicated that both CHX and NaOCl were effective at killing all of the organisms tested, although the results varied with regard to time, vehicle, concentration, and mechanical agitation of the irrigant. Mechanical agitation improved the antimicrobial properties of the chemical substances tested using a biofilm model. However, compared to Spratt et al. [146], in this study the biofilm has been grown for ten instead of 2 days, which may explain the greater biofilm resistance.

Bryce et al. [148] investigated the relative disruption and bactericidal effects of root canal irrigants on single- and dual-species biofilms of root canal isolates. Biofilms of *S. sanguinis*, *E. faecalis*, *F. nucleatum*, and *Porphyromonas gingivalis* were grown on nitrocellulose membranes for 72 h and exposed to NaOCl, EDTA, chlorhexidine, or iodine for 1, 5, or 10 min. The organisms in the dual-species biofilms included *S. sanguinis* and *F. nucleatum*. The ratio of each organism was 1:2 (absorbance of 0.2 and 0.4 at 540 nm) for the *S. sanguinis* and *F. nucleatum*, respectively, and these were incubated anaerobically. The Gram-negative obligate anaerobe species were more susceptible to cell removal than Gram-positive facultative anaerobes. The majority of the cells were killed after the first minute of exposure; however, the extent varied according to the agent and species. Biofilm disruption and cell viability were influenced by the species, their co-association in dual-species biofilms, the test agent, and the duration of exposure. Jiang et al. [149] also investigated a root canal disinfectant on dual-species biofilms. *E. faecalis* with or without *Streptococcus mutans* in biofilms were formed in an active attachment biofilm model for 24 h. This model consisted of a standard 96-well microtiter plate and a lid with an identical number of polystyrene pegs that fit into the wells [150, 151]. The biofilms were then treated with various concentrations of NaOCl for 1 min. The resistance of dual-species biofilms to NaOCl was 30-fold higher than in single-species *E. faecalis* biofilms. The resistance to NaOCl of single-species *S. mutans* biofilms was comparable to that of the dual-species biofilms. The maturation status of the cells in biofilms is a possible reason for their higher resistance [152]. It is also possible that the antimicrobial resistance is related to the amount of biofilm biomass rather than the bacterial interactions in the biofilms. Single-species *E. faecalis* biofilms contain less biomass than the single-species *S. mutans* biofilms and the dual-species biofilms, which may explain the highest sensitivity [153]. Recently, Du et al. [154] evaluated the in vitro killing activity of modified nonequilibrium plasma with CHX against *E. faecalis* and multi-species biofilms on bovine dentin discs. Sterile bovine dentin discs were incubated with *E. faecalis* or a mixture of bacteria from human dental root canal infections to form 1- and 3-week-old biofilms. The results showed that there were only small differences in the susceptibility between the single-species *E. faecalis* biofilm and the multi-species biofilm. This may also be regarded as an indication that biofilm features such as maturation and extracellular polymeric substance are more important in determining the biofilm resistance than its detailed composition.

The development of in vitro multi-species biofilm models is challenging. However, they are necessary to better simulate interactions that take place, e.g., in root canal biofilms. Over the past years, biofilm research in endodontics has used both single-species [155, 156] and multi-species models [39, 157]. Chávez de Paz [158] investigated the ability of four root canal bacteria to establish a multi-species biofilm community and to characterize the main structural, compositional, and physiological features of their communities. The clinical isolates from infected root canals included *Actinomyces naeslundii*, *Lactobacillus salivarius*, *Streptococcus gordonii*, and *E. faecalis* which were grown together in a miniflow cell system. Suspensions of the four microorganisms were mixed in equal proportions to create the mixed-species biofilm inoculums. The species tested were able to form stable biofilm communities. The biofilms formed in rich medium generally showed continuous growth over time; however, the absence of glucose resulted in significantly smaller biofilm volumes. A high proportion of viable cells (>90 %) was generally observed, and biofilm growth was correlated with high metabolic activity of cells. The community structure of biofilms formed in a rich medium did not change considerably over the 120-h period, during which *E. faecalis*, *L. salivarius*, and *S. gordonii* were most abundant.

A bovine tooth biofilm model system was developed by Lundström et al. [133] for the testing of different irrigation protocols. Permanent bovine incisors were coated with mucin and anaerobically inoculated with standardized suspensions of *Streptococcus sanguinis*, *Actinomyces viscosus*, *Fusobacterium nucleatum*, *Peptostreptococcus micros*, or *Prevotella nigrescens*. Teeth were randomly divided into four groups and rinsed for 3 min with 15 mL of irrigant. Biofilms were harvested and spiral-plated on selective media. The results provided strong evidence of a significant difference in the levels of bactericidal activity associated with the type of irrigant for all five bacterial species tested. Levels of antibacterial activity by NaOCl were significantly higher than by stabilized chlorine dioxide (ClO_2) for *S. sanguinis*, *A. viscosus*, and *P. nigrescens*. The differences for *F. nucleatum* and *P. micros* were not significant.

Physiological Status of the Biofilm Bacteria

Biofilm bacteria are frequently encountered in challenging ecological environments in which they can best survive by activating various stress-responding mechanisms [67, 159]. A necrotic root canal represents a challenging environment in which bacteria face toxic substances such as bacteriocins and where they often have limited access to nutrients and certain key elements such as iron. This will force the bacteria to use various survival strategies such as reduced metabolic activity or in extreme situation transform into the "viable but non-culturable" (VBNC) state [157].

The physiological state of bacteria greatly affects the outcome of antimicrobial treatment. However, in most published studies, the biofilms have been grown for 1–7 days [37, 38, 160], while only occasionally have longer times up to several months been used [41, 43]. Few studies have compared the susceptibility of the biofilms to disinfecting agents at different stages of maturation. The importance of oral biofilm age and nutrition on biofilm behavior was recently demonstrated by Shen et al. [41], who exposed young and old biofilms (from 2 days to 12 weeks) to two different types of CHX preparations for 1, 3, or 10 min. The results of this study indicated that biofilms which were 2 weeks old and younger were much more sensitive to the antibacterial agents than biofilms grown for 3 weeks or more. It can be speculated that mature biofilms develop localized environments that dictate the metabolic activities of cells and better protect them against harmful effects of the environment. It must be recognized, however, that nutrients can produce changes within the environment of mature biofilms, such as variations in pH [161], so that the ability to survive or adapt to nutritional and other changes within mature biofilms remains an important aspect of the ecology of biofilm microbes. The results from this study [41] demonstrated that if only young biofilms of a few hours or even up to 2 weeks are used to assess the antibacterial efficacy of disinfecting agents, the results are likely to give a far too optimistic picture of their effectiveness. It is therefore important to understand the maturation curve of each biofilm model used and use mature biofilms when evaluating, e.g., the antibacterial efficacy of endodontic irrigants and other antibacterial materials.

New evidence of the effects of oral biofilm maturation on resistance to disinfecting agents was presented by Stojicic et al. [44], who, using the design described earlier [41], examined the effect of the source of biofilm bacteria, the level of biofilm maturation, and the type of disinfecting agent on the susceptibility of the biofilm bacteria to antibacterial agents. Multi-species biofilms from plaque bacteria of six donors were grown for up to 8 weeks on collagen-coated HA discs. After 1, 2, 3, 4, or 8 weeks of growth, the biofilms were exposed to 1 % NaOCl, 0.2 or 0.4 % iodine potassium iodide, or 2 % chlorhexidine for 1 or 3 min. The results showed that all 1- and 2-week-old biofilms were moderately or very sensitive to the tested disinfecting agents, which killed 20–99 % of the biofilm bacteria. After 3 weeks of growth, the biofilms became much more resistant to the same agents and only 10–30 % of the bacteria were killed using the same agents and exposure times. The same pattern of the effect of biofilm age (maturation) on the resistance of bacteria was observed in all six biofilms and with all three disinfecting agents. It is of interest that although the three disinfecting agents exert their antibacterial effect by different mechanisms, the development of biofilm resistance occurred similarly between 2 and 3 weeks of biofilm maturation for all three agents. The result emphasizes the importance of understanding the maturation timeline of each biofilm model which is used for testing the effectiveness of endodontic disinfecting agents against biofilm bacteria. So far, there has been little emphasis on this important aspect in the research on endodontic biofilms. With short biofilm maturation times, the results from these experiments will give too optimistic picture of the ability of the antibacterial agents to kill bacteria in the biofilms.

Persistent and recurrent apical periodontitis have been a focus of interest in endodontic research for a long time [161–165]. The primary cause of posttreatment apical periodontitis is acknowledged to be the continuing presence of bacteria within the root canal system [109, 166–169]. A histopathological investigation reported biofilm structures in the great majority (74 %) of cases of posttreatment apical periodontitis [168].

A variety of methods such as autoradiography; traditional colony count; 5-cyano-2,3-ditolyl-tetrazolium chloride (CTC); and LIVE/DEAD BacLight staining have been used to evaluate microbial viability. Traditional colony counting can only detect bacteria that are able to initiate cell division at a sufficient rate to form colonies and whose growth requirements are supported by the culture medium used. The bacteria can be sensitive to culture conditions (temperature, media, duration of incubation) [169]. The two-component BacLight staining has gained popularity because of its several potential advantages. It is a rapid and relatively easy-to-use test, and it yields both viable and total counts in one step. The two stains differ in their ability to penetrate normal and damaged bacterial cells. As a result, live bacteria with intact membranes fluoresce green (SYTO9), whereas dead bacteria fluoresce red, supposing that their membrane is damaged allowing penetration of the propidium iodine stain, which is responsible for the red fluorescence (Fig. 4.8). One recent study [157] examined cell culturability and viability using the two methods of bacterial detection in order to better understand bacterial behavior in a multispecies biofilm and to examine the possibility of the presence of the VBNC bacteria under

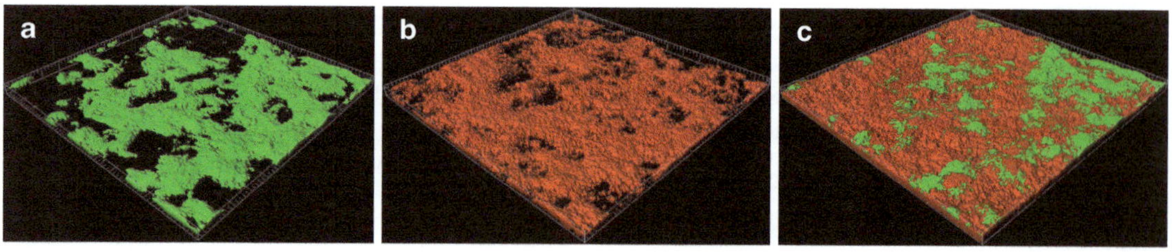

Fig. 4.8 Three-dimensional constructions of confocal laser scanning microscope scans of 3-week-old multispecies biofilms after treatment with CHX-Plus® for 3 min. (**a**) Live bacteria (*green*); (**b**) dead bacteria (*red*); and (**c**) a combination of live and dead bacteria

long-lasting nutrient deprivation. The multi-species biofilm was grown from plaque bacteria on collagen-coated hydroxyapatite discs in BHI broth for 3 weeks (phase I) with a weekly addition of nutrients. This was followed by a 9-week nutrient-deprivation phase (phase II) with just one monthly addition of nutrients, after which the biofilm was reactivated again by weekly additions of fresh BHI medium for 4 weeks (phase III). The number and proportion of live bacteria in biofilm were assessed both by culturing and by confocal laser scanning microscopy using a LIVE/DEAD viability stain throughout the experiment. The results showed that the CFU counts dropped more than four logarithmic steps during phase II (nutrient deprivation), whereas the viability staining and confocal microscopy indicated only a 25 % drop in viability. Interestingly, the CFU counts started increasing during phase III when nutrient addition was changed back from once a month to once a week, but it took 4 weeks for the CFU counts to return (several logarithmic steps) close to the original CFU numbers. Cell viability, as indicated by the staining, improved from 75 % close to the original 95 %. The results strongly indicated that oral bacteria in a multi-species biofilm grown under nutrient deprivation remained viable but became unculturable. Interestingly, the bacteria could be recovered by renewed, more frequent access to fresh nutrients while still inside the biofilm. Viability staining thus seemed to better reflect the true viability of the biofilm bacteria than culturing during the long starvation phase. If this is the situation of in vivo biofilms in root canals with limited nutrition available to the bacteria, the results of this study may have an impact on the interpretation of results of cultural studies on root canal microbiology/biofilms in vivo.

Biofilms: Static Versus Dynamic

A number of different in vitro devices can be used to grow biofilms under continuous flow of fresh culture medium. Such in vitro devices are used to grow dynamic biofilms. The flow cell system is one of the most utilized in dynamic biofilm models. It has a transparent chamber of fixed depth through which the growth medium flows. The inlet tubing supplies growth medium and the outlet tubing drains the medium to a waste reservoir. The growth medium is passed through the cell with the aid of a peristaltic pump, which controls the flow rate of the medium. Prefabricated flow cell systems are available commercially or they can be custom-made based on any particular application. Fluid flow is considered to be a principal determinant of biofilm structure [170]. It provides nutrient exchange [171], influences density and strength [172, 173], and affects the dispersal of cells from the biofilm [174]. In a tooth with apical periodontitis, an exudate may move in and out of the root canal. This fluid exchange provides proteins, glycoproteins, and other nutrients to the bacteria growing as a biofilm in the root canal. However, despite the fluid/nutrient exchange, the flow rate is likely to be so low that it does not create shear forces that would have more than a minimal effect on the developing biofilms in the root canal. Therefore, it can be assumed that a static rather than dynamic biofilm model is a more realistic representation of the true situation of biofilms in the root canal.

The static model represents biofilms that have used up much of the available nutrients during growth and maturation. The key characteristics of such models are that numerous biofilms can be examined at any given time, and they can be used as a high-throughput system for biofilm analysis [175].

Inaccessible Root Canal Areas

Inaccessible regions of the root canal system (e.g., fins, accessory canals, and isthmi) cannot be examined by conventional microbiological sampling methods. The efficacy of passive ultrasonic irrigation at cleaning uninstrumentable recesses of the root canal system has been using artificially created grooves in both simulated root canals in plastic blocks [176, 177] and in extracted human teeth [178–180]. The grooves were packed with dentin debris followed by irrigation. Digital photographs were then taken and evaluated for the amount of residual debris. It should be emphasized though that these studies assessed the efficacy of the irrigation techniques on the visual cleanliness of the artificial grooves rather than the removal of bacteria, particularly those in biofilms.

Recently, Lin et al. [181] using extracted teeth with an artificial apical groove published a standardized biofilm model to quantify the efficacy of hand, rotary nickel–titanium and self-adjusting file (SAF) instrumentation in biofilm bacteria removal. Each tooth with an oblong canal was split longitudinally and a 0.2-mm-wide groove was placed in the apical 2–5 mm of the canal. After growing the polymicrobial biofilm inside the canal under anaerobic condition, the split halves were reassembled in a custom block, creating an apical vapor lock. Teeth were randomly divided into three treatment groups using a K-file, a conventional rotary NiTi file, or SAF. Irrigation was done using 10 mL of 3 % NaOCl and 4 mL 17 % EDTA. Areas inside and outside the groove were examined using SEM. Before treatment, a thick layer of biofilm was detected in the canals after 4 weeks of growth. Inside the groove, a smaller area remained occupied by bacteria after the use of SAF system rather than after the rotary file or hand K-file (3.25, 19.25, 26.98 %). For all groups, significantly more bacteria were removed outside the groove than inside, while no statistically significant differences were found outside the groove. The study demonstrated that none of the instrumentation techniques with irrigation was able to remove all bacteria from the studied area. This biofilm model represents a potentially useful tool for future studies of root canal cleaning in hard-to-reach areas.

Improved Models to Study Biofilms in Dentin Canals

Earlier approaches to establish the presence of bacteria in dentin canals have been based on culturing methods in which bacteria are grown in a liquid medium in the root canals of extracted teeth. Experience has shown, however, that only a low number of dentin canals are invaded by bacteria even after several weeks of incubation, and there are great variations from one area to another [99, 182, 183]. Producing comparable dentin infections with a predictable, heavy presence of bacteria has been difficult, making it challenging to determine the proportion of bacteria after exposure to various antibacterial irrigating solutions and other materials. A new dentin infection model was recently developed by producing a much more standardized infection deep in the dentin, by forcing *E. faecalis* into the dentinal tubules using a series of centrifugations at low and moderate speed [64, 184, 185] (Fig. 4.9). Before centrifugation, the opening of the dentin canals was enlarged by NaOCl and citric acid. Root surface cement was removed before the centrifugation to allow liquid (and bacterial) flow through the tubules. This dentin infection model

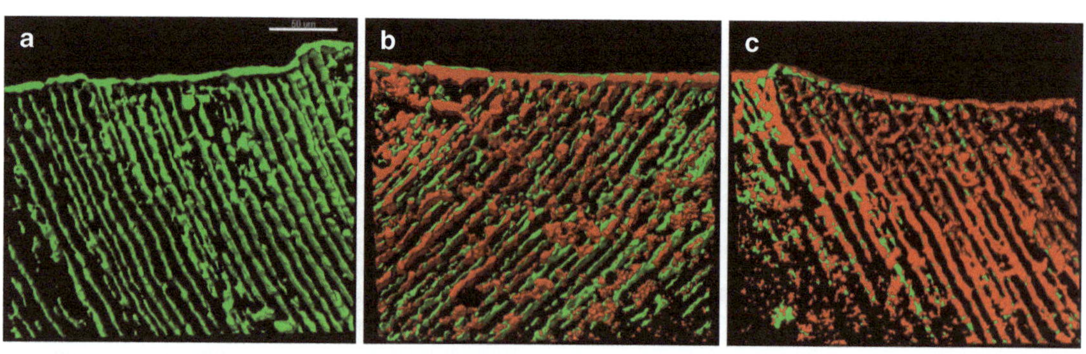

Fig. 4.9 Three-dimensional reconstructions of confocal laser scanning microscope images of *E. faecalis*-infected dentinal tubules treated by different concentrations of sodium hypochlorite (NaOCl) for 3 min, stained with viability staining. (**a**) Infected dentin treated with sterile water showing almost no dead bacteria; (**b**) dentin treated with 2 % NaOCl for 3 min shows moderate killing; and (**c**) dentin treated with 6 % NaOCl for 3 min shows high level of killing

not only provides a natural dentin canal environment for the bacteria to grow, but it also establishes a predictable presence of bacteria and model to quantitatively measure, using fluorescent viability staining and CLSM, the dynamics of bacterial killing after exposure to a variety of disinfecting agents. Negative controls with sterile water showed that *E. faecalis* survives the impact of centrifugation as the number of dead cells was similar to the number found in non-treated biofilms in which centrifugation was not used [184]. One of the limitations of these studies so far is that only a single-species biofilm model has been used instead of a polymicrobial biofilm model. On the other hand, *E. faecalis* is commonly found in persistent cases of endodontic infections, even in pure culture.

Killing experiments using planktonic cultures often show differences of even several logarithmic steps between different medicaments or times of exposure. In biofilms, this is not the case, and typically the differences are within 10–50 % units only. Culturing, on the other hand, is not a sensitive enough method to reliably detect small differences in growth. The new dentin infection model with the high resolution of CLSM and viability stain makes it possible to detect significant differences even within the same logarithmic step, unlike in cultural studies of infected dentin. The percentage of killing of bacteria has been consistent from one study to another, and significant differences have been demonstrated between endodontic irrigation solutions and materials in these studies [64, 184, 185]. The studies have also demonstrated a great difference in sensitivity to disinfecting agents between young and mature biofilms in dentin canals [185]. The new standardized dentin infection model is a promising approach to study dentin disinfection not only by irrigating solutions but also by any material (sealers, cements, etc.) placed on the surface of infected dentin.

Dissolution of Organic Matter in the Root Canal

Sodium hypochlorite (NaOCl) is the most commonly used solution in endodontic irrigation because of its antimicrobial and tissue-dissolving activities. The ability of sodium hypochlorite to dissolve organic substances and thus to dissolve pulp fragments and debris is well known and documented. Tissues from a number of different sources have been used in studies assessing the tissue-dissolving ability of sodium hypochlorite [186]. Porcine muscle tissue [186–188], rabbit liver [189], rat connective tissue [190], pig palatal mucosa [191], bovine muscle tissue [192], bovine pulp [193], and pig pulp [194] have been used to determine the dissolution ability of different irrigants. There are a couple of methods to evaluate the dissolution in an in vitro study. One way is to measure the time of visualizing the end point of sample dissolution. However, it is difficult to determine the end point of complete dissolution of the tissue because of the large number of bubbles (resulting from the saponification reaction) attached to the sample surface. Therefore, fixed time has been used instead, and the samples have been weighed before and after exposure. Other methods have used different approaches, for example, measuring the changes in the solutions, such as the amount of available chlorine after completed dissolution [189] or the amount of hydroxyproline in the residual tissue after incubation with the solution [194].

The effectiveness of sodium hypochlorite relies on its concentration, volume, and contact time but also on the surface area of the exposed tissue [189]. High concentration NaOCl has a stronger effect, but it is also potentially more toxic to periapical tissue [195–197] in case of extrusion. Changes in dentin mechanical properties such as microhardness and roughness have also been reported after long-term exposure to sodium hypochlorite in concentrations of 2.5 and 5.25 % [198]. In one study [199] the authors reported that a 24-min exposure time to 2.5 % NaOCl caused a significant drop in flexural strength, while the modulus of elasticity was not affected during this time. Other authors found a decline of both flexural and elastic strength after a 2-h submersion of dentin bars in NaOCl [200]. The loss of calcium ions appears to be dependent on both the NaOCl concentration (5 % showing the greatest amount of decalcification) and the exposure time [201]. However, one of the shortcomings in models used in many of the studies of the effect on dentin properties by NaOCl and other solutions is that the natural anatomy/structure of dentin is often changed before the exposure. Dentin bars cut from the root dentin are usually devoid of the cement layer, thus allowing rapid penetration of the solutions through the entire thickness of the dentin pieces. In reality in the root canal, hypochlorite penetration into the surrounding root dentin is much more limited. Some studies have used powdered dentin which has been exposed to the irrigating solutions. The process of powdering may remove some of the hydroxyapatite protection around collagen fibers, possibly allowing more dramatic effects to occur. Therefore, new models where the structural integrity of the root dentin is preserved before the exposure are needed to secure a realistic understanding of the effects of endodontic irrigating solutions on dentin.

There are several ways to improve the efficacy of hypochlorite in tissue dissolution. These include increasing the pH [17] and the temperature of the solutions, ultrasonic activation, and prolonged working time [13]. Despite a general consensus that increased temperature enhances the effectiveness of hypochlorite solutions, relatively few articles have been published of the topic [20, 22, 202]. Preheating low-concentration solutions improves their tissue-dissolving capacity with no effect on their short-term stability. Also, systemic toxicity is lower compared with the higher-concentration solutions (at a lower temperature) with the same efficacy [22]. The impact of mechanical agitation of the hypochlorite solutions on tissue dissolution has been suggested to be important [188]. The study emphasized the great impact of violent fluid flow and shearing forces caused by ultrasound on the ability of hypochlorite to dissolve tissue [188]. However, the mechanisms involved are not completely understood [13]. Negative pressure irrigation was introduced to endodontic treatment several years ago as a safe method to effectively irrigate the most apical canals. Recently, a novel technology, the Multisonic Ultracleaning System (Sonendo Inc, Laguna Hills, CA), has been developed for cleaning of the root canal system. The system uses sound energy to create cavitation within the solution to remove soft tissue and bacteria inside root canals. Haapasalo et al. [203] compared the tissue-dissolving effectiveness of the Multisonic Ultracleaning System with conventional methods of irrigation using NaOCl in concentrations ranging from 0.5 to 6 % and at different temperatures (21 and 40 °C) of the irrigating solution. The results showed that the Multisonic Ultracleaning System demonstrated the by far fastest tissue dissolution. Tissue dissolution was more than eight times faster than the second fastest device tested, the Piezon Master 700 ultrasonic system. For all irrigation devices tested, the rate of tissue dissolution increased with a higher concentration and temperature of the NaOCl solution.

Sodium hypochlorite has a relatively low surface tension. Some investigators [204] have proposed adding a surfactant to sodium hypochlorite, in order to lower its surface tension and improve its ability to penetrate the principal canal, lateral canals, and tubules of dentin and predentin. The addition of surfactant would lower the surface tension by 15–20 %. The effect of the surface active agent to hypochlorite was first shown by Cameron [205] who demonstrated that the addition of the surface modifiers enhanced the ability of sodium hypochlorite to dissolve organic material. Clarkson et al. [186] tested the dissolution ability of three different brands of sodium hypochlorite available in Australia and reported that the products with surfactants dissolved porcine pulp in a shorter time than regular sodium hypochlorite at the same concentration. However, Jungbluth et al. [206] and Clarkson et al. [193] found no improvement in pulp tissue dissolution by NaOCl solutions containing surfactant compared with similar solutions without surfactant. The differences may be due to the study design and evaluation method. It should be noted that these investigations were all performed in the in vitro environment. Results may therefore not be directly extrapolated to the clinical situation. The active compound in NaOCl is the chlorine. NaOH-stabilized NaOCl has been suggested to have a stronger tissue-dissolving effect compared with the standard preparation [207]. The reason for this is that the OCl^-/HOCl equilibrium adjusts itself exceedingly fast in non-stabilized solutions [207].

A study of 100 permanent molars revealed that 79 % had lateral/accessory foramina with diameters ranging from 10 to 200 μm [107]. The largest diameter was smaller than the mean diameters reported for the main apical foramen [208–210]. Therefore, disinfection of lateral canals in cases of pulp necrosis and apical and/or lateral periodontitis should be considered an important goal of the treatment, although it is difficult to achieve with current procedures. A model allowing the quantitative assessment of necrotic pulp tissue dissolution in simulated accessory canals was developed by Al-Jadaa et al. [211] to compare the efficacy of passive ultrasonic irrigation with that of sonic irrigation. Transparent root canal models were made from epoxy resin. Simulated accessory root canals (SACs) of 0.2-mm diameter were placed at defined angles and positions in the mid-canal and apical area. SACs were filled with necrotic bovine pulp tissue. The results showed that the location or angulation of simulated accessory canals had no effect on tissue dissolution by passive ultrasonic irrigation (PUI). However, it is important to acknowledge that epoxy resin is a completely different material from human dentin, and caution should be exercised when extending conclusions to the clinical situation.

De Gregorio et al. [88] developed a model that used artificially created lateral canals and cleared teeth to evaluate the efficacy of irrigant penetration. The effect of several irrigation and activation systems on the penetration of NaOCl into artificial lateral canals and to working length in a closed system was evaluated using the model [212]. The results showed apical negative pressure irrigation efficiently reached the entire root canal system up to working length in all samples tested. However, apical negative pressure irrigation demonstrated limited effect in the lateral canals. This limitation could be explained by the osmotic drawing effect described by Pashley et al. [213]. In conclusion, passive ultrasonic activation has demonstrated significantly more penetration of irrigant into lateral canals than negative pressure irrigation.

Gutarts et al. [82] compared the in vivo debridement efficacy of hand/rotary canal preparation versus a hand/rotary/ultrasound technique in mesial root canals of vital mandibular molars. The teeth were prepared with a hand/rotary technique followed by 1 min of ultrasonic irrigation. After extraction and histological preparation, 0.5-μm cross sections, taken every 0.2 mm from the 1- to 3-mm apical levels, were evaluated for percentage of tissue removal. Burleson et al. [83] compared the effectiveness of removal of biofilm/necrotic tissue by a hand/rotary technique versus a hand/rotary/ultrasound technique in the mesial roots of necrotic, human mandibular molars in vivo. Significantly cleaner canals and isthmi were found in teeth cleaned with ultrasonic irrigation than with hand/rotary instrumentation. These studies used a 60-s activation time but did not mention of depth of irrigant delivery. Molar teeth were used but no attempt was made to measure the width of the isthmus prior to tooth selection. Both studies reported debris only in "very narrow isthmi." This kind of in vivo studies is extremely valuable; however, control of confounding factors is often more difficult than in the in vitro studies for practical and ethical reasons.

Mathematical Virtual Simulation Models

Clinical trials and laboratory experiments are both important and complement each other in providing evidence for the development of best clinical practice. However, bridging the gap between the clinical reality and the well-controlled in vitro experiments is challenging. The gap between these studies may be narrowed by a class of experiments that give specific information of the underlying physical processes. Such experiments often require mathematical abstraction of the clinical setting and the isolation of the physical processes that dominate the flow field. This allows a general model of these processes to be developed and then applied to specific circumstances [214]. Computational fluid dynamics (CFD) is a relatively new approach in endodontic research to improve understanding

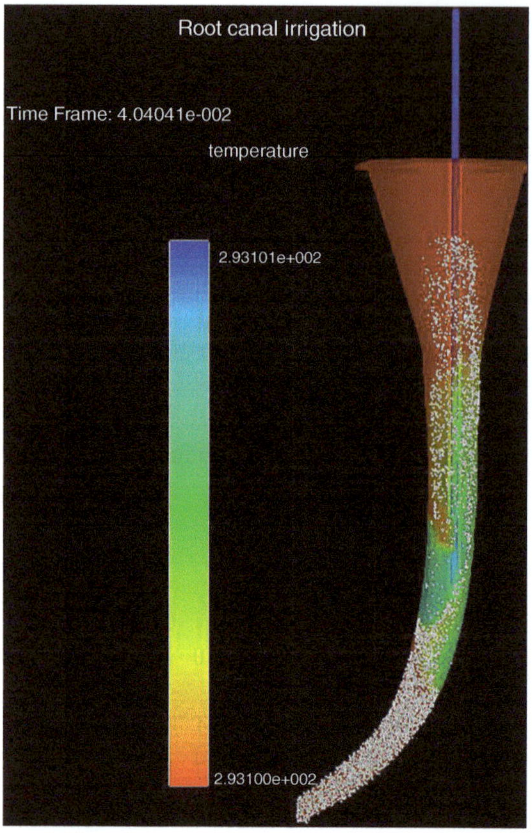

Fig. 4.10 Particle tracking during irrigation simulated by a computational fluid dynamics model. The needle is a side-vented, "safety-designed" needle

of fluid dynamics in the root canal (Fig. 4.10). Fluid flow is commonly studied in one of three ways: experimental fluid dynamics, theoretic fluid dynamics, and computational fluid dynamics. CFD is the science that focuses on predicting fluid flow and related phenomena by solving the mathematical equations that govern these processes. Numerical and experimental approaches play complementary roles in the investigation of fluid flow. Experimental studies, on the other hand, have the advantage of physical realism; once the numerical model is validated by experiments, it can be used to mathematically simulate various conditions and perform parametric investigations [214]. CFD can be used to evaluate and predict specific parameters, such as the streamline, velocity distribution of irrigant flow in various parts of the root canal, wall flow pressure, and wall shear stress on the root canal wall, all of which are practically impossible to measure in vivo because of the size and anatomy of the root canals.

CFD has been used to show turbulence in the canal during irrigation with different injection velocities [11, 108, 215]. The selection of the most suitable turbulence model for a particular application is still an open question because no single model is accepted universally as being superior to others and applicable to all cases [216]. Each model has its strengths and weaknesses, with some being designed purely for one type of flow regimen [216]. Recently, a three-dimensional CFD model of root canal irrigation, based on the geometry and physical characteristics of an in vitro model of syringe irrigation, was developed and validated [79]. In this study, the transparent simulated canal enabled the observation of the flow during irrigation and the direct visual assessment of the magnitude of the "dead water" zone, thus providing useful references for the CFD model. Physical data (e.g., velocity, geometry) of real-world processes are used in CFD models, and CFD solutions can only be as accurate as the physical models on which they are based [217]. The Instron mechanical testing machine provided constant irrigant velocity for the CFD model. Accurate measurements of needle parameters performed on SEM micrographs facilitated for detailed CAD reconstruction of the needle and its opening. The precise CAD solid model of the instrumented canal was obtained by reverse engineering techniques based on micro-CT images of the real model. Following this approach, a CFD model was obtained that replicated the in vitro irrigation model with a great degree of similarity and incorporated all of its geometry and physical parameters. In CFD studies, the use of an unsuitable turbulence model may lead to potential numerical errors in CFD results [218]. In a study by Gao et al. [108], four turbulent models [low Reynolds k-ε, low Reynolds renormalization group k-ε, transitional flow k-ω, and transitional flow shear stress transport (SST) k-ω] were used to simulate root canal irrigation because these turbulent models are suitable for studying flow with low Re. The results showed that the SST k-ω turbulence model appeared to be the most suitable for the problem investigated. While many data are difficult to extract in the in vitro irrigation system (e.g., the distribution of pressure and velocity and turbulent parameters), CFD allows examination of a large number of locations in the region of interest and yields a comprehensive set of flow parameters for analysis. CFD modeling also offers the flexibility of easily modifying the parameters, such as the canal geometry (shape and dimension), the diameters and placement depth of the needle, the needle tip design, and the irrigant flow rates. It also makes possible to observe and measure flow characteristics of the flow region [108, 218].

Particle Image Velocimetry

Particle image velocimetry (PIV) is a well-established technique outside endodontics for the measurement of fluid flow characteristics in a specific environment. Small tracer particles are added to a fluid and visualized, e.g., by reflecting light to facilitate recording by a high-speed camera [219]. Micro-PIV is a modification of PIV to access the small scales of microfluidic devices. High-speed imaging experiments have been performed in the past to visualize and analyze the action of endodontic irrigation systems inside simulated root canals [220]. Boutsioukis et al. [221] developed an unsteady CFD model to evaluate the effect of off-center positioning of the needle inside the root canal. The authors compared the detailed flow field resulting from CFD and micro-PIV was performed to assess the validity of the CFD model. In this micro-PIV setup, an objective lens with a small depth of focus and a continuous light source were used instead of a laser sheet. The main advantage of this setup was that the recording speed was not restricted by the amount of light emitted from fluorescent particles and the recordings could be made both at high recording speeds and for a prolonged time. The results showed that high-speed imaging experiments together with PIV analysis of the flow inside a simulated root canal have good agreement with the velocity field as calculated by a CFD model, even though the flow was unsteady. Small lateral displacements of the needle inside the canal had a limited effect on the flow field. Recently, Koch et al. [222] measured the flow around a rotary file more generally to demonstrate quantitative fluid velocity measurements using the fluorescent particle PIV technique in an in vitro study. The study found that fluid velocities can be much higher than the velocity of the file because of the shape of the file. PIV is an experimental tool that may be valuable to researchers in root canal irrigation. It can provide qualitative insight and quantitative measurements that may be useful for understanding the complex fluid dynamics and transport processes in root canal irrigation and for validating CFD models in dental research.

Irrigation Pressure in the Apical Canal

Apical pressure during irrigation is an important question in clinical endodontics, yet it is an area with few if any well-founded answers. Recently, Park et al. [223] developed a piezoresistive pressure transducer model to measure apical pressure during root canal irrigation using an in vitro human tooth method. The tooth was placed in an airtight custom fixture coupled to a piezoresistive pressure transducer. Pressure waves generated at the root apex propagated through the incompressible fluid and were sensed by the pressure transducer. The pressure range of the setup was −258 to 258 mmHg. A strain gage signal conditioner was connected to the pressure transducer to sample the pressure measurements, and the output was sent to an oscilloscope (BK Precision, Yorba Linda, CA), providing 250 measurements per second. The range of apical pressures generated during positive pressure irrigation in this study showed excellent agreement with the range of pressures calculated for simulated irrigation at 6 mL/min using CFD analysis with the SST k-ω model in a previous study [108]. If the minimum and maximum apical pressure measurements calculated in this CFD study are converted into the pressure units used by Park et al. [223] for a similar needle design and size, the apical pressure range is similar. The CFD study range was 8–12 mmHg [108], in comparison to 5–15 mmHg in the direct measurement study [223]. Thus, the new method of direct measurement of apical pressure seems reproducible and represents a direct approach to validating CFD estimations. There is potential to use this method to assess the safety of current and new irrigating conditions and techniques.

Wall Shear Stress/Wall Velocity

Biofilm and smear layer are removed by both the chemical action and physical shear stress on the canal wall generated by fluid flow during irrigation. Wall shear stress is a difficult parameter to measure directly, but will depend on the flow velocity gradient at the wall. CFD studies have evaluated the effect of root canal taper [224] and apical preparation size [225] on irrigant flow inside a root canal during final irrigation. The results indicated that an increase in root canal taper improved irrigant replacement and wall shear stress while reducing the risk for irrigant extrusion. Irrigant flow in a minimally tapered root canal with a large apical preparation size also showed better irrigant replacement and wall shear stress and reduced the risk for irrigant extrusion than in canals with a smaller apical preparation size. A similar finding has been reported in an ex vivo study by Huang et al. [226], who undertook a systematic evaluation of the influence of canal size and geometry and irrigant volume on the fraction of simulated biofilm (a biomolecular film) removed. A closed-end, single side-opening needle was used with the direction of the single side-opening location fixed in all of the tests on single-rooted extracted teeth with single canals. The bacterial biofilm was simulated using dyed rattail collagen. The authors reported that the efficacy of the removal of the collagen film was improved by increasing the apical size and taper of the canal, increasing the volume of irrigant used, and changing the orientation of the side-opening of the needle [227]. The percentage of canal surface coverage with residual collagen increased from the apex coronally. Complete removal was not achieved in any of the samples.

Needle Design

Different needle types have been proposed to increase the efficiency of syringe irrigation [8, 227–232]. A recent study [108] investigated the effect of irrigation needle tip design on irrigant flow pattern by using the CFD model (Fig. 4.11). The results showed that when different types of needles (beveled, notched, side-vented open-end, and side-vented closed-end needles) were placed 3 or 5 mm from the apex, irrigant velocities on canal walls were very low (0–0.7 m/s) compared to that within the needle lumen (~7 m/s) and varied as a function of needle tip design. Apical pressure was highest with the beveled needle and lowest with the side-vented closed-end needle. For the side-vented needles, the flow on the opposite side to the vent/opening was very low, approaching zero for the side-vented closed-end needle. This result is in accordance with an earlier study which showed that the root canal surface facing the side vent of the needle was significantly cleaner than the opposite side [226]. The results indicate that improving safety by decreasing the apical wall pressure might have a negative impact on the effectiveness of irrigation in some areas of the canal and emphasize the importance of continuing research on needle tip design.

In summary, the computational fluid dynamics models enable estimation of the pressure and thereby provide an assessment of the risk factors for irrigant extrusion through the apex. The three-dimensional streamlines in the CFD models provide a snapshot of the current state of the velocity vectors in a three-dimensional view, helping to visualize features of the measured flow velocity field such as velocity distribution, and predict the exchange of root canal irrigant as a whole in various parts of the root canal.

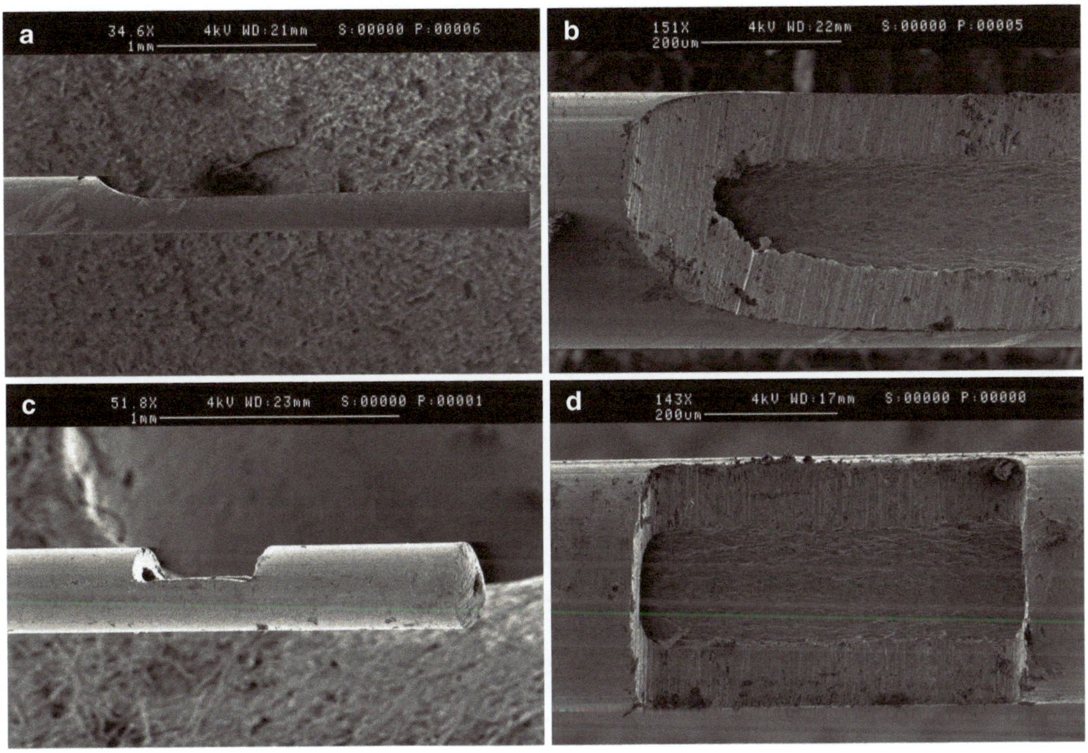

Fig. 4.11 (**a–d**) SEM of two different needle tip designs, (**a**, **c**) low magnification; (**b**, **d**) high magnification

Conclusions

Instrumentation and irrigation are the most important parts of root canal treatment. Irrigation has several key functions, the most important of which are tissue dissolution, killing of microorganisms, and removal of the biofilms. Apical irrigation poses a special challenge with regard to effectiveness and safety. During the past few years, a variety of ex vivo biofilm models have been developed and used in endodontic research on irrigation, but the full potential of biofilm experimentation has not yet been fully exploited. Several new different irrigation models have been developed in recent years and used for a variety of experimental purposes. Future research will hopefully help to optimize the models for each research problem. Generally, models that best can reproduce the in vivo conditions should be preferred. Today, as there is still no ideal irrigation model for all purposes, the challenge continues for the development more accurate and realistic models to study and improve the effectiveness and safety of root canal irrigation.

References

1. Sjögren U, Hägglund B, Sundqvist G, Wing K. Factors affecting the long-term results of endodontic treatment. J Endod. 1990;16:498–504.
2. Shuping GB, Ørstavik D, Sigurdsson A, Trope M. Reduction of intracanal bacteria using nickel–titanium rotary instrumentation and various medications. J Endod. 2000;26:751–5.
3. Card SJ, Sigurdsson A, Ørstavik D, Trope M. The effectiveness of increased apical enlargement in reducing intracanal bacteria. J Endod. 2002;28:779–83.
4. Fariniuk LF, Baratto-Filho F, da Cruz-Filho AM, de Sousa-Neto MD. Histologic analysis of the cleaning capacity of mechanical endodontic instruments activated by the ENDOflash system. J Endod. 2003;29:651–3.
5. Skidmore AE, Bjorndal AM. Root canal morphology of the human mandibular first molar. Oral Surg Oral Med Oral Pathol. 1971;32:778–84.

6. Vertucci FJ. Root canal anatomy of the human permanent teeth. Oral Surg Oral Med Oral Pathol. 1984;58:589–99.
7. Peters OA, Laib A, Rüegsegger P, Barbakow F. Three-dimensional analysis of root canal geometry using high-resolution computed tomography. J Dent Res. 2000;79:1405–9.
8. Moser JB, Heuer MA. Forces and efficacy in endodontic irrigation systems. Oral Surg Oral Med Oral Pathol. 1982;53:425–8.
9. Chow TW. Mechanical effectiveness of root canal irrigation. J Endod. 1983;9:475–9.
10. Sedgley CM, Nagel AC, Hall D, Applegate B. Influence of irrigant needle depth in removing bioluminescent bacteria inoculated into instrumented root canals using real-time imaging *in vitro*. Int Endod J. 2005;38:97–104.
11. Boutsioukis C, Lambrianidis T, Kastrinakis E. Irrigant flow within a prepared root canal using various flow rates: a computational fluid dynamics study. Int Endod J. 2009;42:144–55.
12. Tay FR, Gu LS, Schoeffel GJ, Wimmer C, Susin L, Zhang K, Arun SN, Kim J, Looney SW, Pashley DH. Effect of vapor lock on root canal debridement by using a side-vented needle for positive-pressure irrigant delivery. J Endod. 2010;36:745–50.
13. Zehnder M. Root canal irrigants. J Endod. 2006;32:389–98.
14. Haapasalo M, Shen Y, Qian W, Gao Y. Irrigation in endodontics. Dent Clin North Am. 2010;54:291–312.
15. Bloomfield SF, Miles G. The relationship between residual chlorine and disinfection capacity of sodium hypochlorite and sodium dichloroisocyanurate solutions in the presence of *Escherichia coli* and milk. Microbios Lett. 1979;10:33–43.
16. Cotter JL, Fader RC, Lilley C, Herndon DN. Chemical parameters, antimicrobial activities, and tissue toxicity of 0.1 and 0.5% sodium hypochlorite solutions. Antimicrob Agents Chemother. 1985;28:118–22.
17. Christensen CE, McNeal SF, Eleazer P. Effect of lowering the pH of sodium hypochlorite on dissolving tissue *in vitro*. J Endod. 2008;34:449–52.
18. Cunningham WT, Balekjian AY. Effect of temperature on collagen-dissolving ability of sodium hypochlorite endodontic irrigant. Oral Surg Oral Med Oral Pathol. 1980;49:175–7.
19. Cunningham WT, Joseph SW. Effect of temperature on the bactericidal action of sodium hypochlorite endodontic irrigant. Oral Surg Oral Med Oral Pathol. 1980;50:569–71.
20. Abou-Rass M, Oglesby SW. The effects of temperature, concentration, and tissue type on the solvent ability of sodium hypochlorite. J Endod. 1981;7:376–7.
21. Kamburis JJ, Barker TH, Barfield RD, Eleazer PD. Removal of organic debris from bovine dentin shavings. J Endod. 2003;29:559–61.
22. Sirtes G, Waltimo T, Schaetzle M, Zehnder M. The effects of temperature on sodium hypochlorite short-term stability, pulp dissolution capacity, and antimicrobial efficacy. J Endod. 2005;31:669–71.
23. Giardino L, Ambu E, Becce C, Rimondini L, Morra M. Surface tension comparison of four common root canal irrigants and two new irrigants containing antibiotic. J Endod. 2006;32:1091–3.
24. Lui JN, Kuah HG, Chen NN. Effect of EDTA with and without surfactants or ultrasonics on removal of smear layer. J Endod. 2007;33:472–5.
25. Byström A, Sundqvist G. Bacteriologic evaluation of the efficacy of mechanical root canal instrumentation in endodontic therapy. Scand J Dent Res. 1981;89:321–8.
26. Dalton BC, Ørstavik D, Phillips C, Pettiette M, Trope M. Bacterial reduction with nickel–titanium rotary instrumentation. J Endod. 1998;24:763–7.
27. Siqueira Jr JF, Lima KC, Magalhaes FA, Lopes HP, de Uzeda M. Mechanical reduction of the bacterial population in the root canal by three instrumentation techniques. J Endod. 1999;25:332–5.
28. Siqueira Jr JF, Rôças IN, Favieri A, Lima KC. Chemomechanical reduction of the bacterial population in the root canal after instrumentation and irrigation with 1%, 2.5%, and 5.25% sodium hypochlorite. J Endod. 2000;26:331–4.
29. Gomes BP, Ferraz CC, Vianna ME, Berber VB, Teixeira FB, Souza-Filho FJ. *In vitro* antimicrobial activity of several concentrations of sodium hypochlorite and chlorhexidine gluconate in the elimination of *Enterococcus faecalis*. Int Endod J. 2001;34:424–8.
30. Lynne RE, Liewehr FR, West LA, Patton WR, Buxton TB, McPherson JC. *In vitro* antimicrobial activity of various medication preparations on *E. faecalis* in root canal dentin. J Endod. 2003;29:187–90.
31. Vianna ME, Gomes BP, Berber VB, Zaia AA, Ferraz CC, de Souza-Filho FJ. *In vitro* evaluation of the antimicrobial activity of chlorhexidine and sodium hypochlorite. Oral Surg Oral Med Oral Pathol Oral Radiol Endod. 2004;97:79–84.
32. Haapasalo HK, Sirén EK, Waltimo TM, Ørstavik D, Haapasalo MP. Inactivation of local root canal medicaments by dentine: an *in vitro* study. Int Endod J. 2000;33:126–31.
33. Portenier I, Haapasalo H, Rye A, Waltimo T, Ørstavik D, Haapasalo M. Inactivation of root canal medicaments by dentine, hydroxylapatite and bovine serum albumin. Int Endod J. 2001;34:184–8.
34. Portenier I, Haapasalo H, Ørstavik D, Yamauchi M, Haapasalo M. Inactivation of the antibacterial activity of iodine potassium iodide and chlorhexidine digluconate against *Enterococcus faecalis* by dentin, dentin matrix, type-I collagen, and heat-killed microbial whole cells. J Endod. 2002;28:634–7.
35. Pappen FG, Shen Y, Qian W, Leonardo MR, Giardino L, Haapasalo M. *In vitro* antibacterial action of Tetraclean, MTAD and five experimental irrigation solutions. Int Endod J. 2010;43:528–35.
36. Editorial Board of the Journal of Endodontics. Wanted: a base of evidence. J Endod. 2007;33:1401–2.
37. Dunavant TR, Regan JD, Glickman GN, Solomon ES, Honeyman AL. Comparative evaluation of endodontic

irrigants against *Enterococcus faecalis* biofilms. J Endod. 2006;32:527–31.
38. Williamson AE, Cardon JW, Drake DR. Antimicrobial susceptibility of monoculture biofilms of a clinical isolate of *Enterococcus faecalis*. J Endod. 2009;35:95–7.
39. Shen Y, Qian W, Chung C, Olsen I, Haapasalo M. Evaluation of the effect of two chlorhexidine preparations on biofilm bacteria *in vitro*: a three-dimensional quantitative analysis. J Endod. 2009;35:981–5.
40. Liu H, Wei X, Ling J, Wang W, Huang X. Biofilm formation capability of *Enterococcus faecalis* cells in starvation phase and its susceptibility to sodium hypochlorite. J Endod. 2010;36:630–5.
41. Shen Y, Stojicic S, Haapasalo M. Antimicrobial efficacy of chlorhexidine against bacteria in biofilms at different stages of development. J Endod. 2011;37:657–61.
42. Chávez de Paz LE, Bergenholtz G, Svensäter G. The effects of antimicrobials on endodontic biofilm bacteria. J Endod. 2010;36:70–7.
43. Kishen A, George S, Kumar R. *Enterococcus faecalis-mediated* biomineralized biofilm formation on root canal dentine *in vitro*. J Biomed Mater Res A. 2006;77:406–15.
44. Stojicic S, Shen Y, Haapasalo M. The effect of the source of biofilm bacteria, the level of biofilm maturation, and the type of disinfecting agent on the susceptibility of biofilm bacteria to antibacterial agents. J Endod. 2013;39:473–7.
45. Siqueira Jr JF, Machado AG, Silveira RM, Lopes HP, de Uzeda M. Evaluation of the effectiveness of sodium hypochlorite used with three irrigation methods in the elimination of *Enterococcus faecalis* from the root canal, *in vitro*. Int Endod J. 1997;30:279–82.
46. Bhuva B, Patel S, Wilson R, Niazi S, Beighton D, Mannocci F. The effectiveness of passive ultrasonic irrigation on intraradicular *Enterococcus faecalis* biofilms in extracted single-rooted human teeth. Int Endod J. 2010;43:241–50.
47. Portenier I, Waltimo T, Ørstavik D, Haapasalo M. The susceptibility of starved, stationary phase, and growing cells of *Enterococcus faecalis* to endodontic medicaments. J Endod. 2005;31:380–6.
48. Holland R, Soares IJ, Soares IM. Influence of irrigation and intracanal dressing on the healing process of dogs' teeth with apical periodontitis. Endod Dent Traumatol. 1992;8:223–9.
49. Leonardo MR, Almeida WA, Ito IY, da Silva LA. Radiographic and microbiologic evaluation of posttreatment apical and periapical repair of root canals of dogs' teeth with experimentally induced chronic lesion. Oral Surg Oral Med Oral Pathol. 1994;78:232–8.
50. Tanomaru Filho M, Leonardo MR, da Silva LA. Effect of irrigating solution and calcium hydroxide root canal dressing on the repair of apical and periapical tissues of teeth with periapical lesion. J Endod. 2002;28:295–9.
51. Silva LA, Leonardo MR, Assed S, Tanomaru FM. Histological study of the effect of some irrigating solutions on bacterial endotoxin in dogs. Braz Dent J. 2004;15:109–14.
52. De Rossi A, Silva LA, Leonardo MR, Rocha LB, Rossi MA. Effect of rotary or manual instrumentation, with or without a calcium hydroxide/1% chlorhexidine intracanal dressing, on the healing of experimentally induced chronic periapical lesions. Oral Surg Oral Med Oral Pathol Oral Radiol Endod. 2005;99:628–36.
53. Vivacqua-Gomes N, Gurgel-Filho ED, Gomes BP, Ferraz CC, Zaia AA, Souza-Filho FJ. Recovery of *Enterococcus faecalis* after single- or multiple-visit root canal treatments carried out in infected teeth *ex vivo*. Int Endod J. 2005;38:697–704.
54. Berber VB, Gomes BP, Sena NT, Vianna ME, Ferraz CC, Zaia AA, Souza-Filho FJ. Efficacy of various concentrations of NaOCl and instrumentation techniques in reducing *Enterococcus faecalis* within root canals and dentinal tubules. Int Endod J. 2006;39:10–7.
55. Câmara AC, de Albuquerque MM, Aguiar CM, de Barros Correia AC. *In vitro* antimicrobial activity of 0.5%, 1%, and 2.5% sodium hypochlorite in root canals instrumented with the ProTaper Universal system. Oral Surg Oral Med Oral Pathol Oral Radiol Endod. 2009;108:e55–61.
56. Harrison AJ, Chivatxaranukul P, Parashos P, Messer HH. The effect of ultrasonically activated irrigation on reduction of *Enterococcus faecalis* in experimentally infected root canals. Int Endod J. 2010;43:968–77.
57. Huffaker SK, Safavi K, Spångberg LS, Kaufman B. Influence of a passive sonic irrigation system on the elimination of bacteria from root canal systems: a clinical study. J Endod. 2010;36:1315–8.
58. Gründling GL, Zechin JG, Jardim WM, de Oliveira SD, de Figueiredo JA. Effect of ultrasonics on *Enterococcus faecalis* biofilm in a bovine tooth model. J Endod. 2011;37:1128–33.
59. Kho P, Baumgartner JC. A comparison of the antimicrobial efficacy of NaOCl/Biopure MTAD versus NaOCl/EDTA against *Enterococcus faecalis*. J Endod. 2006;32:652–5.
60. Miller TA, Baumgartner JC. Comparison of the antimicrobial efficacy of irrigation using the EndoVac to endodontic needle delivery. J Endod. 2010;36:509–11.
61. Abdullah M, Ng YL, Gulabivala K, Moles DR, Spratt DA. Susceptibilities of two *Enterococcus faecalis* phenotypes to root canal medications. J Endod. 2005;31:30–6.
62. Radcliffe CE, Potouridou L, Qureshi R, Habahbeh N, Qualtrough A, Worthington H, Drucker DB. Antimicrobial activity of varying concentrations of sodium hypochlorite on the endodontic microorganisms *Actinomyces israelii*, *A. naeslundii*, *Candida albicans* and *Enterococcus faecalis*. Int Endod J. 2004;37:438–46.
63. Waltimo TM, Ørstavik D, Siren EK, Haapasalo MP. *In vitro* susceptibility of *Candida albicans* to four disinfectants and their combinations. Int Endod J. 1999;32:421–9.

64. Ma J, Wang Z, Shen Y, Haapasalo M. A new noninvasive model to study the effectiveness of dentin disinfection by using confocal laser scanning microscopy. J Endod. 2011;37:1380–5.
65. Distel JWD. Biofilm formation in medicated root canals. J Endod. 2002;28:689–93.
66. Chávez de Paz LE. Redefining the persistent infection in root canals: possible role of biofilm communities. J Endod. 2007;33:652–62.
67. George S, Kishen A, Song KP. The role of environmental changes on monospecies biofilm formation on root canal wall by *Enterococcus faecalis*. J Endod. 2005;31:867–72.
68. Johnson SA, Goddard PA, Iliffe C, Timmins B, Rickard AH, Robson G, Handley PS. Comparative susceptibility of resident and transient hand bacteria to para-chloro-meta-xylenol and triclosan. J Appl Microbiol. 2002;93:336–44.
69. Costerton JW, Lewandowski Z, DeBeer D, Caldwell D, Korber D, James G. Biofilms, the customized microniche. J Bacteriol. 1994;176:2137–42.
70. Peters OA, Laib A, Göhring TN, Barbakow F. Changes in root canal geometry after preparation assessed by high-resolution computed tomography. J Endod. 2001;27:1–6.
71. Mannan G, Smallwood E, Gulabivala K. The influence of access cavity design on filing of canals in anterior teeth. Int Endod J. 2001;34:176–83.
72. Peters OA, Schönenberger K, Laib A. Effects of four Ni–Ti preparation techniques on root canal geometry assessed by micro computed tomography. Int Endod J. 2001;34:221–30.
73. Peters OA, Peters CI, Schönenberger K, Barbakow F. ProTaper rotary root canal preparation: effects of canal anatomy on final shape analysed by micro CT. Int Endod J. 2003;36:86–92.
74. Hübscher W, Barbakow F, Peters OA. Root-canal preparation with FlexMaster: canal shapes analysed by micro-computed tomography. Int Endod J. 2003;36:740–7.
75. McComb D, Smith DC, Beagrie GS. The results of *in vivo* endodontic chemomechanical instrumentation—a scanning electron microscope study. J Br Endod Soc. 1976;9:11–8.
76. von Arx T. Frequency and type of canal isthmuses in first molars detected by endoscopic inspection during periradicular surgery. Int Endod J. 2005;38:160–8.
77. Gu L, Wei X, Ling J, Huang X. A microcomputed tomographic study of canal isthmuses in the mesial root of mandibular first molars in a Chinese population. J Endod. 2009;35:353–6.
78. Mannocci F, Peru M, Sherriff M, Cook R, Pitt Ford TR. The isthmuses of the mesial root of mandibular molars: a micro-computed tomographic study. Int Endod J. 2005;38:558–63.
79. Paqué F, Laib A, Gautschi H, Zehnder M. Hard-tissue debris accumulation analysis by high-resolution computed tomography scans. J Endod. 2009;35:1044–7.
80. Endal U, Shen Y, Knut A, Gao Y, Haapasalo M. A high-resolution computed tomographic study of changes in root canal isthmus area by instrumentation and root filling. J Endod. 2011;37:223–7.
81. Usman N, Baumgartner JC, Marshall JG. Influence of instrument size on root canal debridement. J Endod. 2004;30:110–2.
82. Gutarts R, Nusstein J, Reader A, Beck M. *In vivo* debridement efficacy of ultrasonic irrigation following hand-rotary instrumentation in human mandibular molars. J Endod. 2005;31:166–70.
83. Burleson A, Nusstein J, Reader A, Beck M. The *in vivo* evaluation of hand/rotary/ultrasound instrumentation in necrotic, human mandibular molars. J Endod. 2007;33:782–7.
84. Dovgyallo GI, Migun NP, Prokhorenko PP. The complete filling of dead-end conical capillaries with liquid. J Eng Phys Thermophys. 1989;56:395–7.
85. Migoun NP, Azouni MA. Filling of one-side-closed capillaries immersed in liquids. J Colloid Interf Sci. 1996;181:337–40.
86. Pesse AV, Warrier GR, Dhir VK. An experimental study of the gas entrapment process in closed-end microchannels. Int J Heat Mass Transf. 2005;48:5150–65.
87. Senia ES, Marshall FJ, Rosen S. The solvent action of sodium hypochlorite on pulp tissue of extracted teeth. Oral Surg Oral Med Oral Pathol. 1971;31:96–103.
88. de Gregorio C, Estevez R, Cisneros R, Heilborn C, Cohenca N. Effect of EDTA, sonic, and ultrasonic activation on the penetration of sodium hypochlorite into simulated lateral canals: an *in vitro* study. J Endod. 2009;35:891–5.
89. Gu LS, Kim JR, Ling J, Choi KK, Pashley DH, Tay FR. Review of contemporary irrigant agitation techniques and devices. J Endod. 2009;35:791–804.
90. Baumgartner JC, Mader CL. A scanning electron microscopic evaluation of four root canal irrigation regimens. J Endod. 1987;13:147–57.
91. O'Connell MS, Morgan LA, Beeler WJ, Baumgartner JC. A comparative study of smear layer removal using different salts of EDTA. J Endod. 2000;26:739–43.
92. Albrecht LJ, Baumgartner JC, Marshall JG. Evaluation of apical debris removal using various sizes and tapers of ProFile GT files. J Endod. 2004;30:425–8.
93. Johnson M, Sidow SJ, Looney SW, Lindsey K, Niu LN, Tay FR. Canal and isthmus debridement efficacy using a sonic irrigation technique in a closed-canal system. J Endod. 2012;38:1265–8.
94. Carr GB, Schwartz RS, Schaudinn C, Gorur A, Costerton JW. Ultrastructural examination of failed molar retreatment with secondary apical periodontitis: an examination of endodontic biofilms in an endodontic retreatment failure. J Endod. 2009;35:1303–9.
95. Ando N, Hoshino E. Predominant obligate anaerobes invading the deep layers of root canal dentin. Int Endod J. 1990;23:20–7.
96. Peters LB, Wesselink PR, Buijs JF, van Winkelhoff AJ. Viable bacteria in root dentinal tubules of teeth with apical periodontitis. J Endod. 2001;27:76–81.

97. Ricucci D, Pascon EA, Ford TR, Langeland K. Epithelium and bacteria in periapical lesions. Oral Surg Oral Med Oral Pathol Oral Radiol Endod. 2006;101:239–49.
98. Ørstavik D, Haapasalo M. Disinfection by endodontic irrigants and dressings of experimentally infected dentinal tubules. Endod Dent Traumatol. 1990;6:142–9.
99. Haapasalo M, Ørstavik D. *In vitro* infection and disinfection of dentinal tubules. J Dent Res. 1987;66:1375–9.
100. Love RM, Jenkinson HF. Invasion of dentinal tubules by oral bacteria. Crit Rev Oral Biol Med. 2002;13:171–83.
101. Elayouti A, Chu AL, Kimionis I, Klein C, Weiger R, Löst C. Efficacy of rotary instruments with greater taper in preparing oval root canals. Int Endod J. 2008;41:1088–92.
102. Paqué F, Ganahl D, Peters OA. Effects of root canal preparation on apical geometry assessed by micro-computed tomography. J Endod. 2009;35:1056–9.
103. Berutti E, Marini R, Angeretti A. Penetration ability of different irrigants into dentinal tubules. J Endod. 1997;23:725–7.
104. Akpata ES, Blechman H. Bacterial invasion of pulpal dentin wall *in vitro*. J Dent Res. 1982;61:435–8.
105. Dymock D, Weightman AJ, Scully C, Wade WG. Molecular analysis of microflora associated with dentoalveolar abscesses. J Clin Microbiol. 1996;34:537–42.
106. Zou L, Shen Y, Li W, Haapasalo M. Penetration of sodium hypochlorite into dentin. J Endod. 2010;36:793–6.
107. Dammaschke T, Witt M, Ott K, Schäfer E. Scanning electron microscopic investigation of incidence, location, and size of accessory foramina in primary and permanent molars. Quintessence Int. 2004;35:699–705.
108. Gao Y, Haapasalo M, Shen Y, Wu H, Li B, Ruse ND, Zhou X. Development and validation of a three-dimensional computational fluid dynamics model of root canal irrigation. J Endod. 2009;35:1282–7.
109. Ricucci D, Siqueira Jr JF. Fate of the tissue in lateral canals, apical ramifications in response to pathologic conditions and treatment procedures. J Endod. 2010;36:1–15.
110. de Gregorio C, Paranjpe A, Garcia A, Navarrete N, Estevez R, Esplugues EO, Cohenca N. Efficacy of irrigation systems on penetration of sodium hypochlorite to working length and to simulated uninstrumented areas in oval shaped root canals. Int Endod J. 2012;45:475–81.
111. McComb D, Smith DC. A preliminary scanning electron microscopic study of root canals after endodontic procedure. J Endod. 1975;1:238–42.
112. Mader CL, Baumgartner JC, Peters DD. Scanning electron microscopic investigation of the smeared layer on root canal walls. J Endod. 1984;10:477–83.
113. Cengiz T, Aktener BO, Pişkin B. Effect of dentinal tubule orientation on the removal of smear layer by root canal irrigants. A scanning electron microscopic study. Int Endod J. 1990;23:163–71.
114. Aktener BO, Cengiz T, Pişkin B. The penetration of smear material into dentinal tubules during instrumentation with surface active reagents: a scanning electron microscopic study. J Endod. 1989;15:588–90.
115. Eick JD, Wilko RA, Anderson CH, Sorenson SE. Scanning electron microscopy of cut tooth surfaces and identification of debris by use of the electron microprobe. J Dent Res. 1970;49:1359–68.
116. Pashley DH, Tao L, Boyd L, King GE, Horner JA. Scanning electron microscopy of the substructure of smear layers in human dentine. Arch Oral Biol. 1988;33:265–70.
117. Pashley DH. Smear layer: overview of structure and function. Proc Finn Dent Soc. 1992;88 Suppl 1:215–24.
118. Sen BH, Wesselink PR, Türkün M. The smear layer: a phenomenon in root canal therapy. Int Endod J. 1995;28:141–8.
119. Czonstkowsky M, Wilson EG, Holstein FA. The smear layer in endodontics. Dent Clin North Am. 1990;34:13–25.
120. Calt S, Serper A. Time-dependent effects of EDTA on dentine structures. J Endod. 2002;28:17–9.
121. De-Deus G, Reis C, Paciornik S. Critical appraisal of published smear layer-removal studies: methodological issues. Oral Surg Oral Med Oral Pathol Oral Radiol Endod. 2011;112:531–43.
122. Marques AA, Marchesan MA, Sousa-Filho CB, Silva-Sousa YT, Sousa-Neto MD, Cruz-Filho AM. Smear layer removal and chelated calcium ion quantification of three irrigating solutions. Braz Dent J. 2006;17:306–9.
123. Spanó JC, Silva RG, Guedes DF, Sousa-Neto MD, Estrela C, Pécora JD. Atomic absorption spectrometry and scanning electron microscopy evaluation of concentration of calcium ions and smear layer removal with root canal chelators. J Endod. 2009;35:727–30.
124. Mah TF, O'Toole GA. Mechanisms of biofilm resistance to antimicrobial agents. Trends Microbiol. 2001;9:34–9.
125. Svensäter G, Bergenholtz G. Biofilms in endodontic infections. Endod Top. 2004;9:27–36.
126. Ruddle CJ. Cleaning and shaping the root canal system. In: Cohen S, Burns RC, editors. Pathways of the pulp. 8th ed. St. Louis: Mosby Inc.; 2002. p. 231–91.
127. Stepanović S, Cirković I, Ranin L, Svabić-Vlahović M. Biofilm formation by *Salmonella* spp. and *Listeria monocytogenes* on plastic surface. Lett Appl Microbiol. 2004;38:428–32.
128. Haapasalo M, Qian W, Portenier I, Waltimo T. Effects of dentin on the antimicrobial properties of endodontic medicaments. J Endod. 2007;33:917–25.
129. Jagnow J, Clegg S. Klebsiella pneumoniae MrkD-mediated biofilm formation on extracellular matrix- and collagen-coated surfaces. Microbiology. 2003; 149:2397–405.

130. Black C, Allan I, Ford SK, Wilson M, McNab R. Biofilm specific surface properties and protein expression in oral *Streptococcus sanguis*. Arch Oral Biol. 2004;49:295–304.
131. Dewez JL, Lhoest JB, Detrait E, Berger V, Dupont-Gillain CC, Vincent LM, Schneider YJ, Bertrand P, Rouxhet PG. Adhesion of mammalian cells to polymer surfaces: from physical chemistry of surfaces to selective adhesion on defined patterns. Biomaterials. 1998;19:1441–5.
132. De Bruyne MA, De Bruyne RJ, De Moor RJ. Capillary flow porometry to assess the seal provided by root-end filling materials in a standardized and reproducible way. J Endod. 2006;32:206–9.
133. Lundström JR, Williamson AE, Villhauer AL, Dawson DV, Drake DR. Bactericidal activity of stabilized chlorine dioxide as an endodontic irrigant in a polymicrobial biofilm tooth model system. J Endod. 2010;36:1874–8.
134. Camargo CH, Siviero M, Camargo SE, de Oliveira SH, Carvalho CA, Valera MC. Topographical, diametral, and quantitative analysis of dentin tubules in the root canals of human and bovine teeth. J Endod. 2007;33:422–6.
135. Outhwaite WC, Livingston MJ, Pashley DH. Effects of changes in surface area, thickness, temperature and post-extraction time on human dentine permeability. Arch Oral Biol. 1976;21:599–603.
136. Prati C, Pashley DH. Dentine wetness, permeability and thickness and bond strength of adhesive systems. Am J Dent. 1992;5:33–8.
137. Schmalz G, Hiller KA, Nunez LJ, Stoll J, Weis K. Permeability characteristics of bovine and human dentin under different pre-treatment conditions. J Endod. 2001;27:23–30.
138. Forssell-Ahlberg K, Brännström M, Edwall L. The diameter and number of dentin tubules in rat, cat, dog and monkey. A comparative scanning electron microscopic study. Acta Odontol Scand. 1975;33:243–50.
139. Dourda AO, Moule AJ, Young WG. A morphometric analysis of the cross-sectional area of dentine occupied by dentin tubules in human third molar teeth. Int Endod J. 1994;27:184–9.
140. Park Y, Park SN, Park SC, Park JY, Park YH, Hahm JS, Hahm KS. Antibiotic activity and synergistic effect of antimicrobial peptide against pathogens from a patient with gallstones. Biochem Biophys Res Commun. 2004;321:631–7.
141. Gottenbos B, Grijpma DW, van der Mei HC, Feijen J, Busscher HJ. Antimicrobial effects of positively charged surfaces on adhering Gram-positive and Gram-negative bacteria. J Antimicrob Chemother. 2001;48:7–13.
142. Tsibouklis J, Stone M, Thorpe AA, Graham P, Peters V, Heerlien R, Smith JR, Green KL, Nevell TG. Preventing bacterial adhesion onto surfaces: the low-surface-energy approach. Biomaterials. 1999;20:1229–35.
143. Pozarowska D, Pozarowski P. Benzalkonium chloride (BAK) induces apoptosis or necrosis, but has no major influence on the cell cycle of Jurkat cells. Folia Histochem Cytobiol. 2011;49:225–30.
144. Jaramillo DE, Arriola A, Safavi K, Chávez de Paz LE. Decreased bacterial adherence and biofilm growth on surfaces coated with a solution of benzalkonium chloride. J Endod. 2012;38:821–5.
145. Kishen A, Haapasalo M. Biofilm models and methods of biofilm assessment. Endod Top. 2010;22:58–78.
146. Spratt DA, Pratten J, Wilson M, Gulabivala K. An *in vitro* evaluation of the antimicrobial efficacy of irrigants on biofilms of root canal isolates. Int Endod J. 2001;34:300–7.
147. Sena NT, Gomes BP, Vianna ME, Berber VB, Zaia AA, Ferraz CC, Souza-Filho FJ. *In vitro* antimicrobial activity of sodium hypochlorite and chlorhexidine against selected single-species biofilms. Int Endod J. 2006;39:878–85.
148. Bryce G, O'Donnell D, Ready D, Ng YL, Pratten J, Gulabivala K. Contemporary root canal irrigants are able to disrupt and eradicate single- and dual-species biofilms. J Endod. 2009;35:1243–8.
149. Jiang LM, Hoogenkamp MA, van der Sluis LW, Wesselink PR, Crielaard W, Deng DM. Resazurin metabolism assay for root canal disinfectant evaluation on dual-species biofilms. J Endod. 2011;37:31–5.
150. Ceri H, Olson ME, Stremick C, Read RR, Morck D, Buret A. The Calgary Biofilm Device: new technology for rapid determination of antibiotic susceptibilities of bacterial biofilms. J Clin Microbiol. 1999;37:1771–6.
151. Hoogenkamp MA, Crielaard W, ten Cate JM, Wever R, Hartog AF, Renirie R. Antimicrobial activity of vanadium chloroperoxidase on planktonic *Streptococcus mutans* cells and *Streptococcus mutans* biofilms. Caries Res. 2009;43:334–8.
152. Ito A, Taniuchi A, May T, Kawata K, Okabe S. Increased antibiotic resistance of *Escherichia coli* in mature biofilms. Appl Environ Microbiol. 2009;75:4093–100.
153. Davies D. Understanding biofilm resistance to antibacterial agents. Nat Rev Drug Discov. 2003;2:114–22.
154. Du T, Shi Q, Shen Y, Cao Y, Ma J, Lu X, Xiong Z, Haapasalo M. Effect of modified nonequilibrium plasma with chlorhexidine digluconate against endodontic biofilms *in vitro*. J Endod. 2013;39:1438–43.
155. Arias-Moliz MT, Ferrer-Luque CM, Espigares-Garcia M, Baca P. *Enterococcus faecalis* biofilms eradication by root canal irrigants. J Endod. 2009;35:711–4.
156. Arias-Moliz MT, Ferrer-Luque CM, González-Rodríguez MP, Valderrama MJ, Baca P. Eradication of *Enterococcus faecalis* biofilms by cetrimide and chlorhexidine. J Endod. 2010;36:87–90.
157. Shen Y, Stojicic S, Haapasalo M. Bacterial viability in starved and revitalized biofilms: comparison of viability staining and direct culture. J Endod. 2010;36:1820–3.
158. Chávez de Paz LE. Development of a multispecies biofilm community by four root canal bacteria. J Endod. 2012;38:318–23.

159. Heim S, Lleo MM, Bonato B, Guzman CA, Canepari P. The viable but nonculturable state and starvation are different stress responses of *Enterococcus faecalis*, as determined by proteome analysis. J Bacteriol. 2002;184:6739–45.
160. Clegg MS, Vertucci FJ, Walker C, Belanger M, Britto LR. The effect of exposure to irrigant solutions on apical dentin biofilms *in vitro*. J Endod. 2006;32:434–7.
161. Aas JA, Paster BJ, Stokes LN, Olsen I, Dewhirst FE. Defining the normal bacterial flora of the oral cavity. J Clin Microbiol. 2005;43:5721–32.
162. Sjögren U, Happonen RP, Kahnberg KE, Sundqvist G. Survival of *Arachnia propionica* in periapical tissue. Int Endod J. 1988;21:277–82.
163. Nair PNR, Sjögren U, Kahnberg KE, Krey G, Sundqvist G. Intraradicular bacteria and fungi in root-filled, asymptomatic human teeth with therapy-resistant periapical lesions: a long-term light and electron microscopic follow-up study. J Endod. 1990;16:580–8.
164. Figdor D, Sjögren U, Sörlin S, Sundqvist G, Nair PN. Pathogenicity of *Actinomyces israelii* and *Arachnia propionica*: experimental infection in guinea pigs and phagocytosis and intracellular killing by human polymorphonuclear leukocytes *in vitro*. Oral Microbiol Immunol. 1992;7:129–36.
165. Ricucci D, Siqueira Jr JF, Bate AL, Pitt Ford TR. Histologic investigation of root canal-treated teeth with apical periodontitis: a retrospective study from twenty-four patients. J Endod. 2009;3:493–502.
166. Sundqvist G. Bacteriological studies of necrotic dental pulps. Odontological Dissertations, No. 7. Umea: University of Umea; 1976.
167. Siqueira Jr JF, Lopes HP. Bacteria on the apical root surfaces of untreated teeth with periradicular lesions: a scanning electron microscopy study. Int Endod J. 2001;34:216–20.
168. Ricucci D, Siqueira Jr JF. Biofilms and apical periodontitis: study of prevalence, association with clinical and histopathologic findings. J Endod. 2010;36:1277–88.
169. McFeters GA. Enumeration, occurrence and significance of injured indicator bacteria in drinking water. In: McFeters GA, editor. Drinking water microbiology: progress and recent developments. Madison: Science Technology; 2009.
170. Purevdorj B, Costerton JW, Stoodley P. Influence of hydrodynamics and cell signaling on the structure and behavior of *Pseudomonas aeruginosa* biofilms. Appl Environ Microbiol. 2002;68:4457–64.
171. Stoodley P, Dodds I, Boyle JD, Lappin-Scott HM. Influence of hydrodynamics and nutrients on biofilm structure. J Appl Microbiol. 1998;85 Suppl 1:19S–28.
172. Liu Y, Tay JH. Metabolic response of biofilm to shear stress in fixed-film culture. J Appl Microbiol. 2001;90:337–42.
173. Stoodley P, Jacobsen A, Dunsmore BC, Purevdorj B, Wilson S, Lappin-Scott HM, Costerton JW. The influence of fluid shear and AICI3 on the material properties of *Pseudomonas aeruginosa* PAO1 and *Desulfovibrio* sp. EX265 biofilms. Water Sci Technol. 2001;43:113–20.
174. Stoodley P, Cargo R, Rupp CJ, Wilson S, Klapper I. Biofilm material properties as related to shear-induced deformation and detachment phenomena. J Ind Microbiol Biotechnol. 2002;29:361–7.
175. Merritt JH, Kadouri DE, O'Toole GA. Growing and analyzing static biofilms. Curr Protoc Microbiol. 2005;22:Chapter 1:Unit 1B.1.
176. Lee SJ, Wu MK, Wesselink PR. The efficacy of ultrasonic irrigation to remove artificially placed dentine debris from different-sized simulated plastic root canals. Int Endod J. 2004;37:607–12.
177. van der Sluis LW, Wu MK, Wesselink PR. The efficacy of ultrasonic irrigation to remove artificially placed dentine debris from human root canals prepared using instruments of varying taper. Int Endod J. 2005;38:764–8.
178. van der Sluis LW, Wu MK, Wesselink PR. A comparison between a smooth wire and a K-file in removing artificially placed dentine debris from root canals in resin blocks during ultrasonic irrigation. Int Endod J. 2005;38:593–6.
179. van der Sluis LW, Gambarini G, Wu MK, Wesselink PR. The influence of volume, type of irrigant and flushing method on removing artificially placed dentine debris from the apical root canal during passive ultrasonic irrigation. Int Endod J. 2006;39:472–6.
180. van der Sluis LW, Wu MK, Wesselink PR. The evaluation of removal of calcium hydroxide paste from an artificial standardized groove in the apical root canal using different irrigation methodologies. Int Endod J. 2007;40:52–7.
181. Lin J, Shen Y, Haapasalo M. A comparative study of biofilm removal with hand, rotary nickel–titanium and self-adjusting file instrumentation using a novel *in vitro* biofilm model. J Endod. 2013;39:658–63.
182. Nagayoshi M, Kitamura C, Fukuizumi T, Nishihara T, Terashita M. Antimicrobial effect of ozonated water on bacteria invading dentinal tubules. J Endod. 2004;30:778–81.
183. Zapata ROBC, Moraes IG, Bernardineli N, Gasparoto TH, Graeff MS, Campanelli AP, Garcia RB. Confocal laser scanning microscopy is appropriate to detect viability of *Enterococcus faecalis* in infected dentin. J Endod. 2008;34:1198–201.
184. Wang Z, Shen Y, Ma J, Haapasalo M. The effect of detergents on the antibacterial activity of disinfecting solutions in dentin. J Endod. 2012;38:948–53.
185. Wang Z, Shen Y, Haapasalo M. Effectiveness of endodontic disinfecting solutions against young and old *Enterococcus faecalis* biofilms in dentin canals. J Endod. 2012;38:1376–9.
186. Clarkson RM, Moule AJ, Podlich H, Kellaway R, Macfarlane R, Lewis D, Rowell J. Dissolution of porcine incisor pulps in sodium hypochlorite solutions of varying compositions and concentrations. Aust Dent J. 2006;51:245–51.

187. Hasselgren G, Olsson B, Cvek M. Effects of calcium hydroxide and sodium hypochlorite on the dissolution of necrotic porcine muscle tissue. J Endod. 1988;14:125–7.
188. Moorer WR, Wesselink PR. Factors promoting the tissue dissolving capability of sodium hypochlorite. Int Endod J. 1982;15:187–96.
189. Hand RE, Smith ML, Harrison JW. Analysis of the effect of dilution on the necrotic tissue dissolution property of sodium hypochlorite. J Endod. 1978;4:60–4.
190. Naenni N, Thoma K, Zehnder M. Soft tissue dissolution capacity of currently used and potential endodontic irrigants. J Endod. 2004;30:785–7.
191. Türkün M, Cengiz T. The effects of sodium hypochlorite and calcium hydroxide on tissue dissolution and root canal cleanliness. Int Endod J. 1997;30:335–42.
192. Okino LA, Siqueira EL, Santos M, Bombana AC, Figueiredo JA. Dissolution of pulp tissue by aqueous solution of chlorhexidine digluconate and chlorhexidine digluconate gel. Int Endod J. 2004;37:38–41.
193. Clarkson RM, Kidd B, Evans GE, Moule AJ. The effect of surfactant on the dissolution of porcine pulpal tissue by sodium hypochlorite solutions. J Endod. 2012;38:1257–60.
194. Koskinen KP, Stenvall H, Uitto VJ. Dissolution of bovine pulp tissue by endodontic solutions. Scand J Dent Res. 1980;88:406–11.
195. Mehra P, Clancy C, Wu J. Formation of a facial hematoma during endodontic therapy. J Am Dent Assoc. 2000;131:67–71.
196. Gernhardt CR, Eppendorf K, Kozlowski A, Brandt M. Toxicity of concentrated sodium hypochlorite used as an endodontic irrigant. Int Endod J. 2004;37:272–80.
197. Barnhart BD, Chuang A, Lucca JJ, Roberts S, Liewehr F, Joyce AP. An *in vitro* evaluation of the cytotoxicity of various endodontic irrigants on human gingival fibroblasts. J Endod. 2005;31:613–5.
198. Ari H, Erdemir A, Belli S. Evaluation of the effect of endodontic irrigation solutions on the microhardness and the roughness of root canal dentin. J Endod. 2004;30:792–5.
199. Marending M, Paqué F, Fischer J, Zehnder M. Impact of irrigant sequence on mechanical properties of human root dentin. J Endod. 2007;33:1325–8.
200. Grigoratos D, Knowles J, Ng YL, Gulabivala K. Effect of exposing dentine to sodium hypochlorite and calcium hydroxide on its flexural strength and elastic modulus. Int Endod J. 2001;34:113–9.
201. Sayin TC, Cehreli ZC, Deniz D, Akcay A, Tuncel B, Dagli F, Gozukara H, Kalayci S. Time-dependent decalcifying effects of endodontic irrigants with antibacterial properties. J Endod. 2009;35:280–3.
202. Rossi-Fedele G, De Figueiredo JA. Use of a bottle warmer to increase 4% sodium hypochlorite tissue dissolution ability on bovine pulp. Aust Endod J. 2008;34:39–42.
203. Haapasalo M, Wang Z, Shen Y, Curtis A, Patel P, Khakpour M. Tissue dissolution by a novel multisonic ultracleaning system and sodium hypochlorite. J Endod. 2014;40:1178–81.
204. Childer H, Yee FS. Canal debridement and disinfection. In: Cohen S, Burns RC, editors. Pathways of the pulp. 3rd ed. St. Louis: The C.V. Mosby Company; 1984. p. 175.
205. Cameron JA. The effect of a fluorocarbon surfactant on the surface tension of the endodontic irrigant, sodium hypochlorite. A preliminary report. Aust Dent J. 1986;31:364–8.
206. Jungbluth H, Peters C, Peters O, Sener B, Zehnder M. Physicochemical and pulp tissue dissolution properties of some household bleach brands compared with a dental sodium hypochlorite solution. J Endod. 2012;38:372–5.
207. Jungbluth H, Marending M, De-Deus G, Sener B, Zehnder M. Stabilizing sodium hypochlorite at high pH: effects on soft tissue and dentin. J Endod. 2011;37:693–6.
208. Kuttler Y. Microscopic investigation of root apexes. J Am Dent Assoc. 1955;50:544–52.
209. Ponce EH, Vilar Fernández JA. The cemento-dentino-canal junction, the apical foramen, and the apical constriction: evaluation by optical microscopy. J Endod. 2003;29:214–9.
210. Green D. A stereomicroscopic study of the root apices of 400 maxillary and mandibular anterior teeth. Oral Surg Oral Med Oral Pathol. 1956;9:1224–32.
211. Al-Jadaa A, Paqué F, Attin T, Zehnder M. Necrotic pulp tissue dissolution by passive ultrasonic irrigation in simulated accessory canals: impact of canal location and angulation. Int Endod J. 2009;42:59–65.
212. de Gregorio C, Estevez R, Cisneros R, Paranjpe A, Cohenca N. Efficacy of different irrigation and activation systems on the penetration of sodium hypochlorite into simulated lateral canals and up to working length: an *in vitro* study. J Endod. 2010;36:1216–21.
213. Pashley EL, Birdsong NL, Bowman K, Pashley DH. Cytotoxic effects of NaOCl on vital tissue. J Endod. 1985;11:525–8.
214. Gulabivala K, Ng YL, Gilbertson M, Eames I. The fluid mechanics of root canal irrigation. Physiol Meas. 2010;31:R49–84.
215. Shen Y, Gao Y, Qian W, Ruse ND, Zhou X, Wu H, Haapasalo M. Three-dimensional numeric simulation of root canal irrigant flow with different irrigation needles. J Endod. 2010;36:884–9.
216. Banks J, Bressloff NW. Turbulence modeling in three-dimensional stenosed arterial bifurcations. J Biomech Eng. 2007;129:40–50.
217. Vogel M, Franke J, Frank W, Schroten H. Flow in the well: computational fluid dynamics is essential in flow chamber construction. Cytotechnology. 2007;55:41–54.
218. van Ertbruggen C, Corieri P, Theunissen R, Riethmuller ML, Darquenne C. Validation of CFD predictions of flow in a 3D alveolated bend with experimental data. J Biomech. 2008;41:399–405.

219. Raffel M, Willert C, Wereley S, Kompenhans J. Particle imaging velocimetry—a practical guide. 2nd ed. Berlin: Springer; 2007. p. 1–448.
220. de Groot SD, Verhaagen B, Versluis M, Wu MK, Wesselink PR, van der Sluis LW. Laser-activated irrigation of the root canal: cleaning efficacy and flow visualization. Int Endod J. 2009;42:1077–83.
221. Boutsioukis C, Verhaagen B, Versluis M, Kastrinakis E, van der Sluis LW. Irrigant flow in the root canal: experimental validation of an unsteady Computational Fluid Dynamics model using high-speed imaging. Int Endod J. 2010;43:393–403.
222. Koch JD, Smith NA, Garces D, Gao L, Olsen FK. In vitro particle image velocity measurements in a model root canal: flow around a polymer rotary finishing file. J Endod. 2014;40:412–6.
223. Park E, Shen Y, Haapasalo M. Apical pressure and extent of irrigant flow beyond the needle tip during positive pressure irrigation in an *in vitro* root canal model. J Endod. 2013;39:511–5.
224. Boutsioukis C, Gogos C, Verhaagen B, Versluis M, Kastrinakis E, Van der Sluis LW. The effect of root canal taper on the irrigant flow: evaluation using an unsteady Computational Fluid Dynamics model. Int Endod J. 2010;43:909–16.
225. Boutsioukis C, Gogos C, Verhaagen B, Versluis M, Kastrinakis E, Van der Sluis LW. The effect of apical preparation size on irrigant flow in root canals evaluated using an unsteady computational fluid dynamics model. Int Endod J. 2010;43:874–81.
226. Huang TY, Gulabivala K, Ng YL. A bio-molecular film *ex vivo* model to evaluate the influence of canal dimensions and irrigation variables on the efficacy of irrigation. Int Endod J. 2008;41:60–71.
227. Goldman M, Kronman JH, Goldman LB, Clausen H, Grady J. New method of irrigation during endodontic treatment. J Endod. 1976;2:257–60.
228. Goldman LB, Goldman M, Kronman JH, Lin PS. Scanning electron microscope study of a new irrigation method in endodontic treatment. Oral Surg Oral Med Oral Pathol. 1979;48:79–83.
229. Kahn FH, Rosenberg PA, Gliksberg J. An *in vitro* evaluation of the irrigating characteristics of ultrasonic and subsonic handpieces and irrigating needles and probes. J Endod. 1995;21:277–80.
230. Yamamoto A, Otogoto J, Kuroiwa A, Maeda M, Yamaguchi H, Yamada H, Anzai M, Kasahara E. The effect of irrigation using trial-manufactured washing needle. Jap J Conserv Dent. 2006;49:64–70.
231. Vinothkumar TS, Kavitha S, Lakshminarayanan L, Gomathi NS, Kumar V. Influence of irrigating needle-tip designs in removing bacteria inoculated into instrumented root canals measured using single-tube luminometer. J Endod. 2007;33:746–8.
232. Hülsmann M, Rödig T, Nordmeyer S. Complications during root canal irrigation. Endod Top. 2009;16:27–63.

Update of Endodontic Irrigating Solutions

5

Bettina Basrani and Gevik Malkhassian

Abstract

Successful root canal therapy depends on thorough debridement of pulpal tissue, dentin debris, and infective microorganisms. Currently, it is impossible to predictably eradicate intraradicular infection with mechanical instrumentation alone. Therefore, irrigants are required to be used as an important addition in the disinfection process. This chapter analyzes the main irrigating solutions used during the endodontic treatment and their actions and interactions among them. Explanation of their mechanism of action and effect on dentin structure and on biofilm is also described. A clinical protocol is proposed at the end of the chapter.

The goal of endodontic treatment is to prevent or cure apical periodontitis. Apical periodontitis is an inflammatory process in the periradicular tissues caused by microorganisms in the infected root canal [84]. It is well known that shaping, cleaning, and obturating the root canal system provide the strategy for successful treatment. The principle to reach favorable outcomes in endodontic infection management requires the recognition of the problem and the removal of the etiological factors.

B. Basrani, DDS, MSc, RCDC (F), PhD (✉)
Associate Professor, Director M.Sc.
Endodontics Program, Faculty of Dentistry,
University of Toronto, 348C-124 Edward Street,
Toronto, ON M5G1G6, Canada
e-mail: Bettina.Basrani@dentistry.utoronto.ca

G. Malkhassian, DDS, MSc, FRCD(C)
Assistant Professor, Discipline of Endodontics,
Faculty of Dentistry, University of Toronto,
Toronto, ON, Canada

In endodontic disinfection, there are two main challenges which are important to be recognized the anatomical challenge and the microbiological challenge [42].

The anatomical challenge can be divided into complexity of the root canal system, dentin structure, and dentin constituents.

Anatomical Complexities (also see Chap. 2): Root canal is an enclosed complex space with intricate configurations and apical constriction it is important to mention here that more than 35 % of the root canal surface is left untouched by conventional instrumentation [35, 64] (Fig. 5.1). Also, common instrumentation techniques accumulate debris in isthmus areas. Paque et al. showed explained that when rotary files are used in canal with a round cross section, the dentine particles that are cut from the canal wall are car-

B. Basrani (ed.), *Endodontic Irrigation: Chemical Disinfection of the Root Canal System*,
DOI 10.1007/978-3-319-16456-4_5

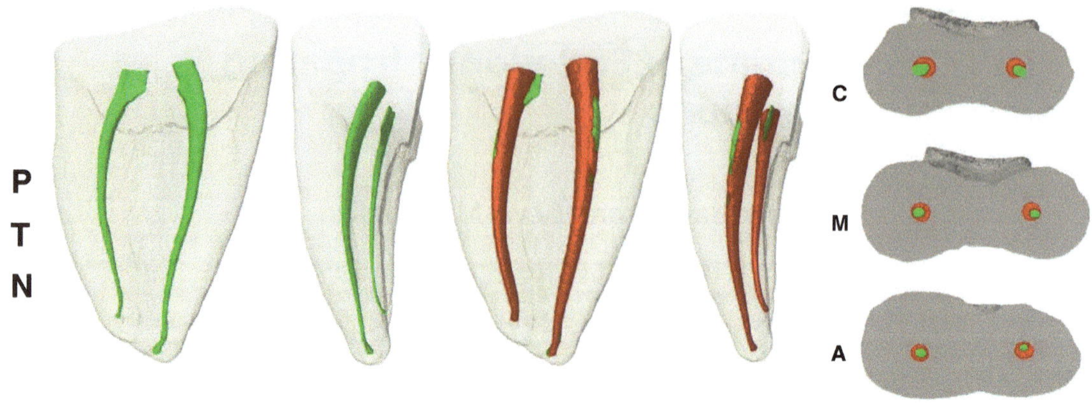

Fig. 5.1 MicroCT scan of pre- and post-instrumentation in a lower molar. Note the amount of walls not touch by the instruments. Lateral view of representative 3D reconstructions of the internal anatomy of a mesial roots of a mandibular molar, before (*in green*) and after (*in red*) canal preparation *C* Coronal, *M* Middle, *A* Apical, (Courtesy of Dr Gagliardi, Versiani and Sousa-Neto)

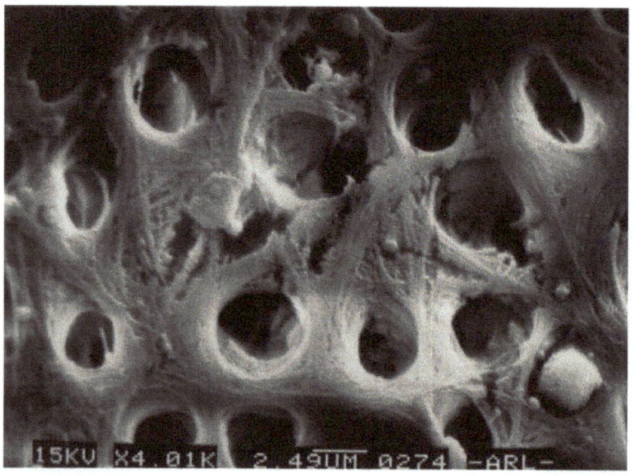

Fig. 5.2 SEM of dentin structure showing irregularities of dentin tissue

ried coronally by the flutes of the file, in a manner similar to that of a common mechanical spiral drill. This removal is apparently less effective when the file has no dentine wall on one side, as is the case of a canal adjacent to an isthmus. Rather than being carried coronally or being contained and packed in the file's flute space, the debris was most probably actively packed into the area with the least resistance, namely into the isthmus [62].

Dentin Structure Physiologically and anatomically, the dentin is a complex structure. Type I collagen is the major protein of intertubular dentin (90 %), whereas no collagen fibrils are observed in the peritubular dentin. The structure is a porous configuration with dentinal tubules that allow bacterial invasion and adherence, making dentin disinfection a challenging step (Fig. 5.2).

Dentin Constituents The effectiveness of antimicrobial irrigants is known to be compromised under in vivo conditions [77]. In recent studies it has been reported that dentin powder, serum albumin, and dentin matrix can inhibit the antibacterial effect of commonly used irrigants [29, 66, 67]. Interestingly, it has been also reported that even the antibacterial effect of advance disinfection techniques like chitosan nanoparticles and photoactivation disinfection can also be neutralized by the dentin constituents [77].

The microbiological challenge is well covered in Chap. 1. It is important to understand that the endodontic problem is a biofilm-related diseases and access, disruption, or penetration of the biofilm should be our disinfection aim [43].

Endodontic irrigants have three major objectives: chemical, biological, and mechanical. Mechanical objectives include to rinse out debris and lubricate the canal; chemical objectives include to soften and dissolve organic and inorganic tissues, prevent the formation of a smear layer during instrumentation, and dissolve smear layer once it has formed; and biological objectives are related to their antiseptic and nontoxic effects such as efficacy against anaerobic facultative microorganisms (planktonic and biofilms), ability to inactivate endotoxin, nontoxic and noncaustic, and little potential to cause anaphylaxis.

The ideal irrigating solution to disinfect the root canal system should be a biocompatible bactericidal agent, tissue solvent, lubricant, and smear layer remover capable of physically flushing debris, with sustained effect but without affecting the physical properties of the dentin.

The irrigating solutions in endodontics can be classified as antimicrobial solutions, chelating solutions (strong or weak), combinations (antibacterial and chelating solutions combined), and solutions with detergent.

Antimicrobial effects: antiseptic solutions, topical antibiotics, bacteriostatic solutions, and bactericidal solutions.

Antiseptic Solutions

Sodium Hypochlorite

Surveys from around the world [17, 23, 94] reported that sodium hypochlorite is the most common irrigating solution used in endodontics. Figure 5.3 shows the percentage of responders who utilize each irrigant as their primary disinfectant agent in a survey by the American Association of Endodontists. It is an effective antimicrobial and proteolytic agent [48, 49], excellent organic tissue solvent [60], and lubricant with fairly quick effects. NaOCl is both an oxidizing agent and a hydrolyzing agent. Commercial sodium hypochlorite solutions are strongly alkaline and hypertonic and typically have nominal concentrations of 10–14 % available chlorine.

Mode of Action

Sodium hypochlorite has a pH of 11. Figure 5.4 shows the schematic interaction of the mechanism of action of NaOCl (Reproduced with permission from Estrela et al., *Brazilian Endodontic Journal*).

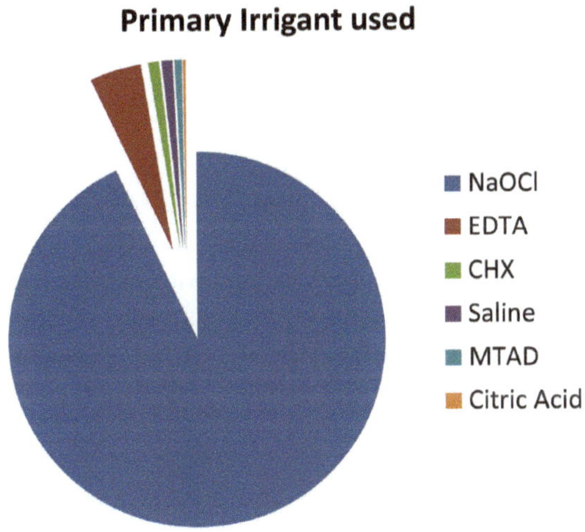

Fig. 5.3 Percentage of responders who utilize each irrigant as their primary disinfectant agent (Reproduced with permission JOE [17])

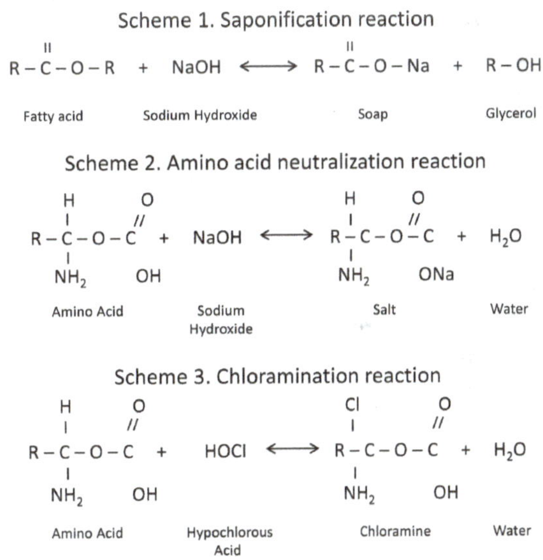

Fig. 5.4 Schematic drawing of NaOCl mechanism of action (Reproduced with permission from [20])

Estrela [20] reported that sodium hypochlorite exhibits a dynamic balance:

1: Saponification reaction:
Sodium hypochlorite acts as an organic and fat solvent that degrades fatty acids and transforms them into fatty acid salts (soap) and glycerol (alcohol), reducing the surface tension of the remaining solution.

2: Neutralization reaction:
Sodium hypochlorite neutralizes amino acids by forming water and salt. With the exit of hydroxyl ions, the pH is reduced.

3: Hypochlorous acid formation:
When chlorine dissolves in water and it is in contact with organic matter, it forms hypochlorous acid. It is a weak acid with the chemical formula HClO that acts as an oxidizer. Hypochlorous acid ($HOCl^-$) and hypochlorite ions (OCl^-) lead to amino acid degradation and hydrolysis.

4: Solvent action:
Sodium hypochlorite also acts as a solvent, releasing chlorine that combines with protein amino groups (NH) to form chloramines (chloramination reaction). Chloramines impede cell metabolism; chlorine is a strong oxidant and inhibits essential bacterial enzymes by irreversible oxidation of SH groups (sulfhydryl group) [20].

5: High pH:
Sodium hypochlorite is a strong base (pH>11). The antimicrobial effectiveness of sodium hypochlorite, based on its high pH (hydroxyl ion action), is similar to the mechanism of action of calcium hydroxide. The high pH interferes in cytoplasmic membrane integrity due to irreversible enzymatic inhibition, biosynthetic alterations in cellular metabolism, and phospholipid degradation observed in lipidic peroxidation [20].

Concentration

In the literature, it can be found that NaOCl can be used in a concentration that ranges from 0.5 to 6 %. It was proven that the lower and higher concentrations are equally efficient in reducing the number of bacteria in infected root canal system but the tissue-dissolving effect is directly related to the concentration [26].

Grossman observed pulp tissue dissolution capacity and reported that 5 % sodium hypochlorite dissolved this tissue in between 20 min and 2 h. The dissolution of bovine pulp tissue by sodium hypochlorite (0.5, 1.0, 2.5, and 5.0 %) was studied in vitro under different conditions (Estrela). It was concluded that:

1. The velocity of dissolution of the bovine pulp fragments was directly proportional to the concentration of the sodium hypochlorite solution and was greater without the surfactant.
2. Variations in surface tension, from beginning to end of pulp dissolution, were directly proportional to the concentration of the sodium hypochlorite solution and greater in the solutions without surfactant. Solutions without surfactant presented a decrease in surface tension and those with surfactant an increase.
3. In heated sodium hypochlorite solutions, dissolution of the bovine pulp tissue was more rapid.
4. The greater the initial concentration of the sodium hypochlorite solutions, the smaller the reduction of its pH (Estrela).

Volume

Volume is more critical for disinfection than its concentration. Frequent exchange with fresh NaOCl is important and the use of large amount of irrigant compensates for the low concentration. It should be kept in mind that the NaOCl will inactivate its components very fast, so fresh irrigating solution should be added to the canal system constantly. (Please see chapter on irrigation dynamics to learn more about the volume.)

Time

How long does NaOCl need to kill bacteria? This question can be misinterpreted in the literature. Some articles will show bacterial killing in 30 min when 0.5 % NaOCl is used, while higher concentrations will need only 30 s to do the same job. Interpretation of results needs to be taken with caution because it will depend on the methods used to test the time. It is important to remember that the presence of organic matter, inflammatory exudates, tissue remnants, and microbial biomass consumes NaOCl and weakens its effect.

The chlorine ion, which is responsible for the dissolving and antibacterial capacity of NaOCl, is unstable and consumed rapidly during the first phase of tissue dissolution, probably within 2 min [57], which provides another reason for continuous replenishment. This should especially be considered in view of the fact that rotary root canal preparation techniques have expedited the shaping process. The optimal time that a hypochlorite irrigant at a given concentration needs to remain in the canal system is an issue yet to be answered [96].

Effect on the Dentin

As it was stated before, the dentin is composed of 22 % organic material by weight. Most of this consists of type I collagen, which contributes considerably to the mechanical properties of the dentin. NaOCl solutions may affect mechanical dentin properties via the degradation of organic dentin components.

Depth of Penetration

The depth of NaOCl penetration varied between 77 and 300 μm, and it depends on concentration, time, and temperature [99]. Figure 5.5 illustrates a microscopic view of stained root section treated by 1 % sodium hypochlorite for 2 min (Published with permission).

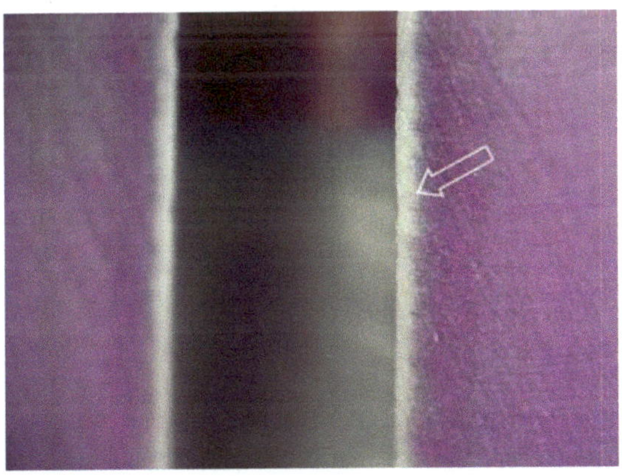

Fig. 5.5 A microscope view of stained root section treated by 1 % sodium hypochlorite for 2 min (*arrow*) (Reproduced with permission [99])

Effect on Biofilms

Clegg et al. [12] demonstrated that 6 % NaOCl was the only agent capable of both physically removing artificial biofilm and killing bacteria. There was a dose-dependent effect of NaOCl against bacteria, as higher concentrations were more antibacterial. Figure 5.6 illustrates the effect of different irrigants on dentin biofilm elimination. In summary, 3 % and 6% NaOCl showed absence of biofilm, 1 % NaOCl showed disruption of biofilm, and 2 % CHX showed intact biofilm (Fig. 5.6).

Limitations

Unfortunately, even though NaOCl has many ideal properties, it has some limitations such as being toxic [39, 48] (see more details in Chap. 7), nonsubstantive, ineffective in smear layer removal and corrosive. It may cause discoloration [40] and has unpleasant odor. When NaOCl is used as a final rinse, bonding of the sealer to the dentin may be altered [72].

Clinical Recommendation

NaOCl in concentrations between 2.5 and 6 % should be used during the whole cleaning and shaping procedure. Pulp chamber should be used as a reservoir of fresh irrigant. Once the mechanical preparation is finished and a master apical file is determined, the protocol of irrigation should start with the activation of fresh NaOCl in each canal [27].

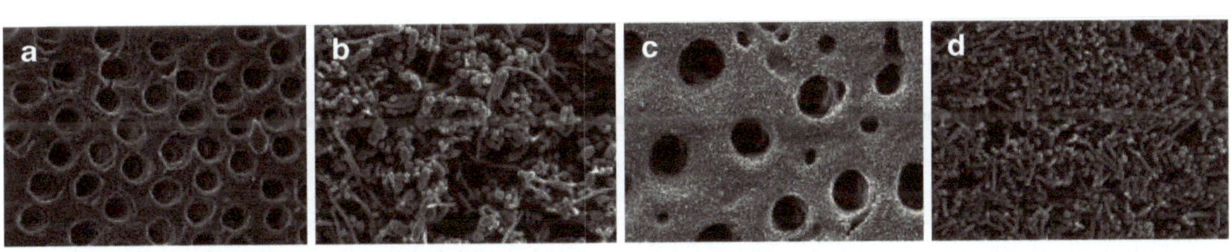

Fig. 5.6 (**a**) Scanning electron micrograph (SEM) of bacteria-free dentin on negative control specimen (original magnification ×3,000). (**b**) SEM of positive control reveals cocci, rods, and filamentous organisms (original magnification ×5,000). (**c**) SEM of dentin section treated with 6 % NaOCl. No bacteria are visible (original magnification ×5,000). (**d**) SEM of dentin section treated with 2 % CHX. The biofilm is intact with no visible disruption (original magnification ×5,000) (Reproduced with permission from JOE [12])

Chlorhexidine Gluconate (CHX) [6]

Molecular Structure

CHX is a strongly basic molecule with a pH between 5.5 and 7 that belongs to the polybiguanide group and consists of two symmetric four-chlorophenyl rings and two biguanide groups connected by a central hexamethylene chain. CHX digluconate salt is easily soluble in water and is very stable [25].

Mode of Action

Chlorhexidine, because of its cationic charges, is capable of electrostatically binding to the negatively charged surfaces of bacteria [14], damaging the outer layers of the cell wall and rendering it permeable [33, 36, 37]. CHX is a wide-spectrum antimicrobial agent, active against gram-positive and gram-negative bacteria and yeasts [16].

Depending on its concentration, CHX can have both bacteriostatic and bactericidal effects. At high concentrations, CHX acts as a detergent and exerts its bactericidal effect by damaging the cell membrane and causes precipitation of the cytoplasm. At low concentrations, CHX is bacteriostatic, causing low-molecular-weight substances (i.e., potassium and phosphorous) to leak out from the cell membrane without the cell being permanently damaged.

Substantivity

Due to the cationic nature of the CHX molecule, it can be absorbed by anionic substrates such as the oral mucosa and tooth structure [54, 73, 92]. CHX is readily adsorbed onto hydroxyapatite and teeth. Studies have shown that the uptake of CHX onto the teeth is reversible [34]. This reversible reaction of uptake and release of CHX leads to substantive antimicrobial activity and is referred to as *substantivity*. This effect depends on the concentration of CHX. At low concentrations of 0.005–0.01 %, only a constant monolayer of CHX is adsorbed on the tooth surface, but at higher concentrations, a multilayer of CHX is formed on the surface, providing a reservoir of CHX which can rapidly release the excess into the environment as the concentration of CHX in the surrounding environment decreases [19]. Time and concentration of CHX can influence the antibacterial substantivity and the conclusions are inconsistent. Some studies demonstrated that 4 % CHX has greater antibacterial substantivity than 0.2 % after 5 min application (332). Other studies stated that CHX should be left for more than 1 h in the canal to be adsorbed by the dentin [50]. Komorowski et al. [45] suggested that a 5-min application of CHX did not induce substantivity, so the dentin should be treated with CHX for 7 days. However, when Paquette et al. [63] and Malkhassian et al. [55] in their in vivo studies medicated the canals with either liquid or gel forms of CHX for 1 week, neither of them could achieve total disinfection. Therefore, residual antimicrobial efficacy of CHX in vivo still remains to be demonstrated.

Chlorhexidine as an Endodontic Irrigant

CHX has been extensively studied as an endodontic irrigant and intracanal medication, both in vivo (Barbosa, Linkgog, Manzur, Paquette, Malkhassian) and in vitro [4, 5, 9, 10, 51, 56].

The antibacterial efficacy of CHX as an irrigant is concentration dependent. It has been demonstrated that 2 % CHX has a better antibacterial efficacy than 0.12 % CHX in vitro ([10]). When comparing its effectiveness with NaOCl, controversial results can be found. NaOCl has an obvious advantage over CHX with the dissolution capacity of organic matter that CHX lacks; therefore, even though in vitro studies suggest some advantages with the use of CHX, as soon as organic and dental tissue is added, NaOCl is clearly preferable.

The antibacterial effectiveness of CHX in infected root canals has been investigated in several in vivo studies. Investigators [70] reported that 2.5 % NaOCl was significantly more effective than 0.2 % CHX when the infected root canals were irrigated for 30 min with either of the solutions.

In a controlled and randomized clinical trial, the efficacy of 2 % CHX liquid was tested against saline using culture technique. All the teeth were initially instrumented and irrigated using 1 % NaOCl. Then either 2 % CHX liquid or saline was applied as a final rinse. The authors reported a further reduction in the proportion of positive cultures in the CHX group. Their results showed a better disinfection of the root canals using CHX compared to saline as a final rinse [95].

In a recent study, the antibacterial efficacy of 2 % CHX gel was tested against 2.5 % NaOCl in teeth with apical periodontitis, with the bacterial load assessed using real-time quantitative polymerase chain reaction (RTQ-PCR) and colony-forming units (CFU). The bacterial reduction in the NaOCl group was significantly greater than the CHX group when measured by RTQ-PCR. Based on culture technique, bacterial growth was detected in 50 % of the CHX group compared to 25 % in the NaOCl group [93]. On the other hand, another study based on this culture technique revealed no significant difference between the antibacterial efficacy of 2.5 % NaOCl and 0.12 % CHX liquid when used as irrigants during the treatment of infected canals [80].

In a recent systematic review, Ng et al. [59] demonstrated that abstaining from using 2 % CHX as an adjunct irrigant to NaOCl was associated with superior periapical healing.

Unlike NaOCl, CHX lacks a tissue-dissolving property. Therefore, NaOCl is still considered the primary irrigating solution in endodontics.

Allergic Reactions to Chlorhexidine

Allergic responses to CHX are rare, and there are no reports of reactions following root canal irrigation with CHX [2, 39]. The sensitization rate has been reported in several studies to be approximately 2 % [47]. However, some allergic reactions such as anaphylaxis, contact dermatitis, and urticaria have been reported following direct contact to mucosal tissue or open wounds [18, 65, 74, 81].

Limitations

The limitations of using CHX as a primary and sole endodontic irrigant are the following: the inability to dissolve organic matter, no action on smear layer, and minor effect on biofilm disruption.

Clinical Recommendations

The clinical recommendation to use CHX during endodontic treatment:

1. In teeth with open apices or perforation where there is a risk to extrude NaOCl.
2. When maximal antimicrobial effect is desirable as a final rinse after EDTA to further facilitate disinfection and to improve dentin bonding (where relevant) [30].

Decalcifying Agents

Debris is defined as dentin chips or residual vital or necrotic pulp tissue attached to the root canal wall. Smear layer was defined by the American Association of Endodontists in 2003 as a surface film of debris retained on the dentin or other surfaces after instrumentation with either rotary instruments or endodontic files; it consists of dentin particles, remnants of vital or necrotic pulp tissue, bacterial components, and retained irrigants. While it has been viewed as an impediment to irrigant penetration into dentinal tubules, there is still a controversy about the influence of smear layer on the outcome of endodontic treatment. Some researchers emphasize the importance of removing the smear layer to allow irrigants, medications, and sealers to penetrate into the dentinal tubules and improve disinfection. On the other hand, other researchers focused on keeping the smear layer as a protection for bacterial invasion, apical and coronal microleakage, bacterial penetration of the tubules, and the adaptation of root canal materials. The majority of the conclusions on smear layer are based on in vitro studies. A recent clinical study by Ng et al.[59] found that the use of EDTA significantly increased the odds of success of retreatment cases by twofold.

The chelating agents can be classified as strong or weak. Strong chelating agents are EDTA, citric acid, and chitosan nanoparticles, while weak chelating agent is HEBP or etidronate.

Ethylenediaminetetraacetic Acid

Ethylenediaminetetraacetic acid, widely abbreviated as EDTA, is an aminopolycarboxylic acid, and a colorless, water-soluble solid. EDTA is often suggested as an irrigant because it can chelate and remove the mineralized portion of the smear layer. It is a polyaminocarboxylic acid with the formula $[CH_2N(CH_2CO_2H)_2]_2$. Its prominence as a chelating agent arises from its ability to sequester di- and tricationic metal ions such as Ca^{2+} and Fe^{3+}. After being bound by EDTA, metal ions remain in solution but exhibit diminished reactivity.

History

The compound was first described in 1935 by Ferdinand Munz, who prepared the compound from ethylenediamine and chloroacetic acid. Chelating agents were introduced into endodontics as an aid for the preparation of narrow and calcified root canals in 1957 by Nygaard-Østby [38]. Today, EDTA is mainly synthesized from ethylenediamine (1, 2-diaminoethane), formaldehyde (methanal), and sodium cyanide [38].

Mode of Action

On direct exposure for extended time, EDTA extracts bacterial surface proteins by combining with metal ions from the cell membrane which can eventually lead to bacterial death [38]. Chelators such as EDTA form a stable complex with calcium. When all available ions have been bound, equilibrium is formed and no further dissolution takes place; therefore, EDTA is self-limiting [38].

Applications in Endodontics

EDTA alone normally cannot remove the smear layer effectively; a proteolytic component, such as NaOCl, must be added to remove the organic components of the smear layer [22]. For root canal preparation, EDTA has limited value alone as an irrigation fluid [22]. EDTA is normally used in a concentration of 17 % and can remove the smear layer when in direct contact with the root canal wall for less than 1 min.

Although citric acid appears to be slightly more potent at similar concentration than EDTA, both agents show high efficiency in removing the smear layer. In addition to their cleaning ability, chelators may detach biofilms adhering to root canal walls [28]. This may explain why an EDTA irrigant proved to be highly superior to saline in reducing intracanal microbiota despite the fact that its antiseptic capacity is relatively limited [28].

The effect of chelators in negotiating narrow, tortuous, calcified canals to establish patency depends on both canal width and the amount of active substance available, since the demineralization process continues until all chelators have formed complexes with calcium [38, 98]. Therefore, studies should be read with caution because one study can show demineralization up to a depth of 50 μm into the dentin [38], but other reports demonstrated significant erosion after irrigation with EDTA [89, 91]. The sequence in which root canal wall dentin is exposed to NaOCl and EDTA has an impact on the level of dentin erosion on the main root canal wall.

In the study reported by Qian et al. [69] no erosion was detected when demineralizing agents were used as a final rinse after NaOCl. However, the erosion of peritubular and intertubular dentin was detected when EDTA was used first followed by 5.25 % NaOCl.

EDTA had a significantly better antimicrobial effect than saline solution. It exerts its strongest effect when used synergistically with NaOCl [32, 78].

Interaction Between CHX and NaOCl

The combination of NaOCl and CHX produces a change of color and a precipitate. The reaction is dependent of the concentration of NaOCl. The higher the concentration of NaOCl, the larger the precipitate is if 2 % CHX is used [7] (Fig. 5.7). Furthermore, concerns have been raised that the color change may have some clinical relevance causing staining of the tooth. Also the resulting precipitate might interfere with the seal of the root canal obturation. Basrani et al. [7] evaluated the chemical nature of this precipitate and reported the formation of 4-chloroaniline (PCA). Furthermore, a recent study [44] (Fig. 5.8) using TOF-SIMS analysis showed the penetration of PCA inside dentinal tubules. PCA has been shown to be toxic in humans with short-term exposure, resulting in cyanosis, which is a manifestation of methemoglobin formation. The interaction should be avoided by using EDTA or other irrigants after NaOCl and before CHX or alternatively, the canals can be dried using paper points before the final rinse [98].

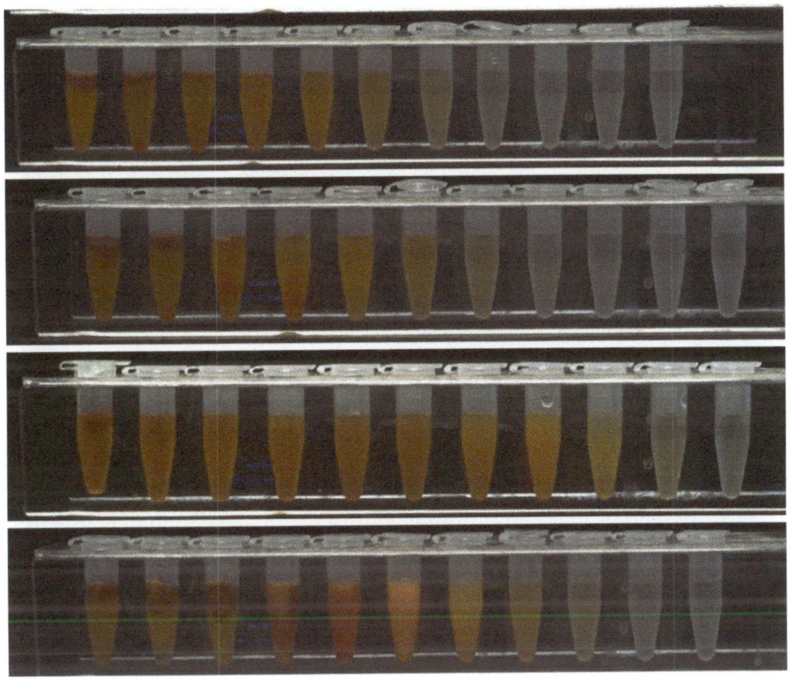

Fig. 5.7 Interaction between different concentrations of NaOCl and 2.0 % CHX. Note that the higher the concentration of NaOCl, the higher the amount of precipitate [7]

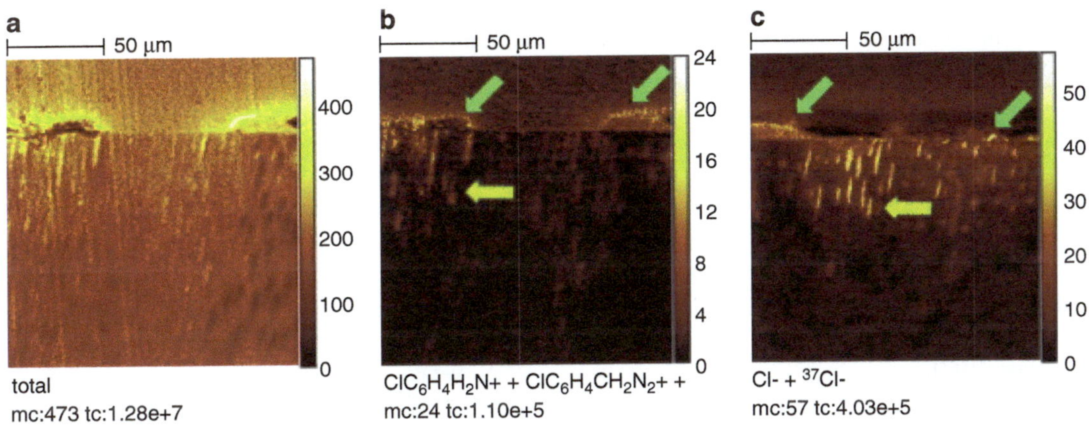

Fig. 5.8 Dentin treated with CHX and NaOCl and analyzed by High-spatial-resolution TOF-SIMS images of ion distribution in longitudinal sections of dentin: Pulp space is on topmost and dentin bottom-most in each image. Note irregular precipitate on surface (*green arrows*), the extension of PCA and CHX breakdown products, in addition to chlorine, into Dentinal tubules (*yellow arrows*). (**a**) "Total" shows raw image; ClC6H4 H_2N+ + $ClC_6H_4CH_2N_2$+ show distribution of PCA and CHX breakdown products, and Cl _+ ^{37}Cl_ show distribution of chlorine. (**b**) Positive ion of CHX group. (**c**) Negative ion of CHX group [44]

Interaction Between CHX and EDTA

The combination of CHX and EDTA produces a white precipitate, so a group of investigators [70] did a study to determine whether the precipitate involves the chemical degradation of CHX. The precipitate was produced and redissolved in a known amount of dilute trifluoroacetic acid. Based on the results, CHX was found to form a salt with EDTA rather than undergoing a chemical reaction (Fig. 5.9).

Interaction Between EDTA and NaOCl

Investigators [24] studied the interactions between EDTA and NaOCl. They concluded that

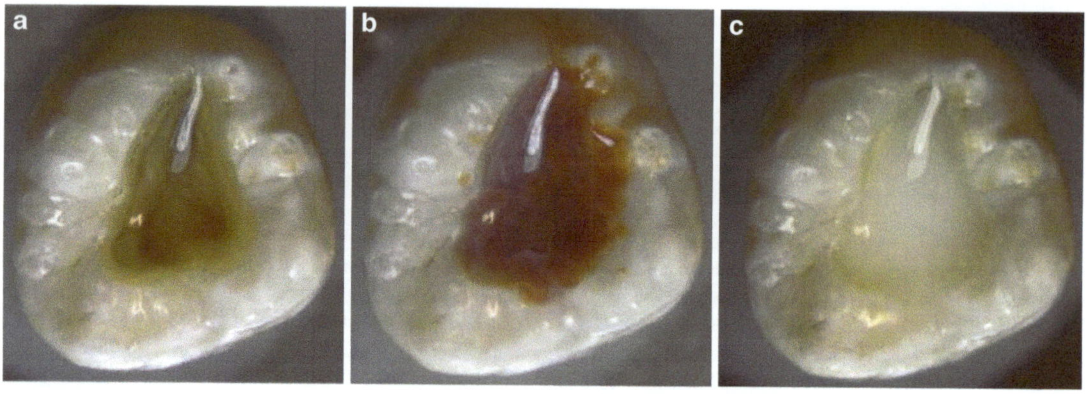

Fig. 5.9 Endodontic access cavities containing CHX mixed with various irrigants. (**a**) Water, (**b**) NaOCl, and (**c**) EDTA. Note that NaOCl and EDTA cause CHX to form a precipitate (Reproduced with permission from [70])

EDTA retained its calcium-complex ability when mixed with NaOCl, but EDTA caused NaOCl to lose its tissue-dissolving capacity, with virtually no free chlorine detected in the combinations. Clinically, this suggests that EDTA and NaOCl should be used separately. In an alternating irrigating regimen, copious amounts of NaOCl should be administered to wash out remnants of the EDTA. In modern endodontics, EDTA is used once the cleaning and shaping is completed for around 1 min. It can be ultrasonically activated for better penetration in dentinal tubules. It should be taken into consideration that a rise on the temperature of EDTA is not desirable. Chelators have a temperature range wherein they can work at their best. When EDTA is heated from 20 to 90°, the calcium-binding capacity decreases [97].

Figure 5.10 (Prado et al.) showed a visual aspect of different interactions between commonly used irrigants (Fig. 5.10).

Clinical Recommendations

After NaOCl was used throughout the cleaning and shaping procedure, irrigation with EDTA for 1 min should be used to remove smear layer. EDTA can be activated for a couple of seconds to improve penetration. Because NaOCl and EDTA may interact negatively, we need to be careful to remove the NaOCl with large amount of EDTA.

EDTA will leave a layer of collagen on the surface of the root canal lumen, and collagen can be important for the binding of bacteria; therefore, a final rinse with a low concentration of NaOCl can be applied at this time. Note that larger concentration may produce dentin erosion [69].

Any collagen and/or other proteins left exposed by EDTA would be removed by a short exposure to sodium hypochlorite [83].

HEBP

Etidronic acid, a substance that prevents bone resorption, has been used in medicine for patients suffering from osteoporosis or Paget's disease and was suggested as a substitute for traditional chelators due to fewer effects observed on dentin structure [85]. It is considered the unique chelator that can be mixed with NaOCl without interfering with its antimicrobial property [98].

A weak chelating agent, such as 2.5 % NaOCl/9 % etidronic acid (HEBP), has been proposed to eliminate debris impaction in the anatomical irregularities. This irrigant has the ability to remove the smear layer similar to that of EDTA or citric acid, and it can be mixed with NaOCl without any loss of the NaOCl antimicrobial activity [98]. A recent report has shown that the tissue dissolution ability of NaOCl is not diminished when mixed with HEBPT also known as 1-hydroxyethylidene-1, 1-bisphosphonate (HEBP) or etidronate [86]. Besides, this combination reduces AHTD and prevents smear layer formation during rotary root canal instrumentation to a similar extent as with the conventional use of NaOCl during instrumentation followed by EDTA [52]. Consequently, the NaOCl/HEBP

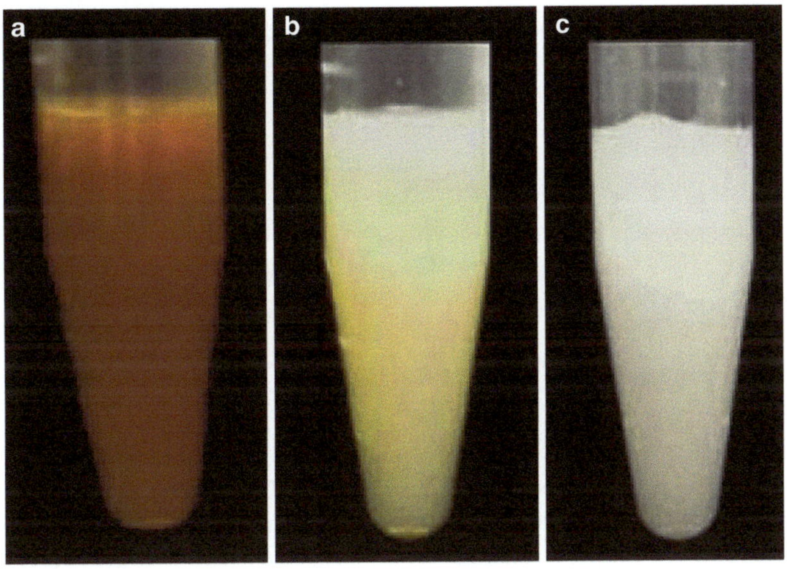

Fig. 5.10 Visual aspect of the interactions between the following: (**a**) 5.25 % NaOCl and 2 % CHX; (**b**) 0.16 % NaOCl and 2 % CHX; (**c**) 17 % EDTA and 2 % CHX (Reproduced with permission from Prado et al. JOE 2007 [68])

solution could be used as a single irrigant during and after instrumentation, replacing the final rinse with a chelating agent [1].

Effect of Temperature

NaOCl + Heat

Increasing the temperature of low-concentration NaOCl solutions improves their immediate tissue-dissolution capacity [98]. Furthermore, heated hypochlorite solutions remove organic debris from dentin shavings more efficiently. There are various devices to preheat NaOCl syringes; however, it was demonstrated that as soon as the irrigant touches the root canal system, the temperature reaches the body temperature [98]. Therefore, in situ heating of NaOCl is recommended by some authors. This can be done by activating ultrasonic or sonic tips to the NaOCl inside the root canal for a couple of minutes. Cavitation is the formation of vapor cavities in a liquid that are the consequence of forces acting upon the liquid. It usually occurs when a liquid is subjected to rapid changes that cause the formation of cavities where the pressure is relatively low. When subjected to higher pressure, the voids implode and can generate an intense shockwave http://en.wikipedia.org/wiki/Cavitation. Macedo et al.[53] state that the efficacy of NaOCl on the dentin is improved by refreshment, ultrasonic activation, and exposure time. In this investigation, a 10 °C temperature rise during ultrasonic activation was insufficient to increase the reaction rate. However, to our knowledge, there are no clinical studies available at this point to support the use of heated NaOCl.

EDTA + Heat

The ultrasonic activation and heat production of chelating agents with an ultrasonic tip are also of questionable value. While the streaming of the solution will be enhanced, the generation of heat and the possibility of cavitation may not be beneficial. Chelators have a clear temperature range at which they work best. Heating from 20 to 90 °C will decrease the calcium-binding capacity of EDTA and citric acid from 219 to 154 and from 195 to 30 mg CaO/g, respectively [97].

CHX + Heat

The use of ultrasonic energy to enhance the efficacy of irrigants is a new trend in clinical endodontics. Cameron [11] reported that an increase

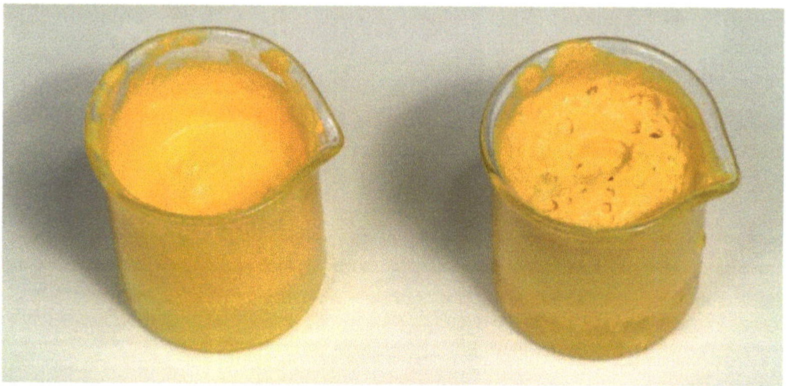

Fig. 5.11 Tubes with PCA and the NaOCl/CHX precipitate turned yellow after heating them to 45°, indicating that the amine (PCA) was present [8]

in the intracanal temperature from 37 to 45 °C occurred close to the tip of the instrument when the NaOCl solution was ultrasonically activated for 30 s without replenishment. In 2009, our group (Basrani) published a paper showing that CHX at room temperature and at 37 °C did not result in a yellow end product when diazotized, therefore indicating that there is no aromatic amine present. However, when CHX that was heated to 45 °C was diazotized, the result was a yellow end product, indicating the presence of PCA or another aromatic amine. These findings might be clinically relevant because PCA has been shown to be toxic. Considering that CHX can break down to form PCA by exposure to heat, it is not recommended to elevate the temperature of the CHX [8]. Figure 5.11 shows that the end products of the PCA, NaOCl/CHX precipitate, and 2.0 % CHX at 45 °C were yellow, indicating that an aromatic amine was present in all samples. However, CHX at room temperature or heated at 37 °C turned white, indicating that no aromatic was present.

Combinations and Solutions with Detergents

The irrigant flow can be affected by density, viscosity, contact angle, and wetting behavior of the irrigant. Even though density and viscosity always affect the flow, surface tension only affects the flow when 2 immiscible (incapable of mixing) fluids are present. Because the dentin is hydrophilic and dentinal tubules always contain water, there is no need in endodontic irigants to add detergents (see Dynamics chapter for more details).

Some added detergents in the market are:

- SmearClear: EDTA + detergents
- Chlor-XTRA: NaOCl + detergents
- CHX-Plus: CHX + detergents
- Tetraclean: 50 mg/mL doxycycline + polypropylene glycol + citric acid
- MTAD: 3 % doxycycline hyclate + 4.25 % citric acid + Tween 80
- QMiX: CHX + EDTA + detergent

BioPure MTAD and Tetraclean

Two new irrigants based on a mixture of antibiotics, citric acid, and a detergent have been developed. These irrigants are capable of removing both the smear layer and organic tissue from the infected root canal system [89, 91]. MTAD, introduced by Torabinejad and Johnson [90] at Loma Linda University in 2003, is an aqueous solution of 3 % doxycycline, a broad-spectrum antibiotic; 4.25 % citric acid, a demineralizing agent; and 0.5 % polysorbate 80 detergent (Tween 80) [89, 91]. It is mixed as a liquid and powder prior to use. MTAD has been recommended in clinical practice as a final rinse after completion of conventional chemomechanical preparation [75, 89, 91].

Tetraclean (Ogna Laboratori Farmaceutici, Muggio, Italy) is a combination product similar to MTAD. The two irrigants differ in the concentration of antibiotics (doxycycline 150 mg/5 ml for MTAD and 50 mg/5 ml for Tetraclean) and the kind of detergent (Tween 80 for MTAD, polypropylene glycol for Tetraclean).

Mode of Action

All tetracyclines are derivatives of four-ringed nucleus that differ structurally in regard to the chemical groups at 2, 5, 6, and 7 positions. These derivatives exhibit different characteristic such as absorption, protein binding, metabolism, excretion, and the degree of activity against susceptible organism [31]. Tetracyclines inhibit protein synthesis by reversibly binding to the 30S subunit of bacterial ribosome in susceptible bacteria. It is effective against *Aa. capnocytophaga*, *P.gingivalis*, and *P. intermedia* and affects both gram-positive and gram-negative (more gram-negative effect). Tetracycline is a bacteriostatic antibiotic, but in high concentrations, tetracycline may also have a bactericidal effect. Doxycycline, citric acid, and Tween 80 together may have a synergistic effect on the disruption of the bacterial cell wall and on the cytoplasmic membrane.

Smear Layer Removal

In two studies, the efficacy of MTAD or EDTA in the removal of the smear layer was confirmed, but no significant difference between these two solutions was reported [87, 88].

Antibacterial Efficacy

Earlier in vitro research on MTAD showed its antimicrobial efficacy over conventional irrigants [15, 87, 88]. Torabinejad et al. [15] found that MTAD was effective in killing *E. faecalis* up to 200× dilution. Shabahang and Torabinejad [76] showed that the combination of 1.3 % NaOCl as a root canal irrigant and MTAD as a final rinse was significantly more effective against *E. faecalis* than other regimens [75]. A study using extracted human teeth contaminated with saliva showed that MTAD was more effective than 5.25 % NaOCl in disinfection of the teeth. In contrast to the previously mentioned studies, later research suggested less than optimal antimicrobial activity of MTAD [21, 41]. Krause et al. [46], using bovine tooth sections, showed that 5.25 % NaOCl was more effective than MTAD in disinfection of dentin disks inoculated with *E. faecalis* [76, 79].

Clinical Trials

Malkhassian et al.[55] in a controlled clinical trial of 30 patients reported that the final rinse with MTAD did not reduce the bacterial counts in infected canals beyond levels achieved by chemomechanical preparation using NaOCl alone.

Protocol for Use

MTAD was developed as a final rinse to disinfect the root canal system and remove the smear layer. The effectiveness of MTAD to completely remove the smear layer is enhanced when a low concentration of NaOCl (1.3 %) is used as an intracanal irrigant before placing 1 ml of MTAD in a canal for 5 min and rinsing it with an additional 4 ml of MTAD as the final rinse [79].

QMiX

QMiX was introduced in 2011; it is one of the new combination products introduced for root canal irrigation. It is recommended to be used at the end of instrumentation, after NaOCl irrigation. According to the patent (195), QMiX contains a CHX analog, triclosan, (*N*-cetyl-*N*,*N*,*N*-trimethylammonium bromide), and EDTA as a decalcifying agent; it is intended as a antimicrobial irrigant as well as to be used in the removal of canal wall smear layers and debris.

Protocol

QMiX is suggested as a final rinse. If sodium hypochlorite was used throughout the cleaning and shaping, saline can rinse out NaOCl to prevent the formation of PCA.

Smear Layer Removal

Stojicic et al. [82] investigated the effectiveness of smear layer removal by QMiX using scanning electron microscopy. QMiX removed smear layer equally well as EDTA. Dai et al. [13] examined the ability of two pH versions of QMiX on removal of canal wall smear layers and debris using an open-canal design. Within the limitations of an open-canal design, the two experimental QMiX versions are as effective as 17 % EDTA in removing canal wall smear layers after the use of 5.25 % NaOCl as the main rinse.

Antibacterial Efficacy and Effect on Biofilms

Stojicic et al. [82] assessed, in a laboratory experimental model, the efficacy of QMiX against *Enterococcus faecalis* and mixed plaque bacteria in planktonic phase and biofilms. QMiX and 1 % NaOCl killed all planktonic *E. faecalis* and plaque bacteria in 5 s. QMiX and 2 % NaOCl killed up to 12 times more biofilm bacteria than 1 % NaOCl ($P<0.01$) or 2 % CHX ($P<0.05$; $P<0.001$). Wang et al. compared the antibacterial effects of different disinfecting solutions on young and old *E. faecalis* biofilms in dentin canals using a novel dentin infection model and confocal laser scanning microscopy. Six percent NaOCl and QMiX were the most effective disinfecting solutions against the young biofilm, whereas against the 3-week-old biofilm, 6 % NaOCl was the most effective followed by QMiX. Both were more effective than 2 % NaOCl and 2 % CHX. Morgental et al. [58] showed that QMiX was less effective than 6 % NaOCl and similar to 1 %NaOCl in bactericidal action. According to their in vitro study, it appears that the presence of dentin slurry has the potential to inhibit most current antimicrobials in the root canal system.

Moreover, Ordinola-Zapata et al. [61] found that several endodontic irrigants containing antimicrobial compounds such as chlorhexidine (QMiX), cetrimide, maleic acid, iodine compounds, or antibiotics (MTAD) lacked an effective antibiofilm activity, when the dentin was infected intraorally. The irrigant solutions 4 % peracetic acid and 2.5–5.25 % sodium hypochlorite decreased significantly the number of live bacteria in biofilms, providing also cleaner dentin surfaces ($P<0.05$). They concluded that several chelating agents containing antimicrobials could not remove nor kill significantly biofilms developed on intraorally infected dentin, with the exception of sodium hypochlorite and 4 % peracetic acid. Dissolution ability is mandatory for an appropriate eradication of biofilms attached to the dentin.

Clinical Trials

The efficacy and biocompatibility of QMiX were demonstrated via nonclinical in vitro and ex vivo studies. Further clinical research from independent investigators is needed to corroborate the findings.

Disinfection Protocol Suggested

Recommended irrigation protocol for root canal treatment: Many protocols are suggested in the modern endodontic literature. The following steps are the most commonly used:

1. 2.5–5 % NaOCl throughout the instrumentation procedure until final shape of the canal is achieved (adequate size and taper).
2. Activation and heating of the fresh NaOCl (such as ultrasonic, sonic or laser activation) for approx. 30 sec with fresh solution per canal.
3. Apical negative pressure devices are optional to enhance apical irrigation without extrusion (ex. Endovac).
4. Smear layer removal (EDTA, Citric acid, etc.) for approx. 1min (activation and/or apical negative pressure optional).
5. Final rinse options:
   a. Fresh NaOCl for approx. 1 min or
   b. CHX, QMiX, or
   c. Alcohol or
   d. Dry with paper points and obturate

References

1. Arias-Moliz MT, Ordinola-Zapata R, Baca P, Ruiz-Linares M, Ferrer-Luque CM. Antimicrobial activity of a sodium hypochlorite/etidronic acid irrigant solution. J Endod. 2014;40(12):1999–2002.
2. Autegarden JE, Pecquet C, Huet S, Bayrou O, Leynadier F. Anaphylactic shock after application of chlorhexidine to unbroken skin. Contact Dermatitis. 1999;40:215–7.
3. Baker NE, Liewehr FR, Buxton TB, Joyce AP. Antibacterial efficacy of calcium hydroxide, iodine

potassium iodide, betadine, and betadine scrub with and without surfactant against E faecalis in vitro. Oral Surg Oral Med Oral Pathol Oral Radiol Endod. 2004;98:359.
4. Barbosa CA, Goncalves RB, Siqueira Jr JF, De Uzeda M. Evaluation of the antibacterial activities of calcium hydroxide, chlorhexidine, and camphorated paramonochlorophenol as intracanal medicament. A clinical and laboratory study. J Endod. 1997;23: 297–300.
5. Basrani B, Ghanem A, Tjäderhane L. Physical and chemical properties of chlorhexidine and calcium hydroxide-containing medications. J Endod. 2004;30: 413–7.
6. Basrani B, Lemonie C. Chlorhexidine gluconate. Aust Endod J. 2005;31:48–52.
7. Basrani BR, Manek S, Sodhi RN, Fillery E, Manzur A. Interaction between sodium hypochlorite and chlorhexidine gluconate. J Endod. 2007;33(8):966.
8. Basrani BR, Manek S, Fillery E. Using diazotization to characterize the effect of heat or sodium hypochlorite on 2.0% chlorhexidine. J Endod. 2009;35(9):1296–9.
9. Basrani B, Santos JM, Tjäderhane L, Grad H, Gorduysus O, Huang J, Lawrence HP, Friedman S. Substantive antimicrobial activity in chlorhexidine-treated human root dentin. Oral Surg Oral Med Oral Pathol Oral Radiol Endod. 2002;94:240–5.
10. Basrani B, Tjäderhane L, Santos JM, Pascon E, Grad H, Lawrence HP, Friedman S. Efficacy of chlorhexidine- and calcium hydroxide-containing medicaments against enterococcus faecalis in vitro. Oral Surg Oral Med Oral Pathol Oral Radiol Endod. 2003;96: 618–24.
11. Cameron JA. The effect of ultrasonic endodontics on the temperature of the root canal wall. J Endod. 1988;14(11):554–9.
12. Clegg MS, Vertucci FJ, Walker C, Belanger M, Britto LR. The effect of exposure to irrigant solutions on apical dentin biofilms in vitro. J Endod. 2006;32: 434–7.
13. Dai L, Khechen K, Khan S, Gillen B, Loushine BA, Wimmer CE, Gutmann JL, Pashley D, Tay FR. The effects of QMiX, an experimental antibacterial root canal irrigant, on removal of canal wall smear layer and debris. J Endod. 2011;37:80–4.
14. Davies A. The mode of action of chlorhexidine. J Periodontal Res. 1973;12:68–9.
15. Davis JM, Maki J, Bahcall JK. An in vitro comparison of the antimicrobial effects of various endodontic medicaments on enterococcus faecalis. J Endod. 2007;33:567–9.
16. Denton G. Chlorhexidine. In: Block SS, editor. Disinfection, sterilization and preservation. 4th ed. Philadelphia: Lea and Febiger; 1991.
17. Dutner J, Mines P, Anderson A. Irrigation trends among American Association of Endodontists members: a web-based survey. J Endod. 2012;38(1):37–40.
18. Ebo DG, Stevens WJ, Bridts CH, Matthieu L. Contact allergic dermatitis and life-threatening anaphylaxis to chlorhexidine. J Allergy Clin Immunol. 1998;101: 128–9.
19. Emilson CG, Ericson T, Heyden G, Magnusson BC. Uptake of chlorhexidine to hydroxyapatite. J Periodontal Res Suppl. 1973;17:17–21.
20. Estrela C, Estrela CR, Barbin EL, Spano JC, Marchesan MA, Pecora JD. Mechanism of action of sodium hypochlorite. Braz Dent J. 2002;13:113.
21. Giardino L, Ambu E, Savoldi E, Rimondini R, Cassanelli C, Debbia EA. Comparative evaluation of antimicrobial efficacy of sodium hypochlorite, MTAD, And Tetraclean against enterococcus faecalis biofilm. J Endod. 2007;33:852–5.
22. Goldman M, Kronman JH, Goldman LB, Clausen H, Grady J. New method of irrigation during endodontic treatment. J Endod. 1976;2:257–60.
23. Gopikrishna V, Pare S, Pradeep Kumar A, Lakshmi Narayanan L. Irrigation protocol among endodontic faculty and post-graduate students in dental colleges of India: a survey. J Conserv Dent. 2013;16(5): 394–8.
24. Grawehr M, Sener B, Waltimo T, Zehnder M. Interactions of ethylenediamine tetraacetic acid with sodium hypochlorite in aqueous solutions. Int Endod J. 2003;36:411–7.
25. Greenstein G, Berman C, Jaffin R. Chlorhexidine. An adjunct to periodontal therapy. J Periodontol. 1986;57:370–5.
26. Grossman L, Meiman B. Solution of pulp tissue by chemical agent. J Am Dent Assoc. 1941;28:223.
27. Gulabivala K, Ng Y-L, Gilbertson M, Eames I. The fluid mechanics of root canal irrigation. Physiol Meas. 2010;31:R49.
28. Gulabivala K, Patel B, Evans G, et al. Effects of mechanical and chemical procedures on root canal surfaces. Endod Top. 2005;10:103–22.
29. Haapasalo HK, Sirén EK, Waltimo TM, Ørstavik D, Haapasalo MP. Inactivation of local root canal medicaments by dentine: an in vitro study. Int Endod J. 2000;33(2):126–31.
30. Haapasalo M. Can I use chlorhexidine as the only irrigating solution in my endodontic treatments? J Can Dent Assoc. 2011;77:b16.
31. Haznedaroglu F, Ersev H. Tetracycline HCl solution as a root canal irrigant. J Endod. 2001;27:738.
32. Heling I, Chandler NP. Antimicrobial effect of irrigant combinations within dentinal tubules. Int Endod J. 1998;31:8.
33. Hennessey TS. Some antibacterial properties of chlorhexidine. J Periodontal Res Suppl. 1973;12: 61–7.
34. Hjeljord LG, Rolla G, Bonesvoll P. Chlorhexidine-protein interactions. J Periodontal Res Suppl. 1973; 12:11–6.
35. Hübscher W, Barbakow F, Peters OA. Root canal preparation with FlexMaster: asessment of torque and force in relation to canal anatomy. Int Endod J. 2003;36(12):883–90.
36. Hugo W, Longworth A. Some aspects of the mode of action of chlorhexidine. J Pharm Pharmacol. 1964; 16:751–8.
37. Hugo WB, Longworth AR. The effect of chlorhexidine on the electrophoretic mobility, cytoplasmic

constituents, dehydrogenase activity and cell walls of excherichia coli and staphylococcus Aureus. J Pharm Pharmacol. 1966;18:569–78.
38. Hülsmann M, Heckendorff M, Lennon A. Chelating agents in root canal treatment: mode of action and indications for their use. Int Endod J. 2003;36(12): 810–30.
39. Hülsmann M, Rödig T, Nordmeyer S. Complications during root canal irrigation. Endod Top. 2007; 16(1):27–63.
40. Jeansonne MJ, White RR. A comparison of 2.0% chlorhexidine gluconate and 5.25% sodium hypochlorite as antimicrobial endodontic irrigants. J Endod. 1994;20:276–8.
41. Kho P, Baumgartner JC. A comparison of the antimicrobial efficacy of naocl/biopure MTAD versus NaOCl/EDTA against enterococcus faecalis. J Endod. 2006;32:652–5.
42. Kishen A. Advanced therapeutic options for endodontic biofilms. Endod Top. 2012;22(1):99–123.
43. Kishen A, Haapasalo M. Biofilm models and methods of biofilm assessment. Endod Top. 2010;22(1):58–78.
44. Kolosowski KP, Sodhi RN, Kishen A, Basrani BR. Qualitative analysis of precipitate formation on the surface and in the tubules of dentin irrigated with sodium hypochlorite and a final rinse of chlorhexidine or QMiX. J Endod. 2014;40:2036–40.
45. Komorowski R, Grad H, Wu XY, Friedman S. Antimicrobial substantivity of chlorhexidine-treated bovine root dentin. J Endod. 2000;26:315–7.
46. Krause TA, Liewehr FR, Hahn CL. The antimicrobial effect of mtad, sodium hypochlorite, doxycycline, and citric acid on enterococcus faecalis. J Endod. 2007; 33:28–30.
47. Krautheim AB, Jermann TH, Bircher AJ. Chlorhexidine anaphylaxis: case report and review of the literature. Contact Dermatitis. 2004;50:113–5.
48. Kuruvilla JR, Kamath MP. Antimicrobial activity of 2.5% sodium hypochlorite and 0.2% chlorhexidine gluconate separately and combined, as endodontic irrigants. J Endod. 1998;24:472.
49. Leonardo MR, Tanomaru Filho M, Silva LA, Nelson Filho P, Bonifacio KC, Ito IY. In vivo antimicrobial activity of 2% chlorhexidine used as a root canal irrigating solution. J Endod. 1999;25:167.
50. Lin S, Zuckerman O, Weiss EI, Fuss Z. Antibacterial efficacy of a new chlorhexidine slow-releasing device to disinfect dentinal tubules. J Endod. 2003;29:416–8.
51. Lindskog S, Pierce A, Blomlof L. Chlorhexidine as a root canal medicament for treating inflammatory lesions in the periodontal space. Endod Dent Traumatol. 1998;14:181–90.
52. Lottanti S, Gautschi H, Sener B, Zehnder M. Effects of ethylenediaminetetraacetic, etidronic and peracetic acid irrigation on human root dentine and the smear layer. Int Endod J. 2009;42:335–43.
53. Macedo R, Verhaagen B, Rivas DF, Versluis M, Wesselink P, van der Sluis L. Cavitation measurement during sonic and ultrasonic activated irrigation. J Endod. 2014;40:580. Teresa Arias-Moliz, DDS, PhD,* Ronald Ordinola-Zapata, DDS, MSc, PhD, † ‡ JOE in press.
54. Magnusson B, Heyden G. Autoradiographic studies of 14c-chlorhexidine given orally in mice. J Periodontal Res Suppl. 1973;12:49–54.
55. Malkhassian G, Manzur AJ, Legner M, Fillery ED, Manek S, Basrani BR, Friedman S. Antibacterial efficacy of MTAD final rinse and two percent chlorhexidine gel medication in teeth with apical periodontitis: a randomized double-blinded clinical trial. J Endod. 2009;35:1483–90.
56. Manzur A, Gonzalez AM, Pozos A, Silva-Herzog D, Friedman S. Bacterial quantification in teeth with apical periodontitis related to instrumentation and different intracanal medications: a randomized clinical trial. J Endod. 2007;33:114–8.
57. Moorer WR, Wesselink PR. Factors promoting the tissue dissolving capability of sodium hypochlorite. Int Endod J. 1982;15:187–96.
58. Morgental RD, Singh A, Sappal H, Kopper PM, Vier-Pelisser FV, Peters OA. Dentin inhibits the antibacterial effect of new and conventional endodontic irrigants. J Endod. 2013;39(3):406–10.
59. Ng YL, Mann V, Gulabivala K. A prospective study of the factors affecting outcomes of nonsurgical root canal treatment: part 1: periapical health. Int Endod J. 2011;44(7):583–609.
60. Ohara P, Torabinejad M, Kettering JD. Antibacterial effects of various endodontic medicaments on selected anaerobic bacteria. J Endod. 1993;19(10): 498–500.
61. Ordinola-Zapata R, Bramante CM, Garcia RB, de Andrade FB, Bernardineli N, de Moraes IG, Duarte MA. The antimicrobial effect of new and conventional endodontic irrigants on intra-orally infected dentin. Acta Odontol Scand. 2013;71(3–4):424–31.
62. Paque F, Laib A, Gautschi H, Zehnder M. Hard-tissue debris accumulation analysis by high-resolution computed tomography scans. J Endod. 2009;35: 1044–7.
63. Paquette L, Legner M, Fillery ED, Friedman S. Antibacterial efficacy of chlorhexidine gluconate intracanal medication in vivo. J Endod. 2007; 33:788–95.
64. Peters OA. Current challenges and concepts in the preparation of root canal systems: a review. J Endod. 2004;30:559.
65. Pham NH, Weiner JM, Reisner GS, Baldo BA. Anaphylaxis to chlorhexidine. Case report. Implication of immunoglobulin e antibodies and identification of an allergenic determinant. Clin Exp Allergy. 2000;30:1001–7.
66. Portenier I, Haapasalo H, Orstavik D, Yamauchi M, Haapasalo M. Inactivation of the antibacterial activity of iodine potassium iodide and chlorhexidine digluconate against Enterococcus faecalis by dentin, dentin matrix, type-I collagen, and heat-killed microbial whole cells. J Endod. 2002;28(9):634–7.
67. Portenier I, Haapasalo H, Rye A, Waltimo T, Ørstavik D, Haapasalo M. Inactivation of root canal medicaments by dentine, hydroxylapatite and bovine serum albumin. Int Endod J. 2001;34(3):184–8.
68. Prado M, Santos Júnior HM, Rezende CM, Pinto AC, Faria RB, Simão RA, Gomes BP. Interactions between

irrigants commonly used in endodontic practice: a chemical analysis. J Endod. 2013;39(4):505–10.
69. Qian W, Shen Y, Haapasalo M. Quantitative analysis of the effect of irrigant solution sequences on dentin erosion. J Endod. 2011;37(10):1437–41.
70. Rasimick BJ, Nekich M, Hladek MM, Musikant BL, Deutsch AS. Interaction between chlorhexidine digluconate and EDTA. J Endod. 2008;34:1521–3.
71. Ringel AM, Patterson SS, Newton CW, Miller CH, Mulhern JM. In vivo evaluation of chlorhexidine gluconate solution and sodium hypochlorite solution as root canal irrigants. J Endod. 1982;8:200–4.
72. Rocha AW, de Andrade CD, Leitune VC, Collares FM, Samuel SM, Grecca FS, de Figueiredo JA, dos Santos RB. Influence of endodontic irrigants on resin sealer bond strength to radicular dentin. Bull Tokyo Dent Coll. 2012;53(1):1–7.
73. Rölla G, Löe H, Schiott CR. The affinity of chlorhexidine for hydroxyapatite and salivary mucins. J Periodontal Res Suppl. 1970;5:90–5.
74. Scully C, Ng YL, Gulabivala K. Systemic complications due to endodontic manipulations. Endod Top. 2003;4:60–8.
75. Shabahang S, Pouresmail M, Torabinejad M. In vitro antimicrobial efficacy of mtad and sodium hypochlorite. J Endod. 2003;450–452.
76. Shabahang S, Torabinejad M. Effect of MTAD on enterococcus faecalis-contaminated root canals of extracted human teeth. J Endod. 2003;29(9):576–9.
77. Shrestha A, Kishen A. The effect of tissue inhibitors on the antibacterial activity of chitosan nanoparticles and photodynamic therapy. J Endod. 2012;38(9):1275–8.
78. Siqueira Jr JF, Batista MM, Fraga RC, de Uzeda M. Antibacterial effects of endodontic irrigants on black-pigmented gram-negative anaerobes and facultative bacteria. J Endod. 1998;24:414.
79. Siqueira Jr JF, Machado AG, Silveira RM, Lopes HP, De Uzeda M. Evaluation of the effectiveness of sodium hypochlorite used with three irrigation methods in the elimination of Enterococcus faecalis from the root canal, in vitro. Int Endod J. 1997;30(4):279–82.
80. Siqueira Jr JF, Rôças IN, Paiva SS, Guimarães-Pinto T, Magalhães KM, Lima KC. Bacteriologic investigation of the effects of sodium hypochlorite and chlorhexidine during the endodontic treatment of teeth with apical periodontitis. Oral Surg Oral Med Oral Pathol Oral Radiol Endod. 2007;104(1):122–30.
81. Snellman E, Rantanen T. Severe anaphylaxis after a chlorhexidine bath. J Am Acad Dermatol. 1999;40:771–2.
82. Stojicic S, Shen Y, Qian W, Johnson B, Haapasalo M. Antibacterial and smear layer removal ability of a novel irrigant, QMiX. Int Endod J. 2012;45:363–71.
83. Sum CP, Neo J, Kishen A. What we leave behind in root canals after endodontic treatment: some issues and concerns. Aust Endod J. 2005;31(3):94–100.
84. Sundqvist G. Bacteriological studies of necrotic dental pulps. Journal: Umae Univ Odontological Dissertations. Jan 1976.
85. Tartari T, Duarte Junior AP, Silva Júnior JOC, Klautau EB, Mario Honorato Silva E Souza Junior; Patrícia de Almeida Rodrigues Silva E Souza. Etidronate from medicine to endodontics: effects of different irrigation regimes on root dentin roughness. J Appl Oral Sci. 2013;21(5):409–15.
86. Tartari BM, Guimarães LS, Amoras MA, Duarte PA, Silva e Souza CM. Bramante Etidronate causes minimal changes in the sodium hypochlorite ability to dissolve organic matter. Int Endod J. 2015;48:399–404.
87. Tay FR, Hosoya Y, Loushine RJ, Pashley DH, Weller RN, Low DC. Ultrastructure of intraradicular dentin after irrigation with BioPure MTAD. II. The consequence of obturation with an epoxy resin-based sealer. J Endod. 2006;32:473.
88. Tay FR, Pashley DH, Loushine RJ, Doyle MD, Gillespie WT, Weller RN, et al. Ultrastructure of smear layer-covered intraradicular dentin after irrigation with BioPure MTAD. J Endod. 2006;32:218.
89. Torabinejad M, Johnson WB, Inventors; US patent and trademark office, assignee. Irrigation solution and methods for use. USA. 2003.
90. Torabinejad M, Johnson WB; inventors. Irrigation solution and methods for use. US Patent 20,030,235,804, 25 Dec 2003.
91. Torabinejad M, Shabahang S, Aprecio RM, Kettering JD. The antimicrobial effect of mtad: an in vitro investigation. J Endod. 2003;29:400–3.
92. Turesky S, Warner V, Lin PS, Soloway B. Prolongation of antibacterial activity of chlorhexidine adsorbed to teeth. Effect of sulfates. J Periodontol. 1977;48:646–9.
93. Vianna ME, Horz HP, Gomes BP, Conrads G. In vivo evaluation of microbial reduction after chemo-mechanical preparation of human root canals containing necrotic pulp tissue. Int Endod J. 2006;39:484–92.
94. Willershausen I, Wolf TG, Schmidtmann I, Berger C, Ehlers V, Willershausen B, Briseño B. Survey of root canal irrigating solutions used in dental practices within Germany. Int Endod J. 2014:1–7.
95. Zamany A, Safavi K, Spangberg LSW. The effect of chlorhexidine as an endodontic disinfectant. Oral Surg Oral Med Oral Pathol Oral Radiol Endod. 2003;96:578–81.
96. Zehnder M. Root canal irrigants. J Endod. 2006;32(5):389–98. Review.
97. Zehnder M, Paque F. Disinfection of the root canal system during root canal re-treatment. Endod Top. 2008;19(1):58–73. Article first published online: 26 MAY 2011.
98. Zehnder M, Schmidlin P, Sener B, Waltimo T. Chelation in root canal therapy reconsidered. J Endod. 2005;31:817–20.
99. Zou L, Shen Y, Li W, Haapasalo M. Penetration of sodium hypochlorite into dentin. J Endod. 2010;36(5):793–6.

Complications of Endodontic Irrigation: Dental, Medical, and Legal

6

Gary Glassman

Abstract

The objective of endodontic treatment is to treat and/or prevent apical periodontitis. Historically, there have been many irrigating agents that have been used to achieve this objective. Sodium hypochlorite, to date, still remains the irrigant of choice to break down the organic tissue of the dental pulp, debride necrotic tissue from the root canal space, and confirm negative bacteria cultures. Sodium hypochlorite while being an excellent endodontic irrigant can also cause devastating complications if extruded past the apex into the periradicular tissues.

This chapter will outline the complications and sequelae that potentially can occur if sodium hypochlorite is accidentally extruded past the apex and into the periradicular tissues. The mechanism of action of the irrigation accident will be detailed as well as preventative measures that can be employed to avoid such occurrences in addition to suggested treatment recommendations should such an accident occur. In addition, the legal and ethical implications with respect to the use and delivery of sodium hypochlorite during endodontic treatment will also be discussed.

Microbial Control: History

G. V. Black [1] recognized the significance of endodontic microbial control over a century ago, and by the mid-1920s, the importance of obtaining a "negative culture" prior to obturation was axiomatic [2]. Unfortunately, the early endodontic pioneers lacked the methods, techniques, and equipment to identify all varieties of microbiota and their symbiotic association within the root canal system. These shortcomings adversely affected the reasoning of many researchers like Bender and Seltzer who by 1964 questioned the need to culture [3, 4]. Fortunately, as microbiology assay methods improved, Sundqvist reestablished the importance of the endodontic microflora [5] and began the scientific path of discovery that would establish endodontic biofilm as the cause of apical periodontitis [6].

G. Glassman, DDS, FRCD(C)
Associate in Dentistry, Graduate, Department of Endodontics, Faculty of Dentistry, University of Toronto, Toronto, ON, Canada

Adjunct Professor of Dentistry, University of Technology, Kingston, Jamaica

Private Practice, Endodontic Specialists, Toronto, ON, Canada
e-mail: gary@rootcanals.ca

B. Basrani (ed.), *Endodontic Irrigation: Chemical Disinfection of the Root Canal System*,
DOI 10.1007/978-3-319-16456-4_6

Table 6.1 While 3 and 6 % NaOCl could eliminate biofilm from the dentinal walls, only 6 % NaOCl could prevent regrowth of the biofilm

Solution	SEM		Culture growth (%)
	Presence of bacteria	Biofilm status	
6 % NaOCl	–	Absent	0
3 % NaOCl	–	Absent	20
1 % NaOCl	+	Disrupted	90
1 % NaOCl/ MTAD	+	Disrupted	0
2 % CHX	+	Intact	0
+ Control	+	Intact	100
– Control	–	Absent	0

From Clegg [8]

Microbial Control: Biofilm and NaOCl

In 2005, Nair reported an abundance of biofilm within the root canal system after using copious amounts of 5.25 % NaOCl during canal preparation [7]. This finding immediately prompted Clegg to investigate the most currently available endodontic irrigation solutions so as to determine their ability to both eradicate biofilm and prevent its regrowth on dentinal walls [8]. His findings conclusively proved that 6 % NaOCl is required to achieve both objectives (Table 6.1). Although chlorhexidine effectively kills biofilm, it lacked the ability to hydrolyze it, thus failing to achieve one of the basic objectives of endodontic treatment – debridement. By default, 6 % NaOCl is the only known endodontic irrigant, to date, capable of addressing the problems associated with endodontic biofilm; therefore, this chapter will only address complications associated with using NaOCl during endodontic treatment.

NaOCl: Cytotoxicity

Unfortunately, the chemical characteristic responsible for complete hydrolysis of biofilm produces devastating effects on living tissue. In a classical 1985 study, Pashley et al. [9] investigated the effect on red blood cells (RBC) and found that 5.25 % NaOCl, when diluted with saline at a ratio of 1:1,000, produced 96.3 % hemolysis of an RBC sample. The study also included the intradermal injection effect using a rat model and 5.25 % NaOCl. The intradermal injections resulted in immediate hemorrhage within the entire area of solution contact, and the affected areas ulcerated after 24 h. Pashley et al. warned: "NaOCl, while a very effective proteolytic solvent, is extremely cytotoxic and should be used judiciously and with caution in endodontic treatment. Even the suggestion that NaOCl, at some dilution, will only affect necrotic tissue should be abandoned." Pashley et al. further noted that one of the serious clinical consequences of using NaOCl is the passage of some of the solution through the foramina, which sometimes occurs when the needle is momentarily wedged tightly into the canal during irrigation. Twenty-eight years after this warning, Pashley coauthored another publication that identified a far simpler and more dangerous cause of the NaOCl extrusion incident – direct intravenous injection via intraosseous infusion [10].

NaOCl: Complications

Complications from NaOCl extrusion includes (1) maxillary sinus incidents [11], (2) severe pain [12], (3) cellulitis [13], (4) life-threatening events [14], (5) permanent facial disfigurement [15], (6) permanent nerve damage [16], (7) secondary infection [17], and (8) acute kidney injury [18]. At the root of the problem is a broad misunderstanding of the reasons NaOCl is extruded from the apical foramen. It is generally believed that apical extrusion of NaOCl happens, as Pashley described, when an irrigation needle is wedged into a canal during irrigation; however, two studies disagree with this belief. First, in a survey of the diplomats of the American Board of Endodontics, only 20 % of the responding diplomats reported they felt the needle was wedged in the canal [19]. Second, in a one-of-a-kind clinical study, Hypaque (a radiopaque dye) was used as an irrigating solution [20]. It is important to note that the Hypaque investigators were aware of the possibility of forceful apical extrusion and reported that care was taken to insure that no irrigation needle was wedged into the walls, yet in both vital and nonvital teeth, apical extrusion of Hypaque was noted (Fig. 6.1). Considering the tissue toxicity of even the smallest amount of NaOCl, it seems reasonable that many patients would feel some degree of postoperative pain or discomfort following traditional endodontic irrigation. Gondim et al. proved this to be a statistically significant fact [21].

NaOCl: Reviewing the Extrusion Incident

A typical NaOCl extrusion is characterized in Fig. 6.2, but if an irrigant can escape the apical foramen as easily as demonstrated in Fig. 6.1, then why are these characteristic signs and symptoms of the NaOCl incident so rare? Furthermore, why isn't the facial area directly superficial to the involved root apex virtually ever affected; while very specific other parts of the face in Fig. 6.2 are usually always affected, and other areas like the cheek are never affected. This is apparent again with the patient shown in Fig. 6.3a. Curiously, almost no ecchymosis is apparent at or near the right alar lobule, and this is the area directly superficial to the apex of the treated tooth (upper right lateral incisor), yet ecchymosis is apparent up to the super palpebral vein (arrow in "A") and down to the angle of the mouth [22]. In July 2013, Boutsioukis et al. [23] published an extensive 16-page review paper that included 105 references and examined 40 case histories and stated: "*There is a lack of clinical studies focusing on irrigant extrusion during root canal irrigation. Currently available case reports provide limited data on the possible factors that may influence irrigant extrusion.*" It is important to note that the Boutsioukis' et al. review was published in July 2013, four months

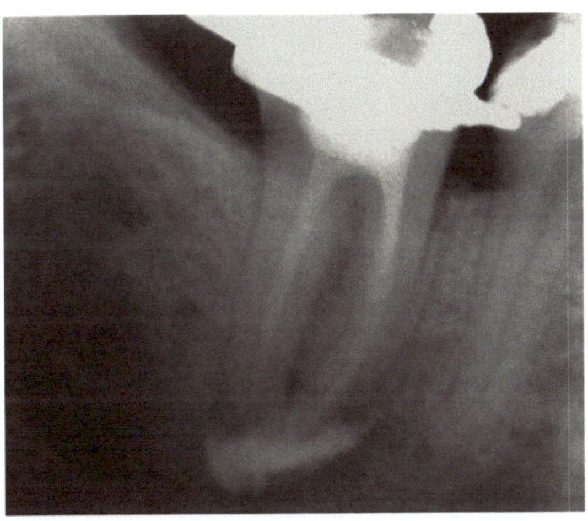

Fig. 6.1 In a unique clinical study, Salzgeber used a radiopaque dye (Hypaque) as an endodontic irrigant delivered judicially and cautiously via a non-binding needle during canal preparation and final irrigation. Despite careful delivery, sometimes regardless of the pulp's vitality, the dye extended into the apical tissues. Regarding nonvital teeth: "When the Hypaque did extend into the periapical tissues in teeth with necrotic pulps, it seemed to respect no boundaries and occupied a random portion of the rarefied area." In a situation as shown here, due to tissue reaction with NaOCl, post-op pain is likely a consequence, a finding supported by Gondim et al. [21] (From Salzgeber and Brilliant [20])

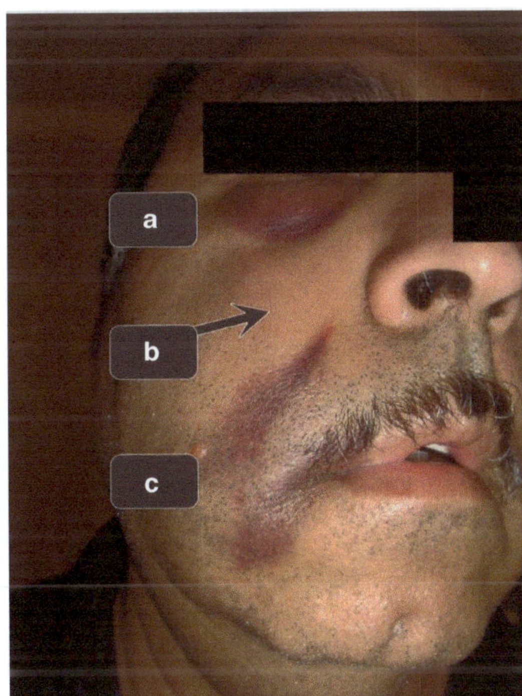

Fig. 6.2 The pathognomonic appearance of a NaOCl extrusion incident typically includes hemifacial edema and ecchymosis involving (*A*) one or both eyelids and (*B*) upper and lower lips beginning at the angle of the mouth but (*C*) never includes the cheek area [18] (With permission from Saudi Journal of Kidney Diseases and Transplantation)

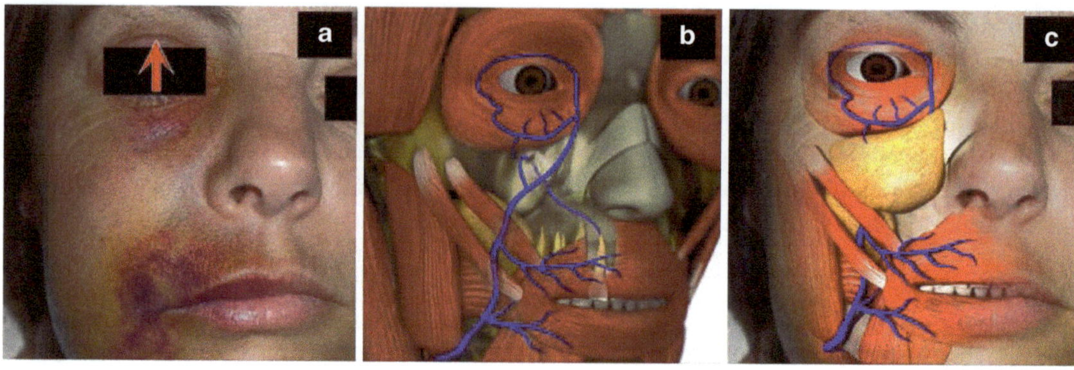

Fig. 6.3 (**a**) The classical pathognomonic facial appearance of NaOCl infusion resulting from the treatment of the maxillary right lateral incisor. Interestingly, although the right superior palpebral vein (*red arrow*) shows the hemorrhagic effect of NaOCl infusion, the midface area just below the eyelids and upper lip is virtually unaffected (From Witton and Brennan [22]). (**b**) The course of the anterior facial vein and its tributaries including the palpebral veins of the eyelids, the superior and inferior labia veins, and, most importantly – *an uncommon connection* [40] – with the superior alveolar vein(s) that normally drains blood from the teeth to the pterygoid plexus of the veins in the infratemporal fossa. (**c**) The area between the eyelids and the angle of the mouth is unaffected because the malar fat pad and the zygomatic muscles cover the anterior facial vein, thus hiding any hemorrhagic effect (Figs. **b & c** with Permission from SybronEndo)

before Pashley et al. described their novel theory of direct intravenous injection via intraosseous infusion.

The article immediately following Boutsioukis' July 2013 review was one of the three ex vivo studies published between April 2013 and May 2014 [24–26]. These ex vivo studies contained a method flaw obviously due to the investigator's lack of knowledge regarding the more recent findings of Pashley et al. The principle investigator with Pashley was Zhu [10], and their work was not referenced in any of Boutsioukis' ex vivo studies [24–26]. Additionally, two extremely important case histories [27, 28] were not included in the Boutsioukis' review; therefore, the method flaw and the case histories will be examined in detail. Finally, the review criticizes the ex vivo study by Desai and Himel [29] as not specifying a research hypothesis or aiming regarding "irrigan[t] extrusion," while in fact Desai stated: "*The specific aim of this in vitro study was to compare the relative safety of various intracanal irrigation systems.*" Furthermore, in Desai's discussion, he stated the following: "*The protocol for this study was designed to maximize the possibility of irrigant extrusion through an unrestricted, yet normal apex. It is understood that in clinical situations several factors might decrease the extent to which these systems extrude solutions. Periapical tissues and bone provide resistance to apical extrusion as well as non-patent canals. If quantities of periapical extrusion occurred clinically such as reported in this article, greater adverse treatment reactions associated with full-strength sodium hypochlorite would most likely occur. The model used most likely correlates, by design, to a canal that is open to atmospheric pressure, such as occurs when the apex of a tooth is extruding into the maxillary sinus with no apical covering or restriction.*"

Maxillary Sinus Considerations

The maxillary sinus is uniquely located in the immediate vicinity to the apices of maxillary teeth. With age, the alveolar bone surrounding these apices becomes thinner to the point where the root tips may project into the maxillary sinus and may not be covered with bony lamina dura or even the schneiderian membrane [30]. Furthermore, the ostium maxillae communicate directly with the nasal cavity and consequently normal atmospheric pressure. Provided the root canal is fully patent during treatment, this unique root canal system and maxillary sinus anatomical relationship offers no resistance to fluid extrusion during endodontic irrigation. Two previously cited studies [25, 29] used similar methods and materials. Each experiment used single straight-rooted teeth with open apical foramen exposed to normal atmospheric pressure. In the Boutsioukis' experiment, the canals were shaped to a #35/.06 and irrigated with open-ended (NaviTip) needles placed at WL – 1 mm with a delivery rate of 15.6 mL/min. Desai's canals were shaped larger to a #50/.04 and also irrigated with an open-ended (NaviTip) needles placed at WL – 1 mm but at a slower delivery rate of 7 mL/min. The percent extrusion was very similar: Boutsioukis ≈60 % and Desai (larger apical size) recorded ≈70 %. In summary, both studies found that an unrestricted apical foramen permits a very high irrigant extrusion escape from the root canal system as in the case of the maxillary sinus situation described earlier [30].

Maxillary Sinus: NaOCl Incident – Case Reports

One of the earliest case histories of NaOCl extruded into the maxillary sinus reported a relatively benign reaction; the authors stated: "The expected deleterious sequelae were not seen" [31]. The authors described a routine endodontic treatment that resulted in the extrusion event and did not report any needle binding nor any dramatic physiological response, just that the patient indicated the taste of NaOCl in his throat during treatment. Treating the extrusion event consisted of flushing sterile water through the palatal canal of the maxillary first molar and out the maxillary sinus via the ostium. Amoxicillin, a decongestant, and Motrin were prescribed for seven days. Except for a mild soreness associated with the tooth and congestion of the associated maxillary sinus and a brownish material expressed when blowing his nose, the patient made a full recovery. Other case reports were not so favorable; Kavanagh and Taylor [32] reported a similar case with a different outcome. During routine treatment of an upper right second bicuspid, NaOCl was inadvertently injected into the maxillary sinus resulting in acute severe facial pain and swelling. A futile attempt was made to aspirate the extruded NaOCl via the endodontic access opening, resulting in the need to admit the patient for a Caldwell-Luc procedure under general anesthesia. The tooth was eventually extracted three months after the hospital procedure. Recently, a never before described sequelae resulting from the extrusion of NaOCl into the maxillary sinus has been reported [33]. Sleiman, who maintains a practice limited to endodontics, was referred to a patient with a chief complaint concerning an uncomfortable feeling relative to her right maxillary molar region where she had received endodontic treatment several months earlier. The clinical examination was normal, and while the radiographic appearance of the molar region revealed that the maxillary first molar had been treated endodontically, the treatment appeared unremarkable having been properly prepared and obturated; the only exception noted radiographically was a vague appearance of something unusual within the maxillary sinus. This vague appearance resulted in a CBCT scan. The panoramic view (Fig. 6.4a) revealed that tissue filled half the volume of the affected maxillary sinus. A close examination of the posterior maxillary sinus wall (Fig. 6.4b) revealed areas of bone loss. Referring to Fig. 6.5 (red arrow), it must be noted that the posterior wall of the maxillary sinus forms part of the anterior boarder of the infratemporal fossa, an area rich with several complex nerves leaving the cranium, and that exposure to NaOCl has been reported to cause permanent nerve damage [16]. Sleiman postulated that *"Potentially, it could be the position of the patient during the root-canal procedure that made NaOCl stagnate on the posterior wall and aggravate[d] the damage."* When the patient was questioned about the procedure, she reported that during the treatment, she "had a chlorine taste in her throat arising from her nose as a liquid was dripping internally," and on her way home from the endodontic treatment,

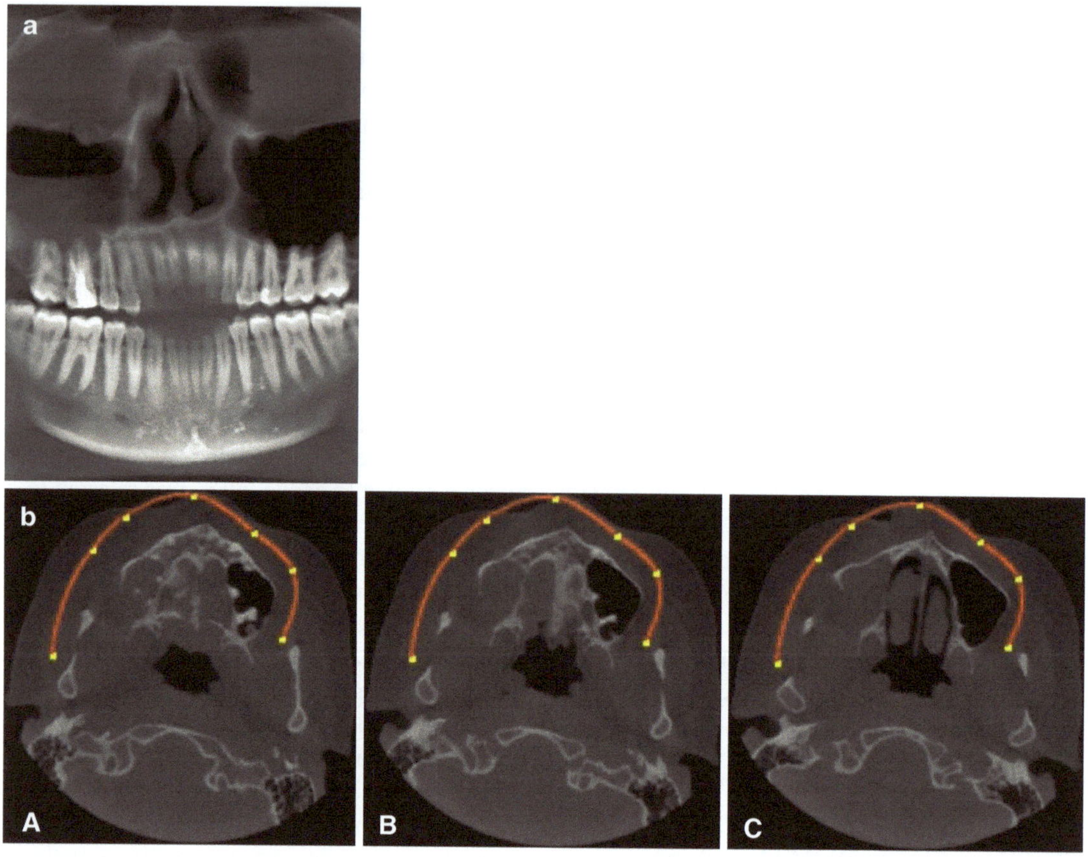

Fig. 6.4 (**a**) Panoramic CBCT scan demonstrates half of the maxillary sinus associated with endodontically treated tooth which is filled with inflammatory tissue (Courtesy of Dr. Philippe Sleiman, Beirut, Lebanon). (**b**) Sectional CBCT scan of same maxillary sinus demonstrates areas of the posterior wall that are nonexistent (Courtesy of Dr. Philippe Sleiman, Beirut, Lebanon)

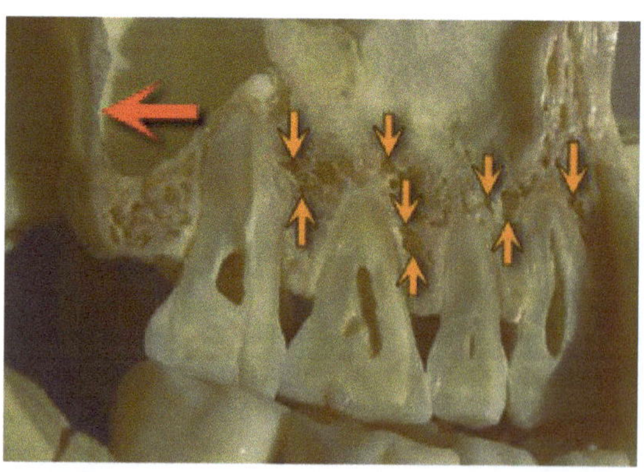

Fig. 6.5 (*Red arrow*) The posterior maxillary sinus wall is a critical anatomical feature because it forms a significant portion of the anterior boarder protecting the infratemporal fossa. In addition to the pterygoid venous plexus, the infratemporal fossa contains the following nerves: mandibular (inferior alveolar, lingual, buccal), plus the otic ganglion and chorda tympani (*Yellow Arrows*). A few of the many abundant sinusoid spaces are identified throughout the maxilla

the strange chlorine type liquid began to drip from her nose. Nothing of further consequence was reported. After viewing the CBCT results, the patient was referred to an otorhinolaryngologist for additional examination and treatment.

Maxillary Sinus: NaOCl Incidents – Treatment and Prevention

These three cited cases represent the spectrum of morbidity associated with extruding NaOCl into the maxillary sinus. Today's imaging technology can, and has revealed heretofore, unknown consequences of extruding NaOCl into the maxillary sinus; therefore, even the most seemingly inconsequential incidents involving extrusion of NaOCl into the maxillary sinus must be approached with caution. The literature universally suggested antibiotic and anti-inflammatory therapeutic treatment in the case of most NaOCl incidents [34, 35]; however, from the CBCT images presented in Fig. 6.4b, it is apparent that in some cases, a consultation with an otorhinolaryngologist may be appropriate in cases involving the maxillary sinus. Regarding prevention, as previously mentioned, the study conducted by Desai was modeled to simulate a root without any resistance to apical extrusion, and balanced to atmospheric as may occur in the maxillary sinus. Desai concluded: "This study concluded that the EndoVac *did not* extrude irrigant after deep intracanal delivery and suctioning the irrigant from the chamber to full working length." In concluding his case study, Sleiman opined: "One of the safest options that we currently have at our disposal is the EndoVac [Apical Negative Pressure] system, which is designed specifically to deliver fresh irrigant all along the root-canal system and, most importantly, to clean the last 3 mm of the root-canal system using the microcannula. It allows us to be certain that no chemicals can go beyond the limits of the root-canal space, nor cause any serious or even minor damage."

Pathognomonic Appearance of NaOCl Extrusion: A Problem

The facial appearance resulting from injecting NaOCl beyond the apical termination of the root canal does not agree with the 1985 Pashley intradermal injection findings. Consider a hypothetical situation whereby excessive amounts of NaOCl exceed the Hypaque extrusion in Fig. 6.1 [20]. If that was the root cause of the NaOCl incident, then according to Pashley in 1985, all of the superficial tissue should be ecchymotic and eventually ulcerate. That doesn't happen. Very specific parts of the face and neck are profoundly affected by ecchymosis: (1) the upper and lower eyelids on one (Fig. 6.6a) [27] or both sides of the face (Fig. 6.6b) [28], (2) the angle of the mouth

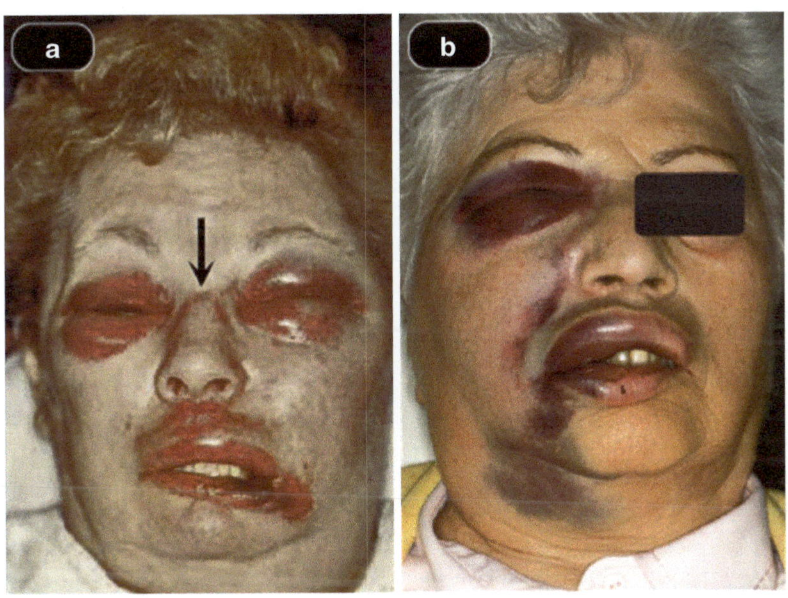

Fig. 6.6 (**a**) Upper left cuspid from Mehra et al. [27]. Most edematous and hemorrhagic effects of published NaOCl incidents are hemifacial. Although bilateral circumorbital ecchymosis is not uncommon, this case clearly demonstrates a vascular connection via superficial nasal veins (*arrow*) between both left and right circumorbital venous complexes suggesting that the NaOCl followed the venous connection across the bridge of the nose. (**b**) Upper right cuspid from Hülsmann [28]. There is no apparent venous connection between the orbits as shown in (**a**); thus, only the right side is affected. However, in this unique case, the anterior facial vein is positioned more toward the medial area of the face. Accordingly, *since part of it is not hidden under the malar fat pad*, the entire course of the anterior facial vein from the circumorbital veins to where it courses under the mandible joins the common facial vein which is apparent (Reproduced with permission of Elsevier)

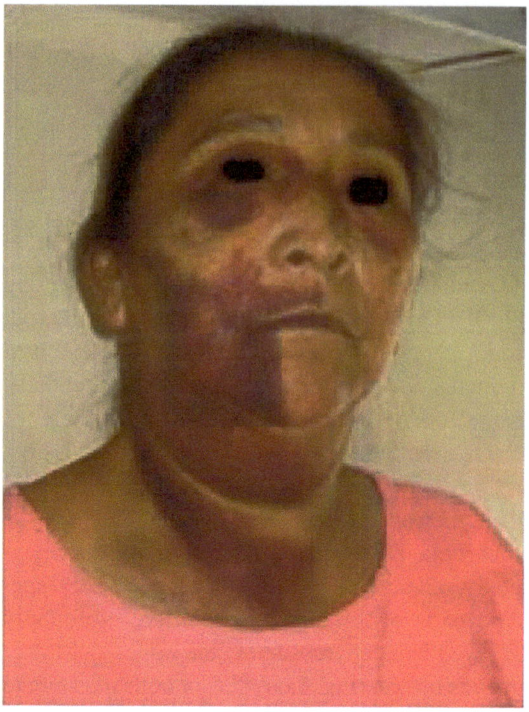

Fig. 6.7 Upper right cuspid from de Sermeño et al. [36]. The ecchymotic pattern of this severe NaOCl incident is classically hemifacial, except where it crosses the bridge of the nose to include left circumorbital area as in Fig. 6.4b. Note the classical absence of ecchymosis in the area of the malar fat pad despite almost all of the middle, lower face and neck being affected

only on the affected side (Fig. 6.6a, b), (3) sometimes the inferior boarder of the mandible only on the affected side (Figs. 6.6b and 6.7) [36], and (4) while other parts of the face, specifically the cheek, are never affected (Fig. 6.7).

Pathognomonic Appearance of NaOCl Extrusion: A New Theory

In 2013 [10], a new theory hypothesized that the NaOCl extrusion incident is not the result of injecting excessive NaOCl into the periapical tissue alone, but rather its direct injection into the venous system, specifically (in most cases) the anterior facial vein and its associated complex of the veins (Fig. 6.3b). This theory evolved from the 1963 study by Rickles et al. [37] initiated by a fatal case history caused by air entering the circulatory system through the root canal space. Their study determined that when the air pressure inside the root canals was increased by using intracanal needles, air would enter the venous system, which would result in a fatal cardiac embolism. Twenty-seven years later, Davies and Campbell [38] reported three fatalities resulting from air entering the vascular system during implant surgery. They specifically stated that "For air embolism to occur there must be an open vessel, a gradient between extravascular and intravascular pressure, and a source of air. Bone tissue is very vascular…." A year prior to the Davies and Campbell paper, Manisali [39] reported an unusual case of canal overfilling (Fig. 6.8). In this unique case report, a radiopaque substance (iodoform paste) was injected into a lower second premolar and was forced out the apical foramen. At first it formed into a disorganized periapical mass similar to the appearance reported by Salzgber, but then within a few millimeters, it formed a second irregular mass that produced a well-defined wavy line extending distally. Manisali opined that the paste could have entered and coursed its way through a vein, not the inferior alveolar canal clearly shown positioned below the wavy line.

A careful examination of Fig. 6.3a shows an ecchymotic threadlike line extending across the upper eyelid. It is clearly the superior palpebral vein that is part of the anterior facial venous network (Fig. 6.3b). A direct vascular connection between the anterior facial vein and the maxillary teeth does, albeit rare, occur [40]. If NaOCl is extruded above a specific pressure gradient through patient's maxillary right lateral incisor, it could enter a vein connected directly to the anterior facial vein and then spread through the venous complex affecting all areas extending from the upper eyelid to the angle of the mouth and beyond to the heart and the entire vascular system. The cheek would not be affected because the cheek fat pad (malar fat pad) and some of the zygomatic muscular fibers cover the anterior facial vein (Fig. 6.3c), therefore masking the hemorrhage. The case shown in Fig. 6.6b is very unique because it exhibits the full course of the anterior facial

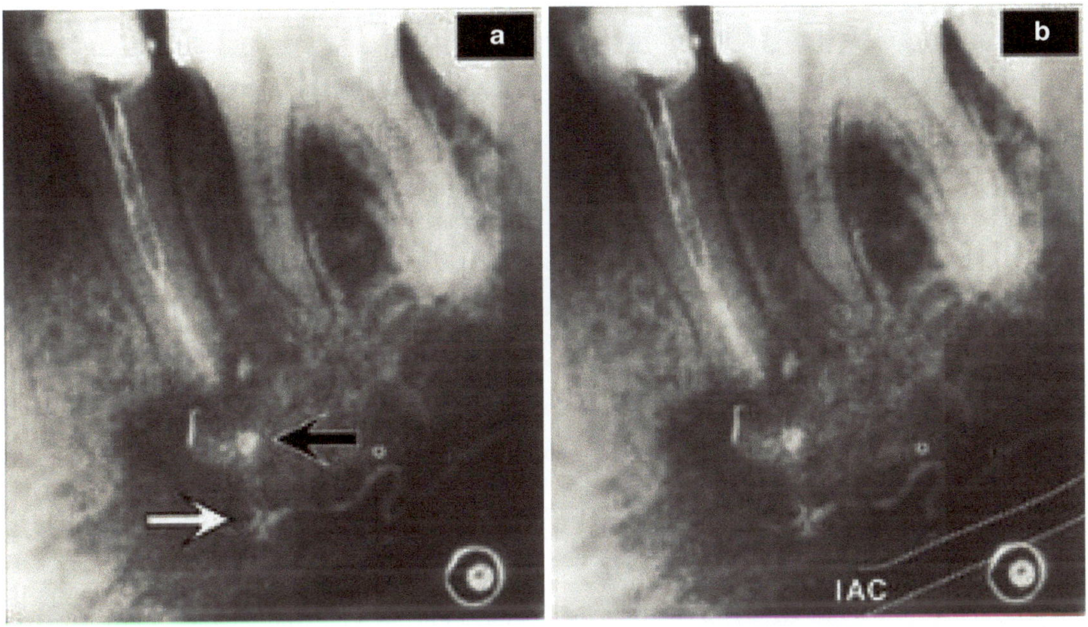

Fig. 6.8 From Manisali et al. [39], this figure shows overfill of iodoform paste which exhibits several unusual features. (**a**) The apical overfill of paste (*black arrow*) initially resembles the disorganized extrusion of Hypaque in Fig. 6.1, but a few millimeters below the initial overfill, a second mass (*white arrow*), appears again as another random mass then forms into a well-organized wavy line. (**b**) This line is not within the inferior alveolar canal (*dotted line*). Also note worthy is the faint radiopacity connecting the two masses. When viewed in its entirety, the paste overfill initially respects no boundaries upon leaving the apical foramen, then it becomes well organized as if running inside a blood vessel as it extends distally above the inferior alveolar canal

venous complex from the eyelids to the area where it courses under the mandible and joins the jugular vein; in this case, the anterior facial vein is positioned more laterally than usual and thus not hidden by the malar fat pad. Except for the inclusion of the other eye, Figs. 6.6a and 6.7 both share the pathognomonic characteristics of Fig. 6.3a including the absence of ecchymosis in the cheek area. Both circumorbital areas apparent in Figs. 6.6a and 6.7 are connected via a complex of superficial veins across the bridge of the nose (black arrow Fig. 6.6a). One apparent flaw in the theory is the fact that veins lack the elasticity of arteries and collapse easily, thus possibly nullifying the theory – but medullary sinusoids do not collapse, and they connect directly to veins. Schoeffel encountered another problem while investigating the uptake of ambient air by a healthy periodontal ligament [41]. He used the lower first premolar of young healthy dogs (Fig. 6.9a) and bonded a 21-gauge needle into a root canal space with an apical foramen prepared to 0.80 mm (Fig. 6.9b), and although the root canal space was pressurized to 175 mmHg above atmospheric pressure, no uptake was measured over 30 min.

Intraosseous Injection

In 1928, Drinker proposed that the intraosseous space be considered a non-collapsible vein [42]. Medullary bone contains thousands of small non-collapsible sinusoids that drain into larger veins [43–45]. The blood pressure in these spaces is approximately 30 mmHg, also known as the ¼ rule or 25 % of normal mammalian blood pressure [46, 47]. Since 1934, the interosseous (IO) space has been used to provide a reliable and safe method for allowing the introduction into systemic circulation [48–56]. Figure 6.10 shows a commercially available device used by the military and civilian medical personnel to establish

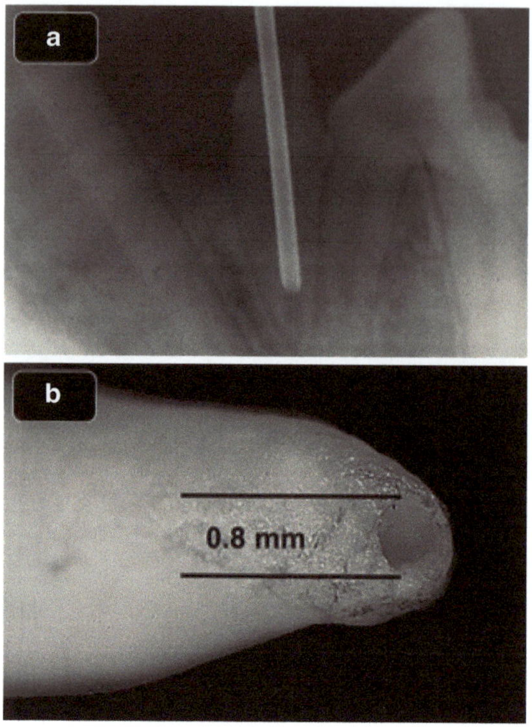

Fig. 6.9 (**a**) Radiograph of 21-gauge needle bonded into the root canal of live dog (From Schoeffel [41]). (**b**) Tooth after extraction demonstrating apical termination opened to 0.8 mm

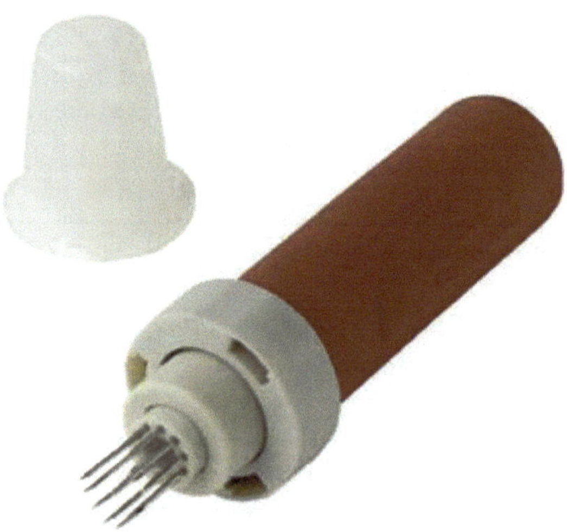

Fig. 6.10 FAST device for interosseous infusion

rapid access to the venous system. Quoting from the FAST patent application 5,360,711: "It has long been recognized that access to the vascular system is available via bone marrow sinuses. See, e.g., Tocantins et al. [55], Turkel and Bethell, A New and Simple Instrument for Administration of Fluids Through Bone Marrow, *War Medicine*, pp. 222–25 (1944). Infusion of drugs or other fluids into the marrow (intraosseous infusion) results in rapid transmission of such fluids into the vascular system. This method of infusion can be quite important when the patient has very low blood pressure or collapsed veins." Additionally, the IO route is used routinely in dentistry to effect profound anesthesia [57]. Accordingly, constructing an ex vivo model as either "open" or "closed" ignores the very well-established medullary bone space anatomy and physiology relative to the circulatory system. Under the correct conditions, intraosseous injection can occur when the pressure gradient exceeds approximately 30 mmHg [10]. Schoeffel's observations in 1980 seem in conflict with Rickles findings, since he was using a model using a pressure gradient (170 mmHg); however, his observations were correct because the pressure approximated a healthy and intact periodontal ligament, not medullary sinusoids.

Pathognomonic Appearance of NaOCl Extrusion: A New Theory – Support

The Peck Case History

Although the pathognomonic features in Fig. 6.2 are indistinguishable from the classical endodontic NaOCl extrusion incident, the NaOCl extrusion was *not* the result of extrusion via the root canal system. This case resulted from the inadvertent injection of NaOCl instead of lidocaine into an anatomical area where a section of the anterior facial vein complex is located – the patient's right infraorbital space. The significant ecchymosis in the lower eyelid is understandable according to Pashley's 1985 findings, but the fact that the ecchymosis skips the cheek area and becomes apparent again at the angle of the mouth is easily explained by Pashley et al. later in 2013 theory of a direct intravenous injection, (Fig. 6.3b). Although Occam's razor proves nothing, it serves as a heuristic device; in this case history, the simplest solution is that NaOCl was injected directly into the anterior facial vein complex near the inferior palpebral vein and followed its natural course toward the heart.

This recent case history also provides a new and alarming insight regarding the systemic effects of a NaOCl extrusion. Due to the immediate facial swelling and hemorrhage, the patient was directed immediately to visit the emergency department of the nearest hospital. A few days after the event, urine microscopy showed the presence of granular casts. Accordingly, the patient was referred for nephrological evaluation that resulted in the diagnosis of acute kidney injury secondary to renal tubular injury. The nephrologists reported: "We speculate that direct tubular epithelial injury occurred as a result of sodium hypochlorite exposure. This is the first report demonstrating that ATN [acute tubular necrosis] is an important diagnosis to consider after systemic sodium hypochlorite exposure during a dental procedure" [18].

Pathognomonic Appearance of NaOCl Extrusion: Multivaried Factors

Although the long-term consequences of NaOCl extrusion have been reported to vary from benign to life-threatening, it is still a rare event. Why? Three conditions must occur together before an intravenous injection can occur: (1) the apical foramen must be patent, (2) an anatomical variation in the venous drainage must exist that directs the blood flow away from the pterygoid plexus of the veins, and (3) the periapical pressure gradient must communicate with and exceed the sinusoidal pressure of approximately 30 mmHg [10]. Excluding wedging the needle in the root canal system, the pressure gradient factor involves its own subset of contributory factors including (1) rate of delivery, (2) location of the irrigation needle relative to the apical foramen, (3) size and shape of the canal relative to the irrigation, (4) design of the irrigation needle, and (5) the use of positive or negative apical pressure. Interestingly, two recent peer-reviewed articles appeared in the April 2013 issue of the Journal of Endodontics, and both cited venous blood pressure as a possible threshold pressure gradient to be avoided [58, 59]. Park et al. opined: "The data of the present study show that it is quite easy to exceed capillary pressure when the needle is close to the working length even at low flow rates."

Pathognomonic Appearance of NaOCl Extrusion – Periapical Pressure

As previously stated, three basic factors must happen simultaneously in order to produce a NaOCl incident: a patent apex, unusual vasculature anatomy, and access to and pressure exceeding the intraosseous space. Periapical pressure presents the most confusion because several basic subfactors influence this issue: canal configuration, type and position of irrigation needle, irrigant delivery rate, and universal misunderstanding of the anatomy and physiology of the periapical region.

Periapical Pressure Gradient: Historical Misconceptions

Until the recent Zhu et al. [10] paper, many fluid dynamic studies modeled their experiments on the premise that "The apical foramen was simulated as a rigid and impermeable wall" [60–64]. More recent ex vivo studies consider the pressure resistance at the apical foramen to be either "low compliant" (atmospheric pressure) or high compliant (incompressible) [24–26]. With the publication of Zhu et al. in 2013, the dental profession has come to realize the efficacy of the intraosseous (IO) fluid delivery method and now must reevaluate safe periapical pressure gradients at the apical foramen by including the interseptal bone spaces that are so abundant in both arches.

Periapical Pressure Gradient: Irrigation Needle Position and Flow Rate

In an ex vivo study, Khan et al. [59] evaluated the apical pressure produced with different 30-gauge open and side-vented irrigation needles located at WL – 1 mm from the apical termination at different flow rates varying from 1 to >8 mL/min. The

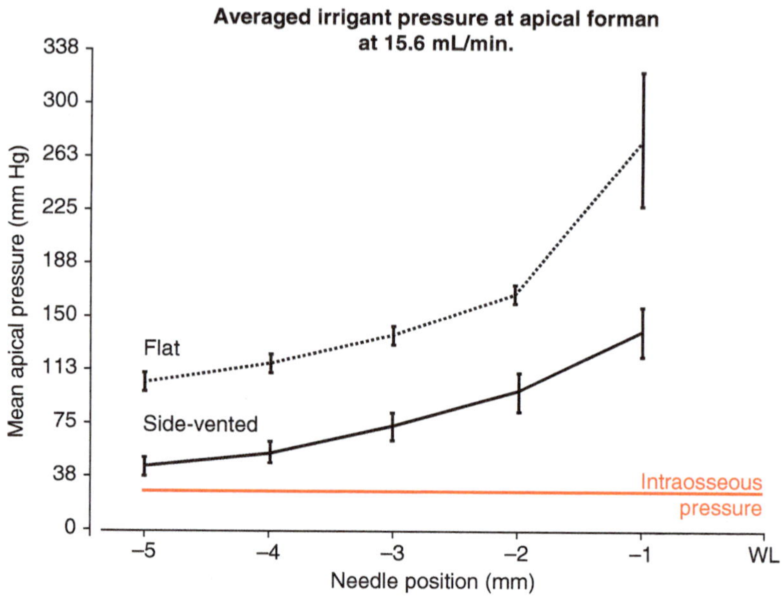

Fig. 6.11 Apical pressures were calculated at a constant *"clinically realistic"* delivery rate (15.6 mL/min.) by using an Unsteady Computational Fluid Dynamics Model. The variables were the depth of needle insertion (WL −1 to −5 mm), and needle configuration - Flat or Side-vented. Note: all pressures recorded exceed normal intraosseous pressure. (From Boutsioukis et al. [63])

Khan study used an ex vivo canal initially shaped to #35/.06 and finally to #40/.02. Boutsioukis et al. [63] employed a similar shape #45/.06 when building their computerized model and positioned their irrigation needles, also 30-gauge open or side-vented, at various working length but at constant flow rate 15.6 mL/min. In both cases, their variables (position or rate of delivery) produced similar results; regardless of needle configuration, the apically directed pressure increased proportionate to either the flow rate or depth of insertion (Figs. 6.11 and 6.12).

Periapical Pressure Gradient: Backflow Resistance – Needle vs. Canal Size

Khan et al. [59] used four different needle types for delivery irrigant via positive pressure; three had an outside diameter of 0.31 mm (Max-i-Probe, NaviTip, and Vpro StreamClean) while one had an outside diameter of 0.38 mm (Vpro EndoSafe). Irrigant was delivered at rates that varied from 1 to >8 mL/min. The recorded pressures are illustrated in Fig. 6.12. All positive pressure needles produced increasing apical >0 mmHg pressure proportionate to the rate of irrigant delivery. The three 0.31 needles produced virtually identical apical pressure, but the 0.38 needle produced dramatically higher apical pressure at the same flow rates, thus proving that resistance to backflow is a direct result of the total surface area available for the irrigant to backflow. The area available for backflow between the canal walls and the tip of a 0.31 needle is .065 mm^2 while the same area for a 0.38 needle is .030 mm^2 or 216 % less surface area. Noting that the thickness of a normal human hair is approximately .07 mm in diameter (the difference between the 0.31 and 0.38 needle), this illustrates that the slightest variation in size or depth of irrigation needles, in critical areas of the root canal, can have profound effects on the final apical pressure.

Periapical Pressure Gradient: Backflow Resistance – Canal Shape

The models used by Boutsioukis et al. [63] and Khan et al. [59] were configured as perfectly round and tapered canals. Although their data was consistent, the models were not representative of the true biological situation. Figure 6.13 demonstrates root canal variations at WL – 1 mm. In the mandibular molar mesial root in Fig. 6.13a, the left canal has limited area for backflow while

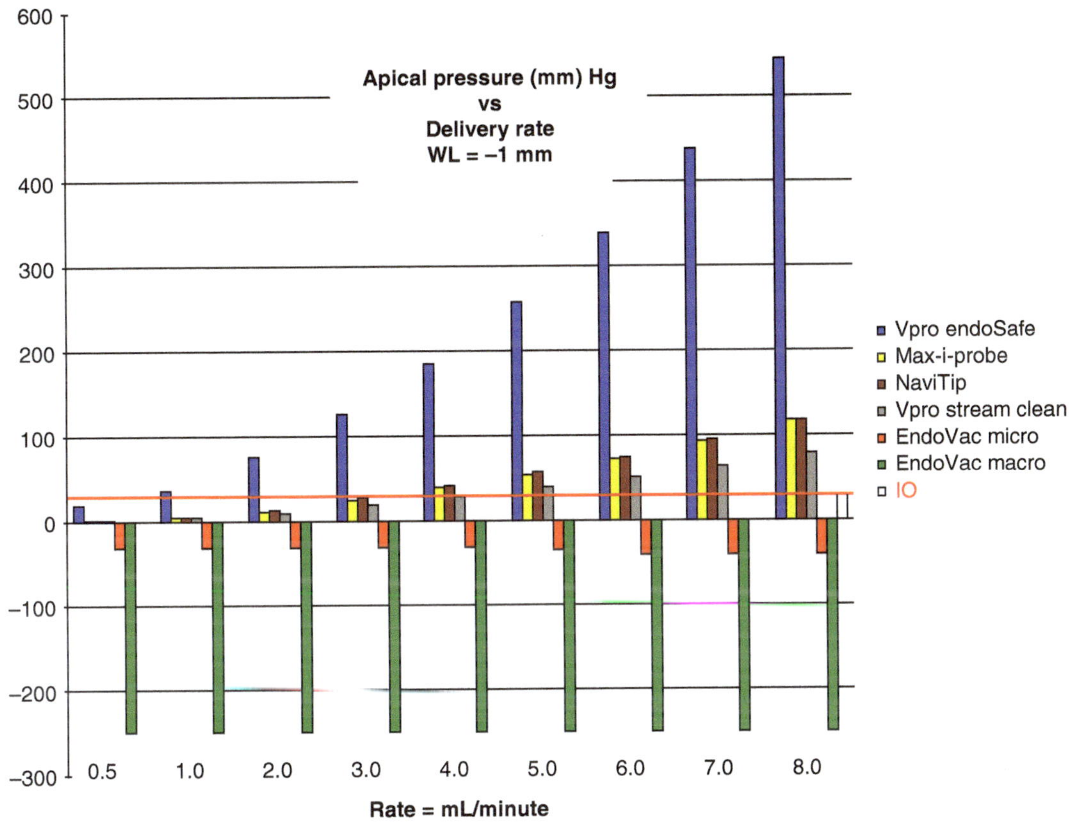

Fig. 6.12 A digital manometer was connected to the apical termination of a root canal model created according to the following parameters: (**a**) material = polycarbonate, (**b**) WL = 17 mm, (**c**) canal preparation #30/.06 followed by #40/.02 at apical seat, and (**d**) needle position = WL – 1 mm [except macro cannula which could not be positioned closer than WL – 4 mm]. Needle designs tested: (1) positive pressure group = Vpro EndoSafe, Max-i-Probe, NaviTip, and Vpro Stream Clean; (2) apical negative pressure group = EndoVac microcannula and macro cannula. In the case of positive pressure, the apical pressure was directly proportionate to increased flow rate. At a flow rate exceeding 3.5 mL/min, all positive pressure needles met or exceed the interosseous (IO) pressure. Conversely, regardless of irrigant flow rates, the negative pressure groups produced a consistent, negative pressures ≈ – 35 mmHg (microcannula) and ≈ – 250 mmHg (macro cannula) (From Khan et al. [59] and Goode et al. [79])

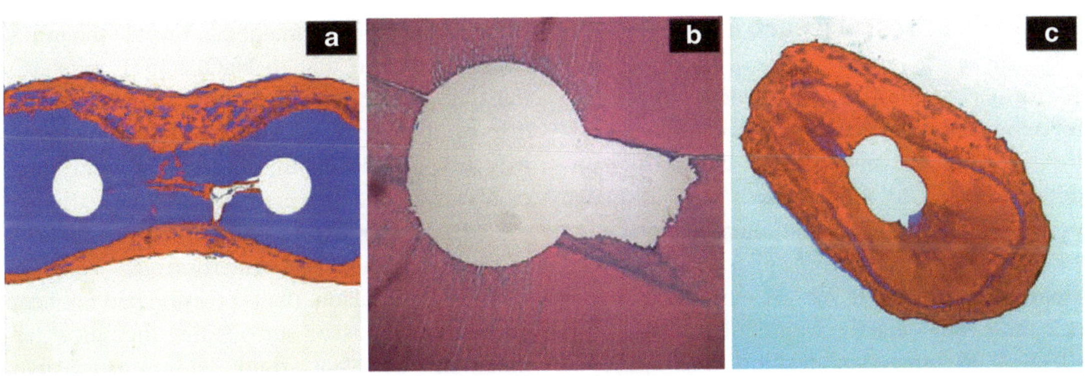

Fig. 6.13 Apical configurations at WL – 1 mm. In keeping with the findings that backflow space affects apical pressure, the intra- and intercanal configurations shown above illustrate different backflow scenarios: (**a**) mesial root lower molar, (**b**) maxillary central incisor, and (**c**) mesial root lower molar

its companion canal demonstrates a fin that obviously increases the backflow area, but if this "fin" is part of an isthmus complex, then entire companion canal could offer a backflow escape route. It is easy to see how two very different apical pressures could be recorded from the same root using the same needle and pressure. In the maxillary anterior root in Fig. 6.13b, although the canal is basically round, a large lateral fin is apparent thus producing a sizeable increased backflow escape area. In mesial root lower molar in Fig. 6.13c, in this situation, both the mesiobuccal and mesiolingual canals converge in the apical millimeter. Irrigant flow directed down either canal at this point will follow the path of least resistance up the companion canal rather than being forced apically. Hess [65] conclusively demonstrated the irregularities of the root canal system, and from the discussion in the previous paragraph, it is apparent that the most seemingly insignificant physical differences in internal anatomical configurations produce profoundly different results even when all other parameters remain constant. Unlike the findings of Boutsioukis and Khan, when reporting their results using human teeth, Park et al. [58] stated: "When the 30-gauge side-vented closed-ended needle was placed at 1 mm from the working length, the apical pressure was unpredictable and oscillated between low and moderate apical pressures."

Periapical Pressure Gradient: Subjective Pressure Factors

A further interesting observation was also reported in the Park experiment. The investigators prepared the mesiobuccal canals of mandibular molars to #35/.06 and used 30-gauge irrigation needles (0.31 mm diameter) placed at −1 mm from WL during one phase of the experiment. Accordingly, at WL − 1 mm, the diameter of the root canal would be 0.41 mm (0.35 + 0.06 mm) thus leaving free space of 0.10 mm (0.41–0.31 mm) and thus making it impossible for binding to occur. However, the investigators noted: "When the needles were placed at 1 mm from the apex, only two needles could be placed at this level in the root canal without binding of the needle tip. These needles included the 30-gauge blunt open-ended (FlexiGlide) needle and the 30-gauge side-vented closed-ended (ProRinse) needle." However, according to the actual preparation geometry vs. the size of the irrigation needle, binding would be physically impossible. The more likely scenario is that the operating clinician experienced the *sensation of binding* as the needles encountered root curvatures, thus demonstrating the highly subjective nature of clinical irrigation methods. It is also important to note that even though Boutsioukis et al. [64] reported an irrigant flow of 15.6 mL/min as a "clinically realistic" flow rate, every one of their apical pressures recording exceeded the intraosseous pressure. Furthermore, in an earlier experiment Boutsioukis et al. [66] surveyed a heterogeneous group of clinicians that included both genders practicing as either endodontists or general dentist and determined that their rates of irrigant delivery varied from 1.2 to 48 mL/min when using a 30-gauge needle, again demonstrating the subjective nature of irrigant delivery techniques.

Preventing the NaOCl Endodontic Incident

The next section will describe treating the NaOCl incident; however, it is imperative to note that since no specific treatment can reverse the initial damages caused due to NaOCl [67], emphasis must be placed on prevention. The previously discussed experiments all proved that flow rates, irrigation needle depth, canal shape, and clinician's subjective delivery technique each affected the periapical pressure. Additionally, until Zhu et al. explained the interosseous route of vasculature infusion, the profession had not been aware that the tissue surrounding the apical termination was not rigid and impermeable. Recalling that Davies and Campbell [38] and Rickles and Joshi [37] reported intravenous air emboli arising from dental procedures as causing patient death, it is important to examine the Bradford et al. [68] study that examined periapical pressures produced via air delivery. Bradford opined in (A) Results: "No needle design or gauge proved safe to use in either round or ovoid canals, regardless of stage of instrumentation" and (B) Discussion: "Vacuum rather than air under pressure, may be a superior means for canal drying."

Several studies have examined vacuum pressure as means of delivering irrigants to the apical termination under various clinical scenarios (Desai, Baumgartner, Khan, and Gondim). In the Desai study, using a totally open apex and equalized atmospheric pressure, no irrigant was expelled during any test. In the Khan study in Fig. 6.12 using a closed system, modeled after Bradford's method, all pressures using apical negative pressure recordings were less than zero meaning not only that irrigants could not be forced *out* of the root canal system but that exudate from the apical area can be aspirated *from* the periapical area (Fig. 6.14).

Treatment of the NaOCl Extrusion Incident

As previously stated, the initial damage from a NaOCl extrusion incident cannot be reversed; therefore, post-extrusion treatment is directed toward preventing further deterioration. Each incident must be evaluated on a case-by-case basis because a multitude of factors must be considered including severity of the incident, allergies to medications, side effects, dosing, and so on. Physiological and systemic concerns must be evaluated on an individual basis, for example, respiratory embarrassment, renal damage, and so on. Accordingly, the following general recommendations are summarized from six sources [28, 69, 70, 33, 18]:

1. Inform the patient regarding the nature of the incident including the possible risks and complications.
2. Hospitalization is required in all cases of respiratory embarrassment or uncontrolled

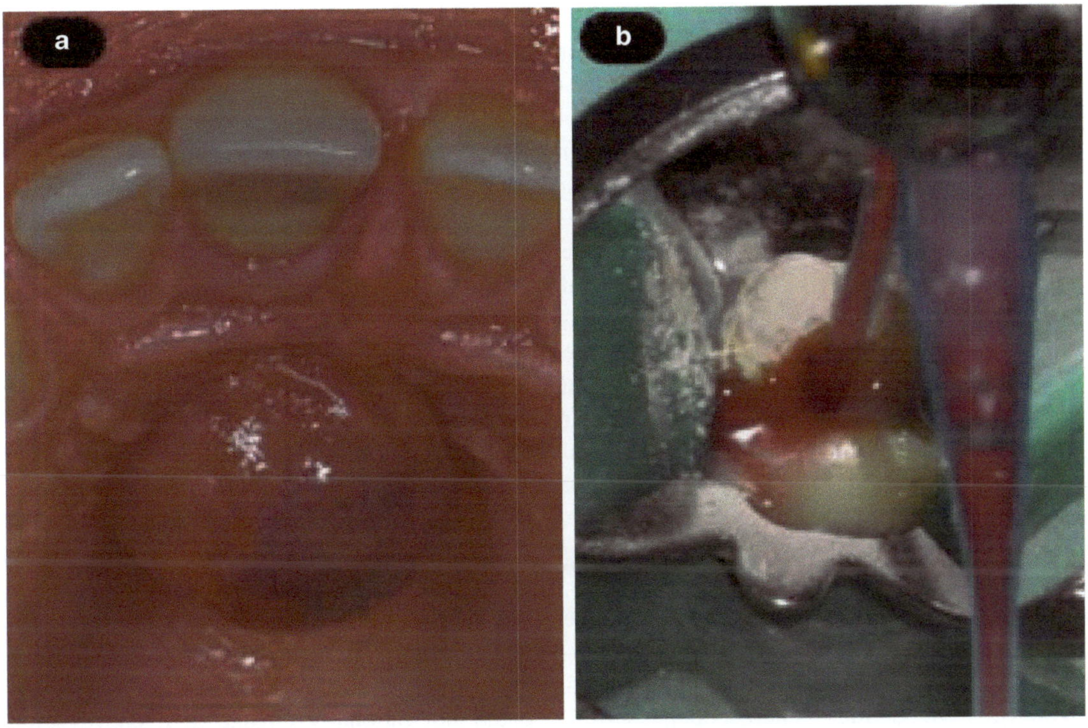

Fig. 6.14 (a) A large palatal lesion filled with purulent exudate is aspirated (b) using apical negative pressure via the root canal system of associated central incisor (Courtesy of Dr. Filippo Santarcangelo, Bari, Italy)

hemorrhage or when the need for intravenous medications is indicated.

3. Pain control can range from local anesthesia to analgesics.
4. Refer to an otolaryngologist when the maxillary sinus is involved or a nephrologist if the urine appears unusually dark.
5. Use external cold compresses for one day to reduce swelling.
6. After the first day, warm mouth rinses will stimulate blood flow.
7. Daily recall is required to monitor recovery.
8. Antibiotics are not always required but are reserved in cases of high risk or evidence of secondary infection.
9. Corticosteroids are often given, but their use is controversial.
10. Further treatment like surgical intervention, tooth extraction, or sinus procedures must be assessed.

Informed Consent

Fifty years ago, John Ingle published the first modern and extremely well-referenced endodontic textbook: *Endodontics* [71]. That all-inclusive work of the day explained the use of silver points, culturing techniques, and all that was known about NaOCl extrusion in a single sentence. "Care must be taken not to seat the needle tightly in the canal or the solution may be forced through the apical foramina and produce a painful apical periodontitis." Nine years later, the first published NaOCl report of apical extrusion through the apex of an upper second premolar was published; the authors described facial swelling and bleeding into the tissue causing the patient discomfort and distress, "However, recovery occurred in a few days" [72]. In the succeeding decades, endodontics materials, methods, and technology have advanced into the ultramodern age characterized by NiTi instrumentation, electronic apex locators, digital radiography, endodontic microscope, CBCT technology, and the realization that Becker's publication would be followed by NaOCl apical extrusion case histories that included severe sequelae including at least one life-threatening event [14] and some reports of permanent facial nerve damage [16]. In just the last two years, the profession has learned that the direct intraosseous infusion route can deliver NaOCl directly into the circulatory system, without the need to wedge a needle into the root canal [10].

Despite the professions' knowledge concerning the often morbid dangers relative to the NaOCl extrusion incident, it has failed to heed the obligation to warn the patient about the use of NaOCl. Pelka concluded his case history: "Because of this fact and the number of reported cases, it is very important to include the adverse reactions of NaOCl into the normal written information provided to the patient before endodontic treatment. Without such written consent, NaOCl should not be used as an irrigation solution during endodontic therapy." As of this writing, the American Association of Endodontists has a position statement on its website entitled: "Informed Consent Guidelines" [73]. Careful reading of this position paper does not mention a word about the NaOCl extrusion incident; it is quite vague about exactly what the patient needs to know, and it ends with a statement: "These guidelines are not to be considered legal advice. Members should consider their own particular needs and on the basis of those needs, draft forms and procedures for use in their own offices. Recognizing that state statutes regarding informed consent vary, it is recommended that members consult their state statutes when developing their own informed consent forms. A copy of your state statute can be obtained from your attorney or by writing to the local county bar association where you practice or reside."

Like the AAE's position statement, it's beyond this author's, editor's, or publisher's professional field to offer legal advice. That said, the clinician must also understand the therapeutic privilege that permits clinicians to tailor (and even withhold) information when, but only when, its disclosure would so upset a patient that he or she could not rationally engage in a conversation about therapeutic options and consequences. The therapeutic privilege itself can vary from state to state as exemplified in two different opinions. The first is entitled: "Legal and Ethical Myths About Informed Consent" [74]. The second is entitled: "Don't lie, but don't tell the whole truth: The Therapeutic Privilege is it ever justified?" [75]. Accordingly, in order to arrive at a correct and proper informed consent document relative to the NaOCl incident, every practicing dentist must consult his or her own attorney on a state-by-state basis when considering all aspects of informed consent, including the therapeutic privilege. The University of Washington School of Law maintains a convenient resource regarding informed consent laws in the United States on a state-by-state basis [76].

In the alternative to an informed consent document dealing with the NaOCl extrusion incident, Rochelle, an ABOTA [American Board of Trial Advocates], has published an opinion entitled: Has The Doctor's Duty To Warn Been Replaced By the Need For The Doctor To Simply Make The Best Decision For The Patient? The entire text can be read at this website [77]. Rochelle based his opinion on the Johnson v. American Standard, Inc. 43 Cal. 4th 56 (2008) case that recognized the "sophisticated user" doctrine as a defense to both negligence and shift product liability claims based on failure to warn. Rochelle states that the Johnson case is the latest in a trend of decisions that act to relieve the manufacturer of a duty to warn the ultimate user (patient) and places the duty on the doctor to warn the patient. Rochelle's opinion is quoted in Disinfection of Root Canal Systems [78]: "that doctor has the affirmative duty to discuss that product with the patient. Alternatively, has medical science progressed to the degree of specialization that the doctor has the duty to simply select the new, lesser risk device? An example of such a newer medical device recently described in the peer review literature is the EndoVac (Kerr (SybronEndo) Endodontics, Orange, CA) delivery system for endodontic irrigation. Previously, the device utilized for irrigation in the root canal was a simple syringe to introduce sodium hypochlorite into the root canal for irrigation and debridement, an important and standard part of endodontic treatment. While the occurrence of sodium hypochlorite extrusion is uncommon, under any analysis of product liability law, the EndoVac would be the preferred alternative device. It is superior in that, for a minimal cost, it does not sacrifice treatment efficacy and eliminates the risk of severe debilitating injury that can occur from sodium hypochlorite extrusion from positive pressure."

Conclusion

In light of the cytotoxicity of the sodium hypochlorite (NaOCl), its extrusion from the root canal will affect the periapical tissue and may cause the patient a series of complications of variable clinical significance, often beginning with postoperative pain [21].

This does not imply that NaOCl can or should be excluded as an endodontic irrigant; in fact, its use is essential to achieve adequate chemical debridement. What this does imply is that it must be delivered safely.

Apical negative pressure devices such as the EndoVac have been shown to enable irrigants to safely reach the apical one third in voluminous amounts and help overcome apical vapor lock (air entrapment at the apical one third) as well as remove tissue and bacteria throughout the root canal system [80–82].

Apart from being able to avoid air entrapment, the EndoVac system is also advantageous in its ability to deliver irrigants safely to working length without causing their undue extrusion into the periapex [29, 80, 83], as long as manufacturer's recommendations are followed, thereby avoiding NaOCl incidents.

Note and Acknowledgement Figure 11: The pressures recorded for the macro cannula were not reported in the Khan study [59] but were mentioned in Goode [79] as unpublished results. Goode coauthored the Khan study [59].

Dr. John Schoeffel, inventor and royalty recipient (SybronEndo/Kerr Endodontics) of the EndoVac system, originally envisioned the concept of NaOCl traveling in the venous system after scrutinizing the Bradford study [68] and the associated references. I am grateful for his help in explaining the concept of intraosseous fluid delivery and the intracanal fluid dynamics that affect periapical pressure as well as his assistance in organizing the logic path and graphics for this chapter.

Dr. Ovidiu Cioanu (www.ovidiu.ca) produced graphics 4 B and C.

References

1. Black GV. Special dental pathology. Chicago: Medico-Dental Publishing Co; 1915. p. 295.
2. Prinz H. Diseases of the soft structures of the teeth and their treatment. Philadelphia: Lea & Febiger; 1928. p. 225.
3. Bender IB, Seltzer S, Turkenkopf S. To culture or not to culture? Oral Surg Oral Med Oral Pathol. 1964;18:527–40.
4. Seltzer S, Bender IB. Cognitive dissonance in endodontics. Oral Surg Oral Med Oral Pathol. 1965;20:505–16.
5. Spånberg LSW. Editorial. Oral Surg Oral Med Oral Pathol Oral Radiol Endod. 2006;102:577–8.
6. Ricucci D, Siqueira Jr JF. Biofilms and apical periodontitis: study of prevalence and association with clinical and histopathologic findings. J Endod. 2010;36(8):1277–88.
7. Nair PN, Henry S, Cano V, et al. Microbial status of apical root canal system of human mandibular first molars with primary apical periodontitis after "one-visit" endodontic treatment. Oral Surg Oral Med Oral Pathol Oral Radiol Endod. 2005;99:231–52.
8. Clegg MS, Vertucci FJ, Walker C, Belanger M, Britto LR. The effect of exposure to irrigant solutions on apical dentin biofilms in vitro. J Endod. 2006;32(5):434–7.
9. Pashley EL, Birdsong NL, Bowman K, Pashley DH. Cytotoxic effects of NaOCl on vital tissue. J Endod. 1985;11(12):525–8.
10. Zhu WC, Gyamfi J, Niu LN, Schoeffel GJ, Liu SY, Santarcangelo F, Khan S, Tay KC, Pashley DH, Tay FR. Anatomy of sodium hypochlorite accidents involving facial ecchymosis – a review. J Dent. 2013;41(11):935–48.
11. Zairi A, Lambrianidis T. Accidental extrusion of sodium hypochlorite into the maxillary sinus. Quintessence Int. 2008;39(9):745–8.
12. Oreadi D, Hendi J, Papageorge MB. A clinico-pathologic correlation. J Mass Dent Soc. 2010;59(3):44–6.
13. Wang S, Chung M, Cheng J, Chen C, Shieh Y. Sodium hypochlorite accidentally extruded beyond the apical foramen. J Med Sci. 2010;30(2):61–5.
14. Bowden J, Ethunandan M, Brennan P. Life-threatening airway obstruction secondary to hypochlorite extrusion during root canal treatment. Oral Surg Oral Med Oral Pathol Oral Radiol Endod. 2006;101:402–4.
15. Markose G, Cotter CJ, Hislop WS. Facial atrophy following accidental subcutaneous extrusion of sodium hypochlorite. Br Dent J. 2009;206(5):263–4.
16. Pelka M, Petschelt A. Permanent mimic musculature and nerve damage caused by sodium hypochlorite: a case report. Oral Surg Oral Med Oral Pathol Oral Radiol Endod. 2008;106(3):e80–3.
17. Bosch-Aranda ML, Vázquez-Delgado E, Gay-Escoda C. Atypical odontalgia: a systematic review following the evidence-based principles of dentistry. Cranio. 2011;29(3):219–26.
18. Peck BW, Workeneh B, Kadikoy H, Abdellatif A. Sodium hypochlorite-induced acute kidney injury. Saudi J Kidney Dis Transpl. 2014;25(2):381–4.
19. Kleier DJ, Averbach RE, Mehdipour O. The sodium hypochlorite accident: experience of diplomates of the American Board of Endodontics. J Endod. 2008;34(11):1346–50.
20. Salzgeber RM, Brilliant JD. An in vivo evaluation of the penetration of an irrigating solution in root canals. J Endod. 1977;3(10):394–8.
21. Gondim Jr E, Setzer F, dos-Carmo CD, Kim S. Postoperative pain after the application of two different irrigation devices in a prospective randomized clinical trial irrigation devices in a prospective randomized clinical trial. J Endod. 2010;36(8):1295–301.
22. Witton R, Brennan PA. Severe tissue damage and neurological deficit following extravasation of sodium hypochlorite solution during routine endodontic treatment. Br Dent J. 2005;198(12):749–50.
23. Boutsioukis C, Psimma Z, van der Sluis LW. Factors affecting irrigant extrusion during root canal irrigation: a systematic review. Int Endod J. 2013;46(7):599–618.
24. Psimma Z, Boutsioukis C, Vasiliadis L, Kastrinakis E. A new method for real-time quantification of irrigant extrusion during root canal irrigation ex vivo. Int Endod J. 2013;46(7):619–31.
25. Psimma Z, Boutsioukis C, Kastrinakis E, Vasiliadis L. Effect of needle insertion depth and root canal curvature on irrigant extrusion ex vivo. J Endod. 2013;39(4):521–4.
26. Boutsioukis C, Psimma Z, Kastrinakis E. The effect of flow rate and agitation technique on irrigant extrusion ex vivo. Int Endod J. 2014;47(5):487–96.
27. Mehra P, Clancy C, Wu J. Formation of a facial hematoma during endodontic therapy. J Am Dent Assoc. 2000;131(1):67–71.
28. Hülsmann M, Rödig T, Nordmeye S. Complications during root canal irrigation. Endod Topics 2009. 2007;16(1):27–63.
29. Desai P, Himel V. Comparative safety of various intracanal irrigation systems. J Endod. 2009;35(4):545–9.
30. Hauman CH, Chandler NP, Tong DC. Endodontic implications of the maxillary sinus: a review. Int Endod J. 2002;35(2):127–41.
31. Ehrich DG, Brian Jr JD, Walker WA. Sodium hypochlorite accident: inadvertent injection into the maxillary sinus. J Endod. 1993;19(4):180–2.
32. Kavanagh CP, Taylor J. Inadvertent injection of sodium hypochlorite into the maxillary sinus. Br Dent J. 1998;185(7):336–7.
33. Sleiman P. Irrigation for the root canal and nothing but the root canal. Roots. 2012;4:32–33.
34. Mehdipour O, Kleier DJ, Averbach RE. Anatomy of sodium hypochlorite accidents. Compend Contin Educ Dent. 2007;28(10):544–6.
35. Hülsmann M, Hahn W. Complications during root canal irrigation – literature review and case reports. Int Endod J. 2000;33(3):186–93.
36. de Sermeño RF, da Silva LA, Herrera H, Herrera H, Silva RA, Leonardo MR. Tissue damage after sodium hypochlorite extrusion during root canal treatment.

Oral Surg Oral Med Oral Pathol Oral Radiol Endod. 2009;108(1):e46–9.
37. Rickles NH, Joshi BA. A possible case in a human and an investigation in dogs of death from air embolism during root canal therapy. J Am Dent Assoc. 1963;67:397–404.
38. Davies JM, Campbell LA. Fatal air embolism during dental implant surgery: a report of three cases. Can J Anaesth. 1990;37(1):112–21.
39. Manisali Y, Yücel T, Erişen R. Overfilling of the root. A case report. Oral Surg Oral Med Oral Pathol. 1989;68(6):773–5.
40. Drake R, Vogl AW, Mitchell AWM. Gray's anatomy for students. 2nd ed. London: Churchill Livingstone/Elsevier; 2009. Chapter 8.
41. Schoeffel GJ. The dynamic response characteristics of the periodontal ligament at the apical foramen to increased intracanal gaseous pressure. Harvard University Master Thesis, Boston; 1980, A-5.
42. Drinker CK, Drinker KR, Lund CC. The circulation in the mammalian bone marrow. Am J Physiol. 1922;62:1–92.
43. Draenert K, Draenert Y. The vascular system of bone marrow. Scan Electron Microsc. 1980;4:113–22.
44. Oni OO, Stafford H, Gregg PJ. An investigation of the routes of venous drainage from the bone marrow of the human tibial diaphysis. Clin Orthop Relat Res. 1988;230:237–44.
45. de Saint-Georges L, Miller SC. The microcirculation of bone and marrow in the diaphysis of the rat hemopoietic long bones. Anat Rec. 1992;233:169–77.
46. Kofoed H. Intraosseous pressure, gas tension and bone blood flow in normal and pathological situations: a survey of methods and results. Bone Circulation and Vascularization in Normal and Pathological Conditions. NATO ASI Ser. 1993;247:101–11.
47. Gurkan UA, Akkus O. The mechanical environment of bone marrow: a review. Ann Biomed Eng. 2008;36:1978–91.
48. Helm M, Breschinski W, Lampl L, et al. Intraosseous puncture in preclinical emergency medicine. Experiences of an air rescue service. Anaesthesist. 1996;45(12):1196–202.
49. Josefson A. A new method of treatment – intraosseous injections. Acta Med Scand. 1934;81:550–64.
50. Arbeiter HI, Greengard J. Tibial bone marrow infusion in infants. J Pediatr. 1944;25:1–12.
51. Elston JT, Jayne RV, Kaump DH, et al. Intraosseous infusions in infants. Am J Clin Pathol. 1947;17:143–50.
52. Heinild S, Sondergaard T, Tudvad F. Bone marrow infusion in childhood: experiences from a thousand infusions. J Pediatr. 1947;30:400–12.
53. Tocantins LM. Rapid absorption of substances injected into the bone marrow. Proc Soc Exp Biol Med. 1940;45:292–6.
54. Tocantins LM, O'Neil JF. Infusions of blood and other fluids into the general circulation via the bone marrow. Surg Gynecol Obstet. 1941;73:281–7.
55. Tocantins LM, O'Neil JF, Jones HW. Infusions of blood and other fluids via the bone marrow. JAMA. 1941;117:1229–34.
56. Tocantins LM, O'Neil JF. Complications of intraosseous therapy. Ann Surg. 1945;122:266–77.
57. Brown R. Intraosseous anesthesia: a review. J Calif Dent Assoc. 1999;27:785–92.
58. Park E, Shen Y, Khakpour M, Haapasalo M. Apical pressure and extent of irrigant flow beyond the needle tip during positive-pressure irrigation in an in vitro root canal model. J Endod. 2013;39(4):511–5.
59. Khan S, Niu LN, Eid AA, Looney SW, Didato A, Roberts S, et al. Periapical pressures developed by nonbinding irrigation needles at various irrigation delivery rates. J Endod. 2013;39(4):529–33.
60. Boutsioukis C, Lambrianidis T, Kastrinakis E. Irrigant flow within a prepared root canal using various flow rates: a computational fluid dynamics study. Int Endod J. 2009;42(2):144–55.
61. Boutsioukis C, Gogos C, Verhaagen B, Versluis M, Kastrinakis E, Van der Sluis LW. The effect of apical preparation size on irrigant flow in root canals evaluated using an unsteady computational fluid dynamics model. Int Endod J. 2010;43(10):874–81.
62. Boutsioukis C, Gogos C, Verhaagen B, Versluis M, Kastrinakis E, Van der Sluis LW. The effect of root canal taper on the irrigant flow: evaluation using an unsteady computational fluid dynamics model. Int Endod J. 2010;43(10):909–16.
63. Boutsioukis C, Lambrianidis T, Verhaagen B, Versluis M, Kastrinakis E, Wesselink PR, van der Sluis LW. The effect of needle-insertion depth on the irrigant flow in the root canal: evaluation using an unsteady computational fluid dynamics model. J Endod. 2010;36(10):1664–8.
64. Boutsioukis C, Verhaagen B, Versluis M, Kastrinakis E, Wesselink PR, van der Sluis PR. Evaluation of irrigant flow in the root canal using different needle types by an unsteady computational fluid dynamics model. J Endod. 2010;36(5):875–97.
65. Hess W. The anatomy of the root-canals of the teeth of the permanent dentition. New York: Wood; 1925.
66. Boutsioukis C, Lambrianidis T, Kastrinakis E, Bekiaroglou P. Measurement of pressure and flow rates during irrigation of a root canal ex vivo with three endodontic needles. Int Endod J. 2007;40(7):504–13.
67. Tegginmani VS, Chawla VL, Kahate MM, Jain VS. Hypochlorite accident – a case report. Endodontology (Indian Endod Soc). 2011;23:89–94.
68. Bradford CE, Eleazer PD, Downs KE, Scheetz JP. Apical pressures developed by needles for canal irrigation. J Endod. 2002;28(4):333–5.
69. Spencer HR, Ike V, Brennan PA. Review: the use of sodium hypochlorite in endodontics—potential complications and their management. Br Dent J. 2007;202(9):555–9.
70. Hales JJ, Jackson CR, Everett AP, Moore SH. Treatment protocol for the management of a sodium hypochlorite accident during endodontic therapy. Gen Dent. 2001;49:278–81.
71. Ingle JI. Endodontics. Philadelphia: Lea & Febiger; 1965. p. 175–6.

72. Becket GL, Cohen S, Borer R. The sequelae of accidentally injecting sodium hypochlorite beyond the root apex. Oral Surg. 1974;38:633–8.
73. http://www.aae.org/uploadedfiles/publications_and_research/guidelines_and_position_statements/informedconsent.pdf.
74. Meisel A, Kuczewski M. Legal and ethical myths about informed consent. Arch Intern Med. 1996;156(22):2521–6.
75. Edwin AK. Don't lie but don't tell the whole truth: the therapeutic privilege is it ever justified? Ghana Med J. 2008;42(4):156–61.
76. http://uwtortswikimiller.wikifoundry.com/page/California [Note to reader: Opening this website will open on California, but the other states are listed on the left].
77. http://rochellegriffith.com/2009/11/02/has-the-doctors-duty-to-warn-been-replaced-by-the-need-to-simply-make-the-best-decision-for-the-patient-endovac-use-in-root-canals.
78. Cohenca N. Disinfection of root canal systems: the treatment of apical periodontitis. Ames: Wiley; 2014. p. 163.
79. Goode N, Khan S, Eid AA, Niu LN, Gosier J, Susin LF, Pashley DH, Tay FR. Wall shear stress effects of different endodontic irrigation techniques and systems. J Dent. 2013;41(7):636–41.
80. Nielsen BA, Craig Baumgartner J. Comparison of the EndoVac system to needle irrigation of root canals. J Endod. 2007;33:611–5.
81. Ribeiro EM, Silva-Sousa YTC, Souza-Gabriel AE, Sousa-Neto MD, Lorencetti KT, Silva SRC. Debris and smear removal in flattened root canals after use of different irrigant agitation protocols. Microsc Res Tech. 2012;75:781–90.
82. Shin S-J, Kim H-K, Jung I-Y, Lee C-Y, Lee S-J, Kim E. Comparison of the cleaning efficacy of a new apical negative pressure irrigating system with conventional irrigation needles in the root canals. Oral Surg Oral Med Oral Pathol Oral Radiol Endod. 2010;109:479–84.
83. Malentacca A, Uccioli U, Zangari D, Lajolo C, Fabiani C. Efficacy and safety of various active irrigation devices when used with either positive or negative pressure: an in vitro study. J Endod. 2012;38:1622–6.

The Role of the Patency File in Endodontic Therapy

7

Jorge Vera

Abstract

The use of a patency file in endodontics remains a controversial issue. Using a small K file inserted passively and intentionally by 1 mm through the foramen is advocated by some investigators and clinicians as an important procedure designed to help the cleaning and shaping process, to aid in delivering irrigating solutions to "hard to reach areas" of the root canal system, as well as to the apical third. This procedure is even cited as an important step in achieving clinical success. Detractors of the use of the patency file have concerns with the increased extrusion of debris and irrigants through the foramen, higher incidence of postoperative pain, lack of proper studies showing its ability to improve cleaning of the complex anatomy of the root canal system in the apical third, and limited information on the influence of the use of the patency file on the prognosis of the root canal treatment. Histological sections of the apical thirds of teeth that were appropriately cleaned with the use of this procedure and then examined usually show remnants of organic tissue and biofilm. The objective of this chapter is to analyse the current literature that addresses the use of the patency file in endodontic therapy.

Introduction

Proper debridement of the root canal system is essential when attempting to obtain favourable long-term prognosis in endodontics. Elimination of organic tissue and reduction of the microbial bio-burden remain a difficult task, especially in the apical third of the root canal system because of anatomical irregularities that compromise the action of irrigants and the instruments used to shape the canals [16].

Microorganisms residing in these complex areas may develop or perpetuate apical periodontitis if they are able to get sufficient nutrients, either from organic tissue that was not properly removed during the chemo-mechanical preparation of the canal or by getting nutrients from

J. Vera, DDS
Department of Endodontics,
University of Tlaxcala Mexico,
Madrid 4920-101 2A seccion Gabriel Pastor, Puebla
72420, Puebla, Mexico
e-mail: jveraro@yahoo.com.mx

B. Basrani (ed.), *Endodontic Irrigation: Chemical Disinfection of the Root Canal System*,
DOI 10.1007/978-3-319-16456-4_7

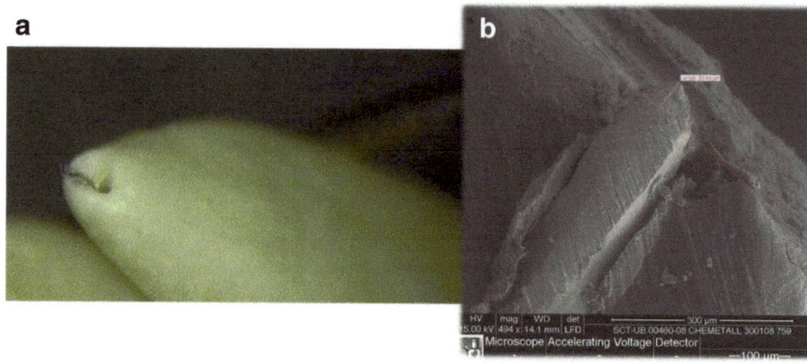

Fig. 7.1 (**a**, **b**) A patency file is a small K file inserted 1 mm through the foramen (Courtesy of Fernando Durán-Sindreu)

periradicular tissues, allowing them to release their by-products [21, 27]

Therefore, it has been established that to successfully clean this apical area, irrigants should be able to penetrate to the full length of the root canal, which should be kept free of packed debris.

One popular method of avoiding accumulation of tissue and debris is by using a *patency file*. This has been described in numerous texts and articles as using a small 10 K file which is inserted passively and intentionally by 1 mm through the foramen, thus preventing ledge formation, blockages, and perhaps perforations in this crucial area [5, 7, 11, 12, 31] (Figs. 7.1 and 7.2).

The patency file would ideally prevent dentin chips from being compacted into the apical portion of the root canal and from blocking access to this area for instruments and irrigants [1], as well as keeping the foramen open in case drainage is needed from the periapical tissues [24].

The use of a patency file remains controversial, however, because (i) there are no studies showing its efficacy in terms of cleaning and shaping, (ii) periradicular tissues may be irritated, and most importantly (iii) there are no controlled studies showing if using it would improve the prognosis of endodontically treated teeth, either vital teeth or teeth with infected pulp and periapical periodontitis (Fig. 7.3).

Until now, only one published study has assessed the prevalence of teaching apical patency in US dental schools [8]. The authors conducted a survey in which they got back 48 responses indicating that only 50 % of the schools were teaching the use of the patency file to their students. At the time of the survey, 16 out of 24 programs were teaching the use of patency to their undergraduate students. Nineteen out of 36 schools that had a graduate program were teaching the patency concept.

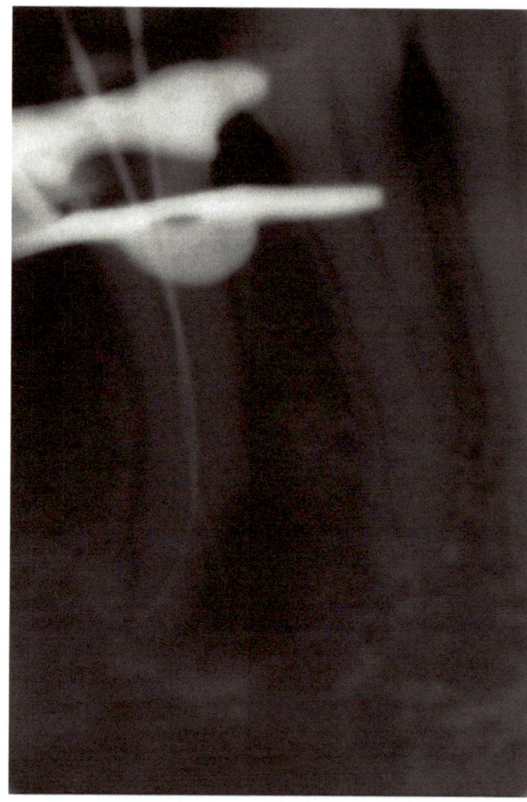

Fig. 7.2 Patency obtained in a two-canal right second lower premolar

Concerning the size of the file used in the schools using patency, the size 10 K file was the most popular file used (42 % of respondents), 33 % taught the use of a size 15 K file, and

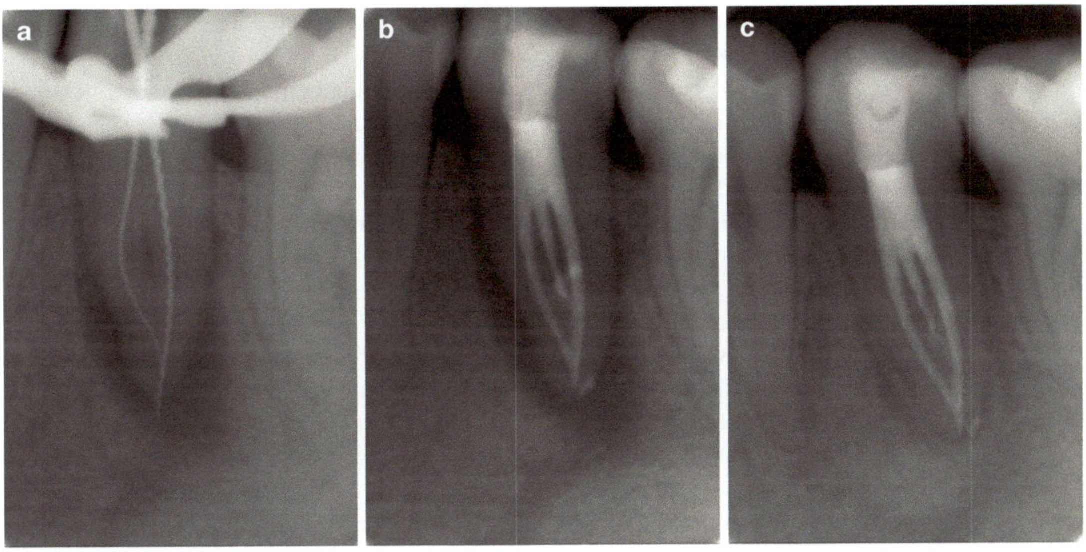

Fig. 7.3 (**a, b**) Treatment of a left second lower premolar. Patency was maintained throughout the cleaning and shaping procedure. (**c**) Two-year follow-up

another 25 % recommended the use of a larger size 20 K file. Another question addressed comments against the use of the patency file. Popular responses included concerns regarding the projection of debris into the periapical tissues with concomitant irritation and the lack of proof of an increased success rate. Thus, the purpose of the present literature review is to dissect studies addressing the use and contraindications for the patency file in endodontics.

Role of the Patency File in Shaping, Irrigating, and Cleaning the Root Canal System

On Apical Transportation

Some authors have evaluated the influence of the patency file on the transportation of the apical root canal or the foramen. Goldberg and Massone [13] evaluated ex vivo the apical transportation caused by #10, #15, #20, and #25 K files in 30 human maxillary lateral incisors. Photographic slides of the foramen were taken after the use of every instrument. Transportation was shown in 18 of the 30 specimens. They proved that transportation occurred even after the use of the small 10 K file in five cases in one of the treatment groups (55.5 %). They further stated that because the foramen commonly exits laterally from the apex, it would not be uncommon that the patency file would lean to one of the walls of the apical foramen, modifying its shape in curved canals. Furthermore, Gutierrez et al. proved that a cementum layer could fracture at the apex after penetration of a 15 K file through the main foramen [15].

By contrast, another ex vivo study found that when a size 08 K-Flexofile or a size 10 stainless steel reamer was used, no transportation was found in the majority of the 102 mesiobuccal canals of maxillary and mandibular molars [30]. The authors evaluated root canal transportation at the major foramen by comparing photographs before and after instrumentation. Similar results were obtained by Tsesis et al. [41]. In their study, 10 K patency files were employed after the use of each instrument with the balanced force technique or the Lightspeed system. The study compared transportation to those similar groups in which patency files were not used and then compared superimposed digital images obtained before and after treatment. The authors not only found that using a patency file helped in maintaining working length but also reported no differences in the degree of apical transportation.

On Extrusion of Irrigants and Debris Through the Apical Foramen

Concerning the extrusion of debris through the foramen during cleaning and shaping procedures, differences in the experimental design between published ex vivo studies as well as differences with what would be in vivo clinical situations make it difficult to extrapolate the results of extrusion from ex vivo studies to clinical reality.

Two studies have shown that even without the use of a patency file, extrusion of debris/irrigants occurs frequently in vitro. Lambrianidis et al. [19] used thirty-three human maxillary incisors in their study in which debris and irrigant were measured after being extruded into a glass vial. All root canals were instrumented to the apical constriction with the step-back technique, but a patency file was not used. The total volume of irrigant used per canal was 10 ml. After this procedure, the apical constriction was further enlarged and the measurement was done again. They found more extrusion when the constriction remained intact and concluded that with more instrumentation, the formation of an apical plug could have helped prevent the extrusion of the irrigant, just as it was shown in a previous study assessing extrusion [20].

Another study used a colour-changing reagent in acrylic receptacles in contact with the root tips of maxillary molars [9]. The authors assessed the extrusion of the irrigant without any instrumentation technique used to flare the canals. In phase one of the study, irrigation was done with 3 ml of NaOCl, placing the needle at the entrance of the canal and injecting without pressure after establishing apical patency. In phase two, size 10 and 15 K-Flexofile were used as patency files; then the canals were irrigated again. The study reported extrusion in 9/17 specimens after the use of the 10 K file for patency from phase one and in all specimens from phase two.

These are examples of how variable the results can be when determining this sensitive issue, because the kind of extrusion reported ex vivo would lead to postoperative pain and flare-ups in the vast majority of cases in vivo. By contrast, clinically postoperative pain after root canal therapy occurs with very low incidence. In addition, not blocking the foramen when using ex vivo specimens would not mimic the in vivo situation, allowing for a larger amount of debris and irrigants to be extruded through the foramen. In vivo, the vapour lock effect present in a closed system would result in different intra-canal hydrodynamics [39].

Conclusions From these results we could conclude that using a small patency file should not alter the anatomy of the apical root canal in a way that could affect clinical results. Further comparative studies with strictly controlled variables should address the influence of a patency file on debris extrusion through the foramen. It is not clear if the use of a patency file would lead to more debris/irrigants being extruded through the apical foramen. Clinically, the use of a patency file helps to maintain working length and to avoid packing debris in the apical third of the complex root canal anatomy.

Role of the Patency File on Irrigant Penetration into the Apical Third of Root Canals

Irrigants should be able to reach the apical third with enough concentration and contact time so that they can dissolve organic tissue, kill planktonic bacteria, and disturb or eliminate biofilms attached to the dentin in the very complex apical anatomy. Salzgeber and Brilliant showed [29] that irrigants (Hypaque) could not reach the apical third of human root canals that contained vital tissue in vivo. They also showed that if the canals were flared to small apical sizes, the irrigant was detected at the apex and, in some instances, in the periapical lesions in nonvital teeth. Instrumentation techniques used at that time would probably push a larger amount of NaOCl and debris through the foramen because of the "pumping" action of hand files. However, comparative studies in vivo have not been carried out to prove such a statement.

In a recent in vivo study using a radiopaque solution Claritrast 300 (ioversol 678 mg/mL) mixed with 5.25 % NaOCl, which was approximated in density and viscosity to that of NaOCl alone, 40 human root canals considered small (buccal roots of maxillary molars, mesial roots of mandibular molars, and both roots of maxillary first premolars) were irrigated with the solution to within 2 ml from the working length (WL) after the use of every rotary instrument. Then, passive ultrasonic irrigation (PUI) was used in both groups for 1 min at the end of the procedure. In group one, apical patency was maintained during the shaping and cleaning procedure with a 10 K file, but not in group two. A blinded calibrated reader determined the presence or absence of the radiopaque irrigating solution in the apical 2 mm of the treated roots. Statistical analysis showed that there was significantly more irrigant after the use of PUI when a patency file had been used throughout the cleaning and shaping procedure compared to the group where it was not [42] (Fig. 7.4).

In a different study where the same methodology was used [45], penetration of irrigants into the apical 2 mm of 43 large root canals (palatal roots of maxillary molars, distal roots of mandibular molars with one canal, and anterior teeth measuring between 19 and 21 mm) was measured. A 27-G side-vented needle was inserted to 2 ml from the WL with gentle in and out movements and maintaining apical patency, demonstrated a higher incidence of the mixture of NaOCl/radiopaque solution in the apical 2 mm of the root canals compared to those teeth where apical patency was not maintained throughout the cleaning and shaping procedure. It was concluded that the low flow rate used was not very efficient in delivering the irrigant into the apical 2 mm when a patency file was not used.

In both of these studies, the lack of penetration of the irrigant deep into the apical 2 mm could have been caused by the presence of the remaining pulp tissue in the apical anatomy that was not removed adequately by the combination of the cleaning and shaping technique and the dissolving action of NaOCl or the presence of an apical gas bubble or vapour lock effect as proven in

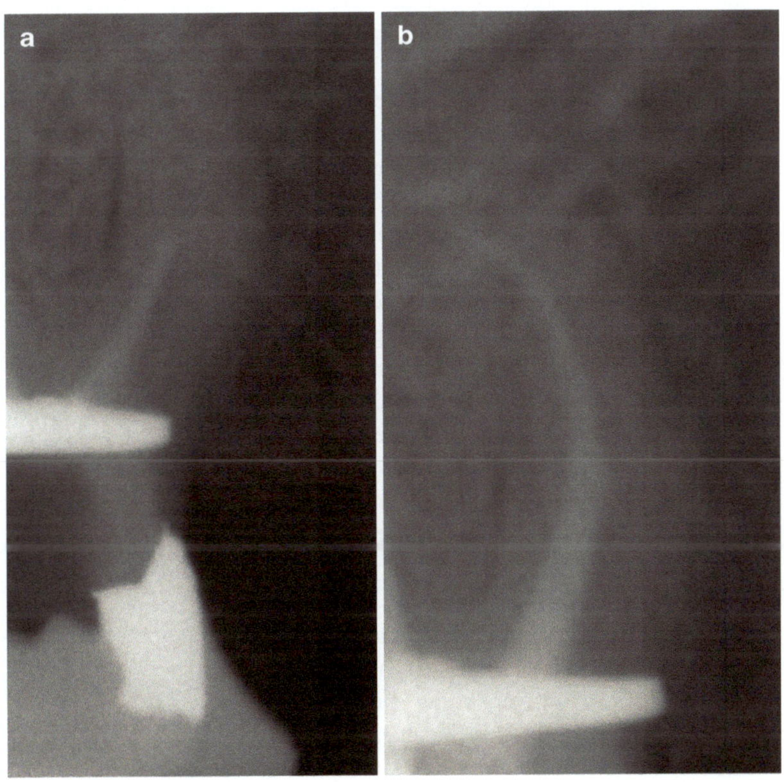

Fig. 7.4 Mixture of a radiopaque solution and NaOCl used as an irrigating solution. (**a**) Passive irrigation without the use of a patency file delivering the solution at 2 mm from the WL. (**b**) After the use of a patency file and passive ultrasonic irrigation

some in vitro studies [39]. Furthermore, the gas bubble could grow larger in size because of the reaction of the irrigant with organic tissue [14]. However, other authors have doubted the presence of a vapour lock if a high enough flow is used while irrigating and by also using an open-ended needle that should be positioned closer to the WL [6]. The advantages and risks involved in irrigating in such a way will be discussed in another chapter of this book.

Besides the role of the patency file in the penetration of irrigants into the difficult-to-reach apical anatomy in human root canals, its influence on the presence of large gas bubbles in the middle and cervical third of human root canals in vivo was evaluated in another study [43]. Apical patency was maintained with a 10 K file in two groups (small and big canals), but not in the other two groups also consisting of both small and large canals. Irrigation was also done using a mixture of 5.25 % NaOCl and the radiopaque solution Claritrast 300, which had been tested in pilot studies to dissolve pulp tissue efficiently. Then, a calibrated reader evaluated the presence of gas bubbles in radiographs that were taken during every step of the cleaning and shaping procedure. It was surprising to note that, when present, these gas bubbles could move in the root canal, but they were not easy to break. Furthermore, when a patency file was not used, the gas bubbles in the middle/cervical third appeared in 40 % of the cases, compared to only in 25 % when the 10 K file was used to maintain patency. Even though the importance of such bubbles may not be much concerning the penetration of the irrigants into the apical third, the consistent presence of these bubbles in the middle and cervical thirds would limit the contact of NaOCl with organic tissue and microorganisms attached to the dentin and hiding in isthmuses and areas where there would be more gas than irrigant during the cleaning and shaping procedure. Some other articles have described this vapour lock effect in closed-ended canals/tubes, preventing irrigating solutions from reaching their apex [10]. However, some studies have mentioned the possibility that the change in composition of the irrigant by mixing NaOCl with a radiopaque solution could also vary the density, and especially its viscosity and surface contact angle, when compared to NaOCl by itself, thus favouring the apical vapour lock effect [6].

Conclusions Using a patency file appears to help irrigants penetrate into the apical 2 mm of the complex anatomy of human root canals both in large and small canals and to prevent gas accumulation in them, at least under the conditions of the aforementioned studies. Whether this in vivo penetration really improves the "cleaning" of the root canal is still not demonstrated and will be discussed further in the following section of this chapter.

The Use and Effect of the Patency File in Cleaning of the Root Canals in Teeth with Vital Pulps

Concerning cleaning and shaping of the apical third, some studies have tested the importance of apical patency during the preparation of the root canal. Some authors have recommended the proper working length to be determined 1–2 mm short of the radiographic apex and avoiding patency [17, 25, 26] (Fig. 7.5).

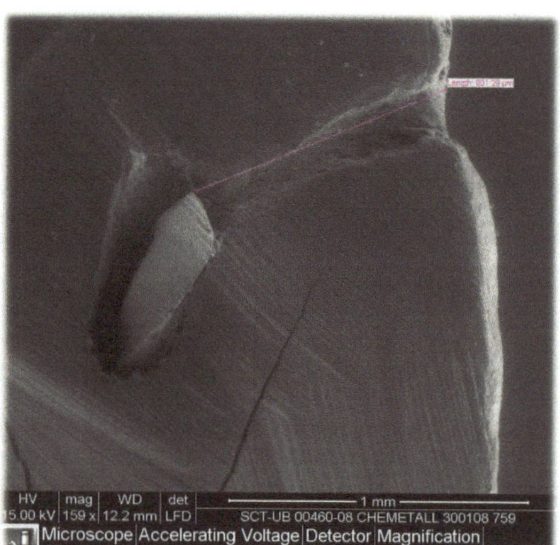

Fig. 7.5 A small K file used short of the foramen. No patency (Courtesy of Fernando Durán-Sindreu)

These authors question and criticize the need for a patency file in cases with vital pulp and actually state that it is contraindicated in cases where there is a clean wound in the apical pulp tissue. A photomicrograph depicting this situation is shown Fig. 7.6, of the buccal root of a maxillary first premolar to be extracted for nonrestorability. The pulp was vital and the canals were instrumented before extraction. Rotary NiTi files were employed, 1 % NaOCl was used as the irrigating solution, and the working length was established 1.5 mm short of the radiographic apex. The section shows an apical delta with undisturbed vital tissue. The use of a patency file in such situations could destroy the connective tissue, impairing or delaying wound healing.

In light of this terminology, it is important to differentiate that the maintenance of apical patency will prevent the blockage of one of the foramens with dentin chips, and not necessarily all of them, because of the complex anatomy of the region (Fig. 7.7). One disadvantage of not using a patency file in noninfected teeth is the possibility of being blocked out or losing working length during instrumentation of the root canal. However, experience and proper use of endodontic instruments should still prevent this accidental procedure. Furthermore, it has been shown clearly that the use of an electronic apex or foramen locator helps determine the ideal position in space for the determination of the optimal working length. The vast majority of studies, as well as indications for the use of different brands of apex locators, recommend advancing the file until the "long" signal is displayed on the screen and then withdrawing it until the display shows "at the foramen" or "slightly short" of the foramen [37]. Therefore, to properly use a device, which is important in modern root canal therapy, a patency file should be used at least once per root canal. The injury that this procedure could potentially inflict on the periapical tissues and the possibility that further use of the patency file two or three more times throughout the shaping and cleaning procedure could increase that injury in a clinically significant manner remain unknown. Interesting discussions on the matter remain academic and possibly without sufficient scientific background to support or avoid the use of this procedure.

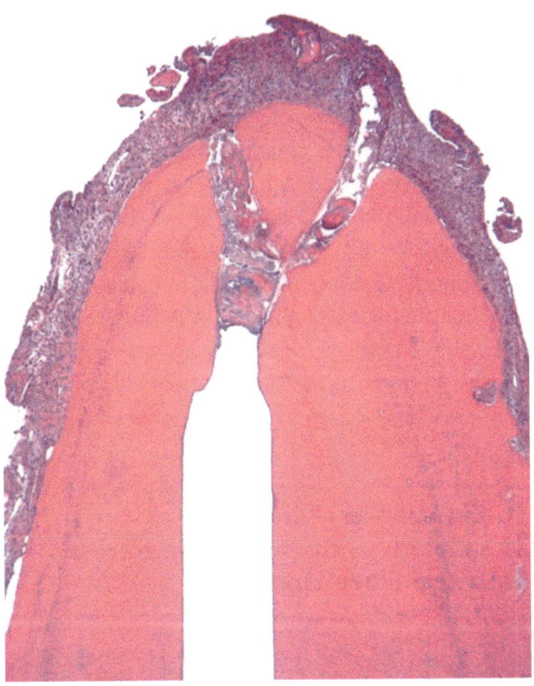

Fig. 7.6 Buccal root of a maxillary first premolar. The pulp was vital and the root canals were instrumented before extraction with NiTi rotary instruments and NaOCl used as the irrigant. WL was established 1.5 mm short of the radiographic apex. Note the apical deltas with undisturbed vital tissue (Courtesy of Domenico Ricucci)

Conclusion The use of a patency file in teeth with noninfected root canals has not proven histologically to aid in cleaning and shaping procedures.

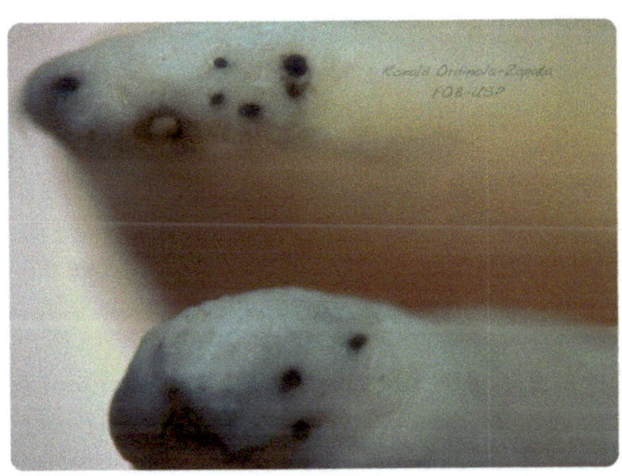

Fig. 7.7 Distal and mesial roots of a mandibular molar showing multiple foramens (Courtesy of Ronald Ordinola-Zapata)

Whether the use of a patency file in such teeth affects healing of the periradicular tissues remains a speculative issue that warrants further histological research. This would be a difficult task since such histology studies could not be performed in humans and animal studies would probably indicate differences from the immunological-inflammatory responses in humans. Nevertheless, achieving patency with a small file is necessary to ensure the proper use of apex locators.

The Use and Effect of the Patency File in Cleaning of the Root Canals in Teeth with Necrotic Pulps and Apical Periodontitis

Some questions have arisen concerning the ability of the patency file to truly clean the foramen. For that, it would have to be instrumented; therefore apical patency and apical cleaning are two procedures that are accomplished differently [36].

The presence of bacteria in the cementum canal [4] is of concern for some authors when attempting to finish the instrumentation technique "short" of the foramen. However, whether the use of a patency file is by itself capable of cleaning these difficult areas has not been demonstrated [44]. In this study, after treating human teeth in vivo and with the use of a patency file in all specimens, masses of amorphous material that included dentin shavings and infected necrotic masses were observed to be packed into the dentin root canal walls and projected in the filling material in all segments of the root canal. Because of the large amount of apical ramifications that remained infected, or contained remnants of organic tissue, as shown in the mentioned study, maintaining one foramen open with the use of the patency file may not help in the cleaning of accessory canals and other foramens present in the same root (Fig. 7.7). Furthermore, in the study by Vera et al., debris and/or bacteria were present in the main foramina in 8 of 13 cases. This clearly shows that in vivo, proper elimination of the bacterial bio-burden and tissue may not depend on the use or lack of use of the patency file. Since there were no teeth that were instrumented without the use of patency, however, proper comparisons could not be made.

In another recent case report in which apical patency was maintained throughout the procedures, with the use of 5 % NaOCl, smear layer removal, and ultrasonic agitation of chlorhexidine, a bacterial biofilm was demonstrated in a network of apical ramifications. This case presents evidence against the concept that patency files are expected to be able to disrupt apical biofilms in vivo; or, at least, these in vivo observations have not been able to demonstrate such a concept [3]. Therefore, some authors have recommended that when pulp necrosis is present, patency should be used only to help maintain proper working length and to avoid packing debris in the apical foramen but that cleaning of the apical foramen be achieved with bigger size files [36]. Other authors have even recommended cleaning the divergent cementum canal with files bigger than the file used to clean the root canal in its apical portion [35]. Whether performing this procedure really helps clean the canal in such a way remains to be demonstrated in histological studies.

Conclusions The use of a patency file has not been proven to aid in the cleaning of accessory canals/foraminas when evaluated histologically. Remnants of tissue and biofilm remain in these "hard to reach areas" despite the use of the patency file. However, it is important to note that the histological information that has been mentioned was obtained either from single cases or from a study where no comparison could be made to cases treated in a similar way but where a patency file had not been used.

The Influence of the Use of a Patency File on Postoperative Pain and Flare-Ups

Controversial results have been presented concerning the possible role of the patency file in causing damage to the periapical tissues [25, 26], in part caused by the file extruding a larger amount of contaminated debris, irrigants, and dentinal chips [19], and, therefore, increasing the incidence of postoperative pain [32].

The use of a patency file is considered by some clinicians as being a non-harmful biologic event because of the great capabilities of the immune and inflammatory system in the periradicular tissues [28]. Some studies or articles have also shown how well these tissues tolerate the use of the file throughout the cleaning and shaping procedures. In fact, one study has shown that contaminated patency files could be disinfected with the NaOCl present in the root canal after irrigation, thus showing that the use of patency would not contaminate or inoculate microorganisms into the periapical tissues [18].

Siqueira et al. [33] evaluated the incidence of postoperative pain. They collected and examined data from 627 teeth that needed to be retreated endodontically or that had necrotic pulps. Only undergraduate students were used as operators, and patients were asked about the occurrence of postoperative pain and its severity. Apical preparation was performed 1 mm short of the root apex with master apical files ranging from #35 to #60. Then, apical patency was confirmed to the radiographic root end with a small file after each larger file. The cleaning and shaping procedures were carried out with 2.5 % NaOCl as the irrigant. The incidence of postoperative pain was calculated for each variable involved in the study, and statistical analysis was applied. Maintaining apical patency did not influence the occurrence of postoperative pain or flare-ups. Torabinejad et al. [40], in a retrospective study, collected and analysed information from 2,000 patients who had undergone root canal therapy and who had been diagnosed as having teeth with necrotic pulps. All 17 operators were endodontists with at least 5 years of practice limited to endodontics. Half of the patients that were treated had reported having had inter-appointment pain or swelling. The other half of the analysed patients reported no pain or complications after the cleaning and shaping procedure. In this study, penetration through the foramen with small instruments during working length determination (in many cases being accidental) had no influence on the incidence of postoperative pain or swelling.

A prospective study on the influence of the patency file on post-endodontic pain was performed by Arias et al. [2]. The incidence, degree, and length of postoperative pain were compared between two groups. In one group of 150 teeth, apical patency was maintained throughout the cleaning and shaping procedures with a size 10 K file, but not in the other group that consisted of 150 teeth in which special care was taken to avoid using any instrument longer than the determined working length. Some other diagnostic factors, including the presence or absence of vitality, preoperative pain, and the location of the tooth in the maxillary or mandibular arch, were taken into consideration. The shaping procedures were performed with the use of Gates-Glidden drills (Dentsply Maillefer) and K-Flexofile instruments (Dentsply Maillefer), and the master apical files used varied from #20 to #30 for small canals and to sizes 25–40 in bigger or wider canals. The working length was confirmed carefully with the use of apex locators. NaOCl was used as the irrigant between all instruments, and all teeth were filled in one appointment. Patients were asked to record the presence or absence of post-endodontic pain and its duration. They were also asked to rate the discomfort as mild, moderate, or severe, using criteria as to whether the discomfort did not require any treatment (mild), the pain was relieved with analgesics (moderate), or the pain did not subside with analgesics (severe). After the patients responded to the questionnaires, 121 teeth were designated as the patency group and 115 as the no patency group. The results were analysed statistically and showed no differences in pain between the patency and the no patency groups. However, some interesting findings were obtained when analysing different variables. For example, when there was preoperative pain present, the number of days in which pain persisted was more in the patency group (up to 3 days more). There was also more postoperative pain in the lower teeth when patency was maintained, and in nonvital teeth the cases where patency was maintained showed less postoperative pain when compared to the non-patency cases.

Conclusions The use of a patency file appears not to increase the incidence of pain or flare-ups when used even in teeth with necrotic pulps or in cases of re-treatment.

The Influence of the Patency File on Prognosis

To some clinicians, the use of a patency file is extremely important. Some clinicians even claim that its use may increase the success rate of endodontic therapy [5, 46]. However, there are few well-controlled studies that have assessed the influence of the patency file in prognosis. Ng et al. [22] investigated the factors involved in the periapical status of teeth following primary or secondary root canal treatment in which radiographic follow-ups were performed in 1170 roots for primary root canal therapy and in 1314 roots for secondary root canal treatment (re-treatment). All teeth were treated by endodontic postgraduate students and follow-ups were performed up to 2–4 years. Cleaning and shaping were done with the use of many different systems and hand files, but if patency was achieved, it was maintained by placing a small file size 8 or 10 to 0.5 mm past the apical terminus, between every instrument used to enlarge the canal. The minimal size to which canals were prepared was a size 30 and flared to different tapers. NaOCl at 2.5–5 % was used as the irrigant.

In the follow-up appointments, many clinical factors were evaluated, including tenderness to percussion or palpation, the quality of the restoration, and, of course, radiographic assessment to detect the presence or absence of radiolucent lesions. In those cases that presented discomfort but where no radiographic evidence of a radiolucent lesion was present, sectional tomography was used. Both pre-calibrated observers were experienced endodontists who were blinded to the treatment procedures used in the cases. In cases where no agreement was achieved, the cases were discussed until an agreement was reached on the outcome, and then statistical analysis was performed. Then, the conditions that improved periapical healing were analysed carefully. Achievement of patency at the canal terminus was found to be one of the significant prognostic factors for root canal treatment. This factor went hand in hand with achieving proper extension of canal cleaning, which needed to be close to the apical terminus. Therefore, despite the fact that the use of a patency file was not compared to those cases reaching proper working length where patency was not maintained, the findings seem to indicate, and agree with previous studies, that teeth where proper working length is not achieved are associated with lower success rates [34, 38].

Concerning tooth survival [23], the event of interest was extraction of the tooth and the time until extraction as measured in months. When entered into the same model, patency at the apical terminus and blockage of the canal during treatment did not have prognostic value when they were analysed together. Interestingly, the authors concluded that the reason may be that canals that get blocked late during the cleaning and shaping procedures may have been cleaned well enough before becoming blocked, thus not affecting the prognosis or survival of those teeth and roots. It was concluded that achieving patency at the apical terminus reduced tooth loss within the first 22 months, but not after that period. It is important to note that no comparison was done between teeth where patency was achieved and then maintained with a small 10 K file going 1 mm long between instruments throughout the cleaning and shaping procedure, versus achieving patency initially and then not using the patency file any further.

Conclusions There are not many scientific studies that have compared the use of a patency file versus not using it, in terms of success in endodontic therapy. Being able to reach the foramen initially does seem to have an impact on the prognosis and survival of endodontically treated teeth. However, no studies have compared, under controlled situations, the prognosis of teeth when using or not using a patency file, as described in the AAE glossary of terms.

References

1. Al-Omari MA, Dummer PM. Canal blockage and debris extrusion with eight preparation techniques. J Endod. 1995;21:154–8.
2. Arias A, Azabal M, Hidalgo JJ, de la Macorra JC. Relationship between postendodontic pain, tooth

diagnostic factors, and apical patency. J Endod. 2009;35:189–92.
3. Arnold M, Ricucci D, Siqueira Jr JF. Infection in a complex network of apical ramifications as the cause of persistent apical periodontitis: a case report. J Endod. 2013;39:1179–84.
4. Baumgartner JC, Falkler WA. Bacteria in the apical 5 mm of infected root canals. J Endod. 1991;17:380–3.
5. Berutti E, Castellucci A. Cleaning and shaping the root canal system. In: Castellucci A, editor. Endodontics, vol. II. 1st ed. Firenze: Il Tridente; 2005. p. 429–57.
6. Boutsioukis C, Kastrinakis E, Lambrianidis T, Verhaagen B, Versluis M, van der Sluis LWM. Formation and removal of apical vapor lock during syringe irrigation: a combined experimental and computational fluid dynamics approach. Int Endod J. 2014;47:191–201. doi:10.1111/iej.12133.
7. Buchanan LS. Cleaning and shaping the root canal system. In: Cohen S, Burns RC, editors. Pathways of the pulp. 5th ed. CV Mosby: St Louis; 1991. p. 166–92.
8. Cailleteau JG, Mullaney TP. Prevalence of teaching apical patency and various instrumentation and obturation techniques in United States dental schools. J Endod. 1997;23:394–6.
9. Camoes IC, Salles MR, Fernando MV, Freitas LF, Gomes CC. Relationship between the size of patency file and apical extrusion of sodium hypochlorite. Indian J Dent Res. 2009;20:426–30.
10. Fazio R, Iacono S. Entrapped gas action for one-dimensional models of capillary dynamics. In: Proceedings of the World Congress on Engineering, July 1–3, 2009, London, vol. II. London: World Congress of Engineering; 2009.
11. Flanders DH. Endodontic patency. How to get it. How to keep it. Why it is so important. N Y State Dent J. 2002;68:30–2.
12. Glossary of endodontic terms. 7th ed. Chicago: American Association of Endodontists; 2003.
13. Golberg F, Massone EJ. Patency file and apical transportation: an in vitro study. J Endod. 2002;28:510–1.
14. Gu L, Kim JR, Ling J, Choi K, Pashley D, Tay F. Review of contemporary irrigant agitation techniques and devices. J Endod. 2009;35:791–804.
15. Gutierrez JH, Brizuela C, Villota E. Human teeth with periapical pathosis after over instrumentation and overfilling of the root canals: a scanning electron microscopic study. Int Endod J. 1999;32:40–8.
16. Haapasalo M, Endal U, Zandi H, Coil JM. Eradication of endodontic infection by instrumentation and irrigation solutions. Endod Top. 2005;10:77–102.
17. Holland R, Sant'anna Júnior A, Souza V, Dezan Junior E, Otoboni Filho JA, Bernabé PFE, Nery MJ, Murata SS. Influence of apical patency and filling material on healing process of dogs' teeth with vital pulp after root canal therapy. Braz Dent J. 2005;16:9–16.
18. Izu KH, Thomas SJ, Zhang P, Izu AE, Michalek S. Effectiveness of sodium hypochlorite in preventing inoculation of periapical tissues with contaminated patency files. J Endod. 2004;30:92–4.
19. Lambrianidis T, Tosounidou E, Tzoanopoulou M. The effect of maintaining apical patency on periapical extrusion. J Endod. 2001;27:696–8.
20. Myers GL, Montgomery SA. Comparison of weights of debris extruded apically by conventional filing and canal master techniques. J Endod. 1991;17:275–9.
21. Nair PN, Henry S, Cano V, Vera J. Microbial status of apical root canal system of human mandibular first molars with primary apical periodontitis after "one-visit" endodontic treatment. Oral Surg Oral Med Oral Pathol Oral Radiol Endod. 2005;99:231–52.
22. Ng YL, Mann V, Gulabivala K. A prospective study of the factors affecting outcomes of nonsurgical root canal treatment: part 1: periapical health. Int Endod J. 2011;44:583–609.
23. Ng YL, Mann V, Gulabivala K. A prospective study of the factors affecting outcomes of non-surgical root canal treatment: part 2: tooth survival. Int Endod J. 2011;44:610–25.
24. Pantera EA. The balanced force technique. Handout–AAE Meeting Honolulu; Apr 1994.
25. Ricucci D. Apical limit of root canal instrumentation and obturation, part 1. Literature review. Int Endod J. 1998;31:384–93.
26. Ricucci D, Langeland K. Apical limit of root canal instrumentation and obturation, part 2. A histological study. Int Endod J. 1998;31:394–409.
27. Ricucci D, Siqueira JF. Fate of the tissue in lateral canals and apical ramifications in response to pathologic conditions and treatment procedures. J Endod. 2010;36:1–15.
28. Ruddle CJ. Cleaning and shaping the root canal system. In: Cohen S, Burns RC, editors. Pathways of the pulp. 8th ed. St Louis: The C.V. Mosby Company; 2002. p. 231.
29. Salzgeber RM, Brilliant JD. An *in vivo* evaluation of the penetration of an irrigating solution in root canals. J Endod. 1977;3:394–8.
30. Sanchez JA, Duran-Sindreu F, Matos MA, Carabaño TG, Bellido MM, Castro SM, Cayón MR. Apical transportation created using three different patency instruments. Int Endod J. 2010;43:560–4.
31. Shilder H. Cleaning and shaping the root canal. Dent Clin N Am. 1974;18:269–96.
32. Siqueira Jr JF. Microbial causes of endodontic flare-ups. Int Endod J. 2003;36:453–63.
33. Siqueira JF, Rocas IN, Favieri A, et al. Incidence of postoperative pain after intracanal procedures based on antimicrobial strategy. J Endod. 2002;28:457–60.
34. Sjögren U, Hägglund B, Sundqvist G, Wing K. Factors affecting the long-term results of endodontic treatment. J Endod. 1990;16:498–504.
35. Souza RA. Endodontia clínica. São Paulo: Santos; 2003.
36. Souza RA. The importance of apical patency and cleaning of the apical foramen on root canal preparation. Braz Dent J. 2006;17:6–9.
37. Stöber EK, de Ribot J, Mercadé M, Vera J, Bueno R, Roig M, Duran-Sindreu F. Evaluation of the raypex 5 and the mini apex locator: an *in vivo* study. J Endod. 2011;10:1349–52.

38. Strindberg LZ. The dependence of the results of pulp therapy on certain factors – an analytical study based on radiographic and clinical follow-up examinations. Acta Odontol Scand. 1956;14:1–175.
39. Tay FR, Gu LS, Schoeffel GJ, et al. Effect of vapor lock on root canal debridement by using a side-vented needle for positive-pressure irrigant delivery. J Endod. 2010;36:745–50.
40. Torabinejad M, Kettering JD, McGraw JC, Cummings RR, Dwayer TG, Tobias TS. Factors associated with endodontic interappointment emergencies of teeth with necrotic pulps. J Endod. 1988;14:261–6.
41. Tsesis I, Amdor B, Tamse A, Kfir A. The effect of maintaining apical patency on canal transportation. Int Endod J. 2008;41:431–5.
42. Vera J, Arias A, Romero M. Effect of maintaining apical patency on irrigant penetration into the apical third of root canals when using passive ultrasonic irrigation: an *in vivo* study. J Endod. 2011;37:1276–8.
43. Vera J, Arias A, Romero M. Dynamic movement of intracanal gas bubbles during cleaning and shaping procedures: the effect of maintaining apical patency on their presence in the middle and cervical thirds of human root canals: an *in vivo* study. J Endod. 2012;38:200–3.
44. Vera J, Siqueira Jr JF, Ricucci D, et al. One- versus two-visit endodontic treatment of teeth with apical periodontitis: a histobacteriologic study. J Endod. 2012;38:1040–52.
45. Vera J, Hernandez EM, Romero M, Arias A, van der Sluis LW. Effect of maintaining apical patency on irrigant penetration into the apical two millimeters of large root canals: an *in vivo* study. J Endod. 2012;38:1340–3.
46. West JD, Roane JB, Goerig AC. Cleaning and shaping the root canal system. In: Cohen S, Burns RC, editors. Pathways of the pulp. 6th ed. St. Louis: The C.V. Mosby Company; 1994. p. 179.

Manual Dynamic Activation (MDA) Technique

8

Pierre Machtou

Abstract

Highest canal disinfection has to be achieved in endodontics in order to expect a predictable successful outcome. So far, following chemomechanical preparation, passive irrigation followed by some type of activation technique has proved to be effective to reduce bacteria counts. Data on the efficiency of current activation systems are inconclusive. Therefore, until a new activation protocol has proven to be the best and although MDA may be perceived by some clinicians as laborious, it is a fast, cost-effective, safe, and convenient method to perform irrigant agitation at the end of the shaping procedure.

Static Versus Dynamic Irrigation

The aim of endodontic treatment is to prevent or treat apical periodontitis which is the result of a bacterial infection of the root canal system. It has been shown that using an antiseptic irrigant during chemo-mechanical preparation plays a major role to help eradicate intracanal bacteria [7]. Nevertheless, despite long efforts to develop new irrigation devices and solutions and new instrumentation techniques, complete sterilization of the root canal systems is currently impossible to achieve. Therefore, the clinical goal is to reduce at best the threshold of the bacterial load to allow the host defenses to repair [33]. When it comes to select an endodontic irrigant, so far, nothing is as efficient as sodium hypochlorite (NaOCl) [42]. In a recent survey among AAE members, more than 90 % of them use it as the primary irrigant [15]. To be effective, NaOCl must be used in large amounts [37], be in contact with the tissues [38], be *mechanically agitated* [26], and be exchanged [2]. Furthermore, NaOCl has to penetrate the full extent of the root canal space since the bacteria involved in the development and continuation of apical periodontitis are located in the last apical 2 ml [25, 27]. But, according to experimental available data, the apical third appears to be the most difficult area to clean [32], implying that irrigant penetration and exchange with the syringe are not easy to occur in this area. It is obvious that a better knowledge of the behavior

P. Machtou, DDS, MS, PhD
Endodontie, UFR d'Odontologie Paris 7-Denis Diderot, Paris Ile de France, France
e-mail: Prpierre.machtou@gmail.com

B. Basrani (ed.), *Endodontic Irrigation: Chemical Disinfection of the Root Canal System*,
DOI 10.1007/978-3-319-16456-4_8

of root canal irrigation is needed and all current research tends toward this goal. However, Yana [41] in an *in vivo* study was the first to distinguish the two different modalities of the irrigation process: static (or passive) irrigation and dynamic (or active) irrigation. At this stage, a clear definition of both terms is required:

- Static (the term "passive" is inappropriate because it implies the result of an action) irrigation occurs when the solution is delivered with the syringe and depends on the depth of penetration of the irrigating needle.
- Dynamic irrigation includes two parts:
  - The penetration depth of the irrigant during the use of any type of instrument which is a function of the size of the instrument and the *motion* applied to the instrument
  - The exchange of irrigant which is a function of the taper and the size of the canal, both parameters being related with the depth of penetration of the endodontic needle

The Vapor Lock Effect

The root canal is similar to a closed system, and in such a situation, a so-called vapor lock effect has been recently described when the irrigating solution is delivered with the syringe. In fact, before irrigating the canal for the first time, a column of air (or gas bubbles) is entrapped in the apical part of the canal and restricts or blocks irrigant penetration [11, 28, 31, 36, 39]. Surprisingly, this phenomenon has first been mentioned by Luks in 1974 [22] and precisely described by Machtou [23] (Fig. 8.1a–d) who recommended, for relevance of in vitro studies, that the tip of the root must be closed with soft modeling wax prior to any investigation (Fig. 8.2). This vapor lock phenomenon can be described as the difficulty of dispersion and mixing of irrigant in a confined geometry [19].

Removal of an apical vapor lock may be challenging so additional techniques like activation or the use of apical negative pressure (ANP) are considered useful adjuncts to overcome the problem [18, 31]. However, a recent study by Boutsioukis et al. [5] has shown that the vapor lock does not exist in all situations and the insertion of a fine needle close to the working length is able to prevent or remove it. This result was expected as shown in an earlier study using digital subtraction to assess irrigant penetration and renewal during the final irrigation regimen [6]. In this study, the needle tip insertion depth was the main factor affecting irrigant penetration followed by apical taper, needle tip design, and volume of the irrigant. As a result, it is possible to admit that total irrigation of the root canal is clinically feasible at the end of the shaping procedure with static irrigation either with the syringe

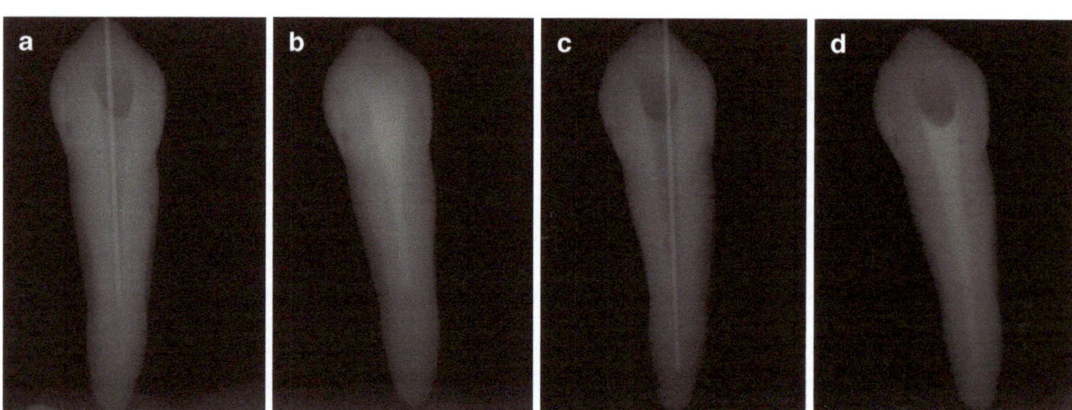

Fig. 8.1 (**a–d**) Vapor lock phenomenon: penetration of the needle and extent of penetration of irrigant (Hypaque) in a closed system (1980)

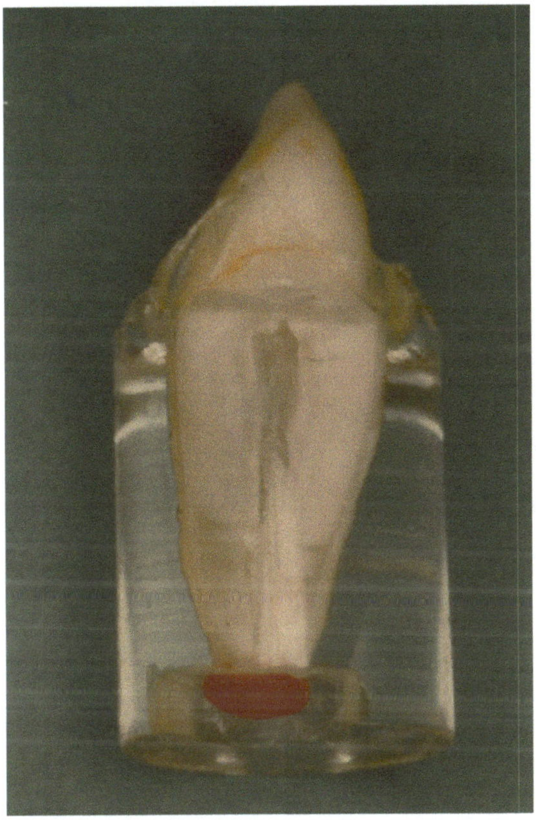

Fig. 8.2 Tooth model with closed apex using soft modeling wax (1980)

and a fine needle [6, 23, 41] or ANP. But additional agitation of the solution is needed if the final goal is to distribute and exchange irrigants into the intricacies of the apical anatomy.

Manual Dynamic Activation Technique

For better cleaning, disinfection, and elimination of biofilm, several activation techniques and devices are available including manual dynamic activation (MDA), intermittent passive ultrasonic irrigation (IPUI), continuous ultrasonic irrigation (CUI), passive ultrasonic irrigation (PUI), sonic irrigation (EndoActivator, Vibringe), hydrodynamic activation (RinsEndo), plastic finishing file (PFF), self-adjusting file (SAF), photoactivated disinfection (PAD), and laser activation (Er: YAG, PIPS). All these techniques and devices have been extensively tested and compared, but it is currently impossible to interpret their results and draw reliable conclusions from the literature. Indeed, results are inconclusive because of different models, mainly plastic and extracted teeth; different evaluation methodologies; different tapers; different apical sizes; and different volumes and time. But, whatever the activation technique, it must be remembered that agitation is a critical factor to help distribute and exchange the solution within the canal space and enhance antiseptic and solvent effectiveness. Hence, a general agreement exists about the benefit of using irrigant activation at the end of the canal preparation which appears to improve canal cleaning and disinfection in comparison with syringe delivery [6].

Manual dynamic irrigation can be performed with hand files [14], brushes [18], or a well-fitting tapered gutta-percha point. It must be realized that MDA starts early during canal preparation when the first scouting hand file is placed inside the canal. It is the apical progression of the instrument that moves irrigant beyond the tip, and once the working length has been reached, the vertical reciprocating movement used allows the solution to involve the entire canal space (Fig. 8.3a–c). But, obviously, at this stage of the procedure, the amount of irrigant is small. During canal shaping, a repeated use of a patency file after each active shaping instrument helps break up the gas bubbles and moves fresh irrigant into the apical last millimeters [39] mixing it with the stagnant solution of the "dead zone" [6, 16]. The frequency of replenishment of the coronal irrigant with the syringe along with the progressive shaping of the root canal and the repeated use of patency files are factors that allow the delivery of irrigant further and further apically.

In 1980, following a series of investigations on endodontic irrigation, it made sense for the author to propose the systematic use of a well-fitting tapered master cone at the end of the shaping procedure to agitate the irrigating solution and enable it to involve the entire length of the root canal [23]. MDA is a simple yet cost-effective way to help the irrigant to get in contact with the canal walls, reach the apical portion of

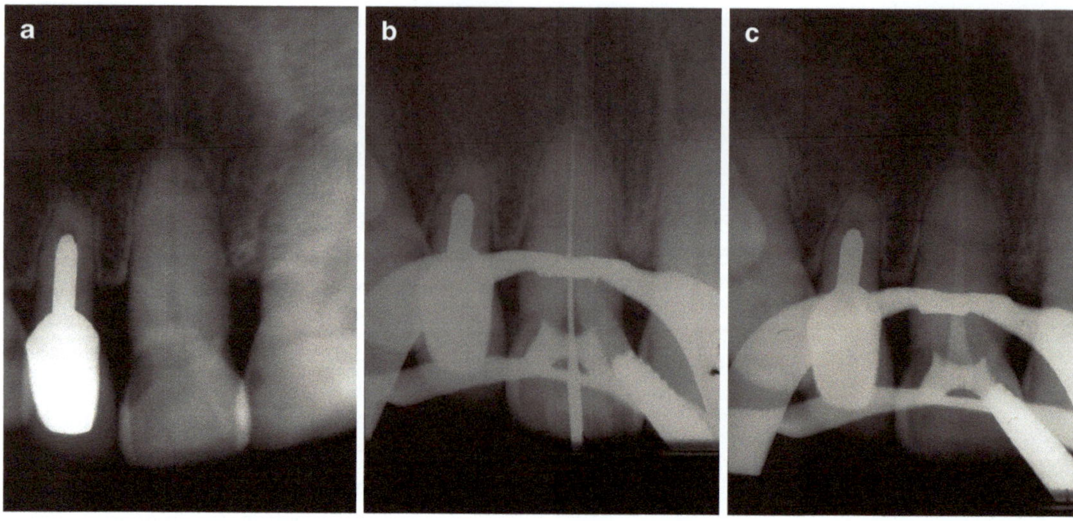

Fig. 8.3 (**a**) Preoperative X-ray. (**b**) Working length determination with $K \neq 15$ file. (**c**) Dynamic irrigation after ≠1#5 file use (irrigant used: Hypaque) (Courtesy of Dr Y. Yana)

the canal, and dislodge the vapor lock effect. It generates higher intracanal pressure changes during the in-and-out movement of the GP cone, and the frequency of the strokes creates turbulences and enhances diffusion by shear stresses. The presence of a thin reflux space between the cone and the canal walls is critical to allow the irrigant to flow back along the cone and induce an effective hydrodynamic effect (Fig. 8.4). Finally, MDA facilitates the mixing of fresh solution with the stagnant solution in the apical millimeters [6].

The efficiency of the technique was confirmed by several studies. Huang et al. [20] who used a dyed collagen biofilm model showed that manual agitation of the master cone was significantly more effective in removal of stained collagen from canal surfaces than static irrigation. Using the same model McGill et al. [24] found that the hydrodynamic device RinsEndo® was significantly less effective than MDA although another study using scanning electron microscopy (SEM) could not find a difference between the two methods in the removal of debris from the root canal walls [40]. One group conducted a series of studies to compare ANP (EndoVac) and MDA. In the first experiment, canal debridement efficiency was tested for both techniques in a closed and an open system [28]. Results showed that a sealed apical foramen adversely affected debridement when using MDA but not ANP. The same group [35] compared canal and isthmus debris debridement efficacies of MDA and ANP in mesial root of the mandibular first molars with narrow isthmi and closed apices. It was shown that both techniques did not completely remove debris from the isthmus region although ANP removed more debris. For the authors, the good debridement efficiency of ANP was the result of wall shear stresses [17]. In contrast, Jiang et al. [21] who compared MDA with tapered and non tapered gutta-percha cones, the Safety irrigator, Continuous Ultrasonic Irrigation (CUI) and ANP found, CUI being the most effective technique in this study. Moreover, the authors [21] emphasized the importance of the reflux space between a well-matching GP cone and the canal walls, a factor described in detail by Machtou [23] and Bronnec et al. [6]. In a recent SEM study, the use of MDA in a well-shaped canal with sufficient apical taper produced very cleaned apical regions and the absence of smear layer in severely curved canals of mandibular molars [9]. Good results of MDA on smear layer removal were confirmed by Saber Sel and Hashem [30] and Andrabi et al. [1]. In 2013, Capar and Aydinbelgehave [8] had shown that final irrigation activation protocols including MDA did not alter the mineral level of root dentine surface.

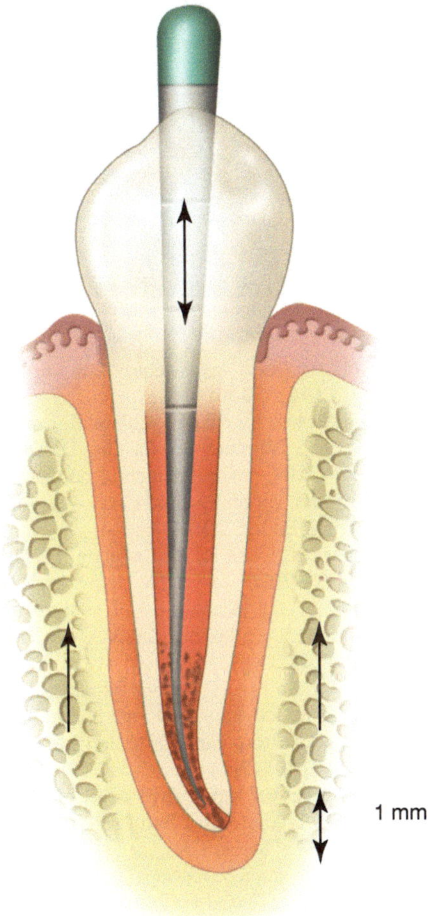

Fig. 8.4 GP cone agitation, reflux space, and disruption of vapor lock

Some other studies can be found where MDA and different activation systems are compared [12, 29], but, as stated earlier, their results must be interpreted with caution.

The main concern during irrigant activation is the risk of apical extrusion. According to available data [3, 4, 13], all tested devices included MDA appear to extrude some irrigant except ANP which is the safest (but ANP should be seen more as a delivery device rather than an activation system). However, it is noteworthy to notice that in a clinical situation, the resistance of the periapical tissues plays a role in limiting the occurrence of extrusion. Irrigant extrusion can be prevented with an accurate use of the MDA technique.

MDA Mode of Use

- A well-matching GP master cone whose taper is slightly less than the taper of the canal is selected. A snug fit is sought after at the working length.
- Then 1 ml is trimmed at the tip of the cone in order to get tug-back 1 ml shorter than the canal terminus.
- After suction of the primary irrigant NaOCL, the canal is filled with 1 ml of EDTA delivered with a 30 gauge NiTi needle (either Navy tip from Ultradent or Stropko NiTi Flexi-Tips from SybronEndo or CanalPro Flex-Tips from Coltene/Whaledent).
- Manual agitation of the master cone is started with an up and down motion and a 2 mm amplitude at a frequency of 100 strokes during approximately 1 min (Fig. 8.5a–b). After that, 1 ml of EDTA is delivered with the irrigating needle to flush out debris. EDTA is then suctioned to eliminate any residual chelating action.
- The canal is flushed with 1 ml of NaOCl, and the same protocol is repeated using 50 in and out strokes during 30 s. A final flush is performed with 3 ml of NaOCl.

This protocol has proven very effective in removing the smear layer and producing very cleaned canals in the apical area [9].

Following the same agitation protocol, QMix (Dentsply), a chlorhexidine-based solution with a weak chelator and surfactant, may alternatively replace both EDTA and NaOCl for final irrigation of the root canal system [10, 34]. A 1 min agitation protocol is recommended, but further scientific data is needed to support and validate the product efficiency.

Conclusion

Highest canal disinfection has to be achieved in endodontics in order to expect a predictable successful outcome. So far, passive irrigation followed by some types of activation technique has proved to be effective to reduce intracanal bacteria counts. Therefore, until a new activation protocol has proven to be the

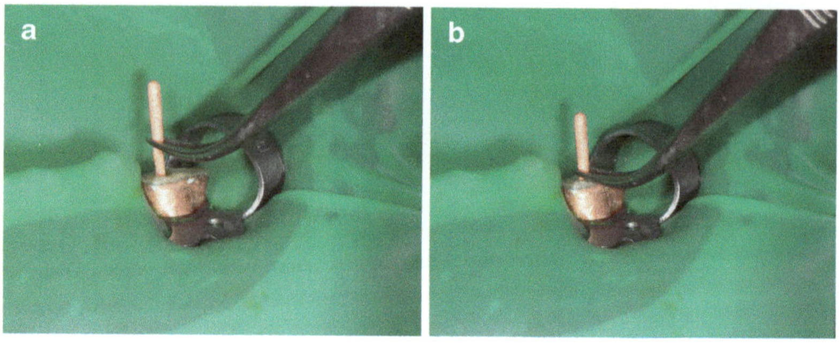

Fig. 8.5 (**a, b**) Clinical MDA technique: agitation of the GP cone with a 2 mm amplitude

best and although MDA may be perceived by some clinicians as laborious, it is a fast, cost-effective, safe, and convenient method to perform irrigant agitation at the end of the root canal preparation.

References

1. Andrabi SM, Kumar A, Mishra SK, Tewari RK, Alam S, Siddiqui S. Effect of manual dynamic activation on smear layer removal efficacy of ethylenediaminetetraacetic acid and SmearClear: an in vitro scanning electron microscopic study. Aust Endod J. 2013;39:131–6.
2. Baumgartner JC, Cuenin PR. Efficacy of several concentrations of sodium hypochlorite for root canal irrigation. J Endod. 1992;18:605–12.
3. Boutsioukis C, Psimma Z, Kastrinakis E. The effect of flow rate and agitation technique on irrigant extrusion ex vivo. Int Endod J. 2014;47:487–96. doi:10.1111/iej.12176.
4. Boutsioukis C, Psimma Z, van der Sluis LW. Factors affecting irrigant extrusion during root canal irrigation: a systematic review. Int Endod J. 2013;46(5):99–618.
5. Boutsioukis C, Kastrinakis E, Lambrianidis T, Verhaagen B, Versluis M, van der Sluis LW. Formation and removal of apical vapor lock during syringe irrigation: a combined experimental and Computational Fluid Dynamics approach. Int Endod J. 2014;47:191–201.
6. Bronnec F, Bouillaguet S, Machtou P. *Ex vivo* assessment of irrigant penetration and renewal during the final irrigation regimen. Int Endod J. 2010;43:663–72.
7. Byström A, Sundqvist G. Bacteriologic evaluation of the effect of 0.5 percent sodium hypochlorite in endodontic therapy. Oral Surg Oral Med Oral Pathol. 1983;55:307–12.
8. Capar ID, Aydinbelge HA. Surface change of root canal dentin after the use of irrigation activation protocols: electron microscopy and an energy-dispersive X-ray microanalysis. Microsc Res Tech. 2013;76:893–6.
9. Caron G, Nham K, Bronnec F, Machtou P. Effectiveness of different final irrigant activation protocols on smear layer removal in curved canals. J Endod. 2010;36:1361–6.
10. Dai L, Khechen K, Khan S, Gillen B, Loushine BA, Wimmer CE, Gutmann JL, Pashley D, Tay FR. The effect of QMix, an experimental antibacterial root canal irrigant, on removal of canal wall smear layer and debris. J Endod. 2011;37:80–4.
11. de Gregorio C, Estevez R, Cisneros R, Heilborn C, Cohenca N. Effect of EDTA, sonic, and ultrasonic activation on the penetration of sodium hypochlorite into simulated lateral canals: an *in vitro* study. J Endod. 2009;35:891–5.
12. Deleu E, Meire MA, De Moor RJ. Efficacy of laser-based irrigant activation methods in removing debris from simulated root canal irregularities. Lasers Med Sci. 2015;30:831–5.
13. Desai P, Himel V. Comparative safety of various intracanal irrigation systems. J Endod. 2009;35:545–9.
14. Druttman AC, Stock CJ. An in vitro comparison of ultrasonic and conventional methods of irrigant replacement. Int Endod J. 1989;22:174–8.
15. Dutner J, Mines P, Anderson A. Irrigation trends among American Association of Endodontists members: a web-based survey. J Endod. 2012;38:37–40.
16. Gao Y, Haapasalo M, Shen Y, Wu H, Li B, Ruse ND, Zhou X. Development and validation of a three-dimensional computational fluid dynamics model of root canal irrigation. J Endod. 2009;35:1282–7.
17. Goode N, Khan S, Eid AA, Niu LN, Gosier J, Susin LF, Pashley DH, Tay FR. Wall shear stress effects of different endodontic irrigation techniques and systems. J Dent. 2013;41:636–41.
18. Gu LS, Kim JR, Ling J, Choi KK, Pashley DH, Tay FR. Review of contemporary irrigant agitation techniques and devices. J Endod. 2009;35:791–804.
19. Gulabivala K, Ng YL, Gilbertson M, Eames I. The fluid mechanics of root canal irrigation. Physiol Meas. 2010;31:R49–84.
20. Huang TY, Gulabivala K, Ng YL. A bio-molecular film ex-vivo model to evaluate the influence of canal dimensions and irrigation variables on the efficacy of irrigation. Int Endod J. 2008;41:60–71.
21. Jiang LM, Lak B, Eijsvogels LM, Wesselink P, van der Sluis LW. Comparison of the cleaning efficacy of different final irrigation techniques. J Endod. 2012;38:838–41.

22. Luks S. Practical endodontics. Philadelphia: JB Lippincott; 1974. p. 82–5.
23. Machtou P. Investigations sur l'irrigation en endodontie. Thèse de doctorat en sciences odontologiques, Université Paris 7, Paris; 1980.
24. McGill S, Gulabivala K, Mordan N, Ng YL. The efficacy of dynamic irrigation using a commercially available system (RinsEndo) determined by removal of a collagen 'bio-molecular film' from an ex vivo model. Int Endod J. 2008;41:602–8.
25. Molven O, Olsen I, Kerekes K. Scanning electron microscopy of bacteria in the apical part of root canals in permanent teeth with periapical lesions. Endod Dent Traumatol. 1991;7:226–9.
26. Moorer WR, Wesselink PR. Factors promoting the tissue dissolving capability of sodium hypochlorite. Int Endod J. 1982;15:187–96.
27. Nair PNR. Pathogenesis of apical periodontitis and the causes of endodontic failures. Crit Rev Oral Biol Med. 2004;15:348–81.
28. Parente JM, Loushine RJ, Susin L, Gu L, Looney SW, Weller RN, Pashley DH, Tay FR. Root canal debridement using manual dynamic agitation or the EndoVac for final irrigation in a closed system and an open system. Int Endod J. 2010;43:1001–12.
29. Ribeiro EM, Silva-Sousa YT, Souza-Gabriel AE, Sousa-Neto MD, Lorencetti KT, Silva SR. Debris and smear removal in flattened root canals after use of different irrigant agitation protocols. Microsc Res Tech. 2012;75:781–90.
30. Saber Sel D, Hashem AA. Efficacy of different final irrigation activation techniques on smear layer removal. J Endod. 2011;37:1272–5.
31. Schoeffel GJ. The EndoVac method of endodontic irrigation: safety first. Dent Today. 2007;26:92, 94, 96.
32. Senia ES, Marshall JF, Rosen S. The solvent action of sodium hypochlorite on pulp tissue of extracted teeth. Oral Surg Oral Med Oral Pathol. 1971;31:96–103.
33. Siqueira Jr JF, Rôças IN. Clinical implications and microbiology of bacterial persistence after treatment procedures. J Endod. 2008;34:1291–301.
34. Stojicic S, Shen Y, Qian W, Johnson B, Haapasalo M. Antibacterial and smear layer removal ability of a novel irrigant, QMiX. Int Endod J. 2012;45:363–71.
35. Susin L, Liu Y, Yoon JC, Parente JM, Loushine RJ, Ricucci D, Bryan T, Weller RN, Pashley DH, Tay FR. Canal and isthmus debridement efficacies of two irrigant agitation techniques in a closed system. Int Endod J. 2010;43:1077–90.
36. Tay FR, Gu LS, Schoeffel GJ, Wimmer C, Susin L, Zhang K, et al. Effect of vapor lock on root canal debridement by using a side-vented needle for positive-pressure irrigant delivery. J Endod. 2010; 36:745–50.
37. The SD. The solvent action of sodium hypochlorite on fixed and unfixed necrotic tissue. Oral Surg Oral Med Oral Pathol. 1979;47:558–61.
38. Trepagnier CM, Madden RM, Lazzari EP. Quantitative study of sodium hypochlorite as an *in vitro* endodontic irrigant. J Endod. 1977;3:194–6.
39. Vera J, Hernández EM, Romero M, Arias A, van der Sluis LW. Effect of maintaining apical patency on irrigant penetration into the apical two millimeters of large root canals: an in vivo study. J Endod. 2012;38:1340–3.
40. Vivan RR, Bortolo MV, Duarte MA, Moraes IG, Tanomaru-Filho M, Bramante CM. Scanning electron microscopy analysis of RinsEndo system and conventional irrigation for debris removal. Braz Dent J. 2010;21:305–9.
41. Yana Y. An *in vivo* comparative study of the penetration of sodium hypochlorite in root canal systems during cleaning and shaping procedures using the B.U. technique and sonic instrumentation. Masters thesis, Boston University, Boston; 1989.
42. Zehnder M. Root canal irrigants. J Endod. 2006;32: 389–98.

Apical Negative Pressure: Safety, Efficacy and Efficiency

9

Gary Glassman and Karine Charara

Abstract

The objective of dentistry is to prevent oral disease and retain the natural dentition, hopefully for the lifetime of the patient. The objective of endodontic treatment is to prevent and/or treat apical periodontitis. In order for an endodontic irrigant delivery system to be mechanically effective and satisfy the objective of endodontics, it must reach the apical terminus, create a current along the root canal wall and have the ability to remove debris, tissue and bacterial contaminants. Currently, the irrigant of choice to achieve this objective is full-strength sodium hypochlorite (NaOCl).

During endodontic irrigation, the organic component of pulpal tissue consumes NaOCl rapidly as the reaction of hydrolysis occurs forming water and releasing ammonia and carbon dioxide as the by-products. In very short order, a column of gas develops at the apical one third of the root canal (apical vapour lock). The conundrum that the clinician faces is to safely and effectively deliver the irrigants to the apical terminus, break the apical vapour lock and allow constant exchange of irrigant and thereby continual hydrolysis of pulpal tissue by the NaOCl, without the risk of apical extrusion.

This chapter will outline the scientific evidence surrounding apical negative pressure as a safe and reliable method to deliver irrigants to the apical terminus, thereby satisfying the objectives of endodontic treatment.

G. Glassman, DDS, FRCD(C) (✉)
Associate in Dentistry, Graduate, Department of Endodontics, Faculty of Dentistry, University of Toronto, Toronto, ON, Canada

Adjunct Professor of Dentistry, University of Technology, Kingston, Jamaica

Private Practice, Endodontic Specialists, Toronto, ON, Canada
e-mail: gary@rootcanals.ca

K. Charara, DMD
Adjunct Professor of Dentistry, Université de Montréal, Montréal, QC, Canada

Private Practice, Clinique Endodontique Mont-Royal, Mont-Royal, QC, Canada

B. Basrani (ed.), *Endodontic Irrigation: Chemical Disinfection of the Root Canal System*,
DOI 10.1007/978-3-319-16456-4_9

The Challenge of Endodontic Debridement

Adequate debridement of the apical one third of the root canal can be very challenging and must not be discounted from providing high-quality endodontic care. Successful endodontic treatment depends on a number of factors, including proper instrumentation, successful irrigation and decontamination of the root canal system to the apices and in areas such as isthmuses and lateral and accessory canals [1]. After traditional nickel–titanium instrumentation and syringe-assisted irrigation, inaccessible areas such as isthmuses, fins, accessory canals and the root canal terminus may remain filled with residual debris and microorganisms [2, 3]. The presence of persistent microbes and their by-products could result in persistent periradicular inflammation [4]. Delivering an endodontic irrigant with a needle and a syringe may be unpredictable, thereby not allowing the irrigant to reach root canal anastomoses and the apical one third of the principal canals. Unless the needle of a positive-pressure delivery system is placed close to the apex, the portion of the canal from the apex to the end of the needle may not be reached by the irrigant [5]. When the needle is placed to a depth that allows the irrigation solution to reach the apex, it is possible the solution may enter the periapical tissues [6]. This can be a source of post-operative pain, and if a significant quantity of a toxic irrigant such as NaOCl is injected into the periapical tissue, the potential to experience a NaOCl accident increases [7]. With debris and bacteria frequently surviving the cleaning and shaping procedures, adjuvant techniques, to the traditional syringe and needle commonly used, may result in superior root canal cleaning [3, 8].

Manual and Machine-Assisted Irrigation Techniques

Root canal irrigation systems can be divided into two categories: manual irrigation techniques and machine-assisted irrigation techniques [9]. Manual irrigation techniques include the positive-pressure syringe fitted with a variety of needle designs and the manual-dynamic agitation using a gutta-percha point. Machine-assisted irrigation techniques include sonics and ultrasonics, as well as newer systems such as the EndoVac, based on apical negative pressure (SybronEndo); the GentleWave (Sonendo), based on multisonic pressure wave formation; the plastic rotary F File (Plastic Endo); the Vibringe (Vibringe); the Rinsendo (Air Techniques); and the EndoActivator (Dentsply Tulsa Dental Specialties). Two important factors that should be considered during the process of irrigation are whether the irrigation systems can deliver the irrigant to the apical terminus and whether the irrigant is capable of debriding areas that could not be reached with mechanical instrumentation, such as lateral/accessory canals, isthmuses and deltas.

Continuous and Intermittent Flushing Techniques

Two flushing methods are currently employed to irrigate root canal systems: the continuous and intermittent. With the intermittent flush technique, the irrigant is injected in the root canal space with a syringe and the irrigant solution can then be activated; the canal is filled several times after each activation cycle. Inversely, the continuous flush techniques provide an uninterrupted supply of fresh irrigation solution into the root canal. This technique can provide more effective results and reduce the time required for final irrigation when compared with intermittent irrigation devices. Taking into consideration that chloride (responsible for dissolving the organic tissues and NaOCl's antibacterial property) is unstable and quickly consumed, a continuous flow of irrigant would make intuitive sense.

Apical Negative Pressure

Pressure is defined as a force per unit area. During root canal treatment, pressure is exerted against the root canal wall when the irrigant solution is delivered into the root canal space. Negative pressure refers to a situation in which an enclosed volume has lower pressure than its surroundings.

Many people use a negative-pressure device on a fairly frequent basis when they use a vacuum cleaner. Negative pressure is also seen in medical quarantine situations where an isolation room will have negative pressure so the outflow of contaminated air is through an opened door or window. This prevents microorganisms from escaping and makes it safer for patients and medical personnel. Oil pipelines also employ negative pressure to prevent the contamination of the environment in the event of a rupture.

In a situation where the pipeline is under the sea and the pipeline's wall breaks off, seawater will flood the pipeline. If the pipeline were positively pressurised, their contents would explode and leak into the ocean, creating a potentially hazardous spill. This chapter will provide a comprehensive review of an apical negative-pressure system for endodontic irrigation, the EndoVac system.

The EndoVac System

The EndoVac system was developed to safely and predictably deliver irrigant to the apical terminus, thereby allowing a better penetration of the irrigation solution into the inherent anatomy and morphology of the root canal system, such as isthmuses, inter-canal and intra-canal communications, curvatures and oval-shaped canals. All these anatomic irregularities make disinfection of the root canal extremely challenging [10] (Fig. 9.1). Apical negative-pressure systems for irrigation have the ability to suction, thereby drawing and delivering the irrigant passively to the apex [9]. The EndoVac system delivers the chosen irrigant passively to the apex [5, 10] and positively addresses the problem of irrigation penetration past the apex into the periapical tissue which may result in treatment complications [6, 11, 12].

The EndoVac apical negative-pressure irrigation system has three active component parts (Fig. 9.2): the Master Delivery Tip (MDT) (Fig. 9.3), the macrocannula and the microcannula. The MDT accommodates a syringe of irrigant, which is expressed through a 20-gauge needle. There is also a plastic suction hood attached around the 20-gauge needle which is connected to clear plastic tubing which inserts into a multiport adaptor which in turn is inserted into the high-volume suction [13]. As such, the MDT can simultaneously deliver and evacuate any excess irrigant that may flow over from the pulp chamber. The macrocannula is used to draw irrigant by way of suction from the chamber to the coronal and middle segments of the canal, while irrigant is simultaneously delivered to the pulp chamber directed towards an axial wall and never towards a canal orifice. The macrocannula or microcannula is connected via clear plastic tubing to the high-speed suction of the dental unit via the multiport adaptor. The plastic macrocannula (Fig. 9.4) has an external diameter of ISO size of 0.55 mm and an internal diameter of ISO size of 0.35 mm. It is made of blue translucent plastic, has a 0.02 taper and is meant for single use only. It is attached snugly

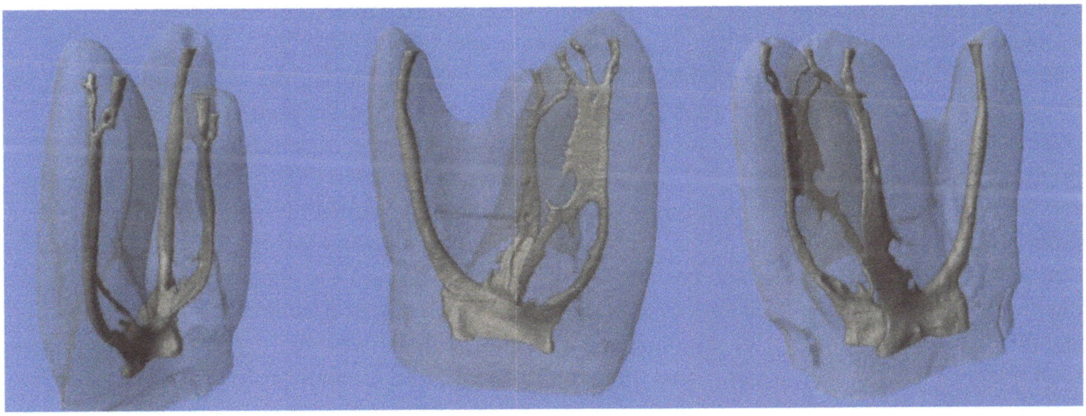

Fig. 9.1 Micro-CT images of a maxillary molar demonstrate the root canal complexity (Courtesy Dr. Ronald Ordinala Zapata)

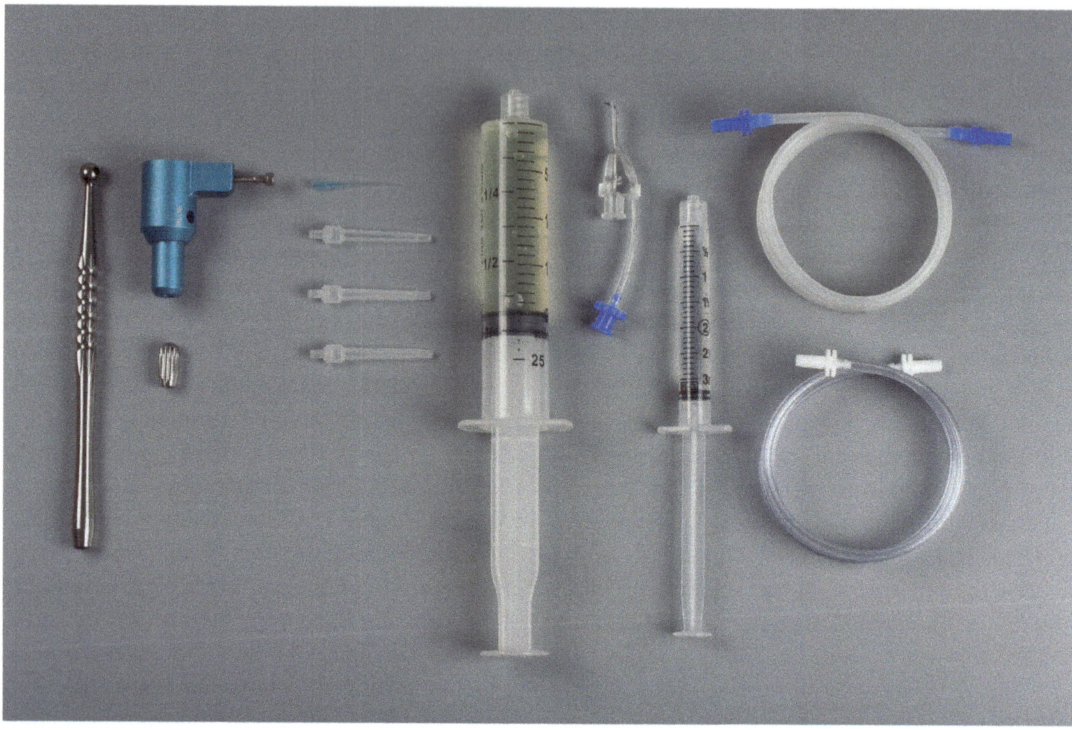

Fig. 9.2 The components of the EndoVac system: the Master Delivery Tip (MDT) accommodates different sizes of syringes filled with irrigant, the macrocannula is attached to the autoclavable aluminium handpiece and the microcannula is attached to an autoclavable aluminium fingerpiece. The macrocannula, the microcannula and the MDT are connected via clear plastic tubing. The tubes are connected to the high-volume suction of the dental chair via the multiport adaptor (Courtesy Dr. John Schoeffel)

to an autoclavable aluminium hand piece (Fig. 9.5) and is used in an up-and-down pecking motion, while irrigant is simultaneously delivered passively to the pulp chamber in the manner mentioned above. It is used to remove the gross debris and tissue left behind during instrumentation. The microcannula (Fig. 9.6) contains 12 microscopic holes and is capable of evacuating debris to full working length [14]. The size of 0.32-mm-external-diameter stainless-steel microcannula of zero taper has four sets of three laser-cut, laterally positioned offset holes adjacent to its closed end, 100 μ in diameter and spaced 100 μ apart. These holes act as filters to prevent the clogging of the internal lumen of the microcannula which has an internal diameter of ISO size of 0.20 mm. The microcannula is attached to an autoclavable aluminium fingerpiece and is used for irrigation of the apical part of the canal when it is positioned at working length. The microcannula has a closed end and should be taken to the full working length to aspirate irrigants and debris. The microcannula can be used in canals that are enlarged with endodontic files to ISO size 35 with 0.04 taper or larger. A non-tapered preparation can also be considered; in this situation the manufacturer recommends an enlargement of the root canal to 40/0.02.

During irrigation, the MDT delivers irrigant to the pulp chamber and siphons off the excess irrigant to prevent overflow. Both the macrocannula and microcannula exert negative pressure that pulls fresh irrigant from the chamber, down the canal to the tip of the cannula, into the cannula and out through the suction hose. Thus, a constant flow of fresh irrigant is delivered by negative pressure to working length, allowing the reaction of hydrolysis to continually occur.

Method of Use

Irrigation begins during rotary instrumentation. The MDT delivers fresh irrigant to the access opening when each instrument is changed in the hand piece. Using the MDT is optional during access and the instrumentation phases of root canal treatment. A normal Monoject syringe may be used to replenish the irrigant in the pulp chamber during instrumentation. This removes instrumentation debris and exchanges irrigant deep within the pulp chamber as subsequent files are brought closer and then finally to

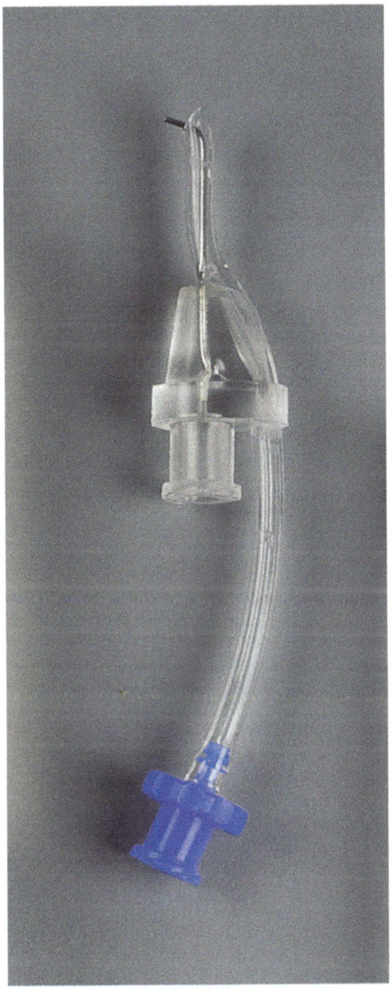

Fig. 9.3 Master Delivery Tip (MDT) composed of a 20-gauge needle and luer lock connectors to connect to the syringe and the high-volume suction of the dental chair (Courtesy Kerr Endodontics (SybronEndo). Orange, California)

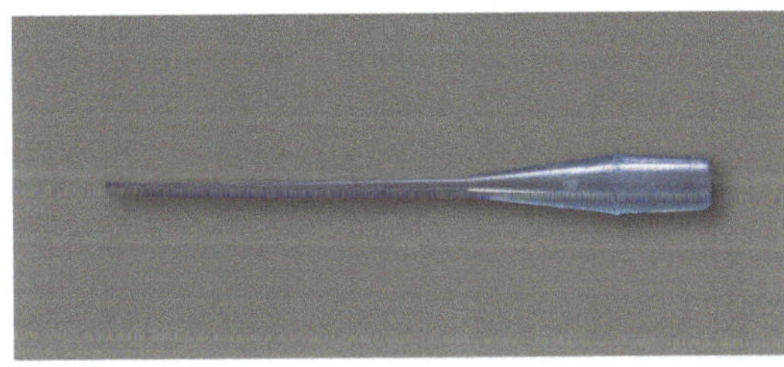

Fig. 9.4 The macrocannula is made of blue translucent plastic and it is attached to an autoclavable aluminium handpiece (Fig. 9.5) (Courtesy Kerr Endodontics (SybronEndo). Orange, California)

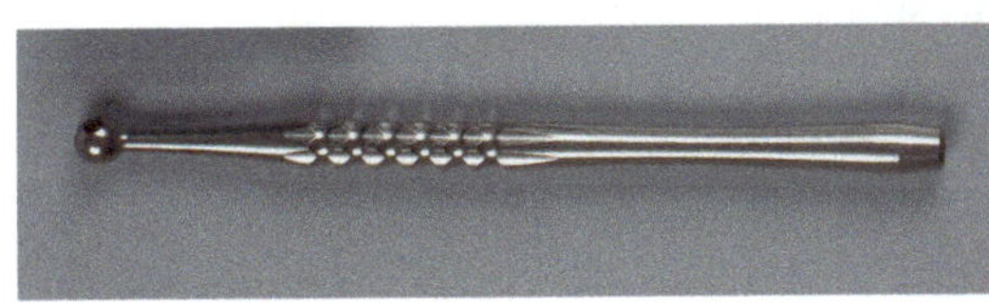

Fig. 9.5 Autoclavable handpiece for the macrocannula (Courtesy Kerr Endodontics (SybronEndo). Orange, California)

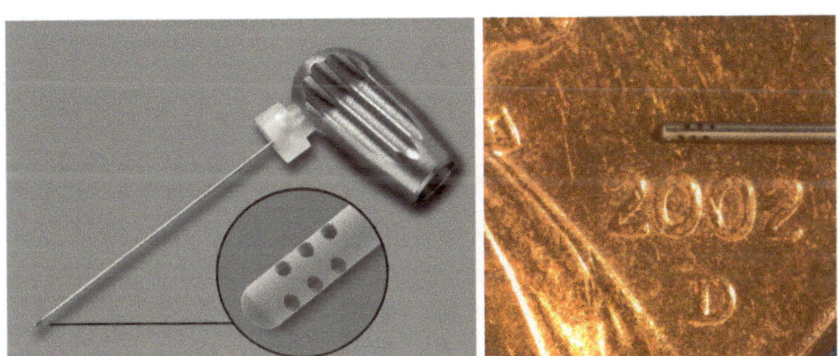

Fig. 9.6 The ISO size of 0.32-mm-external-diameter stainless-steel microcannula of zero taper has four sets of three laser-cut, laterally positioned offset holes adjacent to its closed end, 100 μ in diameter and spaced 100 μ apart (Courtesy Dr. John Schoeffel)

working length. When using the MDT, always direct the irrigant flow against a chamber wall; never direct the flow of irrigant towards a canal's orifice as the pressure of irrigant expression has the potential of causing an irrigation accident in straight and wide canals even when the needle is not placed directly in the orifice or canal.

Following complete instrumentation, the macrocannula is used in each canal for 30 s in a short up-and-down pecking motion as close as possible to working length. Continue to deliver copious NaOCl with the MDT while the macrocannula is moving up and down the canal. Observe the macrocannula for continuous flow and that it does not become blocked with debris. If it does, then remove the plastic tubing from the aluminium handle, place a syringe of water tightly at the end and express the water through the handle and macrocannula to dislodge the blockage. This is carefully done over the sink and not over the patient. This step can also be performed with the microcannula should it get blocked. The use of the macrocannula in the final irrigation protocol will remove the gross debris and tissue left behind during instrumentation. If a shortcut is made and this step is not completed for the full 30 s in each canal, then the microcannula used in the next step may get blocked and slow down the irrigation process.

The next step involves three micro cycles. They are called micro cycles because the microcannula is now used at full working length to remove debris from the canal lumen and isthmus areas. Use a ruler to position the rubber stopper that is placed on the microcannula or score the microcannula with an indelible marker (Fig. 9.7). Delicately guide the microcannula to full working length by holding the fingerpiece. The fingerpiece is then released and the tubing is stabilised. The NaOCl is added with the MDT to the pulp chamber for 10 s (Fig. 9.8). After 10 s the irrigant flow is stopped for just a couple of seconds to allow the gas bubbles formed by hydrolysis to be purged from the canal. The NaOCl is added for another 10 s after which the irrigant flow is stopped again to allow the gas bubbles to be purged from the canal. The NaOCl is then added for the third and final time for another 10 s, but at the end of this time period, the microcannula is removed by the fingerpiece as the MDT continues to deliver NaOCl to the pulp chamber as to not allow its removal from the canal just being treated. This allows the canal to be charged (soaked) with fresh NaOCl for 60 s. The first micro cycle allows the organic com-

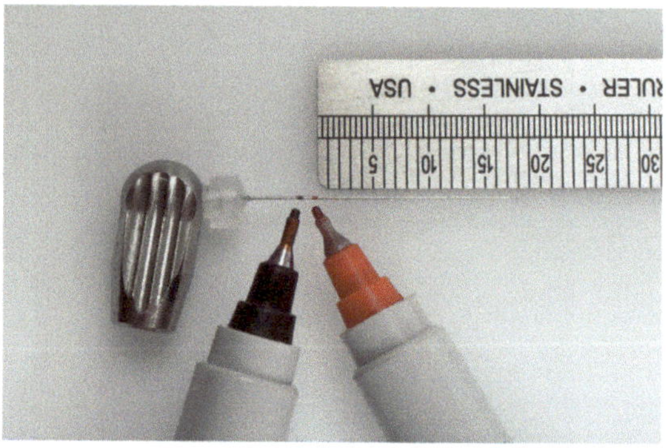

Fig. 9.7 Remove the cap of the microcannula. Use the provided rubber stopper or a marker to indicate working length (Courtesy Kerr Endodontics (SybronEndo). Orange, California)

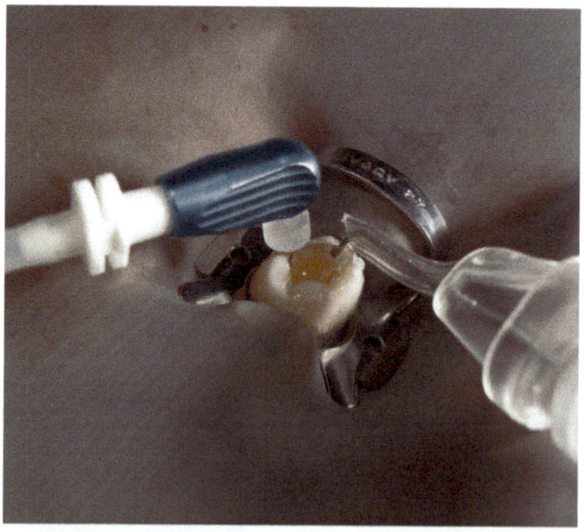

Fig. 9.8 Once the microcannula is placed at full working length, the clinician may leave it in place and proceed with irrigant delivery via the MDT. Put a slight bend on the microcannula if it won't stay in the canal on its own (Courtesy Kerr Endodontics (SybronEndo). Orange, California)

ponent of the smear layer to be removed in addition to any fine debris left behind during instrumentation. The second micro cycle using EDTA removes the inorganic component of the smear layer. The microcannula is again delicately guided to full working length. EDTA is added for 10 s, and then the microcannula is removed allowing the canal to be charged for 60 s. As mentioned, this will remove the inorganic component of the smear layer and expose the dentinal tubules in preparation for the third micro cycle. The third micro cycle is the same as the first micro cycle, two purges and a charge for 60 s. Now that the smear layer has been removed from the root canal walls by the first two micro cycles, this third micro cycle will allow the NaOCl to enter the dentinal tubules via osmosis and dissolve the remaining tissue and microbiota [15]. There is no better way to dry the root canals than to delicately guide the microcannula to full working length for just a moment. This is followed by one or two paper points. The canal(s) is now ready for obturation. Refer to Fig. 9.9 for a flow chart illustrating the final irrigation protocol using the EndoVac system.

Debris Removal

Several studies were carried out to evaluate the EndoVac system's ability to remove debris within the root canal system after instrumentation with rotary files [16–21]. Debridement is a principal objective of root canal treatment and remains a challenge especially in the apical portion of the canal and within the isthmuses and lateral and accessory canals. Debridement is the elimination of organic and inorganic substances as well as microorganisms from the root canal by mechanical and/or chemical means [22]. When compared to traditional syringe and side-vented needle irrigation, the EndoVac system has demonstrated better control to reach the last millimetre of the root canal.

Some in vitro and in vivo studies have demonstrated greater removal of debris from the apical walls and a statistically cleaner result using apical negative-pressure irrigation in closed root canal systems with sealed apices. In an in vivo study of 22 teeth by Siu and Baumgartner, less debris remained at 1 mm from working length using apical negative pressure compared to the use of traditional needle irrigation, while Shin

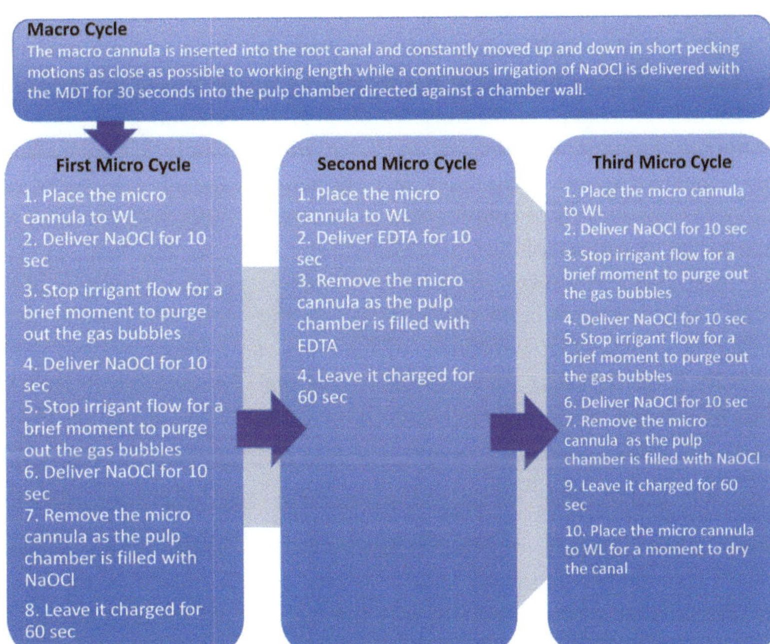

Fig. 9.9 Final irrigation protocol using EndoVac system

et al. found in an in vitro study of 69 teeth comparing traditional needle irrigation with apical negative pressure that these methods both resulted in clean root canals but that apical negative pressure resulted in less debris remaining at 1.5 and 3.5 mm from working length [18, 23, 24]. When comparing root canal debridement using manual-dynamic agitation (using a well-fitted gutta-percha cone in an up-and-down motion in the canal) or the EndoVac system for final agitation in a closed system and an open system, it was found that the presence of a sealed apical foramen adversely affected debridement efficacy when manual-dynamic agitation was used, but did not adversely affect results when the EndoVac system was used. Apical negative-pressure irrigation is an effective method to overcome the fluid-dynamic challenges inherent in closed root canal systems [25, 26]. The ability of the EndoVac system to significantly clean more debris from a mechanically inaccessible recess of the curved in vitro root canal model may be caused by robust bubble formation during irrigant delivery, creating higher wall shear stresses by a two-phase air–liquid flow phenomenon that is well known in other industrial debridement systems [27]. Less debris remained with the EndoVac system at 1 mm from the working length and in isthmuses [18, 20, 21]. To enhance cleanliness of the root canal system, EndoVac system has the ability to safely deliver irrigant to working length [18] by pulling the irrigant into the canal and removing it by negative pressure [18]. This vacuum action enhances the volume of solution and the circulation of the irrigation solution in the apical end of the root canal. Moreover, the negative pressure avoids air entrapment in the apical third [21] and promotes a regular replenishment of the irrigant apically [21]. A recent study demonstrated that the volume of irrigant delivered apically was significantly higher than the volume delivered by conventional syringe needle irrigation within the same period [18] and resulted in significantly more debris removal at 1 mm from working length than did needle irrigation.

One study is not in agreement with those positive outcomes discussed above. Jiang et al. ran a study and evaluated the EndoVac system's ability to remove dentin debris from artificially made grooves in standardised root canals. The model was made of a single tooth root in which an apical groove comparable to an ovoid apical canal was created and packed with dentin debris. They compared several devices to activate the irrigation solution. Once the irrigation regimen was completed, they viewed the grooves through a stereomicroscope to evaluate the residual dentin debris. A score between 0 and 3 was given to each specimen: 0 = the groove is empty, 1 = less than half of the groove is filled with debris, 2 = more than half of the groove is filled with debris and 3 = the complete groove is filled with debris. The specimens irrigated with the EndoVac system had their groove completely filled with debris (score 3) 65 % of the time, while 35 % had less than half filled with debris [17]. It is important to note that Jiang et al. failed to follow the manufacturer's instructions by failing to use the critical macrocannula, an error that could easily cause the microcannula to clog and become ineffective. When the microcannula is blocked by debris, the clinician will experience decreased or complete arrest of irrigant flow. To rectify the situation, the microcannula can be wiped with a 2 × 2 gauze or air and water can be blown into it to unclog it. This can also be done with the macrocannula should it also become clogged during its use (Fig. 9.10). Complete clogging of the microcannula happens very rarely, if the macrocannula is used according to the manufacturer's instructions. The microcannula will continue to work even if several holes are blocked. However, its effectiveness will decrease. To avoid this complication, the macrocannula's main purpose is to remove as much debris as possible before the smaller microcannula is introduced. This will reduce the incidence of it clogging as long as the macrocannula is used according to the manufacturer's recommendation. A weaker capacity of the EndoVac system to remove apical debris could be attributed to the minimal turbulence intensity produced within the canal by the microcannula [28]. This evidence of low wall shear stress values causes a minimum physical interaction between the irrigant and the root canal walls [29]. This absence of

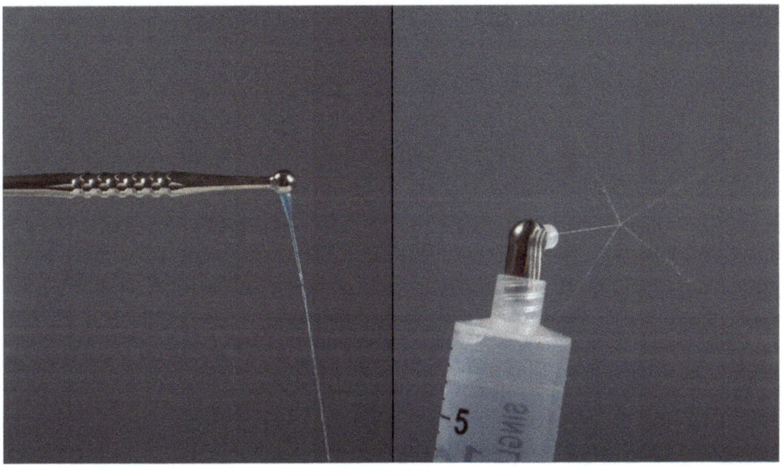

Fig. 9.10 If either cannula becomes clogged, try unclogging it by attaching the back end of either the fingerpiece or handpiece onto a syringe filled with water. Push the plunger; in most instances the hole(s) is immediately cleared (Courtesy Kerr Endodontics (SybronEndo). Orange, California)

interaction may explain the difficulty of the irrigation solution to reach the root canal's lateral canals and anastomoses [5].

Microbial Control

The effective removal of organic and inorganic tissues would logically allow better access and elimination of endodontic pathogens, responsible of apical periodontitis, localised in the root canal system.

Hockett et al. tested the ability of apical negative-pressure irrigation to remove a thick biofilm of *E. faecalis* in mesial roots of mandibular molars, finding that these specimens rendered negative cultures after 48-h incubation, while some of those irrigated using traditional positive-pressure irrigation were positive at 48 h [29]. One in vivo dog study found that apical negative-pressure irrigation with 2.5 % NaOCl resulted in similar bacterial reduction than the use of apical positive-pressure irrigation combined with seven days of intra-canal medication which was the triple antibiotic paste [30]. The triple antibiotic Trimix (metronidazole, ciprofloxacin and minocycline) has been utilised for pulpal regeneration/revascularisation in teeth with incompletely formed apices [31]. The antibiotic medication is applied in regeneration cases to safely kill bacteria. Since the triple antibiotic versus the use of EndoVac with NaOCl was statistically equivalent for mineralised tissue formation and the repair process [30], the study [30] suggests that EndoVac may overcome the need for intra-canal medication. Further research is required to evaluate this potential. Using apical negative pressure with NaOCl also decreases the risk of drug resistance, tooth discoloration and allergic reactions often seen with the administration of antibiotics [32, 33]. A recent randomised controlled clinical trial [34] compared the antimicrobial effectiveness of EndoVac system and the traditional positive-pressure syringe and needle for irrigation. From the 16 mandibular molar treated with the conventional method, negative culture was found in 67 % compared to 100 % among the apical negative-pressure irrigation group. A second clinical study [35] demonstrated a higher frequency of obtaining negative culture with EndoVac system compared to a syringe with regular needle. Unlike Cohenca et al. [34], Pawar et al. [35] did not reach significance between the two clinical groups. However, Pawar et al. added an overriding codicil in their discussion: "The original EndoVac protocol recommends using a concentration of 5.25 % NaOCl. Almost all studies investigating the efficacy of EndoVac have used NaOCl at concentrations ranging from 2.5 to 6 %. The use of 0.5 % NaOCl [a 1,000 % dilution from the manufacturer's instructions] in this study could be considered responsible for the lack of significant differences in antimicrobial efficacy between EndoVac irrigation and standard irrigation" [35].

Smear Layer Removal

The smear layer is created when the dentinal walls of the root canal system interact with endodontic instruments [36]. The smear layer is comprised of inorganic and organic material such as dentin filings and pulp tissue remnants [37]. This deposit can be penetrated by bacteria and may offer protection to biofilms adhering to the root canal walls [38]. Furthermore, the smear layer interferes with the tight adaptation of currently used root canal sealers to dentinal walls and may therefore promote microleakage [39]. Torabinejad et al. [40] suggested that the removal of the smear layer decreases bacteria and improves adaptation of obturation materials to the canal walls. Another study showed that the smear layer produced during root canal preparation promotes adhesion and colonisation of *P. nigrescens* [41] to the dentin matrix and might increase the likelihood of canal reinfection. Removing the smear layer reduces the potential for microleakage [19, 42] and improves sealer penetration in dentinal tubules [43]. When manufacturer's recommendations are followed, EndoVac system delivers a sufficient volume of irrigants which enables to remove smear layer [19, 44, 45] (Fig. 9.11).

Compared to passive ultrasonic irrigation, apical negative-pressure irrigation and manual-dynamic irrigation are more efficient in removing the smear layer in the apical one third [45]. A possible explanation for this is that both techniques reach full working length of instrumented canals, eliminate the apical vapour lock at the apex and hence allow adequate irrigant replacement [44, 45]. When evaluating irrigation of the apical one third, the phenomenon of apical vapour lock should be considered [26, 46, 47].

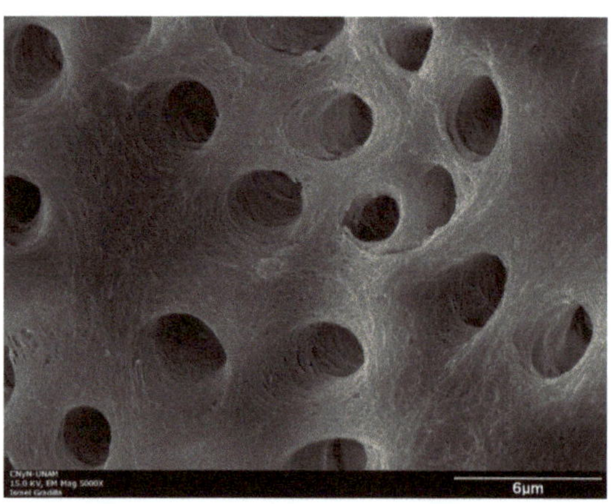

Fig. 9.11 SEM of a clean root canal wall where the smear layer has been removed (Courtesy Dr. Arianna Gomez-Perez)

Apical Vapour Lock

Since roots are surrounded by the periodontium, unless the root canal foramen is open, the root canal behaves like a close-ended channel. This produces an apical vapour lock that resists displacement during instrumentation and final irrigation, thus preventing the flow of irrigant into the apical region and adequate debridement of the root canal system [48, 49]. Apical vapour lock also results in gas entrapment at the apical one third [9]. During irrigation, NaOCl reacts with organic tissue in the root canal system, and the resulting hydrolysis liberates abundant quantities of ammonia and carbon dioxide [50]. This gaseous mixture is trapped in the apical region and quickly forms a column of gas into which further fluid penetration is impossible. Extension of instruments into this vapour lock does not reduce or remove the gas bubble [13], just as it does not enable adequate flow of irrigant.

The phenomenon of apical vapour lock has been confirmed in studies in which roots were embedded in a polyvinyl siloxane impression material to restrict fluid flow through the apical foramen, simulating a close-ended channel [26]. The results in these studies were found to be an incomplete debridement of the apical part of the canal walls with the use of a positive-pressure syringe delivery technique [26]. Micro-CT scanning and histological tests conducted by Tay et al. have also confirmed the presence of apical vapour lock [26]. In fact, studies conducted without ensuring a close-ended channel cannot be regarded as conclusive on the efficacy of irrigants and the irrigant system [51–53]. The apical vapour lock may also explain why in a number of studies investigators were unable to demonstrate a clean apical third in sealed root canals [54–56].

In a paper published in 1983, Chow determined that traditional positive-pressure irrigation had virtually no effect apical to the orifice of the irrigation needle in a closed root canal system [57]. Fluid exchange and debris displacement were minimal. Equally important to his primary findings, Chow set forth an infallible paradigm for endodontic irrigation: "For the solution to be mechanically effective in removing all the particles, it has to: (*a*) reach the apex; (*b*) create a current (force); and (*c*) carry the particles away" [57]. The apical vapour lock and consideration for the patient's safety have always prevented the thorough cleaning of the apical 3 mm. It is critically important to determine which irrigation system will effectively irrigate the apical third, as well as isthmuses and lateral canals [10], and do it in a safe manner that prevents the extrusion of irrigant.

Calcium Hydroxide Removal

As stated previously, the debridement of the root canal system consists of elimination of organic, inorganic and microbial components, thus accomplished by mechanical instrumentation supported by various irrigation regimens and placement of intra-canal medication. Calcium hydroxide is a commonly used intra-canal medicament [58] that has antimicrobial activity proven to contribute to bacterial endotoxin neutralisation [59] and to periapical repair [60]. However, to provide a maximum interface between the root canal walls and the filling material, calcium hydroxide has to be removed [61]; otherwise, the bond strength [62] of the sealer and its penetration into the dentinal tubules could be reduced [63]. Conventional methods for irrigation have demonstrated limited capacity to remove calcium hydroxide from the apical third of the root canal [64]. A scanning electron microscopic evaluation of longitudinally sectioned canines demonstrated that EndoVac system performs better than the traditional syringe irrigation in removing calcium hydroxide from the apical one third of root canals [65]. The results were similar to another study [66] where EndoVac system was compared to the traditional syringe irrigation and the ProUltra® PiezoFlow™ ultrasonic irrigation needle (Dentsply Tulsa, Tulsa, OK, USA). EndoVac system left significantly less calcium hydroxide compared to the traditional syringe irrigation and provided better results than PiezoFlow™, but the difference was not statistically significant [66]. Although the EndoVac system improves the removal of calcium hydroxide, the apical portion of the canal was not completely free of intra-canal medicament. Therefore, the use of the master apical file in combination with the EndoVac system may result in better removal of calcium hydroxide [66].

Sodium Hypochlorite Incidents

In light of the cytotoxicity of the sodium hypochlorite, its extrusion from the root canal will affect the periapical tissue and may cause the patient a series of complications of a variable clinical significance, beginning with the a post-operative pain [7].

Although a devastating endodontic NaOCl incident is rare [67], the cytotoxic effects of NaOCl on vital tissue are well established [68]. The associated sequelae of NaOCl extrusion have been reported to include life-threatening airway obstructions [69], facial disfigurement requiring multiple corrective surgical procedures [70], permanent paraesthesia with loss of facial muscle control [71] and tooth loss [72].

Although the exact aetiology of the NaOCl incident is still uncertain, based on the evidence from actual incidents and the location of the associated tissue trauma, it would appear that an intravenous injection might be the main cause. The patient shown in Fig. 9.12 [73] demonstrates a widespread area of tissue trauma that is in contrast to the characteristics of NaOCl incident trauma reported by Pashley [68]. This extensive trauma, particularly involving the pattern of ecchymosis around the eye, could only have occurred if the NaOCl had been introduced intravenously to a vein close to the root apex through

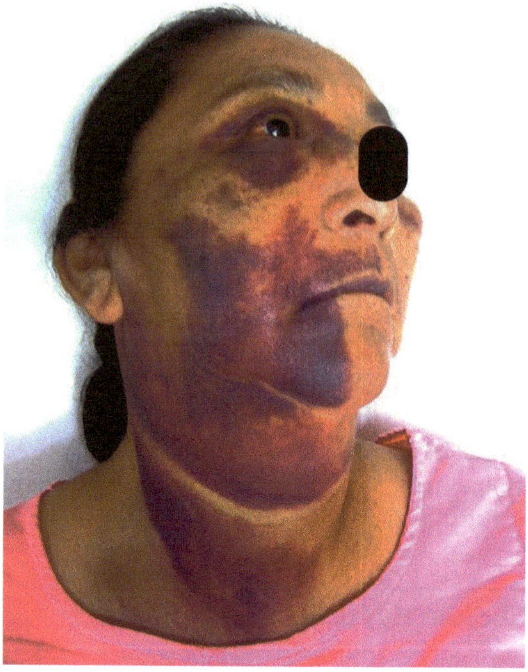

Fig. 9.12 Clinical aspect of emphysema related to extravasation of the sodium hypochlorite solution during endodontic treatment, with ecchymosis and severe swelling of the right side of the face. These symptoms appeared after a root canal treatment of the upper right canine (Reproduced with permission from Elsevier)

which extrusion of the irrigant occurred and the irrigant then found its way into the venous complex. This would require positive pressure apically exceeding the venous pressure, for which the mean value is 5.88 mmHg [12]. In other words, NaOCl extrusion into the venous system is more susceptible to occur when the apical pressure of irrigant is greater than 5.88 mmHg. One in vitro study, where a positive-pressure needle irrigation technique was used to mimic clinical conditions and techniques, demonstrated that the apical pressure generated easily exceeds the value of normal venous pressure [74]. The results of this study suggested that a combination of factors is necessary for a severe NaOCl accident to occur. The hypothesis that involves intravenous infusion of extruded NaOCl into the facial vein via non-collapsible venous sinusoids within the cancellous bone has been suggested [12].

This does not imply that NaOCl can or should be excluded as an endodontic irrigant; in fact, its use is essential to achieve adequate chemical debridement. What this does imply is that it must be delivered safely.

Safety

With traditional root canal irrigation, clinicians must be careful when determining how far an irrigation needle is placed into the canal. Recommendations for avoiding NaOCl incidents include not binding the needle in the canal, not placing the needle close to working length and using a gentle flow rate when using positive-pressure irrigation [75]. In contrast, the EndoVac system pulls irrigant into the canal to working length and irrigant and debris is removed by negative pressure. Apical negative pressure has been shown to enable irrigants to safely reach the apical one third and help overcome apical vapour lock [18, 20].

Apart from being able to avoid air entrapment, the EndoVac system is also advantageous in its ability to deliver irrigants safely to working length without causing their undue extrusion into the periapex [14, 18, 76], thereby avoiding NaOCl incidents. It is important to note that it is possible to create positive pressure in the pulp canal if the MDT is misused, which would create the risk of a NaOCl incident. The manufacturer's instructions must be followed for correct use of the Master Delivery Tip by never directing towards the orifice of a canal.

In order to compare the safety of six current intra-canal irrigation delivery devices, an in vitro test was conducted using the worst-case scenario of apical extrusion, with neutral atmospheric pressure and an open apex [14]. The study concluded that the EndoVac system did not extrude irrigant even after deep intra-canal delivery and suctioning of the irrigant from the chamber to full working length, whereas other devices did. The EndoActivator extruded only a very small volume of irrigant, the clinical significance of which is not known.

Mitchell and Baumgartner tested irrigant (NaOCl) extrusion from a root canal sealed with a permeable agarose gel [11]. Significantly less extrusion occurred using the EndoVac system compared with positive-pressure needle irrigation. A well-controlled study by Gondim et al. found that patients experienced less post-operative pain, measured objectively and subjectively, when apical negative-pressure irrigation was performed (EndoVac system) than with apical positive-pressure irrigation [7]. Furthermore, PiezoFlow™ showed a greater potential to cause apical extrusion compared with EndoVac system's safety. When positioned within the last 5 mm of the root canal, the ultrasonic activated needle could cause apical extrusion of irrigant solution [76].

Conclusion

Traditional endodontic technique advocated placing NaOCl into the root canal space followed by endodontic instruments in the belief that they were carrying the irrigant to the apical terminus. Biological, scanning electron microscopy, light microscopy and other studies have proven this belief to be in error. NaOCl reacts with organic material in the root canal and quickly forms microbubbles at the apical termination that coalesce into a single large apical vapour bubble with subsequent instrumentation. Since the apical vapour lock cannot be displaced via mechanical means, it prevents further NaOCl flow into the apical area. The safest method yet discovered to provide fresh voluminous amounts of NaOCl safely to the apical terminus to eliminate the apical vapour lock is to evacuate it via apical negative pressure. This method has also been proven to be safe because it always draws irrigants to the source via suction—down the canal and simultaneously away from the apical tissue in abundant quantities. When the proper irrigating agents are delivered safely to the full extent of the root canal terminus, thereby removing most of organic tissue and microbial contaminants, success in endodontic treatment may be taken to levels never seen before.

References

1. Friedman S. Prognosis of initial endodontic. Endod Top. 2002;2:59–88.
2. Peters OA, Schönenberger K, Laib A. Effects of four Ni-Ti preparation techniques on root canal geometry assessed by micro computed tomography. Int Endod J. 2001;34:221–30.
3. Cano V, Nair PNR, Henry S, Vera J. Microbial status of apical root canal system of human mandibular first molars with primary apical periodontitis after "one-visit" endodontic treatment. Oral Surg Oral Med Oral Pathol Oral Radiol Endod. 2005;99:231–52.
4. Wu M-K, Dummer PMH, Wesselink PR. Consequences of and strategies to deal with residual post-treatment root canal infection. Int Endod J. 2006;39:343–56.
5. Spoorthy E, Velmurugan N, Ballal S, Nandini S. Comparison of irrigant penetration up to working length and into simulated lateral canals using various irrigating techniques. Int Endod J. 2013;46:815–22.
6. Mitchell RP, Baumgartner JC, Sedgley CM. Apical extrusion of sodium hypochlorite using different root canal irrigation systems. J Endod. 2011;37:1677–81.
7. Gondim E, Setzer FC, Bertelli C, Kim S. Postoperative pain after the application of two different irrigation devices in a prospective randomized clinical trial. J Endod. 2010;36:1295–301.
8. De Gregorio C, Estevez R, Cisneros R, Paranjpe A, Cohenca N. Efficacy of different irrigation and activation systems on the penetration of sodium hypochlorite into simulated lateral canals and up to working length: an in vitro study. J Endod. 2010;36:1216–21.
9. Gu L, Kim JR, Ling J, Choi KK, Pashley DH, Tay FR. Review of contemporary irrigant agitation techniques and devices. J Endod. 2009;35:791–804.
10. De Gregorio C, Paranjpe A, Garcia A, Navarrete N, Estevez R, Esplugues EO. Efficacy of irrigation systems on penetration of sodium hypochlorite to working length and to simulated uninstrumented areas in oval shaped root canals. Int Endod J. 2012;45:475–81.
11. Mitchell RP, Yang S-E, Baumgartner JC. Comparison of apical extrusion of NaOCl using the EndoVac or needle irrigation of root canals. J Endod. 2010;36:338–41.
12. Zhu W, Gyamfi J, Niu L, Schoeffel GJ, Liu S, Santarcangelo F, et al. Anatomy of sodium hypochlorite accidents involving facial ecchymosis – a review. J Dent. 2013;41:935–48.
13. Schoeffel GJ. The EndoVac method of endodontic irrigation, part 2-efficacy [Internet]. Dentistry Today. 2008 [cited 2014 Aug 5]. p. 82, 84, 86–7. Available from: http://www.dentistrytoday.com/endodontics/999.
14. Desai P, Himel V. Comparative safety of various intracanal irrigation systems. J Endod. 2009;35:545–9.
15. Baumgartner JC, Mader CL. A scanning electron microscopic evaluation of four root canal irrigation regimens. J Endod. 1987;13:147–57.
16. Howard RK, Kirkpatrick TC, Rutledge RE, Yaccino JM. Irrigation techniques. J Endod. 2011;37:1301–5.
17. Jiang L-M, Lak B, Eijsvogels LM, Wesselink P, van der Sluis LWM. Comparison of the cleaning efficacy of different final irrigation techniques. J Endod. 2012;38:838–41.

18. Nielsen BA, Craig Baumgartner J. Comparison of the EndoVac system to needle irrigation of root canals. J Endod. 2007;33:611–5.
19. Ribeiro EM, Silva-Sousa YTC, Souza-Gabriel AE, Sousa-Neto MD, Lorencetti KT, Silva SRC. Debris and smear removal in flattened root canals after use of different irrigant agitation protocols. Microsc Res Tech. 2012;75:781–90.
20. Shin S-J, Kim H-K, Jung I-Y, Lee C-Y, Lee S-J, Kim E. Comparison of the cleaning efficacy of a new apical negative pressure irrigating system with conventional irrigation needles in the root canals. Oral Surg Oral Med Oral Pathol Oral Radiol Endod. 2010;109:479–84.
21. Yoo YJ, et al. Multivariate analysis of the cleaning efficacy of different final irrigation techniques in the canal and isthmus of mandibular posterior teeth. Restor Dent Endod. 2013;38:154–9.
22. Glickman GN, Mickel AK, Levin LG, Fouad AF, Johnson W. Glossary of endodontic term. Chicago Am Assoc Endodontists. 2003:1–51.
23. Siu C, Baumgartner JC. Comparison of the debridement efficacy of the EndoVac irrigation system and conventional needle root canal irrigation in vivo. J Endod. 2010;36:1782–5.
24. Park S-Y, Shin S-Y, Yang S-M, Kye S-B. Factors influencing the outcome of root-resection therapy in molars: a 10-year retrospective study. J Periodontol. 2009;80:32–40.
25. Parente JM, Loushine RJ, Susin L, Gu L, Looney SW, Weller RN, et al. Root canal debridement using manual dynamic agitation or the EndoVac for final irrigation in a closed system and an open system. Int Endod J. 2010;43:1001–12.
26. Tay FR, Gu L-S, Schoeffel GJ, Wimmer C, Susin L, Zhang K, et al. Effect of vapor lock on root canal debridement by using a side-vented needle for positive-pressure irrigant delivery. J Endod. 2010;36:745–50.
27. Goode N, Khan S, Eid AA, Niu L, Gosier J, Susin LF, et al. Wall shear stress effects of different endodontic irrigation techniques and systems. J Dent Elsevier Ltd. 2013;41:636–41.
28. Chen JE, Nurbakhsh B, Layton G, Bussmann M, Kishen A. Irrigation dynamics associated with positive pressure, apical negative pressure and passive ultrasonic irrigations: a computational fluid dynamics analysis. Aust Endod J. 2013;40:54–60.
29. Hockett JL, Dommisch JK, Johnson JD, Cohenca N. Antimicrobial efficacy of two irrigation techniques in tapered and nontapered canal preparations: an in vitro study. J Endod. 2008;34:1374–7.
30. Cohenca N, Heilborn C, Johnson JD, Flores DSH, Ito IY, da Silva LAB. Apical negative pressure irrigation versus conventional irrigation plus triantibiotic intracanal dressing on root canal disinfection in dog teeth. Oral Surg Oral Med Oral Pathol Oral Radiol Endod. 2010;109:e42–6.
31. Ding RY, Cheung GS, Chen J, Yin XZ, Wang QQ, Zhang CF. Pulp revascularization of immature teeth with apical periodontitis: a clinical study. J Endod. 2009;35:745–9.
32. Eickholz P, Kim T-S, Burklin T, Schacher B, Renggli HH, Schaecken MT, et al. Non-surgical periodontal therapy with adjunctive topical doxycycline: a double-blind randomized controlled multicenter study. (I). Study design and clinical results. J Clin Periodontol. 2002;29:108–17.
33. De Paz S, Pérez A, Gómez M, Trampal A, Domínguez Lázaro A. Severe hypersensitivity reaction to minocycline. J Investig Allergol Clin Immunol. 1999;9:403–4.
34. Cohenca N, Paranjpe A, Heilborn C, Jd J. Antimicrobial efficacy of two irrigation techniques in tapered and non-tapered canal preparations. A randomized controlled clinical trial. Quintessence Int. 2013;44:2017–28.
35. Pawar R, Alqaied A, Safavi K, Boyko J, Kaufman B. Influence of an apical negative pressure irrigation system on bacterial elimination during endodontic therapy: a prospective randomized clinical study. J Endod. 2012;38:1177–81.
36. McComb D, Smith DC, Beagrie GS. The results of in vivo endodontic chemomechanical instrumentation – a scanning electron microscopic study 1973. J Br Endod Soc. 1976;9:11–8.
37. Gwinnett AJ. Smear layer: morphological considerations. Oper Dent Suppl. 1984;3:2–12.
38. Sen B, Safavi K, Spangberg L. Antifungal effects of sodium hypochlorite and chlorhexidine in root canals. J Endod. 1999;25:1235–8.
39. Clark-Holke D, Drake D, Walton R, Rivera E, Guthmiller JM. Bacterial penetration through canals of endodontically treated teeth in the presence or absence of the smear layer. J Dent. 2003;31:275–81.
40. Torabinejad M, Handysides R, Khademi AA, Bakland LK. Clinical implications of the smear layer in endodontics: a review. Oral Surg Oral Med Oral Pathol Oral Radiol Endod. 2002;94:658–66.
41. Yang S-E, Bae K-S. Scanning electron microscopy study of the adhesion of Prevotella nigrescens to the dentin of prepared root canals. J Endod. 2002;28:433–7.
42. Gençoğlu N, Samani S, Günday M. Evaluation of sealing properties of Thermafil and Ultrafil techniques in the absence or presence of smear layer. J Endod. 1993;19:599–603.
43. White RR, Goldman M, Lin PS. The influence of the smeared layer upon dentinal tubule penetration by endodontic filling materials. Part II. J Endod. 1987;13:369–74.
44. Mancini M, Cerroni L, Iorio L, Armellin E, Conte G, Cianconi L. Smear layer removal and canal cleanliness using different irrigation systems (EndoActivator, EndoVac, and passive ultrasonic irrigation): field emission scanning electron microscopic evaluation in an in vitro study. J Endod. 2013;39:1456–60.
45. Saber SE-D, Hashem AAR. Efficacy of different final irrigation activation techniques on smear layer removal. J Endod. 2011;37:1272–5.
46. Dovgyallo GI, Migun NP, Prokhorenko P. The complete filling of dead-end conical capillaries with liquid. J Eng Phys. 1989;2:563–5.

47. Pesse AV, Warrier GR, Dhir VK. An experimental study of the gas entrapment process in closed-end microchannels. Int J Heat Mass Transf. 2005;48:5150–65.
48. De Gregorio C, Estevez R, Cisneros R, Heilborn C, Cohenca N. Effect of EDTA, sonic, and ultrasonic activation on the penetration of sodium hypochlorite into simulated lateral canals: an in vitro study. J Endod. 2009;35:891–5.
49. Senia ES, Marshall FJ, Rosen S. The solvent action of sodium hypochlorite on pulp tissue of extracted teeth. Oral Surg Oral Med Oral Pathol. 1971;31:96–103.
50. Alouini Z, Seux R. Kinetics and mechanisms of hypochlorite oxidation of α-amino acids at the time of water disinfection. Water Res. 1987;21:335–43.
51. Torabinejad M, Cho Y, Khademi AA, Bakland LK, Shabahang S. The effect of various concentrations of sodium hypochlorite on the ability of MTAD to remove the smear layer. J Endod. 2003;29:233–9.
52. Van der Sluis LWM, Gambarini G, Wu MK, Wesselink PR. The influence of volume, type of irrigant and flushing method on removing artificially placed dentine debris from the apical root canal during passive ultrasonic irrigation. Int Endod J. 2006;39:472–6.
53. Tinaz AC, Alacam T, Uzun O, Maden M, Kayaoglu G. The effect of disruption of apical constriction on periapical extrusion. J Endod. 2005;31:533–5.
54. Fukumoto Y, Kikuchi I, Yoshioka T, Kobayashi C, Suda H. An ex vivo evaluation of a new root canal irrigation technique with intracanal aspiration. Int Endod J. 2006;39:93–9.
55. Usman N, Baumgartner JC, Marshall JG. Influence of instrument size on root canal debridement. J Endod. 2004;30:110–2.
56. Berutti E, Marini R. A scanning electron microscopic evaluation of the debridement capability of sodium hypochlorite at different temperatures. J Endod. 1996;22:467–70.
57. Chow TW. Mechanical effectiveness of root canal irrigation. J Endod. 1983;9:475–9.
58. Siqueira JF, Lopes HP. Mechanisms of antimicrobial activity of calcium hydroxide: a critical review. Int Endod J. 1999;32:361–9.
59. Tanomaru JMG, Leonardo MR, Tanomaru Filho M, Bonetti Filho I, Silva LAB. Effect of different irrigation solutions and calcium hydroxide on bacterial LPS. Int Endod J. 2003;36:733–9.
60. Leonardo MR, Hernandez MEFT, Silva LAB, Tanomaru-Filho M. Effect of a calcium hydroxide-based root canal dressing on periapical repair in dogs: a histological study. Oral Surg Oral Med Oral Pathol Oral Radiol Endod. 2006;102:680–5.
61. Kim SK, Kim YO. Influence of calcium hydroxide intracanal medication on apical seal. Int Endod J. 2002;35:623–8.
62. Erdemir A, Ari H, Güngüneş H, Belli S. Effect of medications for root canal treatment on bonding to root canal dentin. J Endod. 2004;30:113–6.
63. Calt S, Serper A. Dentinal tubule penetration of root canal sealers after root canal dressing with calcium hydroxide. J Endod. 1999;25:431–3.
64. Kenee DM, Allemang JD, Johnson JD, Hellstein J, Nichol BK. A quantitative assessment of efficacy of various calcium hydroxide removal techniques. J Endod. 2006;32:563–5.
65. Türker SA, Koçak MM, Koçak S, Sağlam BC. Comparison of calcium hydroxide removal by self-adjusting file, EndoVac, and CanalBrush agitation techniques: an in vitro study. J Conserv Dent. 2013;16:439–43.
66. Yücel A, Gürel M, Güler E, Karabucak B. Comparison of final irrigation techniques in removal of calcium hydroxide. Aust Endod J. 2011;39:116–21.
67. Mehdipour O, Kleier DJ, Averbach RE. Anatomy of sodium hypochlorite accidents. Compend Contin Educ Dent. 2007;28:544–6, 548, 550.
68. Pashley EL, Birdsong NL, Bowman K, Pashley DH. Cytotoxic effects of NaOCI on vital tissue efecto citotoxico del NaOCI en el tejido vital. J Endod. 1985;11:30–3.
69. Bowden JR, Ethunandan M, Brennan PA. Life-threatening airway obstruction secondary to hypochlorite extrusion during root canal treatment. Oral Surg Oral Med Oral Pathol Oral Radiol Endod. 2006;101:402–4.
70. Markose G, Cotter CJ, Hislop WS. Facial atrophy following accidental subcutaneous extrusion of sodium hypochlorite. Br Dent J. 2009;206:263–4.
71. Pelka M, Petschelt A. Permanent mimic musculature and nerve damage caused by sodium hypochlorite: a case report. Oral Surg Oral Med Oral Pathol Oral Radiol Endod. 2008;106:e80–3.
72. Linden WJ. When irrigation leads to litigation. Oral Health Dent Prod Rep. 2010;101:104.
73. de Sermeño RF, da Silva LA, Herrera H, Herrera H, Silva RA, Leonardo MR. Tissue damage after sodium hypochlorite extrusion during root canal treatment. Oral Surg Oral Med Oral Pathol Oral Radiol Endod. 2009;108:e46–9.
74. Boutsioukis C, Verhaagen B, Versluis M, Kastrinakis E, Wesselink PR, van der Sluis LWM. Evaluation of irrigant flow in the root canal using different needle types by an unsteady computational fluid dynamics model. J Endod. 2010;36:875–9.
75. Hülsmann M, Hahn W. Complications during root canal irrigation–literature review and case reports. Int Endod J. 2000;33:186–93.
76. Malentacca A, Uccioli U, Zangari D, Lajolo C, Fabiani C. Efficacy and safety of various active irrigation devices when used with either positive or negative pressure: an in vitro study. J Endod. 2012;38:1622–6.

Sonic and Ultrasonic Irrigation

10

John M. Nusstein

Abstract

Cleaning and shaping of the root canal with the use of irrigants is a fundamental principle of endodontic therapy. However, current research has shown that needle-delivered irrigation, although effective, is unable to clean and disinfect the root canal system as well as an activated irrigant. This chapter reviews the use of ultrasonic, laser, and sonic-activated irrigation to improve the cleaning and disinfecting of the root canal system. A review of the concepts, systems, and mechanisms will be presented as well as review of the pertinent literature to justify the use of activated endodontic irrigants.

Introduction

The goal of root canal cleaning and shaping is the removal of vital or necrotic tissue, microorganisms, and their by-products and provide space for placing obturating materials. The ultimate goal is the complete removal and disinfection of the root canal space. The question is if that goal is truly achievable utilizing the standard techniques we are currently taught. Almost 100 years ago, Hess [76] showed us the challenges dentists face in cleaning the root canal system (Fig. 10.1). With modern scientific technology, we have been reminded of these facts. According to work by Peters [126], one can see on these overlays (Fig. 10.2) that even with our improved NiTi file systems, all of the walls of the canals are not touched during cleaning and shaping. Hess's original findings on the complexity of root canal anatomy have been reconfirmed. As one looks at a cross section of the mesial root of a mandibular first molar (Fig. 10.3), one sees nice round canal preparations at the 1 mm apical level. However, a great deal of tissue is left behind in the isthmus and along the canal wall irregularities. These findings are the reason why irrigation has taken on a new importance and why there has been an increase in the research on irrigation. Irrigation works at a level that endodontic files cannot reach. Unfortunately the traditional use of needle-only irrigation may not be achieving the results we anticipate.

The ability of an irrigant to dissolve pulp tissue, kill bacteria, and remove smear layer are

J.M. Nusstein, DDS, MS
Division of Endodontics, The Ohio State University College of Dentistry,
Postle Hall, Room 3058, 305 W. 12th Ave.,
Columbus, OH 43210, USA
e-mail: Nusstein.1@osu.edu

B. Basrani (ed.), *Endodontic Irrigation: Chemical Disinfection of the Root Canal System*,
DOI 10.1007/978-3-319-16456-4_10

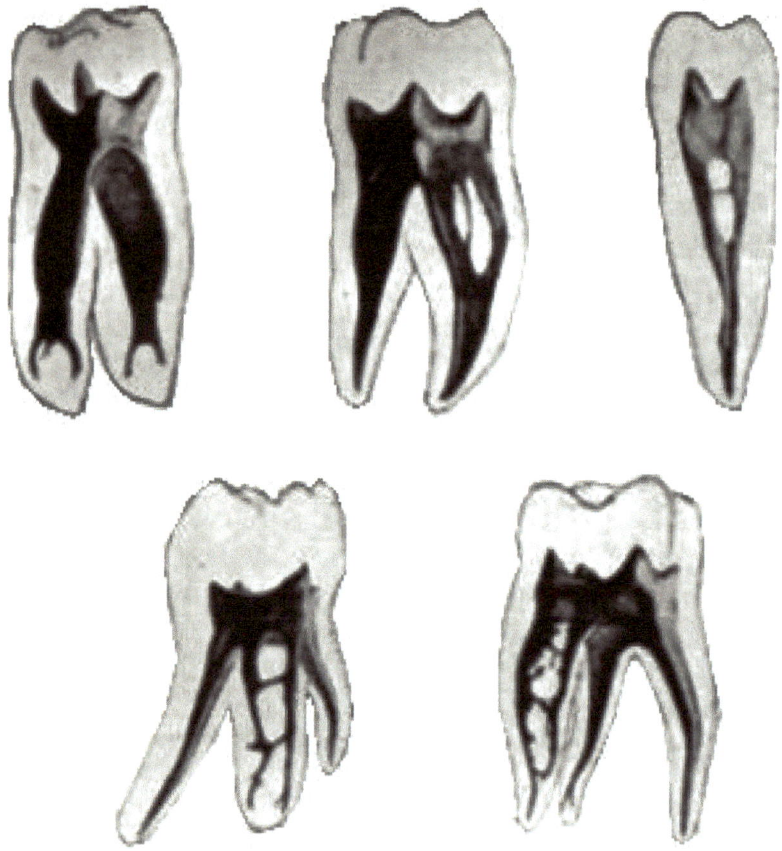

Fig. 10.1 Hess [76] intricacies of canal anatomy

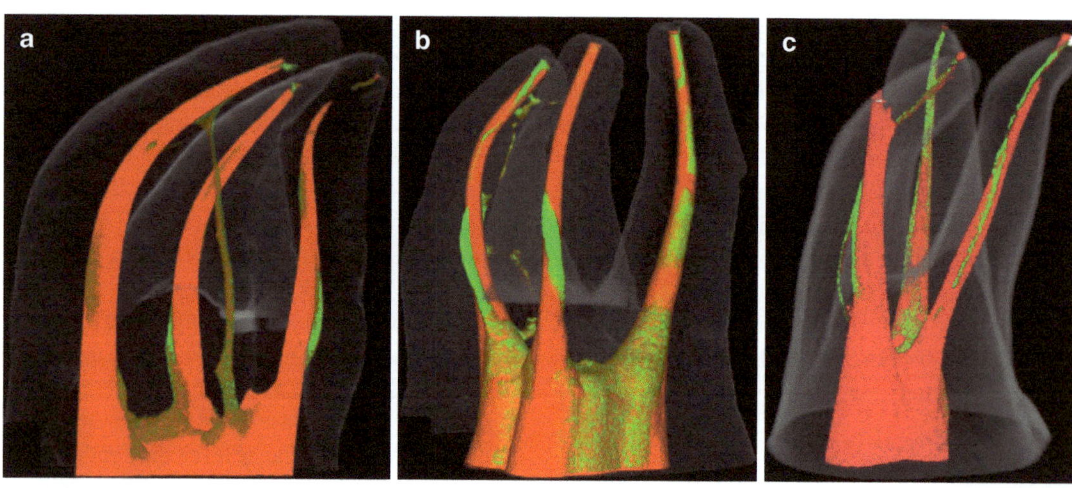

Fig. 10.2 Micro CT scans of canals following rotary file instrumentation (*red*) overlaid preoperative scans (*green*) [126]

well known and reported in the literature. Some irrigants are better suited for some jobs than others. Research has shown that the preparation (hand files and/or rotary NiTi files) of an infected root canal with standard needle irrigation (using sodium hypochlorite – NaOCl) and even

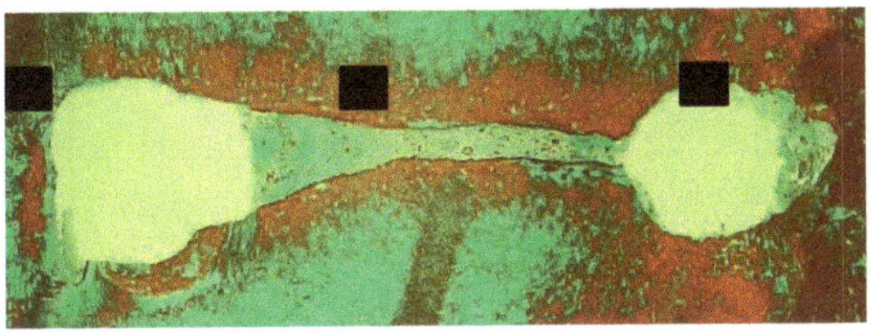

Fig. 10.3 Cross section of mesial root of mandibular molar demonstrating remaining tissue following root canal preparation utilizing NiTi rotary files [73]

placement of calcium hydroxide greatly reduces the number of viable bacteria in the canal [29, 30, 31, 38, 39, 46, 53, 121, 125, 132, 138, 142, 144, 145]. However, it does not eliminate all of them. Removal of biofilm is also limited, especially in the isthmuses and canal ramifications [28].

The flow characteristics of various size and shaped needles (open-ended versus side-vented) have also been described in the endodontic literature. Shen et al. [140] described how the velocity of fluid flow is affected by the needle design. Open-ended or beveled needles deliver fluid at a quicker pace than side-vented needles. This increase in velocity may aid in removing debris from the canal walls. The side-ported needles have their maximum velocity at the site of the port and the energy dissipates apically. Open-ended/beveled needles deliver irrigation solution about 1–2 mm past the end of the needle. This is a benefit if the needle cannot reach the apex of the root canal but a drawback if it does (potential irrigation accident). The side-ported needles allow solution to only reach about 1 mm past the end of the tip and still have similar risks and benefits of the open-ended needles. Shen et al. [140] also calculated the fluid pressure of the irrigant. This pressure may be of benefit in cleaning the canal walls by dislodging material such as biofilm. Of course the three dynamic parameters (fluid flow pattern, velocity, fluid wall pressure) are all affected by the fluid flow rate placed into the needle. Unfortunately, research has continuously shown that traditional needle irrigation fails to clean isthmuses, lateral canals, and cul-de-sacs to any extent ([15, 22, 69, 73, 74, 82, 94, 112, 151, 170]). Activation of the endodontic irrigant appears to be a necessary step in the more complete cleaning of the root canal system. A survey conducted by Dutner et al. [65] on the use of irrigants and adjunctive devices to aid irrigation found that almost 50 % of respondents use some type of irrigation aid. Of that group, 48 % used ultrasonics and 34 % utilized some form of sonic (subsonic) activation.

Ultrasonic Activation

Richman [128] first reported the application of ultrasonics in endodontics. He used a Cavitron® ultrasonic dental unit and concluded that since these cases were treated without untoward post-operative sequelae, the use of ultrasonics in root canal therapy held great promise.

In a series of articles published in the endodontic literature from 1976 to 1985, Martin and Cunningham [48–50, 104–109] reported on the use of ultrasound as a primary method of canal preparation and debridement in root canal therapy. The studies evaluated the efficacy of the endosonic method, its ability to eliminate bacteria from the canal, and its effect on extrusion of debris. Martin and Cunningham [106] concluded that endosonic root canal preparation was superior to hand preparation in mechanical and chemical debridement, disinfection, and final canal shaping. The ultrasonically energized file was reported to rapidly instrument the canal wall more efficiently with less operator fatigue. The "ultrasonically activated" irrigant facilitated cleansing and disinfecting actions within the root canal system.

Other studies of ultrasound as a primary method of instrumentation did not support the claims of Martin and Cunningham [107] that ultrasound removes more tissue from the canal than hand instrumentation. These studies [52, 67, 92, 154] found no difference in tissue removal between ultrasound and hand instrumentation. Also, when antibacterial effects were evaluated, no difference was found between the two instrumentation techniques [16, 60]. The overall performance of ultrasound as a primary method of instrumentation was not found to be superior to hand instrumentation. There was also a reported increase risk in straightening and perforating canals.

Martin and Cunningham [106] attributed the success of ultrasonic instrumentation to the interaction of the ultrasonic energy and the irrigating solution. They called this interaction the "synergistic system." The irrigating solution achieves its active biological-chemical effects when it undergoes ultrasonation. The authors defined the primary effects of ultrasound as being cavitation and acoustic streaming. Transient cavitation was said to occur when the ultrasonic energy creates a bubble which grows to a certain point and then collapses. This collapse creates a pressure-vacuum effect which cleans irregularities in canals and kills microorganisms. The oscillatory effect of the ultrasonic instrument, which vigorously agitates the irrigating solution, is defined as resonant or stable cavitation. Combined with these effects of cavitation is a dispersal of physical energy which leads to physical acoustic (sound wave) streaming. This acoustic streaming purportedly enhances cleansing and disinfection.

When an ultrasonic wave is projected in liquid, negative pressure is created and causes the liquid to fracture, a process known as cavitation. Cavitation creates bubbles that oscillate in the projected ultrasonic waves. As the ultrasonic waves continue, these bubbles grow larger and become very unstable, eventually collapsing in a violent implosion. The implosions radiate high-powered shockwaves that dissipate repeatedly at a rate of 25,000 ~ 30,000 times per second (25–30 kHz). Additionally, the implosion of cavitation bubbles creates temperatures that exceed 5,000 ° C and pressures that exceed 500 atmospheres. The shock waves that are generated by the implosion travel at speeds over 500 mph within the fluid and this current is called acoustic streaming (www.tmasc.com, http://bluewaveinc.com) [21, 157]. Acoustic streaming can also be derived from the ultra-high-frequency oscillation of the ultrasonic tip/file placed in a fluid. Cleaning an object requires dissolving a contaminant (removing substance/object from a wall and putting it into solution) and then displacing the saturated layer of the contaminant so that fresh cleaning solution can come in contact with the unsaturated surface of the contaminant. The ultrasonic cavitation implosion effect is incredibly effective in doing this. The cavitation implosion effect is especially effective on unsmooth and out of reach surfaces that are normally inaccessible through conventional means such as irrigation alone.

To gain an insight into the mechanisms involved in ultrasonic instrumentation, Ahmad et al. [2] investigated the phenomena of cavitation and acoustic streaming as seen within the root canal space. In this initial study, the authors combined the phenomenon of resonant or stable cavitation, as described by Martin and Cunningham [106], with the phenomenon of acoustic streaming. These terms were combined because the rapid vortex-like motion associated with the vibrating file can also be associated with small gas bubbles set into oscillation by the fluctuating pressure field generated by the ultrasonic file. The group looked at transient cavitation using a photometric-sensitive image intensification system. This detection system monitored the light produced by the violent collapse of cavitation bubbles. A rectangular container filled with methylene blue dye and a dispersed film of polystyrene spheres was used to detect acoustic streaming. These spheres were illuminated so that patterns of acoustic streaming could be detected. Forty extracted maxillary anterior teeth were divided into four groups and instrumented either by hand or ultrasonically (Cavi-Endo®), using either water or 2.5 % sodium hypochlorite as an irrigating solution. The teeth were split longitudinally and evaluated for presence of a smear layer using a scanning electron microscope (SEM). It was determined that transient cavitation did not occur with the Cavi-Endo® unit and endosonic files. However, cavitation was produced when a scaler tip was inserted into the unit. The endosonic files produced acoustic streaming. When the amount of remaining debris was evaluated, there was no statistically significant difference between ultrasonic and hand instrumentation when either water or sodium hypochlorite was used as an irrigating solution. The authors concluded that acoustic streaming was more important to cleaning than cavitation. It was also concluded that the recommended technique of ultrasonic instrumentation did not produce sufficient acoustic streaming to effectively clean the canal. Dampening of the files may have caused the limitation in the production of acoustic streaming in the constricted canal system.

Ahmad et al. [3] continued the investigation of ultrasonic debridement by examining acoustic streaming. The authors defined acoustic streaming as the generation of time-independent, steady unidirectional circulation of fluid in the vicinity of a small vibrating object. Using the same method to detect acoustic streaming as described in the previous study [2], different size files were studied at different power settings. The power generated by the files was estimated by measuring the transverse displacement amplitudes that were produced. Transverse displacement amplitude was defined as half of the total distance moved by the pinpoint of light that appeared as a thin transverse line when a file oscillated. Twenty extracted maxillary anterior teeth were divided into two groups and instrumented with the second group using a modified technique in which a #15 endosonic file was allowed to freely vibrate at working length for 5 min. The results showed that each file generated an acoustic streaming field comprised of a primary field consisting of rapidly moving eddies in which the fluid element oscillated about a mean position, and a superimposed secondary field consisting of patterns of relatively slow, time-independent flow (Fig. 10.4). Approximately four clusters of eddies were generated by the #15 and 20 endosonic files. In the primary field, the direction of rotation of the fluid elements in each eddy was opposite to that of its immediate neighbor. The secondary field showed symmetrical longitudinal flows on both sides of the file (Fig. 10.5). Fluid was generally transported from the apical to coronal end of the file. The streaming velocity was greatest at the apical and least at the coronal end of the file. Smaller files generated relatively greater acoustic streaming, the velocity of which increased with increased power. These results were later confirmed by Jiang et al. [83]. Canals instrumented with the modified method were found to exhibit cleaner surfaces. The authors concluded that the freely vibrating file produced hydrodynamic shear stresses large enough to remove debris and the smear layer from the walls of the root canal, resulting in enhanced cleansing action. This hydrodynamic shear stress was proportional to streaming velocity. Therefore, the authors deduced that since streaming velocity was highest at the apical tip of the file, a concentration of stresses in the vicinity of the tip facilitated debridement.

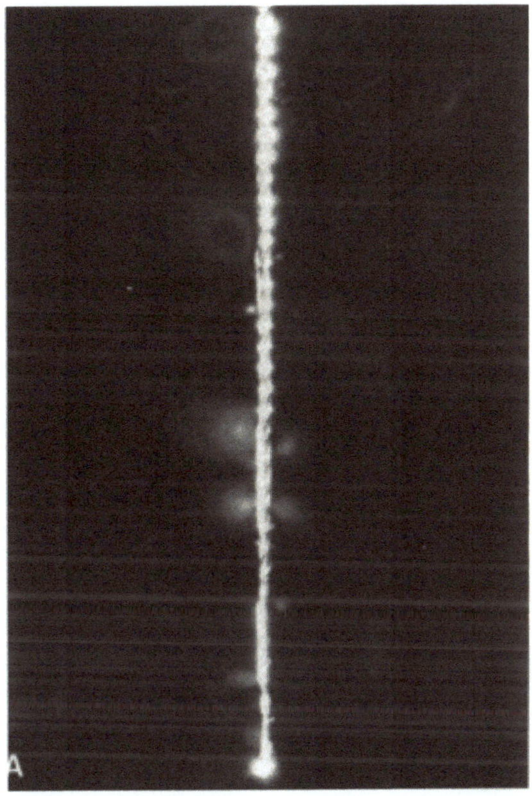

Fig. 10.4 Photo of acoustic streaming around a size 15 endosonic file [3]

In another investigation into the mechanisms of ultrasound, Ahmad et al. [4] examined the effects of acoustic cavitation in debridement of root canals. The authors concluded that cavitation should not be regarded as an important mechanism in root canal debridement. Walmsley [166] also investigated the mechanisms of ultrasound in root canal treatment. His results agreed with Ahmad et al. [2], as he concluded that cavitation had little if any bearing on the debridement

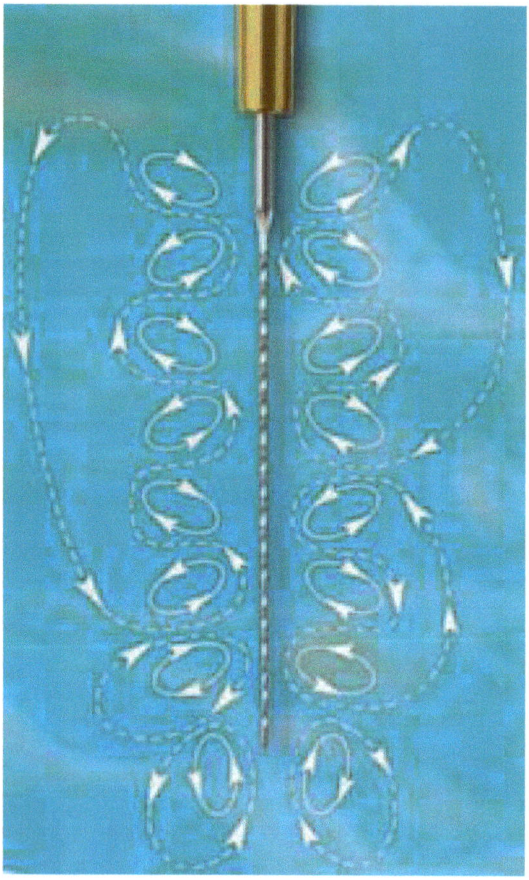

Fig. 10.5 Depiction of the waves generated around the vibrating ultrasonic file (ACTEON North America/ Clinical Research Dental)

activity of ultrasound. This conclusion was based on his postulation that although the displacement amplitudes of the vibrating file were adequate to produce cavitation, the streamlined shape of the endosonic file was not conducive to generating a sound pressure field large enough to produce cavitation. Walmsley [167] also concluded that because of the transverse nature of the vibration pattern of the activated file, the effectiveness of ultrasonic instrumentation is limited by the dampening of the file against the root canal wall. Acoustic streaming is an effective mechanism in disrupting debris within the canals but is reduced when loading occurs against canal walls. Also, the synergistic activity of ultrasound and the irrigating solution does not take place when the file is not allowed to vibrate freely. Recently however, Jiang et al. [83] and Macedo et al. [97] showed that, within a simulated root canal system, cavitation did occur around the tip of an ultrasonically activated file, but that canal size (in relation to the file size) did impact the amount of cavitation produced.

Ahmad et al. [5] also reported that ultrasonic files can generate acoustic streaming both in the free field and in a small channel. Higher-velocity streaming was observed when smaller size files were employed and when the file was precurved (for curved canals). Light file-wall contact did not totally inhibit streaming, while severe file-wall contact inhibited movement of the file and, as a result, no streaming was observed. The positions and length scales of the streaming vortices appeared to be influenced by the presence of boundaries. In the free field, two rows of vortices were situated along the sides of the file (Fig. 10.6a), while in the small channel, the vortices were positioned above the surface of the file (Fig. 10.6b). These results indicated that it is possible for acoustic streaming to occur in a confined space, as in a root canal, provided that severe file-wall contact is avoided. They recommended that allowing the file to freely vibrate during some stage of treatment should be carried out in order to generate streaming in the root canal.

Roy et al. [133] used sonoluminescence as an indicator of transient cavitation activity and photographic analysis was utilized as a means for detecting steady streaming, microstreaming, and stable cavitation with ultrasonic files. Measurements failed to indicate any strong correlation between registered driving power and the propensity to produce transient cavitation. Files that were pitted or possessed salient edges were very effective at generating transient cavitation. When observed, transient cavitation activity generally occurred near the tip of the straight file, provided the wall loading did not inhibit file motion. In all cases studied, steady acoustic streaming and stable cavitation were observed to varying degrees, depending on the amount of file to wall contact. Although the imposition of file-wall contact served to inhibit the production of transient cavitation, this action had relatively

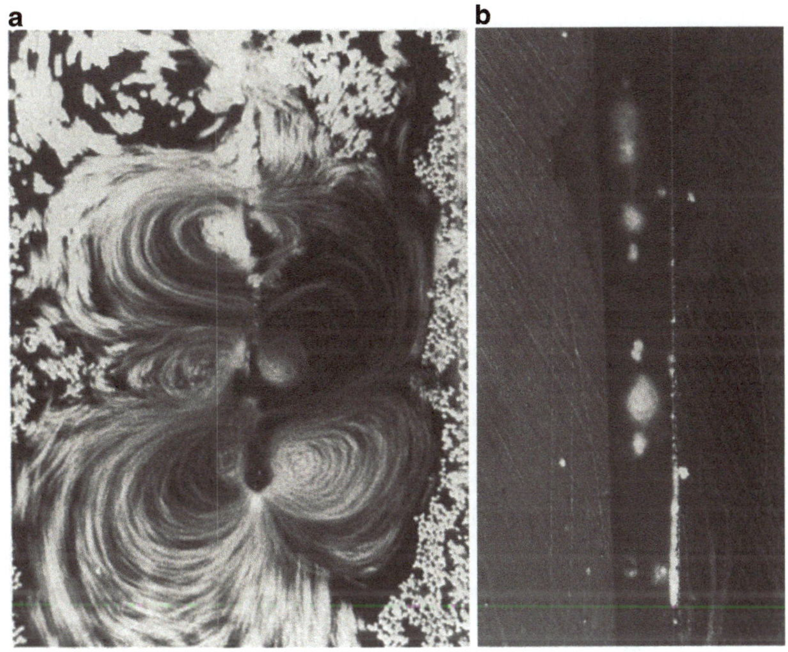

Fig. 10.6 (**a**) Acoustic streaming as generated around a free-moving file and (**b**) within a simulated root canal space [5]

little effect on the ability of a file to produce a nominal level of streaming, microstreaming, and stable cavitation. They concluded that it was not prudent to ascribe enhanced cleaning effects to any one phenomenon, for it is likely that several factors are involved to varying degrees depending on the local conditions of application. Boutsioukis et al. [26] confirmed that an ultrasonically activated file contacts the root canal wall at least 20 % of time during activation. They reported that the depth of penetration of the file, the power utilized to activate the file, and the size of the root canal preparation all affected the amount of contact. However, they did report that cavitation in the fluid was detected even though there was file-wall contact.

Ultrasonic Energy Generation

There are two main types of ultrasonic energy generators used in dentistry which differ in their mode of operations. The magnetostrictive generator utilizes the principle of magnetostriction in which certain materials expand and contract when placed in an alternating magnetic field. Alternating electrical current (AC) from the ultrasonic generator is first converted into an alternating magnetic field through the use of a coil of wire inside the ultrasonic handpiece. The alternating magnetic field is then used to induce mechanical vibrations at an ultrasonic frequency in resonant strips of nickel or other magnetostrictive material that are attached to the surface to be vibrated [45]. Because magnetostrictive materials behave identically to a magnetic field of either polarity, the frequency of the electrical energy applied to the transducer (coiled wire) is half of the desired output frequency. This form of ultrasonic generation requires two transformations of energy: electrical to magnetic and magnetic to mechanical. During these energy transformations, heat is generated as energy is lost. Therefore, the efficiency of this type of generator is affected (as low as 50 %) and cooling measures are required to dissipate the heat generated. The frequency at which magnetostrictive generators operate is also limited. Due to size restrictions, they operate below 30 KHz [45]. To increase the frequency would require enlarging the wire coils and resonant metal strips, as well as increase the need for cooling, to the point of clinical infeasibility.

The piezoelectric generator, on the other hand, converts AC electrical energy directly into mechanical energy through the use of the piezoelectric effect. When electrical energy is applied to ceramic piezoelectric materials (i.e., barium titanate or lead zirconate titanate), there is a conversion and amplification of electrical energy into mechanical energy by way of vibration of the material within the ultrasonic handpiece. This vibration is then directly transmitted into the ultrasonic tip. This method allows piezoelectric transducers to operate well into the megahertz frequency range. Piezoelectric generators are more efficient (95 %) than magnetostrictive units due to the fact that magnetostrictive units require the two conversions of energy [45].

Passive Ultrasonic Irrigation (PUI)/ Ultrasonically Activated Irrigation (UAI)

The terminology for the activation of irrigating fluids in root canals can be a bit confusing. Weller et al. [168] compared the efficacy of ultrasonics as a primary method of instrumentation and as an adjunct to hand instrumentation versus hand instrumentation alone. The authors concluded that ultrasonic instrumentation is not an alternative to hand cleaning but acts as an aid to increase debridement efficacy after hand instrumentation. In this study, the ultrasonic instrument was still used as an adjunct in canal preparation. Later research [12, 36, 69, 74, 82, 94, 112] looked at the use of ultrasonic instrumentation in a more passive manner, that is, it was utilized after hand instrumentation and without the intent to enlarge, instrument, or impact the walls of the root canal. Thus, the term passive ultrasonic irrigation (PUI) came to be. The "passive" portion indicated no active or intentional removal of dentin. Unfortunately, even though no intent is made to contact or alter the root canal walls, contact of the oscillating ultrasonic instrument on the wall occurs (see above). Due to this, the phrase ultrasonically activated irrigation (UAI) was recently suggested by Boutsioukis et al. [26]. Unfortunately the reader must be aware that these terms can and will be used interchangeably in the dental literature and that they represent the same general technique.

Research into PUI/UAI has looked at the ability of the technique to remove tissue and debris, bacteria, biofilm, calcium hydroxide and other medicaments, and smear layer. Research has also looked at the impact of using PUI/UAI in curved canals, the use of a smooth instrument versus an endodontic file, and the effects the size of the instrument and canal preparation size have on cleaning/debridement results. In general, PUI/UAI consists of the use of a size 15 or 20 endodontic-type file or wire attached to an ultrasonic handpiece from which ultrasonic energy is supplied. The depth of the file within the canal and the manner in which irrigating solution is supplied during the process has also been evaluated.

Available products that a clinician can utilize to provide PUI/UAI include file-holder tips (Brasseler). These tips allow for the insertion of a hand file (k-type file, r-type file, spreader, etc.) or a specially designed hand file-type inserts (dia-

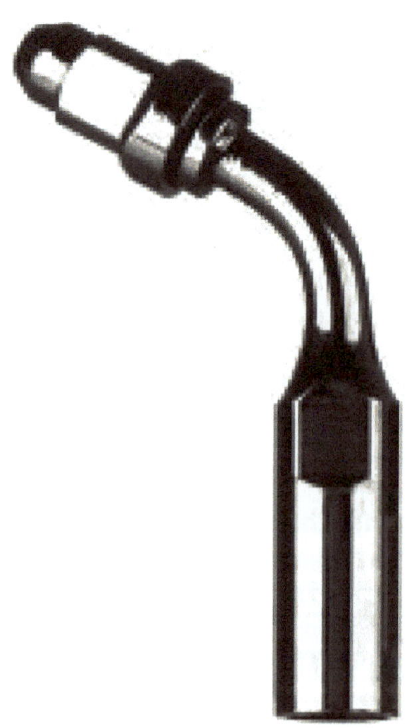

Fig. 10.7 Brasseler file holder E12 (Brasseler)

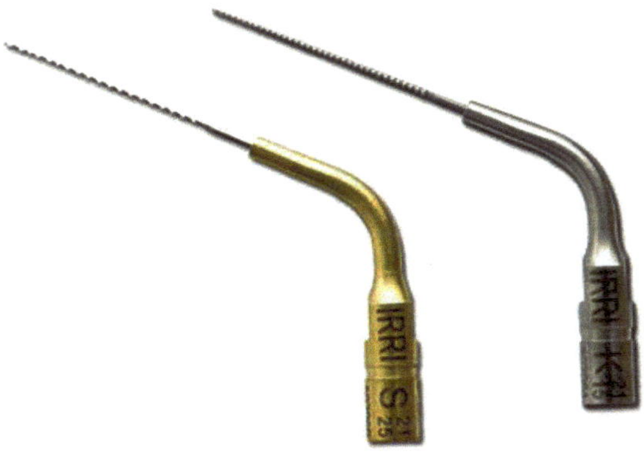

Fig. 10.8 Satelec Acteon Irrisafe™ tips. Note serrated wire with non-cutting sides and irrigation port near attachment hub (Satelec)

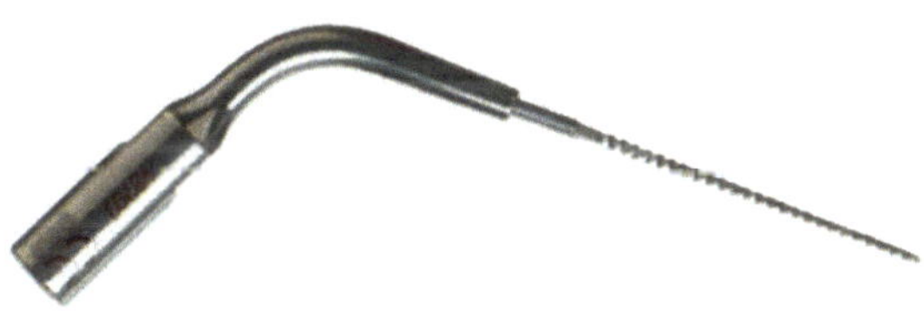

Fig. 10.9 Satelec Sonofile with no irrigation port (Tulsa Dental Products)

mond coated, fluted, smooth-sided, etc.) and secured for use in the canal (Fig. 10.7). Also available is the Irrisafe™ ultrasonic tip (Fig. 10.8) produced by Satelec Acteon which comes in different lengths and diameters and includes a port for the delivery of irrigating fluid, and the Sonofile tips (Fig. 10.9) by Satelec which are similar to the Irrisafe™ files but without the irrigation port.

Debris and Smear Layer Removal

The effectiveness of PUI/UAI following canal preparation to remove tissue and debris has been extensively studied. In general, PUI/UAI has been reported to be more effective than simple syringe and needle irrigation. As previously stated, Weller et al. [168] was the first to report on the benefits of ultrasonic activation of irrigant following hand instrumentation. They reported that the combination was superior to either technique alone. Goodman et al. [69] and Lev at al. [94] reported that the addition of 3 min of PUI/UAI per canal (using NaOCl as an irrigant) significantly improved the cleanliness of the isthmuses of the mesial roots of mandibular molars in vitro at the 1 and 3 mm levels from the canal apex. Metzler and Montgomery [112] found similar results using 2 min of PUI/UAI. Cameron [36] also reported that canals had less tissue and debris following the use of EDTAC/NaOCl and 1.5 min of PUI/UAI in vitro. These studies were followed up by Haidet et al. [74] and Archer et al. [12] who studied the use of 3 min of PUI/UAI per canal in vivo following hand instrumentation and found that isthmus and canal cleanliness was significantly improved at the levels 1–3 mm from the apex as compared to needle irrigation with NaOCl.

Utilizing ex vivo models with artificially prepared grooves, different preparation tapers, and lateral canals filled with dentin debris, various studies have shown that PUI/UAI improved debris removal from the hard-to-reach areas. Looking at the influence of the size of the canal preparation on cleaning with PUI/UAI, Lee et al. [92, 93] and van der Sluis et al. [162] reported that the greater the taper of the canal, the more debris that is removed with the PUI/UAI file. Rödig et al. [129, 130], however, found that apical size had no impact on canal cleanliness when utilizing PUI/UAI. This result contradicted findings that larger apical preparations improved the efficacy of NaOCl [79]. In another study, van der Sluis [163] reported that a smooth wire (such as a finger plugger placed in a file holder) could remove debris as well as a file design. This supported the previous work of Cameron [34] and Goodman et al. [69]. Jiang et al. [84] reported that the direction the ultrasonic file oscillated may affect cleaning. They stated that improved results were achieved when the vibration was directed at the site of a groove to be cleaned. In terms of irrigant penetration, several studies have looked at the ability of PUI/UAI to improve the dispersement of an irrigant into lateral canals. De Gregorio et al. [55] reported that irrigant penetrated artificially made lateral canals much better when PUI/UAI was utilized than needle irrigation or negative pressure irrigation. Spoorthy et al. [148] reported similar results. Al-Jadaa et al. [8] reported similar results (improved debris removal from artificial lateral canals) between PUI/UAI and needle irrigation when controlling for the increase in temperature of the NaOCl irrigant (approximately 30 ° C) caused by the ultrasonic activation.

Clinically, these studies can be translated into improved canal cleanliness in the areas generally untouched by hand and/or rotary files, i.e., isthmuses, lateral canals, canal fins, and cul-de-sacs. In vivo research has indicated that isthmuses and canals are more thoroughly cleaned when PUI/UAI is utilized following canal preparation [12, 74, 112]. Empirically, this increased ability to remove debris and tissue should lead to improved clinical outcomes. An initial study by Liang et al. [95], evaluating 86 patients 10–19 months after root canal treatment, showed an improvement in the reduction and resolution of apical pathosis following the use of PUI/UAI compared to needle irrigation. However, the difference was not found to be significant. More research with longer follow-up times is needed.

In terms of smear layer removal, results have varied with slightly more studies indicating that PUI/UAI helps remove smear layer. These varied results may be due to the use of different types and concentrations of irrigants. When NaOCl was utilized alone, studies have reported almost complete smear layer removal from various levels of the root canal [7, 33, 34, 35, 81, 159]. These studies, again, utilized various concentrations of NaOCl, ranging from 0.5 to 12 %, and different exposure times to the ultrasonic energy (10 s to 5 min). When NaOCl was combined with EDTA, the research has shown a marked improvement in smear layer removal [11, 20, 66, 90]. Several studies, however, did not find PUI/UAI to be very effective in removing smear layer even when NaOCl and EDTA were utilized [1, 42, 44, 134, 156]. The use of water as an irrigant has been reported not to enhance smear layer removal with the addition of PUI/UAI ([33, 34, 75, 159]). This would indicate that the cavitation and acoustic streaming effects alone cannot account for smear layer removal. The difficulty in studying smear layer removal is that it relies on the assessment of SEM images. Only very small portions of a large area of canal wall are evaluated and, often, different conditions can appear on the same image. This makes grading of the images difficult and potentially unreliable depending on the evaluators and the number of images evaluated.

The amount of irrigant, delivery method, and delivery time of irrigants has also been evaluated. Intermittent flushing is a more popular method as compared to external continuous flushing for PUI/UAI. A new method for continuous irrigation utilizing an ultrasonically activated needle was developed and will be discussed later in the chapter. The intermittent flushing process encompasses the use of an irrigating needle/syringe which is utilized to initially fill the root canal and access opening with irrigant and then replenish the irrigant after applications of ultrasonic energy within the canal. This technique is more time consuming due to the stop-and-go process. The need to replenish the irrigant is due to the fact that dentin debris, tissue, bacteria, and biofilm saturate the irrigating solution and increase the viscosity of the solution to the point where no ultrasonic activity may occur in the solution. This effect was reported by Weller [168] and Moorer and Wesselink [115]. Research has shown that refreshing NaOCl during PUI/UAI increases the reaction of NaOCl [98, 161] and improves cleaning of canals. These studies also indicated that an increase in the time of exposure of the canals to PUI/UAI improved cleanliness in ex vivo models.

Continuous flushing of irrigant, as achieved by utilizing the Irrisafe™ tips with its irrigation ports, requires a delivery system that is able to direct irrigant into the tooth and allow for replacement of saturated or contaminated irrigant. Ideally the irrigant replacement should occur to the level of root canal apex. Also, the formation of aerosol as the irrigant contacts the coronal aspect of the ultrasonic file may lead to patient exposure to the NaOCl beyond the rubber dam or by inhalation. Unfortunately research has shown that with this type of system the time of exposure plays a more critical factor since extra time is needed to completely flush the canals in a rather uncontrolled manner [64, 121]. Lev et al. [94]

reported that, in terms of cleaning, 1 min of PUI/UAI per canal was equivalent to 3 min per canal for canal cleanliness, but that 3 min provided cleaner isthmuses when utilizing a continual flushing system. Further research into the effect of time is needed when more standard PUI/UAI techniques are developed. The size of the endodontic access opening may also play a factor in the ability of the irrigant to reach the canal. However, no research has looked at this.

Studies looking at the use of PUI/UAI to remove either calcium hydroxide or other paste fillers from root canals have given mixed results. Complete removal of a medicament is necessary since there is a potential to prevent sealing of the canal due to interference with the filling material by the remaining paste [47, 77, 102]. The addition of PUI/UAI to remove calcium hydroxide and Ledermix was found to improve overall removal, but did not assure complete removal of all material [131]. Wisemann et al. [169] reported similar results. Capar et al. [37] reported that PUI/UAI removed significantly more calcium hydroxide from artificial grooves in the apical third of the root canal as compared to needle irrigation. Complete removal of the paste was not achieved.

The impact of canal curvature on the effectiveness of PUI/UAI has also been reported. Significantly improved cleaning of canals and isthmuses occurred at the apical 5 mm in curved canals versus needle irrigation [69, 82, 112, 135]. Malki et al. [100] report that the flow of irrigant beyond the ultrasonic file tip was not affected by curvature of the canal. Ahmad et al. [5] and Lumley et al. [96] reported improved efficacy when pre-bent files were utilized for PUI/UAI. Amato et al. [10] reported better cleaning of artificially made lateral canals in teeth with PUI/UAI in both straight and curved canals as compared to needle irrigation. However, better cleaning was observed in the straight canals. This could be due to the fact that the ultrasonic file was placed within 1 mm of the apex and contacted the inner wall of the canal at the curvature and the outer wall near the apex therefore leading to diminished or restricted ultrasonic activation of the irrigant. Al-Jadaa et al. [9] reported similar results when comparing the use of straight, pre-bent, and NiTi ultrasonic files placed within 1 mm of the apex of straight and curved canals. In this study, the use of the NiTi file resulted in better debris removal and less transportation versus the straight and precurved stainless steel files/wires.

Bacteria/Biofilm Removal

The removal or reduction in the number of bacteria within the root canal system is one of the primary goals of endodontic therapy. The utilization of ultrasonically activated irrigation to achieve this goal has been researched. A large number of studies have reported a significant reduction in the number of bacteria (as measured by colony forming units – CFU's) following the use of PUI/UAI [6, 16, 32, 60, 81, 103, 146, 147, 158] when compared to needle irrigation. Only one study failed to show an improvement in CFU reduction [143].

The above studies concentrated on the reduction of free bacteria (planktonic) and not the removal of biofilm. The impact of PUI/UAI on removing biofilms has also been evaluated, but to a lesser extent. Bhuva et al. [17] reported no improvement in removal when utilizing an artificially produced biofilm of *E. faecalis*. Shen et al. [140] reported an increase in killing of artificial biofilm when PUI/UAI was utilized with chlorhexidine on dentin discs. Case et al. [40] reported similar results when testing ozone – PUI/UAI helped reduce *E. faecalis* biofilm. Gründling et al. [71] reported that PUI/UAI helped reduce *E. faecalis* biofilm only when NaOCl was used as an irrigant. Joyce et al. [86] looked at the mechanism of action of ultrasonics on biofilm and stated that PUI/UAI caused deagglomeration of the biofilm via the cavitation effect.

Safety

The potential risk of extrusion of debris and irrigant during the use of PUI/UAI has been evaluated. Malki et al. [100] reported that fluid movement and cleaning extends 3 mm beyond the ultrasonic file tip. Munoz et al. [116] reported that the use of PUI/UAI does transport irrigant solution to the apex of the root canal. Vera et al. [164, 165] stated that maintaining apical patency is important to allow irrigant to reach the canal apex during PUI/UAI. Tambe et al. [150] and Mitchel et al. [113] both reported more extrusion of irrigant and debris out the apex of the root canal following the use of PUI/UAI as compared to needle irrigation. Tasdemir et al. [153], however, reported less apical extrusion of irrigant versus needle irrigation. Malentacca et al. [99] reported no extrusion of irrigant out the root apex when the PUI/UAI file was kept at 3 and 5 mm from the apex. However extrusion did occur when the file was placed within 1 mm of the apex. No reports have been made of sodium hypochlorite accidents occurring during the use of PUI/UAI in the literature.

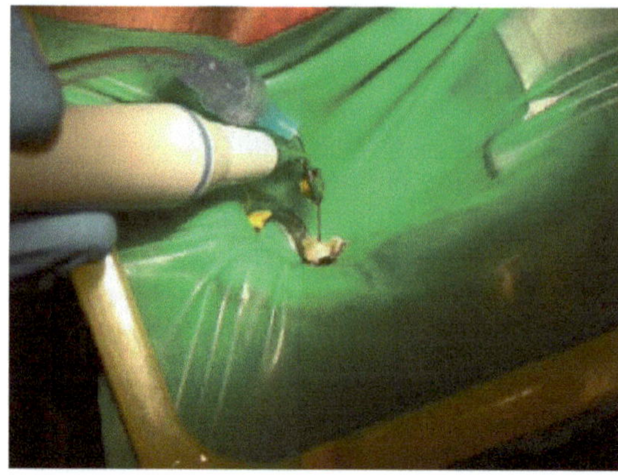

Fig. 10.10 CUI system used by Gutarts et al. [73], Carver et al. [39], Burleson et al. [28]

Continuous Ultrasonic Irrigation (CUI)

As PUI/UAI was reported to improve the cleanliness of root canals and canal isthmuses, the issue of time for the technique and irrigant replenishment became an issue. In vivo studies by Haidet et al. [74] and Archer et al. [12] on mandibular molars utilized 3 min cleaning cycles per canal. This did not include any time utilized to replenish irrigants in the canals and the problems reported with continuous flushing. This 3 min technique could add almost 15 min of treatment time to a mandibular molar. Another problem that was previously noted was the potential for straightening of curved canals and file breakage. These issues lead to the development of an ultrasonically activated irrigating needle which could simultaneously activate and replenish irrigant deep within the canals. This system was designated continuous ultrasonic irrigation (CUI).

Gutarts et al. [73] published the first study using this customized ultrasonic tip (Fig. 10.10). Their in vivo results indicated cleaner canals and canal isthmuses within 3 mm of the canal apex, in vital mandibular molar mesial roots, and irrigating times of 1 min per canal with 5.25 % NaOCl. Placement of the needle was no deeper within the prepared canals (size 30/.04) than 1–2 mm short of binding of the needle. A 25-gauge needle was utilized and 15 ml of irrigant was delivered over the 1 min of continuous ultrasonic activation. This study was followed by Carver et al. [39] who looked at the in vivo removal of planktonic bacteria using the same treatment technique and CUI in necrotic mandibular molars. This group reported a significant increase in negative cultures and reduction of CFU's compared to canal preparation alone with needle irrigation (NaOCl).

Burleson et al. [28] utilized the same device/technique to look at in vivo biofilm removal. Using necrotic mandibular molars, this group prepared and cleaned the mesial root canals similar to Gutarts et al. [73] and extracted, stained, and sectioned the roots from the apical 1–3 mm. They reported significantly cleaner canals and isthmuses following the use of CUI as compared to needle irrigation (Fig. 10.11).

Currently there are two products commercially available for clinical use to provide CUI: Dentsply Tulsa Dental Specialties ProUltra® Piezoflow™ Ultrasonic tip (Fig. 10.12) and Vista Dental Products StreamClean™ Flo-thru tip (Fig. 10.13). The Piezoflow tip is a 25-gauge, blunt-ended stainless steel needle, while the StreamClean™ tip is a 30-gauge blunt-ended NiTi tube with external serrations.

Research utilizing the commercial tips has been rather limited and has looked at the efficacy

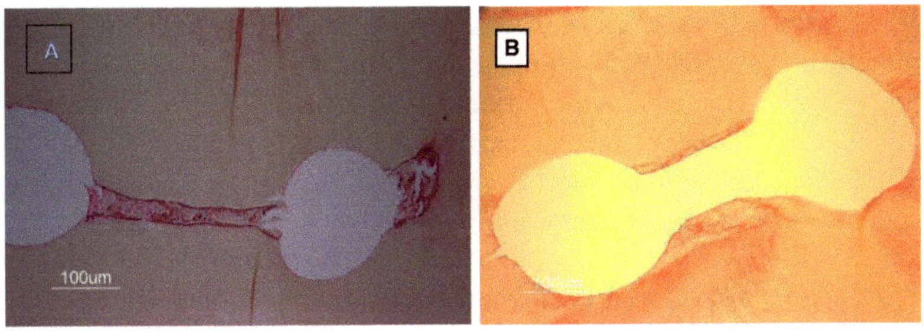

Fig. 10.11 Photomicrograph of cross section at the 2.0 mm level – (**a**) Needle irrigation group (magnification: 100×). (**b**) CUI group (magnification: 40×) (Burleson Master's thesis, 2006)

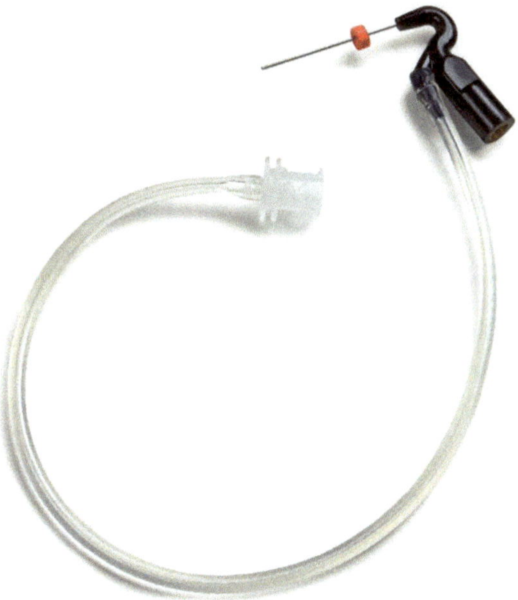

Fig. 10.12 Dentsply Tulsa Dental Specialties ProUltra® Piezoflow™ Ultrasonic tip (Dentsply Tulsa Dental)

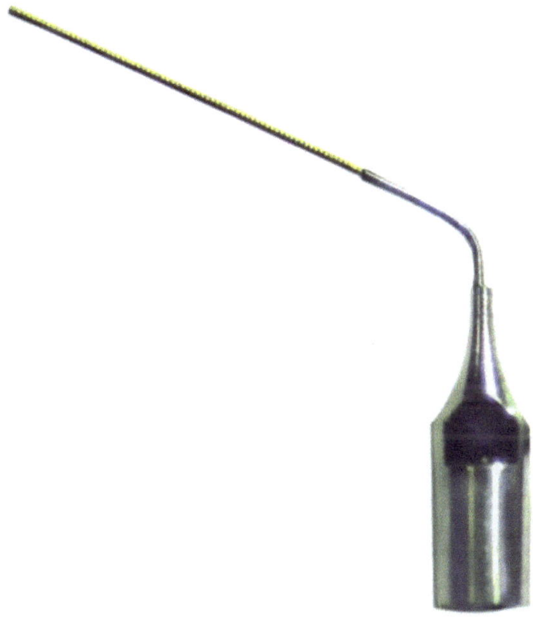

Fig. 10.13 Vista Dental StreamClean™ Flo-thru tip (Vista)

and safety of CUI. Yücel et al. [173] reported that CUI with the Piezoflow™ tip removed calcium hydroxide better than needle irrigation. Yoo et al. [172] reported that CUI with the StreamClean™ tip cleaned canals and isthmuses better than needle irrigation in extracted mandibular molars. Curtis and Sedgley [51] also reported cleaner canals at the 1–3 mm level from the apex using the StreamClean™ tip compared to needle irrigation. Castelo-Baz et al. [41] reported that CUI with the Piezoflow™ tip was more effective than PUI/UAI in getting irrigant into lateral canals. Malentacca et al. [99] reported that CUI with the Piezoflow™ tip removed pulp tissue significantly better than needle irrigation and PUI/UAI. However, Howard et al. [78] reported no differences in debris removal with the Piezoflow™ tip over needle irrigation.

In terms of safety, i.e., extrusion of debris irrigant past the canal apex, Malentacca et al. [99] reported that the use of the Piezoflow™ tip resulted in significant irrigant extrusion beyond the apex when placed within 5 mm of the apex. Placement beyond this length does not follow the manufacturer's recommendations. Utilizing this same system but attaching suction to the ultrasonic tip and placing irrigant in the pulp chamber (similar to the EndoVac system by SybronEndo) proved to be extremely safe [99]. Desai and Himel [61] reported that the use of CUI (using the Burleson et al. set-up) extruded more irrigant out the root apex than needle irrigation. Pafford

[118] reported, in a clinical study using the prototype Piezoflow™ tip, little or no intra- or postoperative treatment pain during and following the use of CUI in vital and necrotic posterior teeth. No sodium hypochlorite accidents have been reported in the literature during the use of a CUI system.

Debate has developed if ultrasonic activation actually is capable of cleaning the apical portions of the root canal due to a phenomenon known as vapor lock. Vapor lock is reported to occur due to the root end being enclosed by the boney socket which results in gas entrapment at its closed end during irrigation. It was first reported in the engineering literature by Dovgyallo et al. [63]. De Gregorio et al. [55] and Tay et al. [155] reported that this effect occurred in the root canal and therefore apical cleaning was impossible (Fig. 10.14). This phenomenon may be a factor that can be controlled in the lab by either sealing the apex of an extracted tooth or by maintaining patency. However, clinically, the debate over an open versus closed system remains. Salzgeber and Brilliant [137] reported that radiopaque dye infused irrigant extruded out the apex of vital and necrotic teeth during hand filing preparation. Vera et al. [164] explained that irrigant can reach the apex of a root (in vivo) when apical patency is maintained with a size 10 file during NiTi rotary preparation of canals with or without the utilization of PUI/UAI. Since there are multiple unfortunate reports of NaOCl accidents in the literature, one may presume that the in vivo status of the root canal system is open unless it becomes blocked with dentin or tissue debris and patency is not maintained. Boutsioukis et al. [24] reported that vapor lock can be removed by increasing the depth of needle penetration, increasing apical preparation size, using an open-ended needle and temporarily increasing fluid flow rate of the irrigant within the root canal.

Laser-Activated Irrigation (LAI)

Activation or agitation of root canal irrigants via the use of lasers is a relatively new concept in endodontics. Previous work with laser has focused on direct canal cleaning and shaping (similar to ultrasonics), disinfection, and smear layer removal. However, issues have arisen in terms of potential damage to the root canal wall dentin, overheating of the root and periodontium, access around the canal curvatures, and the size of the laser tip.

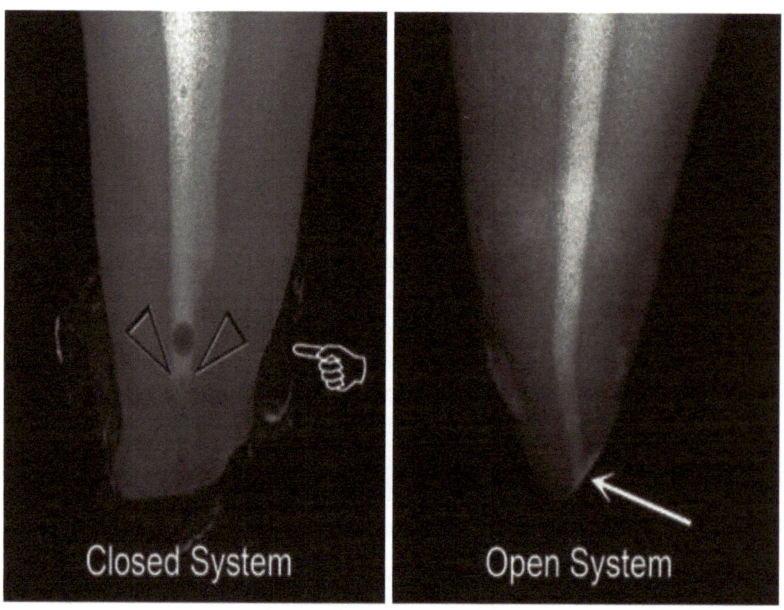

Fig. 10.14 Apical bubble due to vapor lock [155]. *Arrow* shows that the fluid reaches the apex of the root in an open system

Blanken and Verdaasdonk [19] first reported the effects of using an Er,Cr:YSGG (erbium-chromium-yttrium-scandium-garnett) laser on irrigating fluids. They stated that there was immediate fluid movement after each laser pulse and they visualized cavitation (expansion and implosion of gas bubbles) effects. This work was confirmed by Blanken et al. [18], De Moor et al. [57], and Matsumoto et al. [110], who utilized an Er:YAG laser. Matsumoto et al. [110] detailed the cavitational effects by stating that the fluid in the canal (water in their study) instantly vaporized (1 μs) next to the laser tip. The vaporized water expanded forming a void (bubble) as the irradiation continued and heated more water on the inner surface of the void. They reported that this expansion occurred for 700 μs. When the laser pulse ceased, the bubble began to shrink, but the pressure of the surrounding fluid caused a violent collapse resulting in acoustic waves which traveled through the fluid-acoustic streaming (Fig. 10.15). It is these waves (as previously discussed) which result in cleaning of the canal by shearing debris off the walls (Fig. 10.16). Therefore, the cleaning effect of LAI is very similar to that of PUI/UAI and CUI and hence the term laser-activated irrigation. Another term seen in the literature for a similar process is photon-induced photoacoustic streaming (PIPS). The difference in this technique over the LAI techniques is that the laser tip is not placed within the root canal but only placed at the canal orifice [62].

Numerous studies have looked at the cleaning/disinfecting potential of LAI. In terms of bacteria/biofilm removal, most studies utilizing LAI have shown an improvement in the removal of artificially placed biofilms of *E. faecalis*. Ordinola-Zapata et al. [117] reported improved biofilm removal from dentin discs viewed under SEM when compared to PUI/UAI and sonic agitation. Zhu et al. [174] and Sahar-Helft et al. [136] reported the addition of LAI that improved the effects of irrigating solutions (EDTA, NaOCl, chlorhexidine) to remove *E. faecalis* biofilm. However, Zhu et al. [174] found no improvement with LAI (versus needle irrigation) in terms of reducing CFUs. Yavari et al. [171] also reported better results with needle irrigation versus the use of LAI. Seet et al. [139] found that LAI was better at removing *E. faecalis* from dentinal tubules compared to sonic agitation. Peters et al. [127] reported increased disinfection with the use of LAI compared to PUI/UAI, but not complete removal of the biofilm or bacteria.

Debris/material removal from root canals has also benefitted from the use of LAI. Kaptan et al. [88] reported an improvement in calcium hydroxide paste removal following the use of Er:YAG LAI, but the difference in cleaning compared to needle irrigation was not significant. Calcium hydroxide remained in the canals. Deleu et al. [59] reported that the use of Er:YAG laser with a plain tip was the best method to remove dentin debris from artificially prepared canal grooves. De Groot et al. [56] reported LAI with an Er:YAG laser was superior to PUI/UAI in a similar model. Arslan et al. [13] also reported superior debris removal utilizing Er:YAG LAI for 1 min in the

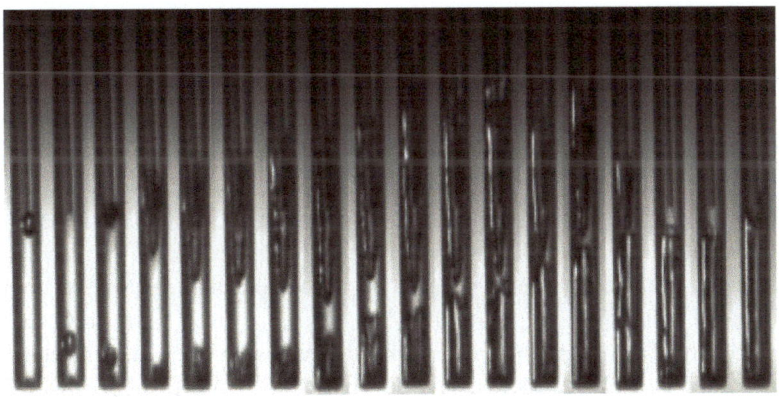

Fig. 10.15 Development of cavitation bubble 750 μs following activation of laser [57]

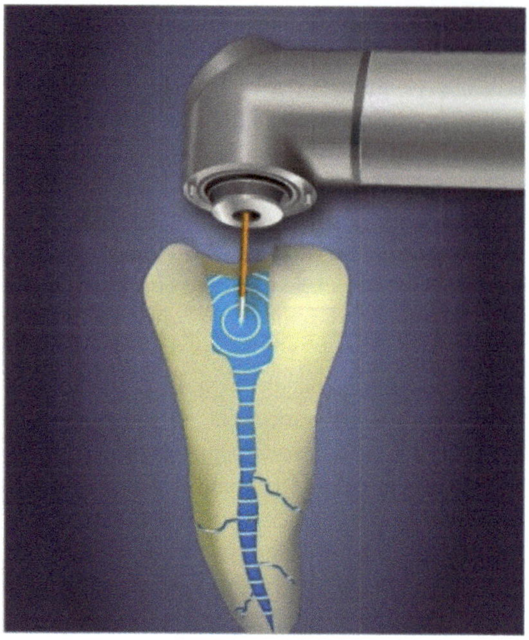

Fig. 10.16 Laser activated irrigation (healthmantra.com)

apical 2–5 mm of the root canal using the same type of model. De Moor et al. [58] looked at both Er:YAG and Er,Cr:YSGG LAI in removing dentin debris and found that both were equal to PUI/UAI utilizing intermittent flushing and irrigant replacement. Peeters and Suardita [124] reported cleaner canals following the use of Er,Cr:YSGG LAI for 60 s in canals prepared to a size 30 file as compared to shorter durations of LAI and smaller canal preparations.

Removing smear layer, DiVito et al. [62] reported that the combination of Er:YAG LAI with EDTA produced very clean dentinal walls with little smear layer remaining. Peeters and Suardita [124] also reported that the combination of Er,Cr:YSGG LAI with EDTA resulted in cleaner dentinal tubules, especially after a 60 s application. The size of the canal preparation was also found to impact the effectiveness of the laser to remove smear layer. Moon et al. [114] reported Nd:YAG LAI with either NaOCl or EDTA equaled the effect of EDTA alone for smear layer removal and hence sealer penetration into the dentinal tubules.

Safety of LAI has also been evaluated. Peeters and Mooduto [123] reported that, in vivo, there was no extrusion of a radiopaque-infused irrigant beyond the apex of the treated tooth following Er,Cr:YSGG LAI. Guidotti et al. [72] reported that the temperature increase, internally, was minimal (less than 4 °C) after use of an Er:YAG laser to perform LAI and an average increase of only 1.3 °C was found on the external root surface.

Sonic Activation

Efficacy of sonic/subsonic activation of irrigants has been evaluated as a manner to improve overall canal cleanliness. Sonic devices generally oscillate at a frequency of 20–20,000 Hz. By definition, sonic frequency is anything in the audible hearing range of a human. The major systems available to produce sonic/subsonic agitation are the Micromega® Sonic Air®1500 handpiece with an attached Rispi-Sonic® file (Medidenta International Inc.) seen in Fig. 10.17; the EndoActivator® system with attached polymer tips (Dentsply Tulsa Dental Specialties) seen in Fig. 10.18; and the Vibringe® sonic irrigation system (Vibringe B.V.) seen in Fig. 10.19.

The Sonic Air® 1500 unit is an air-driven device that produces vibrations ranging from 1,500 to 3,000 Hz (manufacturer data). The Rispi-Sonic® files are stainless steel and have barbs along the length of the file in a spiral design (Fig. 10.17b). This file is designed to cut dentin as well as agitate the irrigant solution with the canal. Irrigant is delivered and refreshed intermittently via needle delivery and not by the handpiece. The EndoActivator® is a battery-operated portable handpiece with a 3-speed electric motor. That handpiece accepts one of three different size, disposable, and polymer tips (15/.02, s5/.04, 35/.04). The polymer tips are smooth sided. Operating frequencies were reported by Jiang et al. [84] to be 160, 175, and 190 Hz. These frequencies are different from the manufacturer reported frequencies of 33, 100, and 167 Hz. The tips agitate the irrigating solution placed in the root canal and access opening via needle irrigation. The Vibringe® irrigation system consists of a battery-operated plunger and thumb ring which

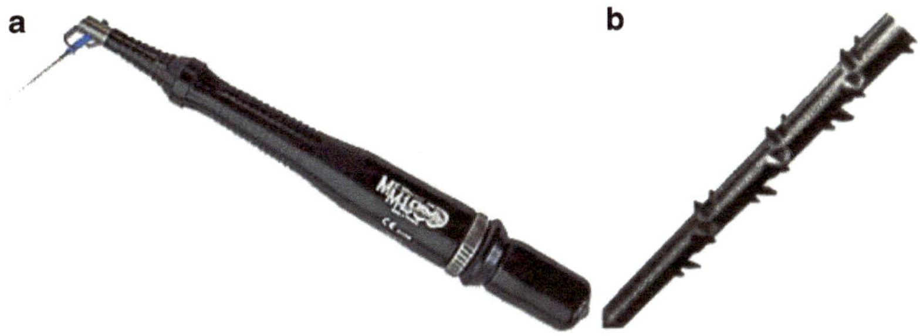

Fig. 10.17 (**a**) Micromega® Sonic Air® 1500 handpiece. (**b**) Rispi-Sonic® file (Micromega)

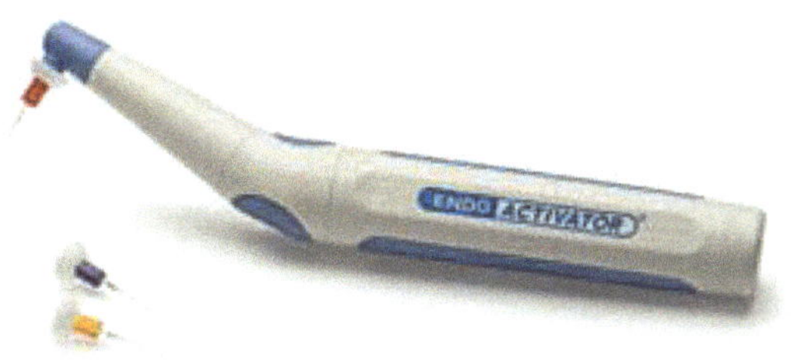

Fig. 10.18 EndoActivator® system with polymer tips (Dentsply Tulsa Dental)

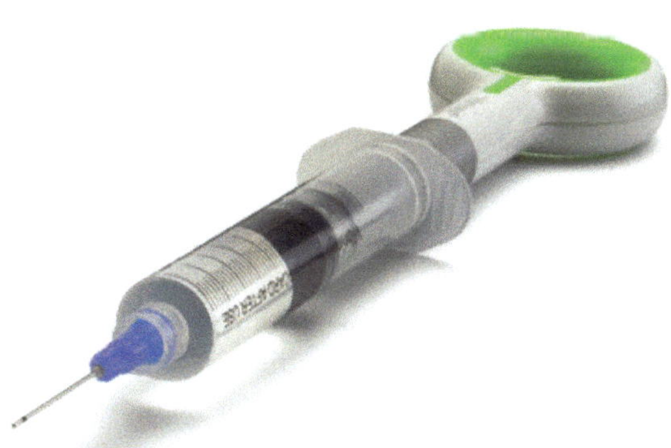

Fig. 10.19 Vibringe irrigation system (Vibringe)

is placed into a disposable, 10 ml, nylon syringe. An endodontic irrigating needle, of varying size depending on the root canal preparation, is attached. As the irrigant is delivered into the root canal, the thumb ring is activated causing vibration of the irrigating needle. The reported frequency of agitation is 150 Hz (manufacturer data).

Debris and Smear Layer Removal

Research into the improved cleaning of the root canal walls, lateral canals, and isthmuses, as well as removal of pastes (mainly calcium hydroxide) and smear layer removal, has provided rather mixed results with sonic activation of irrigants. Stojicic et al. [149] reported on the effect sonic agitation of NaOCl has on dissolution of tissue. They reported that increasing the concentration of the NaOCl had the greatest impact and that agitation (sonic) had the second greatest effect (more than increasing the temperature of the solution). Sabins et al. [135] reported that sonic irrigant activation (using a MicroMega® 1500 system) improved canal cleanliness over needle irrigation alone, but was inferior to PUI/UAI. De Gregorio et al. [54] found that sonic activation with the EndoActivator® equaled the effectiveness of PUI/UAI in getting irrigant solution into lateral canals 2–4.5 mm from the root apex when EDTA was used. In a later study, de Gregorio et al. [55] reported that the EndoActivator® was superior to needle irrigation in getting irrigating solution to the apex of the root canal preparation and into lateral canals. However, it was inferior to PUI/UAI and EndoVac® (SybronEndo) for the same role. Merino et al. [111] stated that PUI/UAI was superior to the EndoActivator® in getting irrigant to the canal apex in variously tapered, curved canals. They found that the taper of the preparation had no impact on the irrigant movement.

Research on debris removal has shown that both Vibringe® and EndoActivator® are superior to needle irrigation in both straight and curved canals. Rödig et al. [129] reported that use of the Vibringe® resulted in a cleaner apical 1/3 of the canal as compared to needle irrigation alone. However, PUI/UAI was superior over the entire length of the root canal. The group attributed the difference in cleanliness to the flow velocity of the irrigant during activation/agitation – a lower flow velocity with sonic activation prevented removal of debris from artificial grooves along the canal wall. In curved canals, debris removal was equivalent between PUI/UAI and EndoActivator®. Kanter et al. [87] reported that the use of the EndoActivator® removed more debris and cleaned lateral canals better than PUI/UAI and needle irrigation. Johnson et al. [85] reported that using Vibringe® cleaned canals and isthmuses filled with artificial collagen to the same degree as needle irrigation although there were some differences at various levels of the canals.

In removing smear layer, sonic activation has also had mixed results. Paragiola et al. [119] reported that the use of EndoActivator® was superior to needle irrigation in removing smear layer, but inferior to PUI/UAI. Uroz-Torres et al. [160] reported no differences between needle irrigation and the use of EndoActivator® in removing smear layer when using EDTA and NaOCl. They stated that no smear layer was removed when only NaOCl was utilized. Rödig et al. [130] reported that the addition of PUI/UAI or EndoActivator® to activate the irrigants (NaOCl and EDTA) in curved canals resulted in superior smear layer removal, especially in the coronal portion of the canal. Blank-Goncalves et al. [20] also showed improved smear layer removal with activation of EDTA in curved canals with EndoActivator®. Bolles et al. [23] compared fluorescent dye-labeled sealer penetration in dentinal tubules following the use of EndoActivator® and Vibringe® on 17 % EDTA. They reported that the use of the activators did not improve sealer penetration (therefore smear layer removal was absent) in the apical 4 mm of the root canal compared to needle irrigation with 17 % EDTA. Mancini et al. [101] reported that the use of the EndoActivator® significantly improved smear layer removal when utilizing 5.25 % NaOCl over PUI/UAI 3–8 mm from the root apex in an SEM study.

Calcium hydroxide and other paste and sealer removal have also been evaluated utilizing sonic activation. Chou et al. [43] evaluated removal of Ledermix®, Doxypaste, Odontopaste®, and Pulpdent® (calcium hydroxide) from root canals. They found that the use of the EndoActivator® resulted in more complete removal of the pastes as compared to needle irrigation. There was no difference in calcium hydroxide removal. Calcium hydroxide was found to be the most difficult product to remove. Grischke et al. [70] evaluated the use of the EndoActivator® to remove set AH Plus sealer from artificial grooves in roots. The group reported that the EndoActivator® scored poorly in removing the sealer with PUI/UAI providing better results. Neither technique, however, was able to remove all of the sealer from the grooves. Goode et al. [68] and Khaleel et al. [89] also studied the efficacy of the EndoActivator® to remove calcium hydroxide from root canals. Both groups reported that no irrigation technique could remove all of the material. Khaleel reported better results with the EndoActivator® and PUI/UAI (similar results) than needle irrigation, while Goode's group reported no difference between the techniques (EndoActivator® versus needle irrigation).

Bacteria and Biofilm Removal

Removal of bacteria from the root canal system has been evaluated utilizing a number of irrigation techniques including sonic activation. Brito et al. [27] reported that the use of the EndoActivator® was similar to needle irrigation (NaOCl as the irrigant) in reducing artificially placed *E. faecalis* counts in extracted teeth. Townsend and Maki [158] utilized *E. faecalis-infected* plastic root canal models to determine the removal efficacy of several irrigating techniques. They reported that sonic activation with the Micromega® 1500 and EndoActivator® systems were similar in results and superior to needle irrigation but inferior to PUI/UAI. Tardivo et al. [152] found no difference in removal of *E. faecalis* between the EndoActivator® and PUI/UAI (Irrisafe™ system) from the root canal system. Neither technique could remove all the bacteria. Pasqualini et al. [120], using similar artificially contaminated root canals, reported that 30 s of EndoActivator® agitation of 5 % NaOCl was superior to needle irrigation (15 and 30 s) and 15 s of sonic agitation. Bago et al. [14] found similar results (EndoActivator® was superior to needle irrigation) and that EndoActivator® agitation was superior to diode laser irradiation in reducing *E. faecalis* counts in root canals. Shen et al. [141] utilized infected hydroxyapatite discs to evaluate chlorhexidine in killing bacteria. They found that the addition of EndoActivator® agitation improved the killing effect of the chlorhexidine, but did not remove biofilm from the disc samples. Huffaker et al. [80], using an in vivo model, reported that use of the EndoActivator® was similar to needle irrigation in reducing bacterial counts in root canals. They stated that the use of calcium hydroxide as an intra-appointment canal medicament gave the best results in reducing bacteria.

In terms of biofilm removal, Ordinola-Zapata et al. [115] looked at its removal in bovine teeth via an SEM study. They reported that EndoActivator® agitation and needle irrigation were similar in results and were both inferior to PUI/UAI and PIPS irrigation techniques. In another SEM study, Seet et al. [139] determined that EndoActivator® agitation decreased bacterial counts and removed *E. faecalis* biofilm from root canal walls but not from dentinal tubules. The sonic activation was better than needle irrigation but not as effective as LAI.

Safety

As with other irrigating techniques, the safety of sonic irrigation has been evaluated in terms of extrusion of the irrigant past the apex of the root canal. Desai and Himel [61] first reported on irrigant extrusion and stated that little-to-no extrusion occurred with the use of the EndoActivator®. Mitchell et al. [113] reported that the use of the EndoActivator® and MicroMega® Sonic Air® 1500 systems did result in extrusion of irrigant but that this occurred less frequently with the EndoActivator®. The MicroMega® unit resulted in similar extrusion patterns as seen with slotted needle irrigation. Boutioukis et al. [25] reported that flow rate of the irrigant had a direct correlation with the amount of irrigant extrusion. They found that the use of the EndoActivator® resulted in significantly less extrusion than manual dynamic agitation (moving a fitted gutta-percha cone up and down in an irrigant-filled canal). The same was true for PUI/UAI.

Summary

The use of an irrigant in endodontic therapy to supplement cleaning and disinfection of the root canal system is a basic requirement. However, the limitations of traditional needle-delivered irrigation have been shown in numerous investigations. Activation of irrigants via sonic, ultrasonic, or laser devices has shown great improvement in the cleaning and disinfection of the root canal system and should be considered an important fundamental step in non-surgical endodontic therapy.

References

1. Abbott PV, Heijkoop PS, Cardaci SC, Hume WR, Heithersay GS. An SEM study of the effects of different irrigation sequences and ultrasonics. Int Endod J. 1991;24:308–16.
2. Ahmad M, PittFord TR, Crum LA. Ultrasonic debridement of root canals: An insight into the mechanisms involved. J Endod. 1987;13:93–101.
3. Ahmad M, PittFord TR, Crum LA. Ultrasonic debridement of root canals: acoustic streaming and its possible role. J Endod. 1987;13:490–9.
4. Ahmad M, PittFord TR, Crum LA. Ultrasonic debridement of root canals: acoustic cavitation and its relevance. J Endod. 1988;14:486–93.
5. Ahmad M, Roy RA, Kamarudin AG. Observations of acoustic streaming fields around an oscillating ultrasonic file. Endod Dent Traumatol. 1992;8:189–94.
6. Ahmad M. Effect of ultrasonic instrumentation on *Bacteroides intermedius*. Endod Dent Traumatol. 1989;5:83–6.
7. Alaçam T, Demirtola N, Misirligil A, Ayhan N, Gökay O. *In vivo* comparison of antimicrobial effectiveness of conventional and ultrasound activated irrigation techniques in root canal therapy. Bull Tokyo Dent Coll. 1987;28:19–22.
8. Al-Jadaa A, Paqué F, Attin T, Zehnder M. Acoustic hypochlorite activation in simulated curved canals. J Endod. 2009;35:1408–11.

9. Al-Jadaa A, Paqué F, Attin T, Zehnder M. Necrotic pulp tissue dissolution by passive ultrasonic irrigation in simulated accessory canals: impact of canal location and angulation. Int Endod J. 2009; 42:59–65.
10. Amato M, Vanoni-Heineken I, Hecker H, Weiger R. Curved versus straight root canals: the benefit of activated irrigation techniques on dentin debris removal. Oral Surg Oral Med Oral Pathol Oral Radiol Endod. 2011;111:529–34.
11. Andrabi SM, Kumar A, Zia A, Iftekhar H, Alam S, Siddiqui S. Effect of passive ultrasonic irrigation and manual dynamic irrigation on smear layer removal from root canals in a closed apex in vitro model. J Investig Clin Dent. 2014;5(3):188–93.
12. Archer R, Reader A, Nist R, Beck M, Meyers WJ. An *in vivo* evaluation of the efficacy of ultrasound after step-back preparation in mandibular molars. J Endod. 1992;18:549–52.
13. Arslan H, Capar ID, Saygili G, Gok T, Akcay M. Effect of photon-initiated photoacoustic streaming on removal of apically placed dentinal debris. Int Endod J. 2014;47(11):1072–77.
14. Bago I, Plečko V, Gabrić Pandurić D, Schauperl Z, Baraba A, Anić I. Antimicrobial efficacy of a high-power diode laser, photo-activated disinfection, conventional and sonic activated irrigation during root canal treatment. Int Endod J. 2013;46:339–47.
15. Baker NA, Eleazer PD, Averbach RE, Seltzer S. Scanning electron microscope study of the efficacy of various irrigating solutions. J Endod. 1975;1:127–35.
16. Barnett F, Trope M, Khoja M, Tronstad L. Bacteriologic status of the root canal after sonic, ultrasonic, and hand instrumentation. Endod Dent Traumatol. 1985;1:228–31.
17. Bhuva B, Patel S, Wilson R, Niazi S, Beighton D, Mannocci F. The effectiveness of passive ultrasonic irrigation on intraradicular *Enterococcus faecalis* biofilms in extracted single-rooted human teeth. Int Endod J. 2010;43:241–50.
18. Blanken J, De Moor RJ, Meire M, Verdaasdonk R. Laser induced explosive vapor and cavitation resulting in effective irrigation of the root canal. Part 1: a visualization study. Lasers Surg Med. 2009;41:514–9.
19. Blanken JW, Verdaasdonk R. Cavitation as a working mechanism of the Er, Cr:YSGG laser in endodontics: a visualization study. J Oral Laser Appl. 2007;7:97–106.
20. Blank-Gonçalves LM, Nabeshima CK, Martins GH, Machado ME. Qualitative analysis of the removal of the smear layer in the apical third of curved roots: conventional irrigation versus activation systems. J Endod. 2011;37:1268–71. http://www.ncbi.nlm.nih.gov/pubmed/?term=blank-goncalves.
21. Hancock J. Ultrasonic cleaning. ASM Handbook® Vol 5: Surface Engineering. 1994;44–7. http://bluewaveinc.com/ultrasonic-cleaning-101/. Accessed 11 Mar 2014.
22. Bolanos OR, Jensen JR. Scanning electron microscopy comparisons of the efficacy of various methods of root canal preparation. J Endod. 1980;6:815–22.
23. Bolles JA, He J, Svoboda KK, Schneiderman E, Glickman GN. Comparison of Vibringe, EndoActivator, and needle irrigation on sealer penetration in extracted human teeth. J Endod. 2013;39:708–11.
24. Boutsioukis C, Kastrinakis E, Lambrianidis T, Verhaagen B, Versluis M, van der Sluis LW. Formation and removal of apical vapor lock during syringe irrigation: a combined experimental and Computational Fluid Dynamics approach. Int Endod J. 2014;47:191–201.
25. Boutsioukis C, Psimma Z, Kastrinakis E. The effect of flow rate and agitation technique on irrigant extrusion *ex vivo*. Int Endod J. 2014;47:487–96.
26. Boutsioukis C, Verhaagen B, Walmsley AD, Versluis M, van der Sluis LW. Measurement and visualization of file-to-wall contact during ultrasonically activated irrigation in simulated canals. Int Endod J. 2013;46:1046–55.
27. Brito PR, Souza LC, Machado de Oliveira JC, Alves FR, De-Deus G, Lopes HP, Siqueira Jr JF. Comparison of the effectiveness of three irrigation techniques in reducing intracanal *Enterococcus faecalis* populations: an *in vitro* study. J Endod. 2009;35:1422–7.
28. Burleson A, Nusstein J, Reader A, Beck M. The in vivo evaluation of hand/rotary/ultrasound instrumentation in necrotic, human mandibular molars. J Endod. 2007;33:782–7.
29. Byström A, Sundqvist G. Bacteriologic evaluation of the efficacy of mechanical root canal instrumentation in endodontic therapy. Scand J Dent Res. 1981;89:321–8.
30. Byström A, Sundqvist G. Bacteriologic evaluation of the effect of 0.5 percent sodium hypochlorite in endodontic therapy. Oral Surg Oral Med Oral Pathol. 1983;55:307–12.
31. Byström A, Sundqvist G. The antibacterial action of sodium hypochlorite and EDTA in 60 cases of endodontic therapy. Int Endod J. 1985;18:35–40.
32. Cachovan G, Schiffner U, Altenhof S, Guentsch A, Pfister W, Eick S. Comparative antibacterial efficacies of hydrodynamic and ultrasonic irrigation systems *in vitro*. J Endod. 2013;39:1171–5.
33. Cameron JA. The use of ultrasonics in the removal of the smear layer: a scanning electron microscope study. J Endod. 1983;9:289–92.
34. Cameron JA. The synergistic relationship between ultrasound and sodium hypochlorite: a scanning electron microscope evaluation. J Endod. 1987;13:541–5.
35. Cameron JA. The use of ultrasound for the removal of the smear layer. The effect of sodium hypochlorite concentration; an SEM study. Aust Dent J. 1988;33:193–200.
36. Cameron JA. The choice of irrigant during hand instrumentation and ultrasonic irrigation of the root

canal: a scanning electron microscope study. Aust Dent J. 1995;40:85–90.
37. Capar ID, Ozcan E, Arslan H, Ertas H, Aydinbelge HA. Effect of different final irrigation methods on the removal of calcium hydroxide from an artificial standardized groove in the apical third of root canals. J Endod. 2014;40:451–4.
38. Card SJ, Sigurdsson A, Ørstavik D, Trope M. The effectiveness of increased apical enlargement in reducing intracanal bacteria. J Endod. 2002;28:779–83.
39. Carver K, Nusstein J, Reader A, Beck M. In vivo antibacterial efficacy of ultrasound after hand and rotary instrumentation in human mandibular molars. J Endod. 2007;33:1038–43.
40. Case PD, Bird PS, Kahler WA, George R, Walsh LJ. Treatment of root canal biofilms of *Enterococcus faecalis* with ozone gas and passive ultrasound activation. J Endod. 2012;38:523–6.
41. Castelo-Baz P, Martín-Biedma B, Cantatore G, Ruíz-Piñón M, Bahillo J, Rivas-Mundiña B, Varela-Patiño P. *In vitro* comparison of passive and continuous ultrasonic irrigation in simulated lateral canals of extracted teeth. J Endod. 2012;38:688–91.
42. Cheung GS, Stock CJ. *In vitro* cleaning ability of root canal irrigants with and without endosonics. Int Endod J. 1993;26:334–43.
43. Chou K, George R, Walsh LJ. Effectiveness of different intracanal irrigation techniques in removing intracanal paste medicaments. Aust Endod J. 2014;40:21–5.
44. Ciucchi B, Khettabi M, Holz J. The effectiveness of different endodontic irrigation procedures on the removal of the smear layer: a scanning electron microscopic study. Int Endod J. 1989;22:21–8.
45. Magnetorestrictive versus piezoelectric transducers for power ultrasonic applications. Cleaning Technologies Group (CTM). http://www.ctgclean.com/blog/technology-library/articles/magnetostrictive-versus-piezoelectric-transducers-for-power-ultrasonic-applications. Accessed 25 Feb 2014.
46. Coldero LG, McHugh S, MacKenzie D, Saunders WP. Reduction in intracanal bacteria during root canal preparation with and without apical enlargement. Int Endod J. 2002;35:437–46.
47. Contardo L, De Luca M, Bevilacqua L, Breschi L, Di Lenarda R. Influence of calcium hydroxide debris on the quality of endodontic apical seal. Minerva Stomatol. 2007;56:509–17.
48. Cunningham WT, Martin H. A scanning electron microscope evaluation of root canal debridement with the endosonic ultrasonic synergistic system. Oral Surg Oral Med Oral Pathol. 1982;53:527–31.
49. Cunningham WT, Martin H, Forrest WR. Evaluation of root canal debridement by the endosonic ultrasonic synergistic system. Oral Surg Oral Med Oral Pathol. 1982;53:401–4.
50. Cunningham WT, Martin H, Pelleu G, Stoops D. A comparison of antimicrobial effectiveness of endosonic and hand root canal therapy. Oral Surg Oral Med Oral Pathol. 1982;54:238–41.
51. Curtis TO, Sedgley CM. Comparison of a continuous ultrasonic irrigation device and conventional needle irrigation in the removal of root canal debris. J Endod. 2012;38:1261–4.
52. Cymerman J, Jerome L, Moodnik R. A scanning electron microscope study comparing the efficacy of hand instrumentation with ultrasonic instrumentation of the root canal. J Endod. 1983;9:327–31.
53. Dalton BC, Ørstavik D, Phillips C, Pettiette M, Trope M. Bacterial reduction with nickel-titanium rotary instrumentation. J Endod. 1998;24:763–7.
54. de Gregorio C, Estevez R, Cisneros R, Heilborn C, Cohenca N. Effect of EDTA, sonic, and ultrasonic activation on the penetration of sodium hypochlorite into simulated lateral canals: an *in vitro* study. J Endod. 2009;35:891–5.
55. de Gregorio C, Estevez R, Cisneros R, Paranjpe A, Cohenca N. Efficacy of different irrigation and activation systems on the penetration of sodium hypochlorite into simulated lateral canals and up to working length: an *in vitro* study. J Endod. 2010;36:1216–21.
56. de Groot SD, Verhaagen B, Versluis M, Wu MK, Wesselink PR, van der Sluis LW. Laser-activated irrigation within root canals: cleaning efficacy and flow visualization. Int Endod J. 2009;42:1077–83.
57. De Moor RJ, Blanken J, Meire M, Verdaasdonk R. Laser induced explosive vapor and cavitation resulting in effective irrigation of the root canal. Part 2: evaluation of the efficacy. Lasers Surg Med. 2009;41:520–3.
58. De Moor RJ, Meire M, Goharkhay K, Moritz A, Vanobbergen J. Efficacy of ultrasonic versus laser-activated irrigation to remove artificially placed dentin debris plugs. J Endod. 2010;36:1580–3.
59. Deleu E, Meire MA, De Moor RJ. Efficacy of laser-based irrigant activation methods in removing debris from simulated root canal irregularities. Lasers Med Sci. 2015;30(2):831–5.
60. DeNunzio MS, Hicks ML, Pelleu GB, Kingman A, Sauber JJ. A bacteriological comparison of ultrasonic and hand instrumentation of root canals in dogs. J Endod. 1989;14:290–3.
61. Desai P, Himel V. Comparative safety of various intracanal irrigation systems. J Endod. 2009;35:545–9.
62. DiVito E, Peters OA, Olivi G. Effectiveness of the erbium:YAG laser and new design radial and stripped tips in removing the smear layer after root canal instrumentation. Lasers Med Sci. 2012;27:273–80.
63. Dovgyallo GI, Migun NP, Prokhorenko PP. The complete filling of dead-end conical capillaries with liquid. J Eng Phys. 1989;56:395–7.
64. Druttman AC, Stock CJ. An in vitro comparison of ultrasonic and conventional methods of irrigant replacement. Int Endod J. 1989;22:174–8.
65. Dutner J, Mines P, Anderson A. Irrigation trends among American Association of Endodontists members: a web-based survey. J Endod. 2012;38:37–40.
66. Goel S, Tewari S. Smear layer removal with passive ultrasonic irrigation and the NaviTip FX: a scanning

electron microscopic study. Oral Surg Oral Med Oral Pathol Oral Radiol Endod. 2009;108:465–70.
67. Goldman M, White R, Moser C, Tenca J. A comparison of three methods of cleaning and shaping the root canal *in vitro*. J Endod. 1988;14:7–12.
68. Goode N, Khan S, Eid AA, Niu LN, Gosier J, Susin LF, Pashley DH, Tay FR. Wall shear stress effects of different endodontic irrigation techniques and systems. J Dent. 2013;41:636–41.
69. Goodman A, Reader A, Beck F, Melfi R, Meyers W. An *in vitro* comparison of the efficacy of the step-back technique versus a step-back ultrasonic technique in human mandibular molars. J Endod. 1985;11:249–56.
70. Grischke J, Müller-Heine A, Hülsmann M. The effect of four different irrigation systems in the removal of a root canal sealer. Clin Oral Investig. 2014;18(7):1845–51.
71. Gründling GL, Zechin JG, Jardim WM, de Oliveira SD, de Figueiredo JA. Effect of ultrasonics on *Enterococcus faecalis* biofilm in a bovine tooth model. J Endod. 2011;37:1128–33.
72. Guidotti R, Merigo E, Fornaini C, Rocca JP, Medioni E, Vescovi P. Er:YAG 2,940-nm laser fiber in endodontic treatment: a help in removing smear layer. Lasers Med Sci. 2014;29:69–75.
73. Gutarts R, Nusstein J, Reader A, Beck M. *In vivo* debridement efficacy of ultrasonic irrigation following hand-rotary instrumentation in human mandibular molars. J Endod. 2005;31:166–70.
74. Haidet J, Reader A, Beck M, Meyers W. An *in vivo* comparison of the step-back technique versus a step-back/ultrasonic technique in human mandibular molars. J Endod. 1989;15:195–9.
75. Heard F, Walton RE. Scanning electron microscope study comparing four root canal preparation techniques in small curved canals. Int Endod J. 1997;30:323–31.
76. Hess W, et al. The anatomy of the root canals of the teeth of the permanent dentition. London: J. Bale, Sons and Danielsson, Ltd; 1925.
77. Hosoya N, Kurayama H, Iino F, Arai T. Effects of calcium hydroxide on physical and sealing properties of canal sealers. Int Endod J. 2004;37:178–84.
78. Howard RK, Kirkpatrick TC, Rutledge RE, Yaccino JM. Comparison of debris removal with three different irrigation techniques. J Endod. 2011;37:1301–5.
79. Huang TY, Gulabivala K, Ng YL. A bio-molecular film ex-vivo model to evaluate the influence of canal dimensions and irrigation variables on the efficacy of irrigation. Int Endod J. 2008;41:60–71.
80. Huffaker SK, Safavi K, Spangberg LS, Kaufman B. Influence of a passive sonic irrigation system on the elimination of bacteria from root canal systems: a clinical study. J Endod. 2010;36:1315–8.
81. Huque J, Kota K, Yamaga M, Iwaku M, Hoshino E. Bacterial eradication from root dentine by ultrasonic irrigation with sodium hypochlorite. Int Endod J. 1998;31:242–50.
82. Jensen SA, Walker TL, Hutter JW, Nicoll BK. Comparison of the cleaning efficacy of passive sonic activation and passive ultrasonic activation after hand instrumentation in molar root canals. J Endod. 1999;25:735–8.
83. Jiang LM, Verhaagen B, Versluis M, Langedijk J, Wesselink P, van der Sluis LW. The influence of the ultrasonic intensity on the cleaning efficacy of passive ultrasonic irrigation. J Endod. 2011;37:688–92.
84. Jiang LM, Verhaagen B, Versluis M, van der Sluis LW. Influence of the oscillation direction of an ultrasonic file on the cleaning efficacy of passive ultrasonic irrigation. J Endod. 2010;36:1372–6.
85. Johnson M, Sidow SJ, Looney SW, Lindsey K, Niu LN, Tay FR. Canal and isthmus debridement efficacy using a sonic irrigation technique in a closed-canal system. J Endod. 2012;38:1265–8.
86. Joyce E, Phull SS, Lorimer JP, Mason TJ. The development and evaluation of ultrasound for the treatment of bacterial suspensions. A study of frequency, power and sonication time on cultured Bacillus species. Ultrason Sonochem. 2003;10:315–8.
87. Kanter V, Weldon E, Nair U, Varella C, Kanter K, Anusavice K, Pileggi R. A quantitative and qualitative analysis of ultrasonic versus sonic endodontic systems on canal cleanliness and obturation. Oral Surg Oral Med Oral Pathol Oral Radiol Endod. 2011;112:809–13.
88. Kaptan F, Karapinar-Kazandag M, Kayahan MB, Bora T, Bayirli G. Potential of an Er:YAG laser in the removal of calcium hydroxide from root canals. Photomed Laser Surg. 2012;30:250–4.
89. Khaleel HY, Al-Ashaw AJ, Yang Y, Pang AH, Ma JZ. Quantitative comparison of calcium hydroxide removal by EndoActivator, ultrasonic and ProTaper file agitation techniques: an *in vitro* study. J Huazhong Univ Sci Technolog Med Sci. 2013;33:142–5.
90. Kuah HG, Lui JN, Tseng PS, Chen NN. The effect of EDTA with and without ultrasonics on removal of the smear layer. J Endod. 2009;35:393–6.
91. Langeland K, Liao K, Pascon E. Work saving devices in endodontics: efficacy of sonic and ultrasonic technique. J Endod. 1985;11:499–510.
92. Lee SJ, Wu MK, Wesselink PR. The effectiveness of syringe irrigation and ultrasonics to remove debris from simulated irregularities within prepared root canal walls. Int Endod J. 2004;37:672–8.
93. Lee SJ, Wu MK, Wesselink PR. The efficacy of ultrasonic irrigation to remove artificially placed dentine debris from different-sized simulated plastic root canals. Int Endod J. 2004;37:607–12.
94. Lev R, Reader A, Beck M, Meyers W. An *in vitro* comparison of the step-back technique versus a step-back/ultrasound technique for one and three minutes. J Endod. 1987;13:523–30.
95. Liang YH, Jiang LM, Jiang L, Chen XB, Liu YY, Tian FC, Bao XD, Gao XJ, Versluis M, Wu MK, van der Sluis L. Radiographic healing after a root canal treatment performed in single-rooted teeth with and without ultrasonic activation of the irrigant: a randomized controlled trial. J Endod. 2013;39:1218–25.

96. Lumley PJ, Walmsley AD, Walton RE, Rippin JW. Effect of precurving endosonic files on the amount of debris and smear layer remaining in curved root canals. J Endod. 1992;18:616–9.
97. Macedo RG, Verhaagen B, Fernandez Rivas D, Gardeniers JG, van der Sluis LW, Wesselink PR, Versluis M. Sonochemical and high-speed optical characterization of cavitation generated by an ultrasonically oscillating dental file in root canal models. Ultrason Sonochem. 2014;21:324–35.
98. Macedo RG, Verhaagen B, Wesselink PR, Versluis M, van der Sluis LW. Influence of refreshment/activation cycles and temperature rise on the reaction rate of sodium hypochlorite with bovine dentine during ultrasonic activated irrigation. Int Endod J. 2014;47:147–54.
99. Malentacca A, Uccioli U, Zangari D, Lajolo C, Fabiani C. Efficacy and safety of various active irrigation devices when used with either positive or negative pressure: an *in vitro* study. J Endod. 2012;38:1622–6.
100. Malki M, Verhaagen B, Jiang LM, Nehme W, Naaman A, Versluis M, Wesselink P, van der Sluis L. Irrigant flow beyond the insertion depth of an ultrasonically oscillating file in straight and curved root canals: visualization and cleaning efficacy. J Endod. 2012;38:657–61.
101. Mancini M, Cerroni L, Iorio L, Armellin E, Conte G, Cianconi L. Smear layer removal and canal cleanliness using different irrigation systems (EndoActivator, EndoVac, and passive ultrasonic irrigation): field emission scanning electron microscopic evaluation in an *in vitro* study. J Endod. 2013;39:1456–60.
102. Margelos J, Eliades G, Verdelis C, Palaghias G. Interaction of calcium hydroxide with zinc oxide-eugenol type sealers: a potential clinical problem. J Endod. 1997;23:43–8.
103. Martin H. Ultrasonic disinfection of the root canal. Oral Surg Oral Med Oral Pathol. 1976;42:92–9.
104. Martin H, Cunningham WT. The effect of endosonic and hand manipulation on the amount of root canal material extruded. Oral Surg Oral Med Oral Pathol. 1982;53:611–3.
105. Martin H, Cunningham WT. An evaluation of postoperative pain incidence following endosonic and conventional root canal therapy. Oral Surg Oral Med Oral Pathol. 1982;54:74–6.
106. Martin H, Cunningham WT. Endosonic endodontics: the ultrasonic synergistic system. Int Dent J. 1984;34:198–203.
107. Martin H, Cunningham WT. Endosonics – the ultrasonic synergistic system of endodontics. Endod Dent Traumatol. 1985;1:201–6.
108. Martin H, Cunningham WT, Norris JP, Cotton WR. Ultrasonic versus hand filing of dentin: a quantitative study. Oral Surg Oral Med Oral Pathol. 1980;49:79–81.
109. Martin H, Cunningham WT, Norris JP. A quantitative comparison of the ability of diamond and K-type files to remove dentin. Oral Surg Oral Med Oral Pathol. 1980;50:566–8.
110. Matsumoto H, Yoshimine Y, Akamine A. Visualization of irrigant flow and cavitation induced by Er:YAG laser within a root canal model. J Endod. 2011;37:839–43.
111. Merino A, Estevez R, de Gregorio C, Cohenca N. The effect of different taper preparations on the ability of sonic and passive ultrasonic irrigation to reach the working length in curved canals. Int Endod J. 2013;46:427–33.
112. Metzler RS, Montgomery S. The effectiveness of ultrasonics and calcium hydroxide for the debridement of human mandibular molars. J Endod. 1989;15:373–8.
113. Mitchell RP, Baumgartner JC, Sedgley CM. Apical extrusion of sodium hypochlorite using different root canal irrigation systems. J Endod. 2011;37:1677–81.
114. Moon YM, Kim HC, Bae KS, Baek SH, Shon WJ, Lee W. Effect of laser-activated irrigation of 1320-nanometer Nd:YAG laser on sealer penetration in curved root canals. J Endod. 2012;38:531–5.
115. Moorer WR, Wesselink PR. Factors promoting the tissue dissolving capability of sodium hypochlorite. Int Endod J. 1982;15(4):187–96.
116. Munoz HR, Camacho-Cuadra K. In vivo efficacy of three different endodontic irrigation systems for irrigant delivery to working length of mesial canals of mandibular molars. J Endod. 2012;38(4):445–8.
117. Ordinola-Zapata R, Bramante CM, Aprecio RM, Handysides R, Jaramillo DE. Biofilm removal by 6 % sodium hypochlorite activated by different irrigation techniques. Int Endod J. 2014;47(7):659–66.
118. Pafford J. In vivo evaluation of intraoperative and postoperative pain of hand/rotary/ultrasound technique in the root canals of vital and necrotic teeth. Master's thesis, The Ohio State University; 2007.
119. Paragliola R, Franco V, Fabiani C, Mazzoni A, Nato F, Tay FR, Breschi L, Grandini S. Final rinse optimization: influence of different agitation protocols. J Endod. 2010;36:282–5.
120. Pasqualini D, Cuffini AM, Scotti N, Mandras N, Scalas D, Pera F, Berutti E. Comparative evaluation of the antimicrobial efficacy of a 5 % sodium hypochlorite subsonic-activated solution. J Endod. 2010;36:1358–60.
121. Passarinho-Neto JG, Marchesan MA, Ferreira RB, Silva RG, Silva-Sousa YT, Sousa-Neto MD. *In vitro* evaluation of endodontic debris removal as obtained by rotary instrumentation coupled with ultrasonic irrigation. Aust Endod J. 2006;32:123–8.
122. Pataky L, Ivanyi I, Grigar A, Fazekas A. Antimicrobial efficacy of various root canal preparation techniques: an *in vitro* comparative study. J Endod. 2002;28:603–5.
123. Peeters HH, Mooduto L. Radiographic examination of apical extrusion of root canal irrigants during cavitation induced by Er, Cr:YSGG laser irradiation: an in vivo study. Clin Oral Investig. 2013;17:2105–12.
124. Peeters HH, Suardita K. Efficacy of smear layer removal at the root tip by using ethylenediaminetet-

raacetic acid and erbium, chromium: yttrium, scandium, gallium garnet laser. J Endod. 2011;37:1585–9.
125. Peters LB, van Winkelhoff AJ, Buijs JF, Wesselink PR. Effects of instrumentation, irrigation and dressing with calcium hydroxide on infection in pulpless teeth with periapical bone lesions. Int Endod J. 2002;35:13–21.
126. Peters OA. Current challenges and concepts in the preparation of root canal systems: a review. J Endod. 2004;30:559–67.
127. Peters OA, Bardsley S, Fong J, Pandher G, Divito E. Disinfection of root canals with photon-initiated photoacoustic streaming. J Endod. 2011;37:1008–12.
128. Richman MJ. The use of ultrasonics in root canal therapy and root resection. J Dent Med. 1957;12:12–8.
129. Rödig T, Bozkurt M, Konietschke F, Hülsmann M. Comparison of the Vibringe system with syringe and passive ultrasonic irrigation in removing debris from simulated root canal irregularities. J Endod. 2010;36:1410–3.
130. Rödig T, Döllmann S, Konietschke F, Drebenstedt S, Hülsmann M. Effectiveness of different irrigant agitation techniques on debris and smear layer removal in curved root canals: a scanning electron microscopy study. J Endod. 2010;36:1983–7.
131. Rödig T, Hirschleb M, Zapf A, Hülsmann M. Comparison of ultrasonic irrigation and RinsEndo for the removal of calcium hydroxide and Ledermix paste from root canals. Int Endod J. 2011;44:1155–61.
132. Rollison S, Barnett F, Stevens RH. Efficacy of bacterial removal from instrumented root canals *in vitro* related to instrumentation technique and size. Oral Surg Oral Med Oral Pathol Oral Radiol Endod. 2002;94:366–71.
133. Roy RA, Ahmad M, Crum LA. Physical mechanisms governing the hydrodynamic response of an oscillating ultrasonic file. Int Endod J. 1994;27:197–207.
134. Saber S-D, Hashem AA. Efficacy of different final irrigation activation techniques on smear layer removal. J Endod. 2011;37:1272–5.
135. Sabins RA, Johnson JD, Hellstein JW. A comparison of the cleaning efficacy of short-term sonic and ultrasonic passive irrigation after hand instrumentation in molar root canals. J Endod. 2003;29:674–8.
136. Sahar-Helft S, Stabholtz A, Moshonov J, Gutkin V, Redenski I, Steinberg D. Effect of Er:YAG laser-activated irrigation solution on *Enterococcus faecalis* biofilm in an *ex-vivo* root canal model. Photomed Laser Surg. 2013;31:334–41.
137. Salzgeber RM, Brilliant JD. An *in vivo* evaluation of the penetration of an irrigating solution in root canals. J Endod. 1977;3:394–8.
138. Schuping GB, Ørstavik D, Sigurdsson A, Trope M. Reduction of intracanal bacteria using nickel-titanium rotary instrumentation and various medications. J Endod. 2000;26:751–5.
139. Seet AN, Zilm PS, Gully NJ, Cathro PR. Qualitative comparison of sonic or laser energisation of 4 % sodium hypochlorite on an *Enterococcus faecalis* biofilm grown *in vitro*. Aust Endod J. 2012;38:100–6.
140. Shen Y, Gao Y, Qian W, Ruse ND, Zhou X, Wu H, Haapasalo M. Three-dimensional numeric simulation of root canal irrigant flow with different irrigation needles. J Endod. 2010;36:884–9.
141. Shen Y, Stojicic S, Qian W, Olsen I, Haapasalo M. The synergistic antimicrobial effect by mechanical agitation and two chlorhexidine preparations on biofilm bacteria. J Endod. 2010;36:100–4.
142. Siqueira JF, Lima KC, Magalhaes FA, Lopes HP, de Uzeda M. Mechanical reduction of the bacterial population in the root canal by three instrumentation techniques. J Endod. 1999;25:232–5.
143. Siqueira JF, Machado AG, Silveira RM, Lopes HP, de Uzeda M. Evaluation of the effectiveness of sodium hypochlorite used with three irrigation methods in the elimination of *Enterococcus faecalis* from the root canal, *in vitro*. Int Endod J. 1997;30:279–82.
144. Siqueira JF, Rôças IN, Favieri A, Lima KC. Chemomechanical reduction of the bacterial population in the root canal after instrumentation and irrigation with 1 %, 2.5 %, and 5.25 % sodium hypochlorite. J Endod. 2000;26:331–4.
145. Siqueira JF, Rôças IN, Santos SRLD, Lima KC, Magalhaes FAC, de Uzeda M. Efficacy of instrumentation techniques and irrigation regimens in reducing the bacterial population within root canals. J Endod. 2002;28:181–4.
146. Sjögren U, Sundqvist G. Bacteriologic evaluation of ultrasonic root canal instrumentation. Oral Surg Oral Med Oral Pathol. 1987;63:366–70.
147. Spoleti P, Siragusa M, Spoleti MJ. Bacteriological evaluation of passive ultrasonic activation. J Endod. 2003;29:12–4.
148. Spoorthy E, Velmurugan N, Ballal S, Nandini S. Comparison of irrigant penetration up to working length and into simulated lateral canals using various irrigating techniques. Int Endod J. 2013;46:815–22.
149. Stojicic S, Zivkovic S, Qian W, Zhang H, Haapasalo M. Tissue dissolution by sodium hypochlorite: effect of concentration, temperature, agitation, and surfactant. J Endod. 2010;36:1558–62.
150. Tambe VH, Nagmode PS, Vishwas JR, P SK, Angadi P, Ali FM. Evaluation of the Amount of Debris extruded apically by using Conv-entional Syringe, Endovac and Ultrasonic Irrigation Technique: An In Vitro Study. J Int Oral Health. 2013;5(3):63–6.
151. Tan BT, Messer HH. The quality of apical canal preparation using hand and rotary instruments with specific criteria for enlargement based on initial apical file size. J Endod. 2002;28:658–64.
152. Tardivo D, Pommel L, La Scola B, About I, Camps J. Antibacterial efficiency of passive ultrasonic versus sonic irrigation. Ultrasonic root canal irrigation. Odontostomatol Trop. 2010;33:29–35.
153. Tasdemir T, Er K, Celik D, Yildirim T. Effect of passive ultrasonic irrigation on apical extrusion of irrigating solution. Eur J Dent. 2008;2:198–203.

154. Tauber R, Morse D, Sinai I, Furst M. A magnifying lens comparative evaluation of conventional and ultrasonically energized filing. J Endod. 1983;9:269–74.
155. Tay FR, Gu LS, Schoeffel GJ, Wimmer C, Susin L, Zhang K, Arun SN, Kim J, Looney SW, Pashley DH. Effect of vapor lock on root canal debridement by using a side-vented needle for positive-pressure irrigant delivery. J Endod. 2010;36:745–50.
156. Tinaz AC, Karadag LS, Alaçam T, Mihçioglu T. Evaluation of the smear layer removal effectiveness of EDTA using two techniques: an SEM study. J Contemp Dent Pract. 2006;7:9–16.
157. The ultrasonic cleaning process: How does an ultrasonic cleaner clean?. TM Associates. http://www.tmasc.com/qa%20process.htm. Accessed 11 Mar 2014.
158. Townsend C, Maki J. An in vitro comparison of new irrigation and agitation techniques to ultrasonic agitation in removing bacteria from a simulated root canal. J Endod. 2009;35:1040–3.
159. Türkün M, Cengiz T. The effects of sodium hypochlorite and calcium hydroxide on tissue dissolution and root canal cleanliness. Int Endod J. 1997;30:335–42.
160. Uroz-Torres D, González-Rodríguez MP, Ferrer-Luque CM. Effectiveness of the EndoActivator System in removing the smear layer after root canal instrumentation. J Endod. 2010;36:308–11.
161. van der Sluis LW, Vogels MP, Verhaagen B, Macedo R, Wesselink PR. Study on the influence of refreshment/activation cycles and irrigants on mechanical cleaning efficiency during ultrasonic activation of the irrigant. J Endod. 2010;36:737–40.
162. van der Sluis LW, Wu MK, Wesselink PR. The efficacy of ultrasonic irrigation to remove artificially placed dentine debris from human root canals prepared using instruments of varying taper. Int Endod J. 2005;38:764–8.
163. van der Sluis LW, Wu MK, Wesselink PR. A comparison between a smooth wire and a K-file in removing artificially placed dentine debris from root canals in resin blocks during ultrasonic irrigation. Int Endod J. 2005;38:593–6.
164. Vera J, Arias A, Romero M. Effect of maintaining apical patency on irrigant penetration into the apical third of root canals when using passive ultrasonic irrigation: an *in vivo* study. J Endod. 2011;37:1276–8.
165. Vera J, Hernández EM, Romero M, Arias A, van der Sluis LW. Effect of maintaining apical patency on irrigant penetration into the apical two millimeters of large root canals: an *in vivo* study. J Endod. 2012;38:1340–3.
166. Walmsley AD. Ultrasound and root canal treatment: the need for scientific evaluation. Int Endod J. 1987;20:105–11.
167. Walmsley AD, Williams AR. Effects of constraint on the oscillatory pattern of endosonic files. J Endod. 1989;15:189–94.
168. Weller RN, Brady JM, Bernier WE. Efficacy of ultrasonic cleaning. J Endod. 1980;6:740–3.
169. Wiseman A, Cox TC, Paranjpe A, Flake NM, Cohenca N, Johnson JD. Efficacy of sonic and ultrasonic activation for removal of calcium hydroxide from mesial canals of mandibular molars: a microtomographic study. J Endod. 2011;37:235–8.
170. Yang SF, Rivera EM, Walton RE, Baumgardner KR. Canal debridement: effectiveness of sodium hypochlorite and calcium hydroxide as medicaments. J Endod. 1996;22:521–5.
171. Yavari HR, Rahimi S, Shahi S, Lotfi M, Barhaghi MH, Fatemi A, Abdolrahimi M. Effect of Er, Cr: YSGG laser irradiation on Enterococcus faecalis in infected root canals. Photomed Laser Surg. 2010;28 Suppl 1:S91–6.
172. Yoo YJ, Lee W, Kim HC, Shon WJ, Baek SH. Multivariate analysis of the cleaning efficacy of different final irrigation techniques in the canal and isthmus of mandibular posterior teeth. Restor Dent Endod. 2013;38:154–9.
173. Yücel AÇ, Gürel M, Güler E, Karabucak B. Comparison of final irrigation techniques in removal of calcium hydroxide. Aust Endod J. 2013;39:116–21.
174. Zhu X, Yin X, Chang JW, Wang Y, Cheung GS, Zhang C. Comparison of the antibacterial effect and smear layer removal using photon-initiated photoacoustic streaming aided irrigation versus a conventional irrigation in single-rooted canals: an in vitro study. Photomed Laser Surg. 2013;31:371–7.

Continuous Instrumentation and Irrigation: The Self-Adjusting File (SAF) System

11

Zvi Metzger and Anda Kfir

Abstract

The recently introduced self-adjusting file (SAF) system is the first of its kind, performing continuous and simultaneous instrumentation and irrigation. As an instrumentation device it adapts itself to the shape of the canal, including its cross section, as opposed to most rotary file systems that machine the canal to the shape of the file. The SAF system removes a uniform dentin layer from all around the canal as opposed to rotary files which are using excessive removal of sound dentin in attempt to include the whole canal within the preparation. Combined with its effective irrigation, it allows a new concept of minimally invasive endodontics. The SAF system is a no-pressure irrigation system combined with an added mechanical scrubbing effect. The effective cleaning of oval canals enables more effective disinfection and better obturation than can be achieved with rotary files. Its scrubbing effect is also useful in the final stage of retreatment as well as in the treatment of root canals of immature teeth.

The Role of Irrigants in Endodontic Treatment

If the simple idea that "the file shapes; the irrigant cleans" was always true, there would be no need for special irrigation systems. Shaping a canal with rotary files to the extent that a thin irrigation needle can be inserted to a working length would always provide clean, ready-to-fill canals. Unfortunately, this simple concept, which may be effective in narrow, straight canals with a round cross section, fails to deliver the desired result in oval canals [23, 59, 72, 77, 100]. Such canals represent 24 % of the total number of root canals, and in certain types of teeth, the incidence of oval canals can reach 90 % [29, 50, 58, 99].

Furthermore, the assumption that the above concept provides adequate cleaning of the whole canal has led to an oversimplified approach to root canal treatment: one only has to machine the canal to a certain shape to accommodate a similarly

Z. Metzger, DMD (✉) • A. Kfir, DMD
Department of Endodontology, The Goldschlager School of Dental Medicine, Tel Aviv University, Ramat Aviv, Tel Aviv 69978, Israel
e-mail: metzger.zvi@gmail.com; dr.andakfir@gmail.com

B. Basrani (ed.), *Endodontic Irrigation: Chemical Disinfection of the Root Canal System*,
DOI 10.1007/978-3-319-16456-4_11

shaped master cone. The irrigant is thus expected to clean the rest of the canal space by its tissue or biofilm-dissolving action [27, 35, 78, 89]. The distance from this simplistic idea to practically reducing the whole endodontic treatment to preparing a space to accommodate a master cone may be small.

Studies indicate that the effective cleaning of oval canals is a challenge that is beyond the ability of syringe and needle irrigation. The action of rotary files in such canals not only fails to clean the buccal and/or lingual "fins" or the isthmus between canals but also actively packs these recesses with dentin particles [63, 66, 67] that are difficult to remove, even with passive ultrasonic irrigation [66].

Such findings led De-Deus et al. to conclude that "the notion that 'the file shapes; the irrigant cleans' represents wishful thinking rather than an established scientific fact, at least in the case of oval canals" [23].

These limitations of syringe and needle irrigation led to a search for and introduction of new irrigation methods that are designed to overcome this barrier, by either (a) affecting the flow or motion of the irrigant at given time points of the procedure or by (b) adding a scrubbing effect to a continuous flow of the irrigant. The first group included negative pressure irrigation systems [36, 60, 69, 81] and sonic and ultrasonic irrigant activation systems [9, 25, 43]. The new self-adjusting file system represents the second approach.

The Self-Adjusting File (SAF) System

The self-adjusting file system is a shaping and cleaning system designed for minimally invasive endodontic treatment. The system consists of a self-adjusting file that is operated with a special RDT handpiece head and an irrigation pump that delivers a continuous flow of irrigant through the hollow file [39, 53–57].

The Self-Adjusting File (SAF)

The SAF is the first file that does not have a solid metal core. The file is designed as a hollow tube, in which the walls are made from a thin nickel-titanium lattice with a rough outer surface. The tube has an asymmetrically positioned tip (Fig. 11.1). The tip is located at the wall of the tube, as opposed to the symmetrically centered tips that may be found in all conventional nickel-titanium rotary files. The file is extremely compressible, such that a 1.5 mm SAF diameter may be compressed into a root canal that only a #20 K file can be inserted into (Fig. 11.2). This compressibility also enables the file to adapt to the shape of the cross section of the canal [39, 53–56]. When inserted into an oval canal with a 0.2 mm mesiodistal diameter, a 1.5 mm SAF will be compressed mesiodistally and thus spread buccolingually, reaching a buccolingual diameter of 2.4 mm [39, 53–57]. This will occur even if the operator is not aware that the canal is oval, hence the name "self-adjusting file." Naturally, such a flattened file cannot rotate while it is in the canal and is operated with in-and-out vibrations that are created by the RDT handpiece head.

The RDT Handpiece Head

The RDT handpiece head (Fig. 11.3) has a dual mechanical function. It transforms the rotation of the micromotor into a trans-line in-and-out vibration with an amplitude of 0.4 mm and contains a clutch mechanism that allows the SAF to rotate slowly when not engaged in the canal but that completely stops the rotation once the file is engaged with the canal walls. The micromotor is operated at 5,000 rpm, which results in 5,000 vibrations/min, and the operator uses pecking motions when using the SAF. Free rotation of the file should occur at the outbound portion of every pecking stroke, when the SAF is disengaged from the canal walls. When the SAF enters the canal during the inbound pecking motion, it should do so at random, with different circular positions, thus ensuring uniform treatment of the canal walls [53–56, 68, 73, 74, 95]. This random circular position also allows the asymmetrical tip of the file to negotiate curvatures that may be found in the root canal. RDT heads may be adapted to a large variety of endodontic motors (Fig. 11.3).

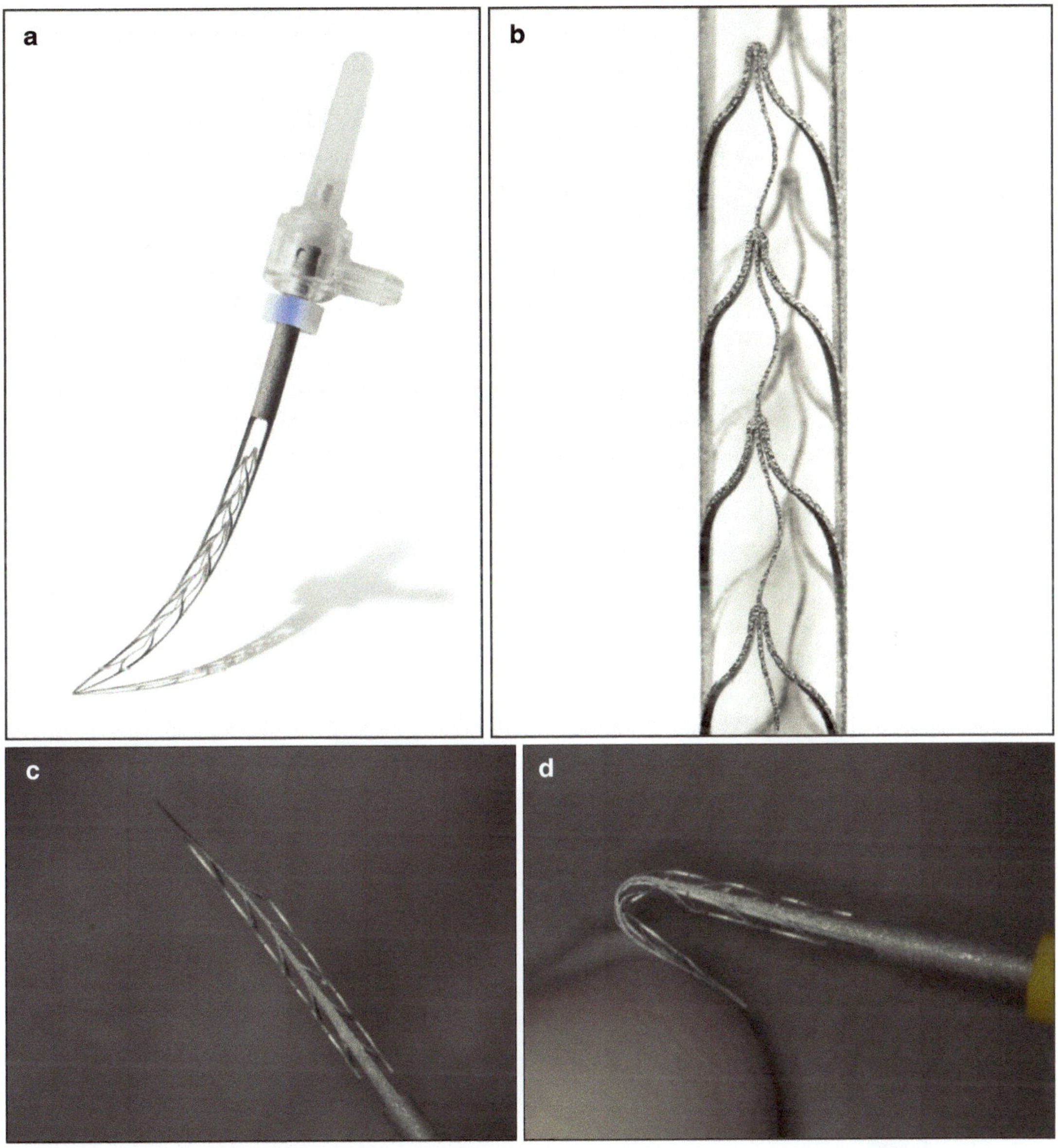

Fig. 11.1 The SAF. (a) The SAF. (b) Structure of the file: two longitudinal beams, connected by a series of arches that are designed to allow maximal compressibility. The arches are harnessed to each other with thin struts that prevent pulling the arches out of the cylinder. (c) The asymmetrically located tip of the file. (d) Extreme flexibility of the SAF. This should be compared to that of the last rotary file that is used in the canal

EndoStation/VATEA Irrigation Pumps

The SAF is provided with a freely rotating hub to which a polyethylene tube is connected (Fig. 11.4), thus allowing the irrigant to flow through the hollow file into the root canal. The irrigant is delivered into the tube by either EndoStation or VATEA irrigation pumps (Fig. 11.5).

The VATEA is a self-contained pump that has a built-in irrigant reservoir of 500 mL and is powered by a rechargeable battery (Fig. 11.1a). The EndoStation is a compound all-in-one machine that can be operated in either rotary or reciprocat-

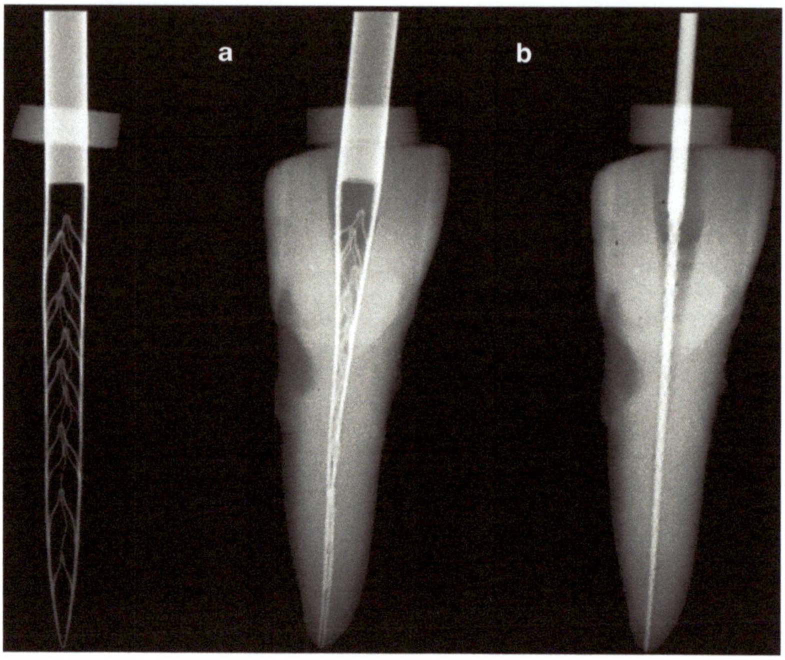

Fig. 11.2 SAF compressed into a narrow canal. *Left*: the SAF in its relaxed form. (**a**) The same SAF inserted into a narrow canal, which was prepared with a # 20 K file. (**b**) A #20 K file that fits into the same canal

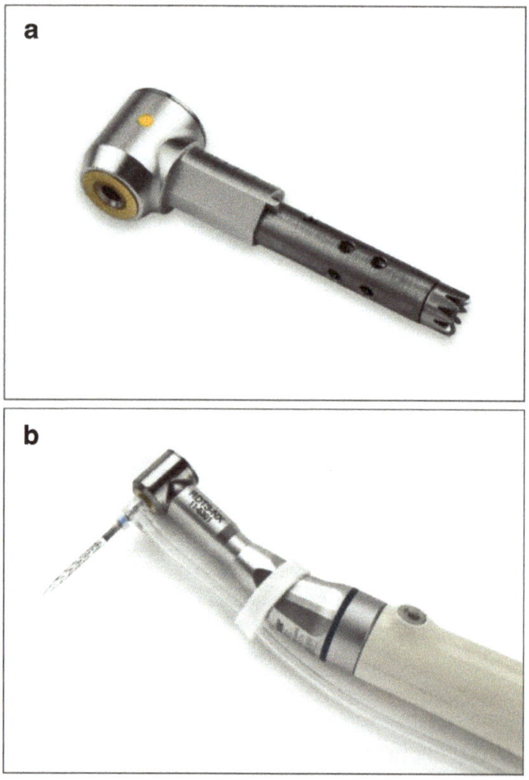

Fig. 11.3 RDT handpiece heads. (**a**) RDT3 handpiece head that may fit into various handpieces. (**b**) RDT3-NX handpiece head attached to an X-smart endomotor through a 1:1 NSK gear/adaptor

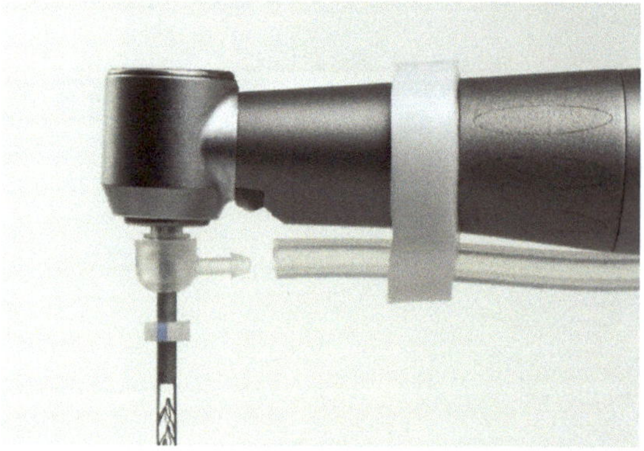

Fig. 11.4 Rotating hub on the SAF for connecting the irrigation tube. The SAF is equipped with a rotating hub that allows it to attach to the irrigation tube, which allows the irrigant to flow from the irrigation pump to the hollow file

ing file modes, using a regular handpiece, or in the SAF mode, which enables continuous irrigation when using a special separate handpiece with an RDT head. The irrigant container of the EndoStation is an external bottle from which a peristaltic pump draws the irrigant into the tube and into the attached file (Fig. 11.5b).

Either irrigation pump delivers the irrigant at an adjustable flow rate of 1–10 mL/min. Because the file is built as a lattice-walled cylinder, no

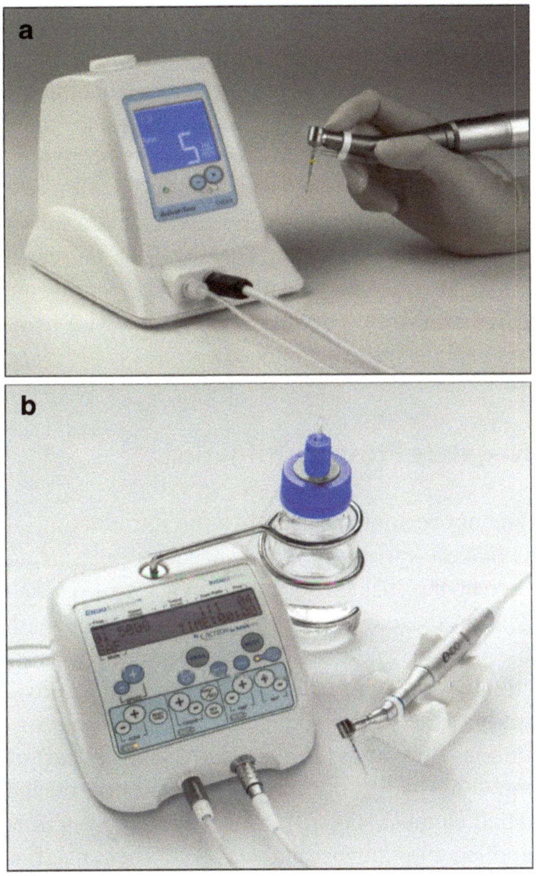

Fig. 11.5 EndoStation and a VATEA pump. (**a**) A VATEA peristaltic pump with irrigant container within the unit. (**b**) EndoStation is an all-in-one endodontic motor that can be operated in either the ASF mode with irrigation using a handpiece with an RDT head or in rotary mode or reciprocating modes using a regular E-type handpiece. The built-in peristaltic pump draws the irrigant from the external bottle container

pressure is generated within the file: any small pressure that is generated by the pump to deliver the irrigant through the tube is eliminated when the irrigant enters the file.

Minimally Invasive Shaping and Cleaning

The concept of minimally invasive shaping and cleaning uses a *different method* of achieving *the same aims* as the conventional, traditional shaping and cleaning procedures. Conventional shaping and cleaning, which uses rotary files, involves (a) the removal of large amounts of sound dentin in attempt to include as much as possible the canal wall within the preparation and to allow effective irrigation at the apical end of the canal and (b) the creation of unnoticeable micro-cracks in the remaining dentin by the rotary files [3, 8, 13, 37, 46, 85, 102]. Both these damaging effects were either accepted so far or ignored, as there was no other effective means to thoroughly clean the root canal.

The minimally invasive concept is aimed at achieving the effective cleaning of a root canal by (a) removing a uniform thin layer of dentin around the entire root canal without the unnecessary excessive removal of sound dentin and without causing micro-cracks and (b) providing a continuous flow of fresh, fully active irrigant that is applied with a scrubbing motion of the walls, all the way to the apical part of the canal.

Conventional shaping procedures involve machining the root canal into a desired shape, with either a sequence of rotary instruments or one reciprocating tool. Such process is used (a) to enable irrigation in the apical part of the canal and (b) to facilitate obturation by using a master cone that has the shape of the machined canal. If the canal is straight and narrow with a round cross section, this concept may work well as it may allow the removal of all the inner layers of dentin with anything that was attached to it, be it pulp tissue or bacterial biofilm. The debris are carried coronally by the flutes or compacted into the flutes, and the subsequent irrigation may remove the leftover debris from the canal.

Nevertheless, if this simplistic view of the process is applied to all canals, it may often be considered as *treating imaginary canals* while ignoring the 3D reality of root canals. MicroCT studies have shown that in oval and curved canals, rotary files fail to remove the inner layer of dentin from all around the canal wall [66, 71]. Furthermore, the discrepancy between the size of the tip of many rotary files (i.e., #25) and the known dimensions and shape of the apical parts of root canals led to the suggestion that a larger apical preparation should be used to include all the apical canal surfaces within the perimeter of the instrumented canal [7, 15, 72]. A larger apical preparation may lead to a further unnecessary removal of sound dentin [44, 52]. All these are avoided when using the minimally invasive concept.

Mode of Irrigation by the SAF System

Positive Pressure Irrigation

The delivery of the irrigant to the apical part of the canal has been traditionally achieved using syringe and needle irrigation [35, 72, 93]. This mode of irrigation applies positive pressure to deliver the irrigant and has several limitations. The irrigant cannot be delivered further than 1–2 mm beyond the tip of the needle; thus, effective irrigation requires the tip of the needle to be 1–2 mm from the working length [10, 16]. The application of positive pressure close to the apical foramen involves the potential risk of pushing the irrigant beyond the apex, commonly termed a "sodium hypochlorite accident" [35]. Consequently, many operators avoid inserting a needle up to the required length, thus compromising the efficacy of the irrigation of the apical cul-de-sac area.

Sonic and Passive Ultrasonic Irrigation

Sonic and passive ultrasonic irrigations are designed to induce agitation or streaming movements of the irrigant to increase the efficiency of its action [18, 47, 48]. Sonic irrigation operates at a low frequency (1–6 kHz) and high amplitude and generates small shear stresses, which have been shown to be efficient for root canal debridement. Studies reported that the sonic instruments may contribute to the cleanliness of the canals but can leave residual debris attached to the canal walls in hard-to-reach areas of long oval canals, isthmuses, and recesses.

Passive ultrasonic irrigation is the use of a smooth metal file that vibrates in the canal at an ultrasonic frequency. The vibrating file induces acoustic streaming, which is a very effective cleaning method [48, 93]. Nevertheless, some studies have not supported these findings. To be effective, the file must have free movement in the canal, without making contact with the canal walls. Consequently, this method may be applied effectively only after canal instrumentation and may be ineffective when applied in curved canals in which the file touches the wall at the canal bend. When either sonic or passive ultrasonic irrigations are used, the canal is filled with irrigant using a syringe and needle.

Negative Pressure Irrigation

The above limitations led to the introduction of irrigation systems that use negative pressure to deliver the irrigant to the desired area [16, 79]. The access cavity is continuously flooded with the irrigant, and a small cannula, through which negative pressure is applied, is inserted in proximity to the working length. This causes the continuous flow of the irrigant into the apical part of the canal while the irrigant is aspirated by the small cannula [60, 79]. This irrigation system is applied after the instrumentation of the canal. For a full effect, this method requires an enlargement of the canal to #40/0.04 or #40/0.06 [12, 26], which makes the method useful in straight canals but of limited value in thin, curved canals in which such enlargement may not be safely achieved.

No-Pressure Irrigation

The SAF may be defined as a no-pressure irrigation system that is applied throughout the instrumentation process [53–57]. Once the irrigant enters the SAF, any pressure that may have existed in the tube disappears due to the lattice structure of the file. The irrigant is continuously delivered into the root canal, and the vibrations of the file, combined with the pecking motion applied by the operator, result in the continuous mixing of the irrigant that is present in the root canal with fresh, fully active irrigant. This mode of action raises two questions: (a) will the freshly applied irrigant be able to reach the apical part of the canal and (b) what is the potential of the pecking motion, which is applied to the working length, to push the irrigant beyond the apex?

The setup in Fig. 11.6a was used to answer the first question. The simulated canal in the transparent block was filled with green liquid, representing the irrigant that is present in the canal (Fig. 11.6b). The SAF was operated with vibrations and pecking motions. At a given time, a red liquid, representing fresh, fully active sodium hypochlorite, was injected into the tube, and the time required for the apical part of the canal to turn completely red was measured. The total replacement of the irrigant in the apical section occurred within 30 s (Fig. 11.6c). When using the SAF system for 4 min, as required by the manufacturer's instructions, the sodium hypochlorite in the apical part of the canal is continuously replaced with a fresh, fully active solution at least 8 times.

The setup in Fig. 11.7 was used to answer the second question. The tooth was mounted at the bottom of a plastic container with its tip protruding below the container. The canal was prepared to a working length with a #20 K file, and the patency of the apical foramen was verified by passing a #15 K file through it (Fig. 11.7a). The SAF was used in the canal for 4 min with continuous irrigation, and the apical foramen was visually checked for any liquid passage. No liq-

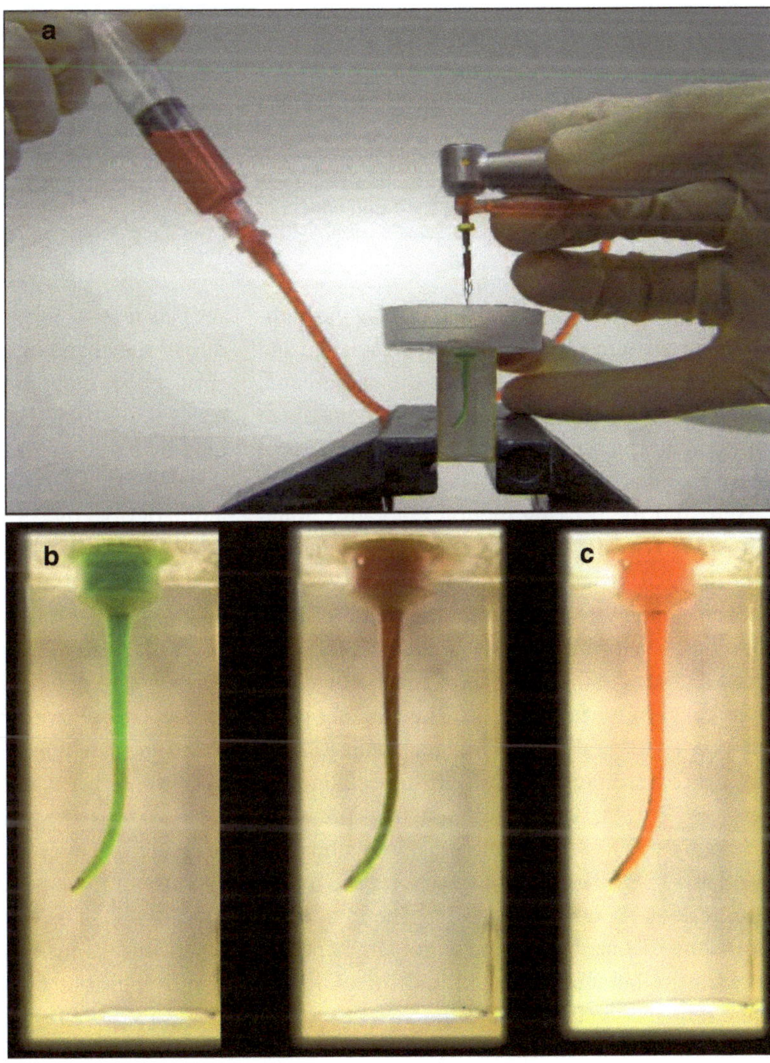

Fig. 11.6 Measuring the time needed for the replacement of the irrigant in the apical part of a simulated canal. A simulated canal was filled with a green liquid, and the SAF was used in this canal. At a given time point, a red liquid was fed into the irrigation tube, and the time required for the liquid in the apical part of the canal to turn red was measured. (**a**) The setup. (**b**) Before SAF operation; (**c**) 30 s after SAF operation. The red liquid represented fresh, fully active sodium hypochlorite. During 4 min of SAF operation, the full replacement of the irrigant at the apical part with fresh, active irrigant occurred eight times

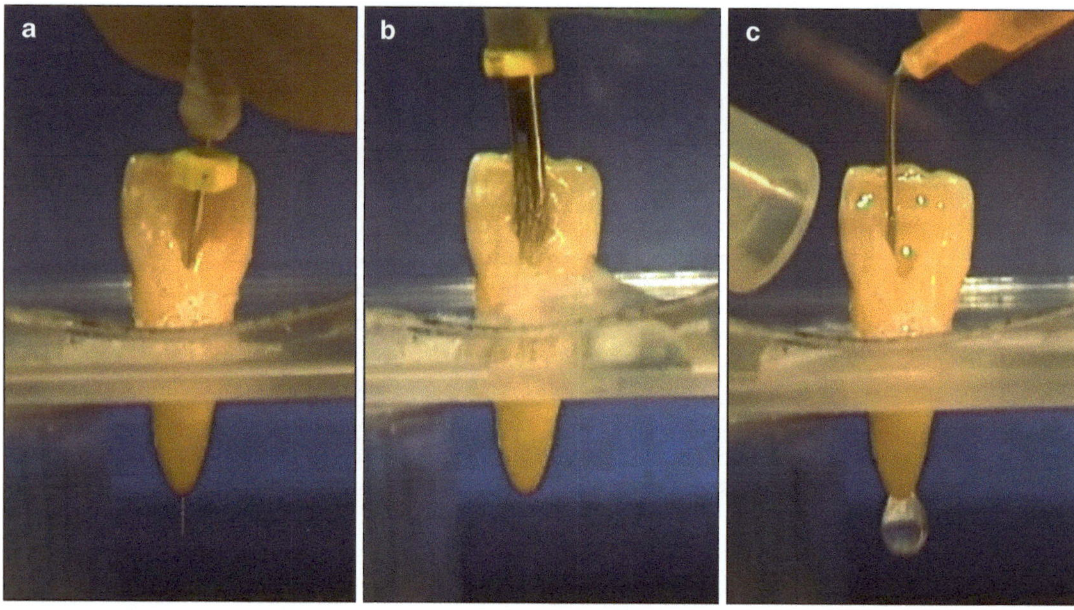

Fig. 11.7 The SAF system *vs.* syringe and needle irrigation. The tooth was prepared with a #15 K file, which passed through the apical foramen (**a**) and with a #20 K file to a working length of 1 mm short of the apical foramen. The SAF was used in the canal for 4 min with continuous irrigation (**b**). No irrigant passed through the apical foramen. (**c**) A short needle was inserted into the canal to a distance of 12 mm from the apical foramen. The needle was free in the canal and did not touch its walls. When irrigated with this needle, a flow of irrigant traveled through the apex, even though the needle was at a distance from the apex and was free in the canal

uid passed through the apical foramen throughout the procedure (Fig. 11.7b). When syringe and needle irrigation was applied in the same canal immediately after the SAF, keeping the needle at approximately 12 mm from WL, the liquid passed freely beyond the apex (Fig. 11.7c).

Why did the pecking motion not cause liquid extrusion? Why did the syringe and needle cause a free flow of irrigant beyond the apex? Fluid mechanics analyses provide the answers to these questions. Even with a much larger apical foramen with a diameter of 0.35 mm, the liquid is contained in the canal by surface tension. The bursting pressure needed to break this surface tension is 832 Pa. The hydrostatic pressure of a 20 mm column of water is 195 Pa, and the stagnating pressure, caused by 5,000 vibrations per min within the liquid, is 196 Pa. The piston pressure caused by the SAF pecking motion is only 3 Pa. The total pressure in the root canal (394 Pa) is not large enough to reach the bursting pressure, and therefore the liquid remained in the canal [39].

The reason for such a low piston pressure is due to the shape of the apical motion of the SAF (Fig. 11.8). Even in the extreme case of a diameter of 0.2 mm in the apical part of the canal (created by a #20 K file), the fully compressed tip of the SAF has a cross section in the shape of a rectangle of 0.16 by 0.12 mm (Fig. 11.8). This leaves 38 % of the canal cross section open for the backflow of irrigant; thus, the potential piston is ineffective [39].

When calculating the pressures caused by syringe and needle irrigation in a canal similar to the one above and keeping the needle in a position in which 38 % of the canal cross section is free for backflow, the syringe and needle create a pressure of more than 1,270 Pa. Such a pressure is generated by the flow of the liquid, even though the needle is not tightly fitted to the canal walls. The total pressure in the canal will reach in this case 1,465 Pa, which is above the eruption pressure and allows the free passage of liquid [39].

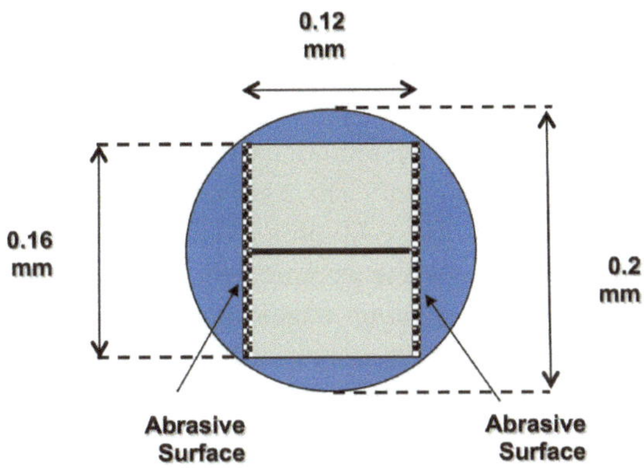

Fig. 11.8 The tip of the SAF within a canal prepared with a # 20 file. A schematic presentation of the tip of a SAF (*rectangle*) when inserted into a canal, which was prepared with a #20 K file (*circle*). Thirty-eight percent of the cross section of the canal is free for backflow. This explains why the SAF is not pushing debris or irrigant through the apical foramen, as presented in Fig. 11.6 (Adapted from Hof et al. [39])

The above experiment (Fig. 11.7) was completed in a canal with an open apical foramen with only air surrounding the apex. One may assume that if no liquid passed through the apex during the operation of the SAF system, even in such conditions, the chance that the irrigant will be pushed beyond the apex under clinical conditions, in which the tissues surround the apex, is low.

In this context, when a #20 hand file is moved toward the apex in a tight canal with a diameter of 0.2 mm, the calculated piston pressure may reach the range of hydraulic pressure: 199,700 Pa. This may explain some of the postoperative pain that patients often experience because such pressures are likely to push small volumes of irrigant and/or debris beyond the apical foramen [39].

Mode of Action of Sodium Hypochlorite

As an irrigant, sodium hypochlorite is used (a) to dissolve vital or necrotic pulp tissue that remained in the recesses of the canal after instrumentation and (b) to kill bacteria that may be present in the canal. However, during this process, sodium hypochlorite is gradually inactivated [14, 19, 34].

When pulp tissue is inserted into a test tube containing sodium hypochlorite, sodium hypochlorite quickly dissolves the tissue [75, 96]. In such conditions, the volume of sodium hypochlorite is infinitely larger than that of the pulp tissue, and the inactivation of the solution may not be noticeable. However, in vivo, in the presence of inflammatory exudate, pulp tissue, and microbial remnants, the action of sodium hypochlorite on such substances may consume, weaken, and inactivate sodium hypochlorite [35].

When placed in a root canal, the volume of the sodium hypochlorite is rather limited (~10 μL in the maxillary central incisors), and when pulp tissue or bacteria are present, sodium hypochlorite may be quickly consumed and inactivated. Therefore, simple flooding the canal with sodium hypochlorite during the procedure may be ineffective. Frequent replacement of the irrigant is commonly suggested to maintain the desired activity [6, 35]. When a syringe and needle irrigation is applied, fresh, fully active sodium hypochlorite may be present during the irrigation process, but only up to 2 mm from the distance at which the needle can be inserted. This implies that as long as the needle cannot be safely inserted to WL, no fully active sodium hypochlorite will be present at the apical part of the canal [64]. Any amount of sodium hypochlorite that seeps into this area will be readily inactivated. Thus during traditional endodontic procedures, with intermittent irrigation, the total time that fully active sodium hypochlorite is present at the apical part of the canal is limited.

When negative pressure irrigation is considered, the size of the canal during the instrumentation process is also a limiting factor. Only when the apical part is sufficiently enlarged and the small cannula is inserted to WL can the fully active sodium hypochlorite reach this area.

Mode of Action of EDTA

EDTA is often used in endodontic treatment protocols. Some use it to soften the dentin walls of the canal to facilitate instrumentation, while others use it at later stages of the cleaning process to remove the smear layer before disinfection and/or obturation of the root canal. For decalcification of dentin by EDTA, the dentin must first be exposed to sodium hypochlorite [6, 31, 33, 61]. Therefore, in areas of the canal that were not effectively exposed to active sodium hypochlorite, the effect of EDTA may be limited. As any mechanical device, the SAF generates a smear layer [54]. Nevertheless, the subsequent use of EDTA and its activation by the vibrations of the SAF effectively remove the smear layer, even in the apical cul-de-sac area. The frequent appearance of lateral canals in SAF-treated cases (Fig. 11.9) may be the result of the removal of the smear layer plugs that otherwise block the lateral canal entrance [83].

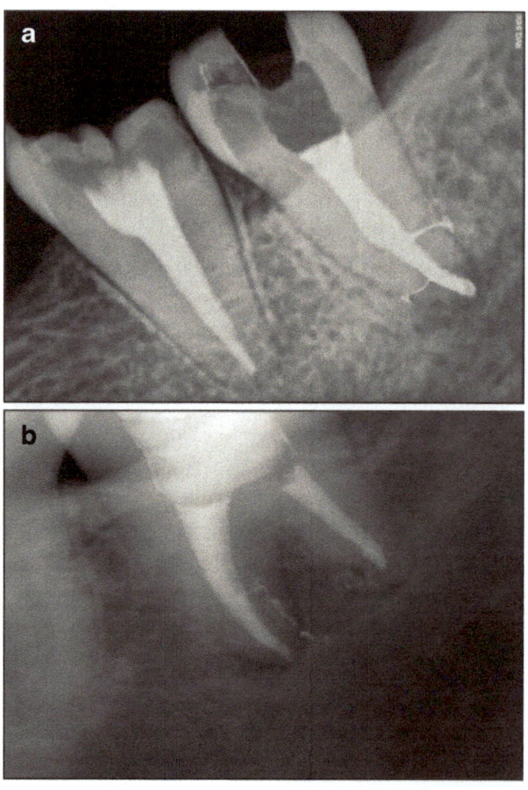

Fig. 11.9 Lateral canals in SAF-treated clinical cases. Lateral canals frequently appear when SAF-treated cases are obturated. (**a**) Courtesy of Dr. Ajinkia Pawar, Mumbai, India; (**b**) Adapted from Solomonov [82]

Mode of Cleaning with the SAF System

When the SAF system is used, the process of delivering fresh, fully active sodium hypochlorite is continuous. The SAF protocol requires a glide path that allows the compressed SAF to reach WL at the *beginning* stages of the procedure. This is different from other instrumentation concepts in which reaching WL represents the *end* of the procedure. The SAF system is then used for 4 min using pecking motions that reach the WL with a simultaneous continuous replenishing flow of fresh, fully active sodium hypochlorite. This may explain the effective cleaning of the apical part of the canal [2, 54, 55, 101] and the cleaning of the canal's recesses and fins [23, 45].

Another important cleaning feature of the SAF system is the *scrubbing* of the canal walls. If pulp tissue or a bacterial biofilm is left in the canal, sodium hypochlorite is commonly expected to dissolve them. However, one should consider the volume and three-dimensional structure of these substances. When the outer layer of the target material is attacked, the inner layers may still be protected from the actions of the sodium hypochlorite. Furthermore, when attacking the outer layers, sodium hypochlorite is inactivated and becomes less potent. The deeper the fin or recess, the more difficult it is to simply dissolve the pulp tissue or biofilm that it may contain.

If the pulp tissue or bacterial biofilm were loosely attached to the canal wall, they could potentially be detached by the flow of irrigant. However, both substances are closely and firmly attached to the canal wall (Fig. 11.10) [59]. Direct mechanical action is often required to remove them from the canal wall [57].

The SAF consists of a metal mesh, which closely adapts around the canal walls, even in oval canals. Continuous movements of this metal mesh over the surface have a scrubbing effect, which is a more effective method of cleaning (Fig. 11.11).

This dual cleaning action of the SAF system, continuous replacement of fresh, fully active sodium hypochlorite, all the way to WL

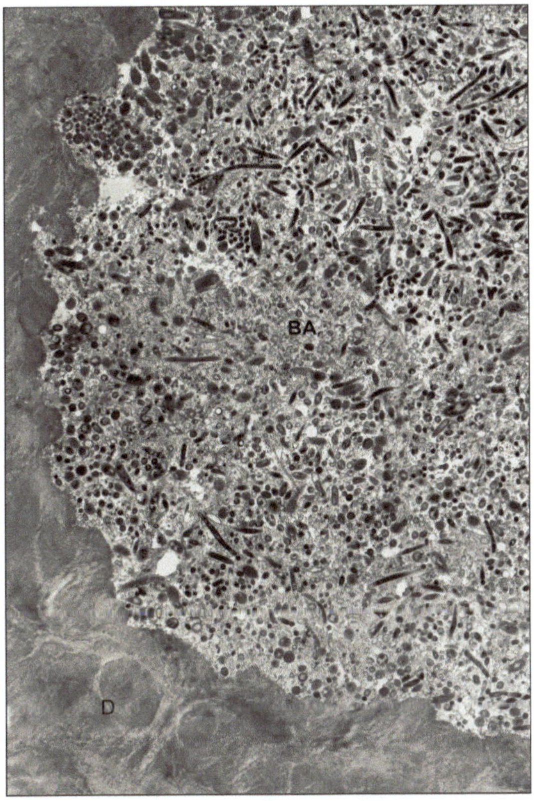

Fig. 11.10 A bacterial biofilm tightly attached to the root canal wall. The mesial root of a mandibular molar was clinically treated, resulting in a satisfactory radiographic result. The apical tip of the root was removed surgically after the procedure and subjected to transmission electron microscopy. The intact biofilm that remained in the isthmus was tightly attached to the dentin wall and was not affected by the copious irrigation with sodium hypochlorite used during the endodontic treatment (Adapted from Nair et al. [59]). *BA* Bacteria, *D* Dentin

throughout the procedure, and the continuous scrubbing of the canal walls may explain the unique cleaning efficacy of the SAF system [54, 56, 57].

When using the SAF system, EDTA may be applied in the canal with a syringe and needle and then agitated for 30 s by the SAF with the irrigation pump turned off. Alternatively, the pump may be turned off and EDTA applied through a special "y" connector that is attached to the irrigation tube close to its connector to the SAF (Fig. 11.12). In such a case, the continuous flow of EDTA is manually controlled by the person holding the syringe.

Cleaning Efficacy of the SAF System

The ultimate tool for evaluating the cleaning efficacy of a root canal is scanning electron microscopy (SEM). Many studies have used this tool to evaluate the cleaning of a root canal [4, 17, 28, 40, 51, 62, 70, 94].

In the majority of these studies, while the coronal and middle parts of the root canal may be effectively cleaned by rotary files and syringe and needle irrigation, the apical part of the canal, with its cul-de-sac shape, presented a greater challenge. In most of these studies, the apical part of the canal contained large amounts of debris and was covered with a smear layer, even after EDTA irrigation [4, 17, 28, 40, 51, 62, 70, 94].

When the SAF system was used, alternating between sodium hypochlorite and EDTA, the apical part of the canal was clean of debris in all of the samples, and in 65 % of the cases, no smear layer was present (Fig. 11.13) [2, 54, 101]. This was likely due to the dual action described above.

Lin et al. recently used a unique model to study the ability of different files and irrigation systems to remove the bacterial biofilm from grooves that were placed in the wall of the root canals, representing fins or other recesses [45]. They found that when hand files were used with copious sodium hypochlorite irrigation applied with syringe and needle, 27 % of the groove area was still covered with biofilm. Rotary files with similar irrigation reduced the area of the groove covered by biofilm to 19 %, while the SAF system with its scrubbing effect and continuous sodium hypochlorite irrigation left only 3 % of the groove area covered with biofilm [45].

Histology is another effective tool to evaluate the efficacy of cleaning root canals. De-Deus et al. used this tool on pair-matched, flat-oval canals of canines with vital pulp, to study the cleaning efficacy of rotary files and syringe and needle irrigation, and compared them to the SAF system [23]. They found that while rotary files left large amounts of pulp tissue in the canal fins (Fig. 11.14), the SAF system was more effective in cleaning and removing the pulp tissue [23].

Both above methods of study involved the interpretation of the observer and can potentially

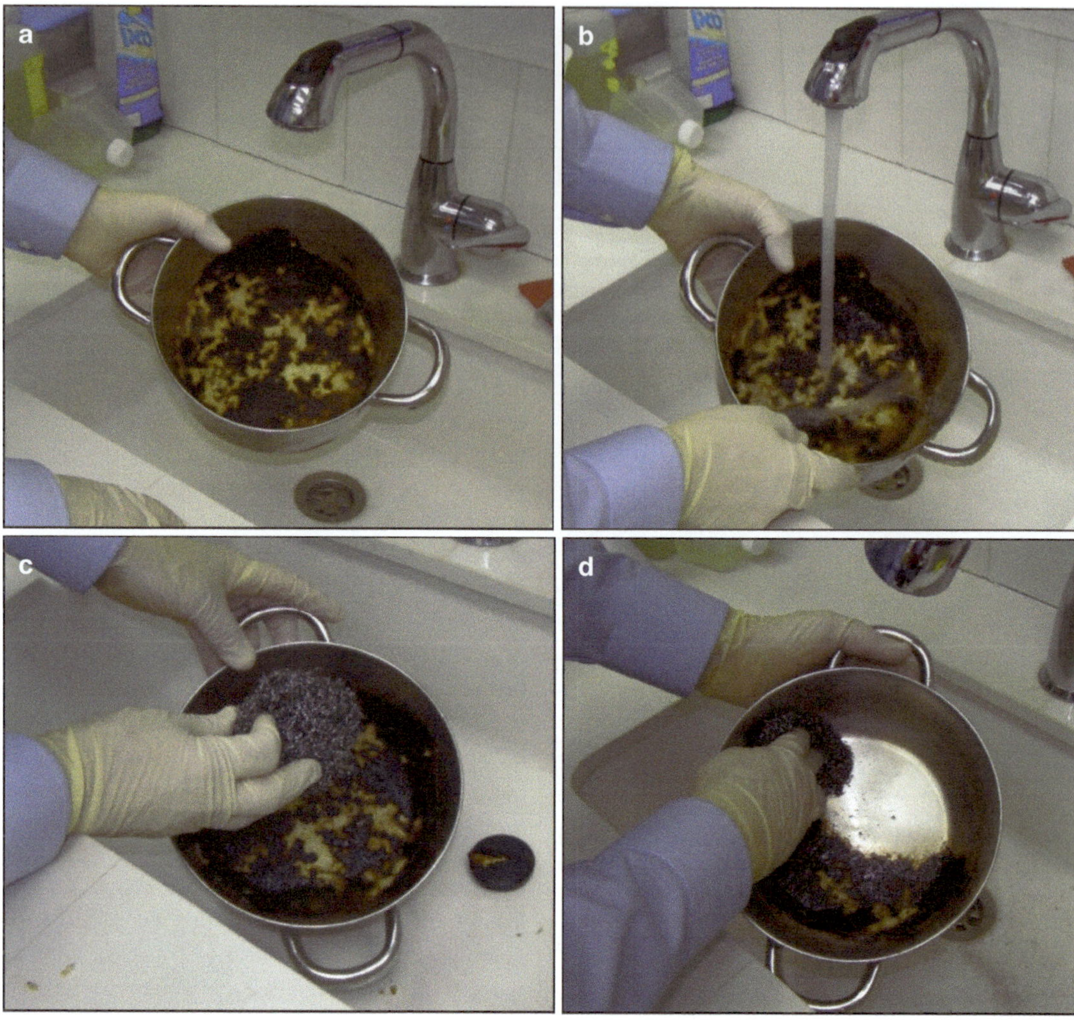

Fig. 11.11 Irrigation *vs*. scrubbing. An illustration of the efficacy of cleaning by scrubbing. (**a**) Burnt forage on the bottom of the pot represents the bacterial biofilm or pulp tissue that is tightly attached to the canal walls. (**b**) Irrigation alone, with no mechanical action, is unlikely to remove such bound material. (**c**) A metal scrubbing cushion, representing the SAF, is much more effective in cleaning off a tightly bound material (**d**)

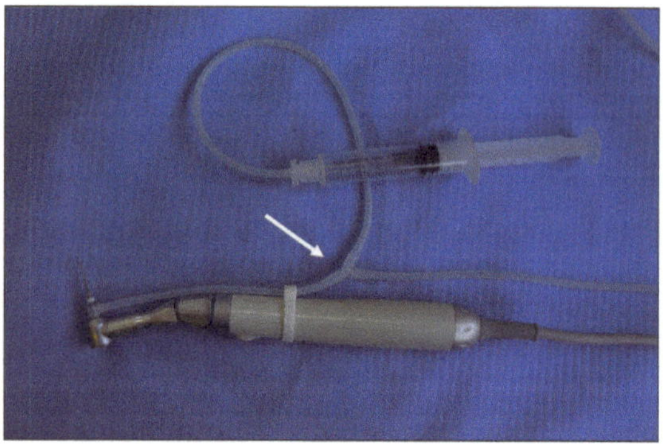

Fig. 11.12 "Y" connector with a syringe containing EDTA. A "Y" connector in the irrigation tube (*arrow*) allows for the attachment of a syringe containing EDTA that may be applied into the SAF during its operation while the irrigation pump is turned off. The tube connecting the "y" connector to the EDTA syringe may be longer, to allow comfortable operation by the dental assistant

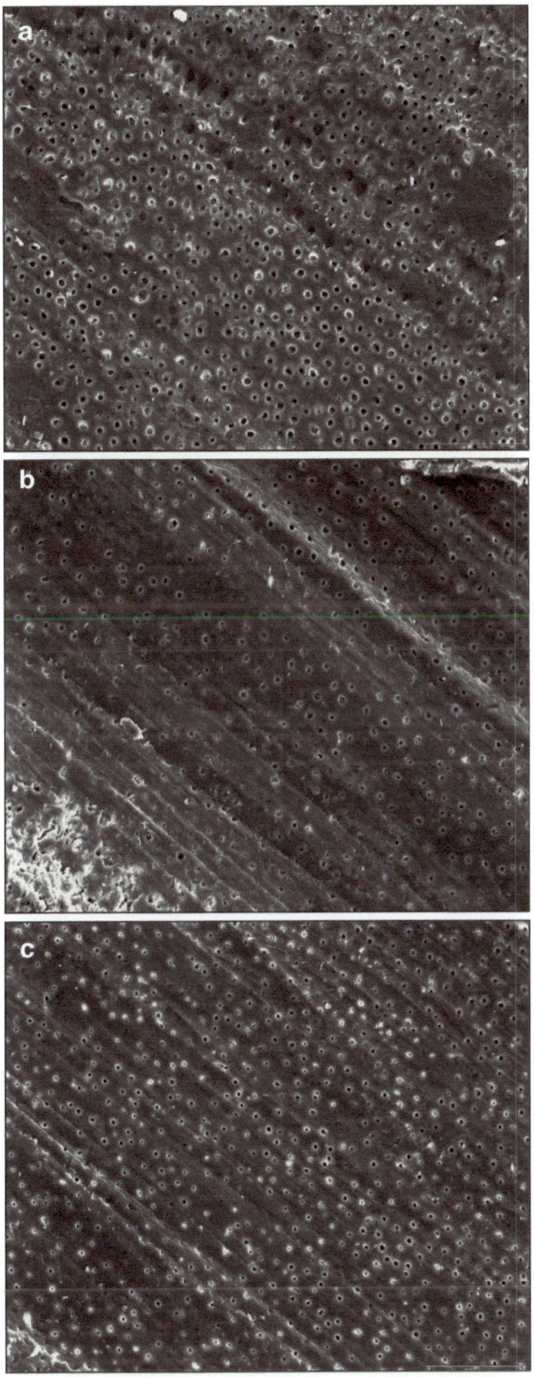

Fig. 11.13 SEM of a root canal treated with the SAF system, alterating between sodium hypochlorite and EDTA. (**a**) Coronal part of the canal. (**b**) Middle part of the canal. (**c**) Apical part of the canal. All of these images are at ×500 times magnification. All of the coronal and mid-root surfaces were clean of debris and of a smear layer. In a study by Metzger et al. [54], all of the apical parts of the canals were free of debris, and in 65 % of the cases, they were also free of a smear layer

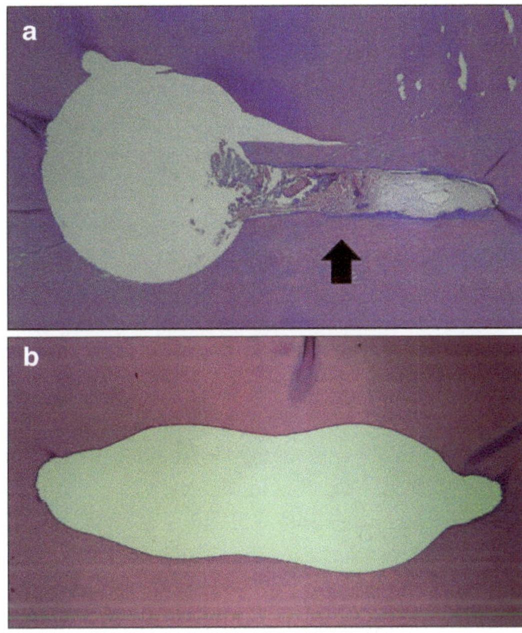

Fig. 11.14 Intact pulp that remained in the "fin" of an oval canal treated with rotary files. (**a**) A rotary file was used in an oval canal with syringe and needle irrigation (3 % sodium hypochlorite). The pulp in the deeper part of the "finlike" recess remained intact. Dentin particles that were packed into the "fin" by the rotating file can be observed (*arrow*). (**b**) Similar oval canal that was treated with the SAF system with a continuous flow of 3 % sodium hypochlorite. Both cases were pair-matched canines, which were vital before extraction (Adapted from De-Deus et al. [24])

be subjected to field selection or section-level selection bias.

MicroCT is a tool that cannot directly evaluate the soft tissue or biofilm remaining in the canal. Nevertheless, it allows an indirect evaluation of the whole canal walls with complete computerized analysis. One may assume that if a layer of dentin was removed from all the root canal surfaces, any material attached to this dentin surface is likely to be removed from these walls [56, 57]. Under this assumption, the efficacy of cleaning root canals may be evaluated three-dimensionally by the microCT tool. When rotary files were used in oval or curved canals, a large percent of the canal wall was unaffected by the procedure. This reached 70 % in oval canals [65] and up to 45–50 % in the curved canal of maxillary molars [71]. When the SAF was used in similar canals, the percent of the canal wall unaffected by the procedure dropped to 23 % [68, 74], indirectly indicating a more effective removal of any material that may have been attached to the canal walls.

Disinfection of Oval Canals

Most endodontic protocols can substantially reduce the amount of bacteria in the canal [5, 11, 86–88]. One of the end points by which the disinfection efficacy of different protocols may be compared is the percentage of canals that presented with negative cultures after the completion of the procedure [5, 11, 86–88]. Such findings do not indicate that the canal is sterile; however, the number of viable bacteria in the canal is lower than the detection level of the assay used. When used in straight round canals, most endodontic protocols do not differ in their disinfection efficacy. The situation may be different when infected oval canals are concerned. Siqueira et al. compared the disinfection efficacy in infected flat-oval canals. Rotary instrumentation combined with syringe and needle irrigation left 55 % of the canals with positive cultures when cleaning and shaping was completed [87]. When the SAF system was used with continuous sodium hypochlorite irrigation, the incidence of positive cultures after the procedure decreased to 20 % [87]. This finding is easily understood when observing the sections of the instrumented canals from this study (Fig. 11.15). In the canal treated with rotary files, the uninstrumented area (arrow in Fig. 11.15b) was likely to serve as a sanctuary in which the sodium hypochlorite could not reach the bacteria. Furthermore, the entrance to this recess was likely blocked by debris packed into it by the rotary file (see below).

Despite this finding in oval canals, narrow isthmuses may represent the limit, even for the SAF system. A recent study by the same group indicated that the SAF was not better than rotary files in terms of the disinfection of infected isthmus-containing mesial root canal systems. All tested systems had a high percent of positive cultures by the end of the procedure [88].

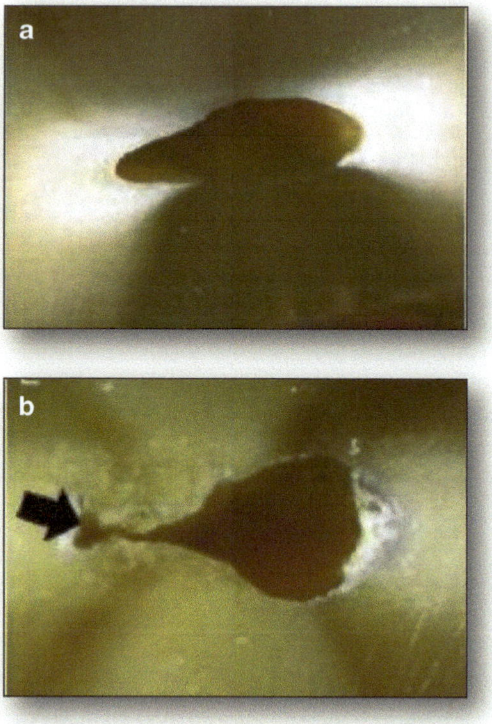

Fig. 11.15 Infected oval root canals treated with SAF vs. rotary files. (**a**) Infected oval root canal treated with the SAF system with continuous irrigation (3 % sodium hypochlorite). (**b**) Infected oval root canal treated with rotary files with syringe and needle irrigation (3 % sodium hypochlorite). Note the uninstrumented area (*arrow*) that most likely served as a sanctuary for bacteria in which they were protected from the action of the irrigant (Adapted from Siqueira et al. [87])

Effect of Cleaning on Obturation

Many root canal obturation systems have been employed for filling root canals after cleaning and shaping. These include warm vertical or lateral compaction, thermoplasticized obturators, cold lateral compaction, and single-cone methods [80]. Common to all of these obturation methods is the assumption that the canal is clean before any obturation is attempted. Straight narrow canals with a round cross section can be effectively cleaned using rotary files and syringe and needle irrigation. They may be well obturated using a single cone, as the canal is often machined to the shape of a given cone [32, 38,

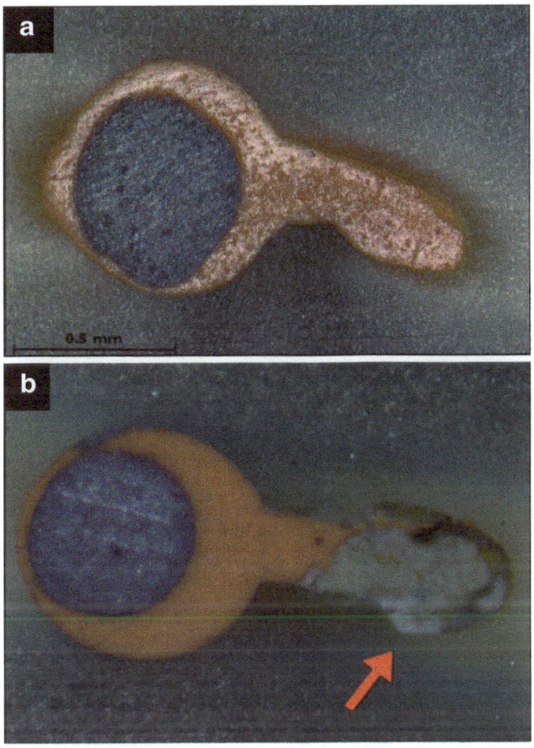

Fig. 11.16 Obturation of oval canals after SAF *vs.* rotary files. Pair-matched oval canals that were treated with either rotary files with syringe and needle irrigation (3 % sodium hypochlorite) or the SAF system with the continuous flow of the same irrigant. Root filling was performed using Thermafil obturators, without sealer. (**a**) SAF-treated canal after obturation. (**b**) Rotary file-treated canal after obturation. Note: The debris (*arrow*) prevented the gutta-percha from flowing into the "finlike" recess of the canal (Adapted from De-Deus et al. [24])

92, 103]. When oval canals are concerned, the task of obturation is often complicated by inadequate cleaning of the root canal by rotary files and syringe and needle irrigation [21, 22, 24, 55].

In a series of studies, De-Deus and his coinvestigators showed that when flat-oval canals were instrumented and cleaned using rotary files and a syringe and needle, gross defects of obturation were found, which might be attributed to debris that was left in the canal or actively packed into the uninstrumented canal recesses [21, 22, 24, 55, 63] (see below). When looking at the images of these studies, debris was present in the recess, preventing even thermoplasticized gutta-percha from flowing in [21]. In a similar study carried in pair-matched teeth with oval canals, the canals that were instrumented and cleaned with the SAF system were free from such debris and could be adequately obturated, while those cleaned with rotary files with syringe and needle irrigation contained debris that prevented adequate obturation (Fig. 11.16) [24].

Metzger et al. studied the correlation between the indirect cleaning parameter of "percent canal wall area unaffected by the procedure" (see above) and the adaptation of a root-filling material to the walls of the same canal [55]. The adaptation of root filling to the canal walls was of limited efficacy in oval canals, which were treated with rotary files and syringe and needle irrigation, and a large percent of the canal wall area was unaffected by the instrumentation. However, in canals that were instrumented and cleaned using the SAF system, the percent of canal wall unaffected by the procedure was much smaller, and the adaptation of the root filling to the canal walls was better [55]. In the first group, large amounts of debris were left or packed into canal recesses (see below), thus limiting the quality of the root filling.

The Challenge of Isthmuses

Isthmuses connecting two canals in the same root represent the greatest challenge to cleaning the root canal space. This results from the inability to adequately instrument these isthmuses, which is further aggravated by the active packing of debris and dentin particles into these isthmuses by the action of rotary files [63, 66, 67].

Paqué and his coworkers studied this phenomenon using microCT [63, 66, 67]. Isthmuses that were radiolucent before instrumentation with rotary files became radiopaque after instrumentation due to the active packing of dentin particles into the isthmus (Fig. 11.17) [63, 66, 67]. Such packing was also found by Nair et al. [59] who noted that the remaining bacterial biofilm in isthmuses treated with rotary files had embedded dentin particles (Fig. 11.18).

These packed particles cannot be completely dislodged or removed from the isthmuses. Even

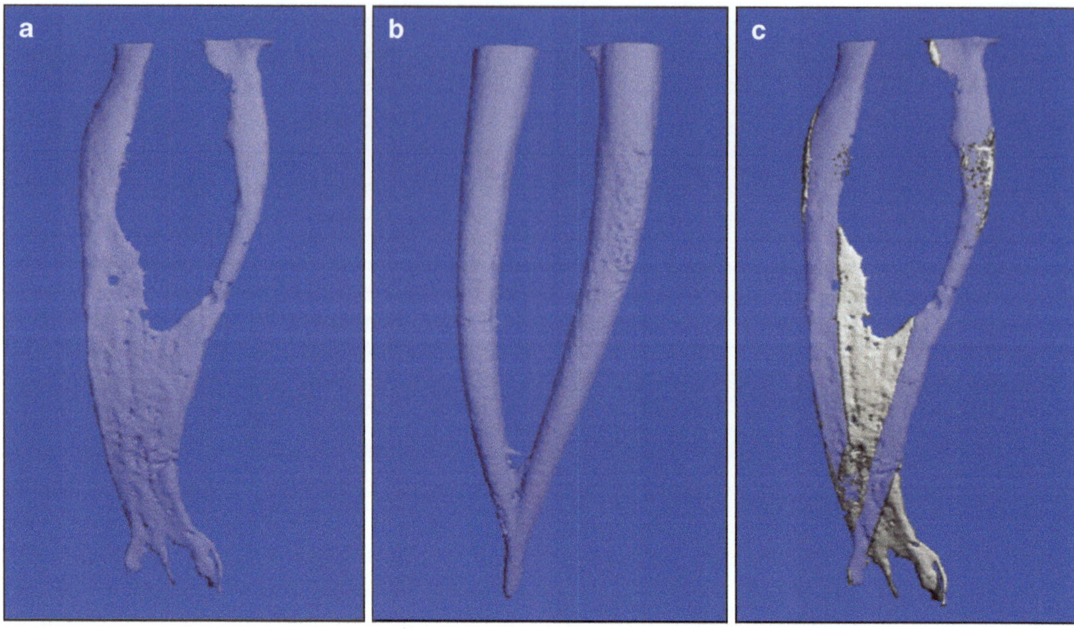

Fig. 11.17 An isthmus packed with dentin particles by a rotary file. (**a**) The root canal space of a mesial root of a mandibular molar, containing an isthmus, before treatment. (**b**) The same root canal space after treatment with rotary files. Note the disappearance of the isthmus. (**c**) White: areas that were radiolucent before treatment and became radiopaque after treatment due to active packing of dentin chips into the isthmus by the rotary files. Reconstructions of the radiolucent space of the root canal from CBCT scans taken before and after treatment (Adapted from Paqué et al. [63])

when using passive ultrasonic irrigation, 50 % of the material could not be removed from the isthmuses [66]. This phenomenon is not limited to isthmuses, as demonstrated by De-Deus et al. [23]. In their histological study, evidence for this type of packing of dentin chips into the fins of oval-shaped canals was also clearly demonstrated (Fig. 11.14).

Avoiding active packing, by using nonrotating tools such as the SAF, may be the solution [67]. A comparative study was conducted in oval canals between rotary files with syringe and needle irrigation and the SAF system. While the material packed into the isthmus by rotary files filled 10 % of the volume of the isthmus, only a limited degree of this phenomenon occurred in the SAF-treated canals, and only 1.7 % of the isthmus contained radiopaque particles [67].

Despite the improved cleaning ability provided by the SAF system, narrow long isthmuses represent a problem for this technology as well. When fully flattened, the SAF's mesiodistal dimension is 0.2 mm [39, 56]. Thus, the SAF cannot enter into and/or clean isthmuses that are thinner than 0.2 mm. A 0.1 mm thick isthmus may contain a substantial bacterial biofilm that is ~100 bacterial cells thick. Cleaning the entrance of the isthmus and avoiding packing debris into this opening are essential as it may allow some effect of sodium hypochlorite to take place. Nevertheless, such narrow isthmuses represent a limit, even for the SAF adaptive technology.

Cleaning of Canals During Retreatment

Retreatment procedures may be roughly divided into two stages: first in which the bulk of root filling is removed and second in which the walls of the canal are cleaned from residues of sealer and gutta-percha and tissue debris and/or bacterial biofilm that such residues may harbor.

The removal of the main bulk of the root filling may be effectively accomplished using rotary files

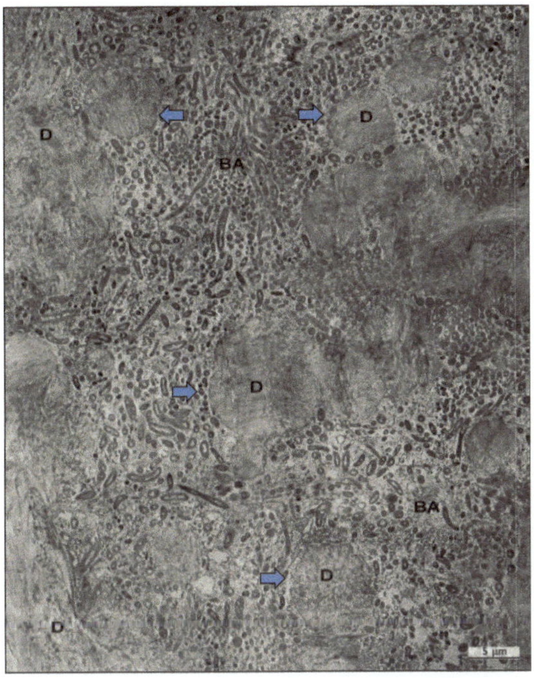

Fig. 11.18 Dentin particles packed into a bacterial biofilm. A mesial root of a mandibular molar was clinically treated with rotary files, resulting in a satisfactory radiographic result. The apical tip of the root was removed surgically after the procedure and was subjected to transmission electron microscopy. The biofilm that remained in the isthmus was packed with dentin particles (*arrows*) by the rotary action of the file (Adapted from Nair et al. [59]). *BA* Bacteria, *D* Dentin

[20, 41, 49, 90, 91]. Many studies indicated that a substantial amount of residue is still attached to the canal walls after using rotary files. Cleaning the canal of the root-filling residue cannot be accomplished by simple irrigation with sodium hypochlorite. Mechanical scrapping of the walls may be required, as the root-filling and sealer residues are strongly attached to the canal walls.

Abramovitz et al. were the first to suggest the use of the scrubbing action of the SAF to remove such root-filling residue [1]. The curved canals of the mesial roots of mandibular molars were initially prepared with #40 K files and were obturated with gutta-percha and AH26 using lateral compaction. After a full setting of the sealer, a retreatment procedure was applied, starting with ProTaper retreatment files D1–D3 [1, 30, 90]. The radiopaque residue was evaluated with buccolingual radiographs. After this first stage, 34.7 % of the area of the apical third of the canal was still covered with radiopaque residue. The most common location of the residue was in the inner side of the curvature, attached to the distal wall of the apical third of the canal (Fig. 11.19). The canals were then dried with paper points, and a drop of chloroform was placed in the canals (~10 µL). The SAF was operated in the canals for 1 min, with the irrigation turned off. Later the irrigation pump was turned on, and the SAF was operated in the canal for an additional 3 min with a continuous flow of sodium hypochlorite. The amount of residue in the apical third of the canal was reduced from 34.7 % after the first stage to 6.7 % after the second stage [1]. This was due to the combination of the softening effect of the chloroform and the scrubbing effect of the SAF.

Similar results were reported by Solomonov et al., who studied the retreatment of distal oval roots of mandibular molars using microCT as the investigation tool [84]. When ProTaper retreatment files were used, followed by F1 and F2 ProTaper instruments, 5.39 % of the original volume of the root filling was still retained in the canal by the end of the procedure. When a ProFile #25.06 instrument was used for the first stage, followed by the SAF in the second stage, the root-filling residue left in the canal after the procedure was only 0.41 % [82, 84]. A third study was performed with no chloroform, using only the scrubbing action of the SAF and a continuous flow of irrigant [97]. The results of this study indicated that using the SAF as a supplementary cleaning device in the retreatment of curved canals of maxillary molars improved the cleaning of the canal. Thus the combination of rotary files that are used to remove the bulk of the root filling followed by cleaning the canal using the scrubbing effect of the SAF is an effective cleaning tool during retreatment.

The Challenge of Immature Teeth

Immature permanent teeth that have lost their vitality due to trauma, caries, or infection of the pulp often present a special cleaning challenge. If these teeth have an open apex and relatively thin

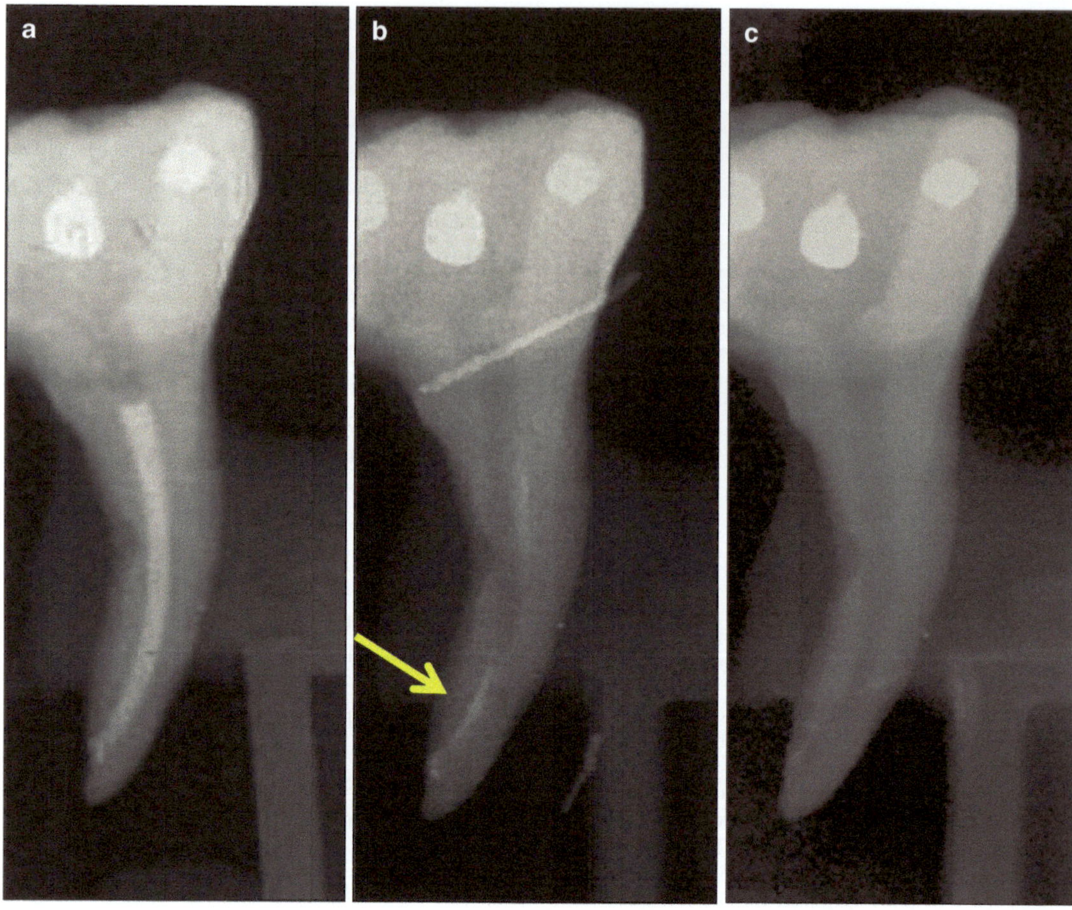

Fig. 11.19 The SAF system in retreatment. The mesial roots of mandibular molars were prepared up to #40 K file and were obturated. (**a**) Radiograph of the root filling. (**b**) Retreatment was performed using ProTaper retreatment files. The radiograph shows residual radiopaque material at the inner side of the curvature of the apical part of the canal. (**c**) Further cleaning of the canal using the SAF system removed the radiopaque residue (Adapted from Abramovitz et al. [1]). *Arrow* Radiopaque residue in the distal side (inner side of the curvature) that remained after use of ProTaper retreatment files

dentin walls, the common instrumentation methods are not suitable for effective and safe cleaning. Here, the goal should be to effectively clean all the canal walls but without a reduction of the thickness in the dentin walls of the root. This is true in both of the cases planned for apexification procedures and revascularization attempts [42, 76, 98].

Some have suggested in such cases that irrigation alone should be used with copious amounts of sodium hypochlorite to reach the abovementioned goal. Nevertheless, the chance of leaving either necrotic tissue or a portion of the bacterial biofilm attached to some areas of the canal wall cannot be ignored.

The SAF system can be used to clean such canal walls without the removal of dentin. The mode of action of the SAF on the canal walls is different than its action in mature, narrow canals. When SAF are used in root canals that are substantially narrower than the thickness of the SAF, the file is compressed and attempts to return to its original, non-compressed form, thus generating light pressure. This pressure allows the removal of a thin uniform layer of dentin around the perimeter of the canal [53, 56]. When the SAF is inserted into a wide canal, the compression of the file is smaller, and the pressure on the walls is limited. Consequently, removal of dentin is no longer effective, even when the SAF is intimately adapted to and touching the canal walls. This phenomenon may be useful in cleaning the walls of immature teeth. In such wide canals, the SAF is likely to scrub the canal walls without removing a layer of dentin. In single-rooted teeth, SAF with a 2.0 mm diameter can be used, while in immature roots of molars, 1.5 mm SAF may be useful.

The continuous flow of sodium hypochlorite without any pressure in the apical direction may also be both useful and safe when treating immature teeth. If syringe and needle irrigation is applied, the pressure generated by the flow from the needle orifice may be sufficient to push sodium hypochlorite beyond the apex. A special risk exists when the periapical tissue contains a cavity of an abscess or a bay cyst. Such pressure is not present when the SAF is used (see above) [39, 56, 57]. The sodium hypochlorite is brought into the canal with continuous flow and with continuous agitation. The combination of a continuous supply of fresh sodium hypochlorite with the scrubbing effect on the walls may provide a unique method to effectively clean the walls of those wide canals without reducing the thickness of their dentin walls. Because many of the canals of immature teeth are rather wide, in several cases, microscopically estimating the cleaning effectiveness of these canals by the SAF system is possible, and the results are impressive.

The use of the SAF for this unique purpose is based on sporadic clinical observations. To the best of our knowledge, no study on this possible use of the SAF has been published thus far, and further exploration of this idea is warranted.

References

1. Abramovitz I, Relles-Bonar S, Baransi B, Kfir A. The effectiveness of a self-adjusting file to remove residual gutta-percha after retreatment with rotary files. Int Endod J. 2012;45:386–92.
2. Adigüzel Ö, Yiğit-Özer S, Kaya S, Uysal I, Ganidaüli-Ayas S, Akkus Z. Effectiveness of ethylenediaminetetraacetic acid (EDTA) and MTAD on debris and smear layer removal using a self-adjusting file. Oral Surg Oral Med Oral Pathol Oral Radiol Endod. 2011;112:803–8.
3. Adorno CG, Yoshioka T, Suda H. Crack Initiation on the apical root surface caused by three different nickel-titanium rotary files at different working lengths. J Endod. 2011;37:522–5.
4. Ahlquist M, Henningsson O, Hultenby K, et al. The effectiveness of manual and rotary techniques in the cleaning of root canals: a scanning electron microscopy study. Int Endod J. 2001;34:533–7.
5. Alves FRF, Almedina BM, Neves MAS, Rôças IN, Siqueira Jr JF. Time-dependent antibacterial effects of the self-adjusting file used with two sodium hypochlorite concentrations. J Endod. 2011;37:1451–5.
6. Basrani B, Haapasalo M. Update on endodontic irrigating solutions. Endo Topics. 2012;27:74–102.
7. Baugh D, Wallace J. The role of apical instrumentation in root canal treatment: a review of the literature. J Endod. 2005;31:333–40.
8. Bier CA, Shemesh H, Tanomaru-Filho M, Wesselink PR, Wu MK. The ability of different nickel-titanium rotary instruments to induce dentinal damage during canal preparation. J Endod. 2009;35:236–8.
9. Blank-Gonçalves LM, Nabeshima CK, Martins GHR, de Lima Machado ME. Qualitative analysis of the removal of the smear layer in the apical third of curved roots: conventional irrigation versus activation systems. J Endod. 2011;37:1268–71.
10. Boutsioukis C, Lambrianidis T, Verhaagen B, Versluis M, Kastrinakis E, Wesselink PR, van der Sluis LWM. The effect of needle-insertion depth on the irrigant flow in the root canal: evaluation using an unsteady computational fluid dynamics model. J Endod. 2010;36:1664–8.
11. Brito PR, Souza LC, Machado de Oliveira JC, Alves FRF, De-Deus G, Lopes HP, Siqueira JF. Comparison of the effectiveness of three irrigation techniques in reducing intracanal Enterococcus faecalis populations: an in vitro study. J Endod. 2009;35:1422–7.
12. Brunson M, Heilborn C, Johnson DJ, Cohenca N. Effect of apical preparation size and preparation taper on irrigant volume delivered by using negative pressure irrigation system. J Endod. 2010;36:721–4.
13. Bürklein S, Tsotsis P, Schäfer E. Incidence of dentinal defects after root canal preparation: reciprocating versus rotary instrumentation. J Endod. 2013;39:501–4.
14. Camps J, Pashley DH. Buffering action of human dentine in vitro. J Adhes Dent. 2000;2:39–50.
15. Card SJ, Sigurdsson A, Ørstavik D, Trope M. The effectiveness of increased apical enlargement in reducing intracanal bacteria. J Endod. 2002;28: 779–83.
16. Chow TW. Mechanical effectiveness of root canal irrigation. J Endod. 1983;9:475–9.
17. Crumpton BJ, Goodell GG, McClanaban SB. Effects on smear layer and debris removal with varying volumes of 17 % REDTA after rotary instrumentation. J Endod. 2005;31:536–8.
18. Cunningham W, Martin H, Forrest W. Evaluation of root canal debridement by the endosonic ultrasonic synergistic system. Oral Surg Oral Med Oral Pathol. 1982;53:401–4.

19. Cupkova V, Sirotkova L, Mlynarcik D, Devinsky F, Lacko I, Kovackova Z. Primary biodegradation of amine oxide and quaternary ammonium amphiphiles. Folia Microbiol. 1993;38:43–8.
20. de Carvalho Maciel AC, Zaccaro Scelza MF. Efficacy of automated versus hand instrumentation during root canal retreatment: an ex vivo study. Int Endod J. 2006;39:779–84.
21. De-Deus G, Gurgel-Filho ED, Magalhães KM, Coutinho-Filho T. A laboratory analysis of gutta-percha filled area obtained using Thermafil, System B and lateral condensation. Int Endod J. 2006;39:378–83.
22. De-Deus G, Reis C, Beznos D, Gruetzmacher-de-Abranches AM, Coutinho-Filho T, Pacionrik S. Limited ability of three commonly used thermoplasticised gutta-percha techniques in filling oval-shaped canals. J Endod. 2008;34:1401–5.
23. De-Deus G, Souza EM, Barino B, Maia J, Zamolyi RQ, Reis C, Kfir A. The self-adjusting file optimizes debridement quality in oval-shaped root canals. J Endod. 2011;37:701–5.
24. De-Deus G, Barino B, Marins J, Magalhães K, Thuanne E, Kfir A. Self-adjusting file cleaning-shaping-irrigation system optimizes the filling of oval-shaped canals with thermoplasticized gutta-percha. J Endod. 2012;38:846–9.
25. de Gregorio C, Estavez R, Cisneros R, Heilborn C, Cohenca N. Effect of EDTA, sonic and ultrasonic activation on the penetration of sodium hypochlorite into simulated lateral canals: an in vitro study. J Endod. 2009;35:891–5.
26. de Gregorio C, Arias A, Navarrete N, del Rio V, Oltra E, Cohenca N. Effect of apical size and taper on volume of irrigant delivered at working length with apical negative pressure at different root curvatures. J Endod. 2013;39:119–24.
27. del Carpio-Perochena AE, Bramante CM, Duarte MAH, Cavenago BC, Villas-Boas MH, Graeff MS, Bernardinieli N, de Andrade FB, Ordinola-Zapata R. Biofilm dissolution and cleaning ability of different irrigant solutions on intraorally infected dentin. J Endod. 2011;37:1134–8.
28. Gambarini G, Laszkiewicz J. A scanning electron microscopic study of debris and smear layer remaining following use of GT rotary instruments. Int Endod J. 2002;35:422–7.
29. Gani O, Visvisian C. Apical canal diameters in the first upper molar at various ages. J Endod. 1999; 25:689–91.
30. Giuliani V, Cocchetti R, Pagavino G. Efficacy of ProTaper universal retreatment files in removing filling materials from root canal. J Endod. 2008;34:1381–4.
31. Goldman M, Kronman JH, Goldman LB, Clausen H, Grady J. New method of irrigation during endodontic treatment. J Endod. 1976;2:257–60.
32. Gordon MPJ, Love RM, Chandler NP. An evaluation of tapered gutta-percha cones for filling of 0.06 taper prepared curved root canals. Int Endod J. 2005;38:87–96.
33. Haapasalo M, Ørstavik D. In vitro infection and disinfection of dentinal tubules. J Dent Res. 1987;66:1375–9.
34. Haapasalo HK, Siren EK, Waltimo TM. Inactivation of local root canal medicaments by dentine: an in vitro study. Int Endod J. 2000;33:126–31.
35. Haapasalo M, Shen Y, Qian W, Gao Y. Irrigation in endodontics. Dent Clin N Am. 2010;54:291–312.
36. Heilborn C, Reynolds K, Johnson JD, Cohenca N. Cleaning efficacy of an apical negative-pressure irrigation system at different exposure times. Quintessence Int. 2010;41:759–67.
37. Hin ES, Wu M-K, Wesselink PR, Shemesh H. Effects of self-adjusting file, Mtwo, and ProTaper on the root canal wall. J Endod. 2013;39:262–4.
38. Hiraishi N, Papacchini F, Loushine RJ, et al. Shear bond strength of resilon to a methacrylate-based root canal sealer. Int Endod J. 2005;38:753–63.
39. Hof R, Perevalov V, Eltanani M, Zary R, Metzger Z. The self-adjusting-file (SAF). Part 2: Mechanical analysis. J Endod. 2010;36:691–6.
40. Hülsmann M, Rümmelin C, Schäfers F. Root canal cleanliness after preparation with different endodontic handpieces and hand instruments: a comparative SEM investigation. J Endod. 1997;23:301–6.
41. Hülsmann M, Bluhm V. Efficacy, cleaning ability and safety of different rotary NiTi instruments in root canal retreatment. Intel Endod J. 2004;37:468–76.
42. Iwaya SI, Ikawa M, Kubota M. Revascularization of an immature permanent tooth with apical periodontitis and sinus tract. Dent Traumatol. 2001;17:185–7.
43. Jiang L-M, Verhaagen B, Versluis M, van der Sluis LWM. Evaluation of a sonic device designed to activate irrigant in the root canal. J Endod. 2009;36(1):143–6.
44. Lertchirakarn V, Palamara JE, Messer HH. Patterns of vertical root fracture: factors affecting stress distribution in the root canal. J Endod. 2003;29:523–8.
45. Lin J, Shen Y, Haapasalo M. A comparative study of biofilm removal with hand, rotary nickel-titanium, and self-adjusting file instrumentation using a novel in vitro biofilm model. J Endod. 2013;39:658–63.
46. Liu R, Kaiwar A, Shemesh H, Wesselink PR, Hou B, Wu M-K. Incidence of apical root cracks and apical dentinal detachments after canal preparation with hand and rotary files at different instrumentation lengths. J Endod. 2013;39:129–32.
47. Martin H. Ultrasonic disinfection of the root canal. Oral Surg Oral Med Oral Pathol. 1976;42:92–9.
48. Martin H, Cunningham W. Endosonics–the ultrasonic synergistic system of endodontics. Endod Dent Traumatol. 1985;1:201–6.
49. Masiero AV, Barletta FB. Effectiveness of different techniques for removing gutta-percha during retreatment. Int Endod J. 2005;38:2–7.
50. Maunger MJ, Schindler WG, Walker WA. An evaluation of canal morphology at different levels of root resection in mandibular incisors. J Endod. 1998;24:607–9.
51. Mayer BE, Peters OA, Barbakow F. Effect of rotary instruments and ultrasonic irrigation on debris and

smear layer scores: a scanning electron microscopic study. Int Endod J. 2002;35:582–9.
52. McCann JT, Keller DL, LaBounty GL. Remaining dentin/cementum thickness after hand or ultrasonic instrumentation. J Endodon. 1990;16:109–13.
53. Metzger Z, Teperovich E, Zary R, Cohen R, Hof R. The Self-Adjusting File (SAF). Part 1: Respecting the root canal anatomy-a new concept of endodontic files and its implementation. J Endod. 2010;36:679–90.
54. Metzger Z, Cohen R, Zary R, Teperovich E, Paqué F, Hülsmann M. The Self-Adjusting File (SAF). Part 3: Removal of debris and smear layer – a scanning electron microscope study. J Endod. 2010;36:697–702.
55. Metzger Z, Zary R, Cohen R, Teperovich E, Paqué F. The quality of root canal preparation and root canal obturation in canals treated with rotary versus self adjusting files: a three-dimensional micro-computed tomographic study. J Endod. 2010;36:1569–73.
56. Metzger Z, Kfir A, Abramovitz I, Weissman A, Solomonov M. The self-adjusting file system. ENDO (Lond Eng). 2013;7:189–210.
57. Metzger Z, Solomonov M, Kfir A. The role of mechanical instrumentation in the cleaning of root canals. Endod Topics. 2013;29:87–109.
58. Milanezi de Almeida M, Bernardineli N, Ordinola-Zapata R, Villas Bôas MH, Amoroso-Silva PA, Brandão CG, Guimarães BM, Gomes de Moraes I, Húngaro-Duarte MA. Micro-computed tomography analysis of the root canal anatomy and prevalence of oval canals in mandibular incisors. J Endod. 2013;39:1529–33.
59. Nair PNR, Henry S, Cano V, Vera J. Microbial status of apical root canal system of human mandibular first molars with primary apical periodontitis after "one-visit" endodontic treatment. Oral Surg Oral Med Oral Pathol Oral Radiol Endod. 2005;99:231–52.
60. Nielsen BA, Baumgartner CJ. Comparison of the EndoVac system to needle irrigation of root canals. J Endod. 2007;33:611–5.
61. Ørstavik D, Haapasalo M. Disinfection by endodontic irrigants and dressings of experimentally infected dentinal tubules. Endod Dent Traumatol. 1990;6:142–9.
62. Paqué F, Musch U, Hülsmann M. Comparison of root canal preparation using RaCeand ProTaper rotary Ni-Ti instruments. Int Endod J. 2005;38:8–16.
63. Paqué F, Laib A, Gautschi H, Zehnder M. Hard-tissue debris accumulation analysis by high-resolution computed tomography scans. J Endod. 2009;35:1044–7.
64. Ram Z. Effectiveness of root canal irrigation. Oral Surg Oral Med Oral Pathol. 1977;44:306–12.
65. Paqué F, Ballmer M, Attin T, Peters OA. Preparation of oval-shaped root canals in mandibular molars using nickel-titanium rotary instruments: a micro-computed tomography study. J Endod. 2010;36:703–7.
66. Paqué F, Boessler C, Zehnder M. Accumulated hard tissue debris levels in mesial roots of mandibular molars after sequential irrigation steps. Int Endod J. 2011;44:148–53.
67. Paqué F, Al-Jadaa A, Kfir A. Hard tissue debris accumulation caused by conventional rotary versus self-adjusting file instrumentation in mesial root canal systems of mandibular molars. Int Endod J. 2012;45:413–8.
68. Paqué F, Peters OA. Micro-computed tomography evaluation of the preparation of long oval root canals in mandibular molars with the self-adjusting file. J Endod. 2011;37:517–21.
69. Pawar R, Alqaied A, Safavi K, Boyko J, Kaufman B. Influence of an apical negative pressure irrigation system on bacterial elimination during endodontic therapy: a prospective randomized clinical study. J Endod. 2012;38:1177–81.
70. Peters OA, Barbakow F. Effects of irrigation on debris and smear layer on canal walls prepared by two rotary techniques: a scanning electron microscopic study. J Endod. 2000;26:6–10.
71. Peters OA, Peters CI, Schönenberger K, Barbakow F. ProTaper rotary root canal preparation: effects of root canal anatomy on final shape analyzed by micro CT. Int Endod J. 2003;36:86–92.
72. Peters OA. Current challenges and concepts in the preparation of root canal systems: a review. J Endod. 2004;30:559–67.
73. Peters OA, Boessler C, Paqué F. Root canal preparation with a novel nickel-titanium instrument evaluated with micro-computed tomography: canal surface preparation over time. J Endod. 2010;36:1068–72.
74. Peters OA, Paqué F. Root canal preparation of maxillary molars with the self-adjusting file: a micro-computed tomography study. J Endod. 2011;37:53–7.
75. Portenier I, Waltimo T, Ørstavik D, et al. The susceptibility of starved, stationary phase, and growing cells of Enterococcus faecalis to endodontic medicaments. J Endod. 2005;31:380–6.
76. Rafter M. Apexification: a review. Dent Traumatol. 2005;21:1–8.
77. Ricucci D, Bergenholtz G. Bacterial status in root-filled teeth exposed to the oral environment by loss of restoration and fracture or caries – a histobacteriological study of treated cases. Int Endod J. 2003;36:787–97.
78. Rôças IN, Siqueira Jr JF. Comparison of the in vivo antimicrobial effectiveness of sodium hypochlorite and chlorhexidine used as root canal irrigants: a molecular microbiology study. J Endod. 2011;37:143–50.
79. Schoeffel GJ. The EndoVac method of endodontic irrigation, part 2–efficacy. Dent Today. 2008:27:82, 84, 86–7.
80. Schilder H. Filling root canals in three dimensions. J Endod. 2006;32:281–90.
81. Shin SJ, Kim HK, Jung IY, Lee CY, Lee SJ, Kim E. Comparison of the cleaning efficacy of a new apical negative pressure irrigating system with conventional irrigation needles in the root canals. Oral

Surg Oral Med Oral Pathol Oral Radiol Endod. 2010;109:479–84.
82. Solomonov M, Paqué F, Fan B, Eilat Y, Berman LH. The challenge of C-shaped canal systems: a comparative study of the self-adjusting file and ProTaper. J Endod. 2012;38:209–14.
83. Solomonov M. Eight months of clinical experience with the self-adjusting file system. J Endod. 2011;37:881–7.
84. Solomonov M, Paqué F, Kaya S, Adıgüzel Ö, Kfir A, Yiğit-Özer S. Self-adjusting files in retreatment: a high-resolution micro-computed tomography study. J Endod. 2012;38:1283–7.
85. Shemesh H, Bier CA, Wu MK, Tanomaru-Filho M, Wesselink PR. The effects of canal preparation and filling on the incidence of dentinal defects. Int Endod J. 2009;42:208–13.
86. Siqueira Jr JF, Lima KC, Magalhães FAC, Lopes HP, de Uzeda M. Mechanical reduction of the bacterial population in the root canal by three instrumentation techniques. J Endod. 1999;25:332–5.
87. Siqueira Jr JF, Alves FRF, Bernardo M, Almeida BM, Machado de Oliveira JC, Rôças IN. Ability of chemomechanical preparation with either rotary instruments or self-adjusting file to disinfect oval-shaped root canals. J Endod. 2010;36:1860–5.
88. Siqueira Jr JF, Alves FLF, Versiani MA, Rôças IN, Almeida BM, Neves MAS, Sousa-Neto MD. Correlative bacteriologic and micro–computed tomographic analysis of mandibular molar mesial canals prepared by self-adjusting file, reciproc, and twisted file systems. J Endod. 2013;39:1044–50.
89. Susin L, Lin Y, Yoon JC, et al. Canal and isthmus debridement efficacies of two irrigant agitation techniques in a closed system. Int Endod J. 2010;43:1077–90.
90. Takahashi CM, Cunha RS, de Martin AS, Fontana CE, Silveira CF, da Silveira Bueno CE. In vitro evaluation of the effectiveness of ProTaper universal rotary retreatment system for gutta-percha removal with or without a solvent. J Endod. 2009;35:1580–3.
91. Taşdemir T, Er K, Yildirim T, Celik D. Efficacy of three rotary NiTi instruments in removing gutta-percha from root canals. Int Endod J. 2008;41:191–6.
92. Tay FR, Loushine RJ, Monticelli F, et al. Effectiveness of resin-coated gutta-percha cones and a dual-cured hydrophilic methacrylate resin-based sealer in obturating root canals. J Endod. 2005;31:659–64.
93. Van der Sluis LWM, Versluis M, Wu MK, Wesselink PR. Passive ultrasonic irrigation of the root canal: A review of the literature. Int Endod J. 2007;40:415–26.
94. Versümer J, Hülsmann M, Schäfers F. A comparative study of root canal preparation using ProFile.04 and Lightspeed rotary Ni-Ti instruments. Int Endod J. 2002;35:37–46.
95. Versiani MA, Pecora JD, de Sousa-Neto MD. Flat-oval root canal preparation with self-adjusting file instrument: a micro–computed tomography study. J Endod. 2011;37:1002–7.
96. Vianna ME, Gomes BP, Berber VB, et al. In vitro evaluation of the antimicrobial activity of chlorhexidine and sodium hypochlorite. Oral Surg Oral Med Oral Pathol Oral Radiol Endod. 2004;97:79–84.
97. Voet KC, Wu M-K, Wesselink PR, Shemesh H. Removal of gutta-percha from root canals using the self-adjusting file. J Endod. 2012;38:1004–6.
98. Weisleder R, Benitez CR. Maturogenesis: is it a new concept? J Endod. 2003;29:776–8.
99. Wu M-K, R'oris A, Barkis D, Wesselink PR. Prevalence and extent of long oval canals in the apical third. Oral Surg Oral Med Oral Pathol Oral Radiol Endod. 2000;89:739–43.
100. Wu MK, Wesselink PR. A primary observation on the preparation and obturation of oval canals. Int Endod J. 2001;34:137–41.
101. Yiğit-Özer S, Adigüzel Ö, Kaya S. Removal of debris and smear layer in curved root canals using self-adjusting file with different operation times. A scanning electron microscope study. Int Dent Res. 2011;1:1–6.
102. Yoldas O, Yilmaz S, Atakan G, Kuden C, Kasan Z. Dentinal microcrack formation during root canal preparations by different Ni-Ti rotary instruments and the self-adjusting file. J Endod. 2012;38:232–5.
103. Zmener O, Pameijer CH, Macri E. Evaluation of the apical seal in root canals prepared with a new rotary system and obturated with a methacrylate based endodontic sealer an in vitro study. J Endod. 2005;31:392–5.

Ozone Application in Endodontics 12

Zahed Mohammadi and Amir Azarpazhooh

Abstract

Ozone is a triatomic molecule consisting of three oxygen atoms. It is applied to oral tissues in the forms of ozonated water, ozonated olive oil, and oxygen/ozone gas. This chapter presents a brief review on the chemistry of ozone as well as its medical and dental applications, in particular in endodontics. Ozone's antimicrobial activity, its effect on dentin bonding, toxicity, and contraindications are also reviewed.

Introduction

Ozone (O_3) is a triatomic molecule consisting of three oxygen atoms. Its molecular weight is 47.98 g/mol. Thermodynamically, it is a highly unstable compound and, depending on system conditions like temperature and pressure, decomposes to pure oxygen with a short half-life [1]. Ozone is 1.6 times denser and 10 times more soluble in water (49.0 mL in 100 mL water at 0 °C) than oxygen. Although ozone is not a radical molecule, it is the third most potent oxidant after fluorine and persulfate. Ozone is an unstable gas that cannot be stored and should be used at once because it has a half-life of 40 min at 20 °C [2]. It is naturally produced by the photodissociation of molecular oxygen (O_2) into activated oxygen atoms, which then react with oxygen molecules. This transient radical anion rapidly becomes protonated, generating hydrogen trioxide (HO_3), which, in turn, decomposes to an even more powerful oxidant, the hydroxyl radical (OH) [2]. It is the fundamental form of oxygen that occurs naturally as a result of ultraviolet energy or lightning, causing a temporary recombination of oxygen atoms into groups of three. In the clinical setting, an oxygen/ozone generator simulates lightning via an electrical discharge

Z. Mohammadi, DMD, MSD
Iranian Center for Endodontic Research (ICER), Research Institute of Dental Sciences, Shahid Beheshti University of Medical Sciences, Tehran, Iran

A. Azarpazhooh, DDS, MSc, PhD, FRCD(C) (✉)
Division of Endodontics, Department of Dentistry, and Clinician Scientist, Lunenfeld-Tanenbaum Research Institute, Mount Sinai Hospital, Toronto, ON, Canada

Dental Public Health and Endodontics, Faculty of Dentistry, University of Toronto, 515-C, 124 Edward St, Toronto, ON M5G 1G6, Canada
e-mail: amir.azarpazhooh@dentistry.utoronto.ca

B. Basrani (ed.), *Endodontic Irrigation: Chemical Disinfection of the Root Canal System*,
DOI 10.1007/978-3-319-16456-4_12

field. Ozone gas has a high oxidation potential and is 1.5 times more powerful than chloride when used as an antimicrobial agent [3, 4].

Applications of Ozone in Medicine

Ozone was discovered by Christian Friedrich Schönbein in 1839 [5]. In 1857, Werner von Siemens designed an ozone generator [6]. Ozone was first used in medicine in 1870 [3]. Medication forms of gaseous ozone are somewhat unusual, and that is why special application techniques have had to be developed for its safe use. According to the European Cooperation of Medical Ozone Societies, direct intravenous injections of ozone/oxygen gas may produce air embolisms [7]. In local applications, as in the treatment of external wounds, ozone application in the form of a transcutaneous gas bath has been established as a practical method – for example, at low (subatmospheric) pressures in a closed system guaranteeing no escape of ozone into the ambient air [8].

Apart from rectal insufflation, principally used in the treatment of intestinal conditions, but also applied systemically, autohemotherapy has established itself as a systemic therapy of choice [2]. A corresponding dosage of ozone gas is passed through or, more correctly, transferred (in the form of microbubbles) to 50–100 ml of the patient's blood in a sealed, pressureless system, thereby assuring the finest possible distribution to reach the greatest possible number of red and white blood cells with the aim of activating their metabolism [1, 2]. In treating pain in the locomotor system, ozone can be applied supportively in the form of intramuscular or intra-articular injections [2]. Ozone can also enhance both lung function and inflammatory airway responses in subjects with preexisting allergic airway diseases [7]. However, its use is contraindicated for the following conditions: acute alcohol intoxication, recent myocardial infarction, hemorrhaging from any organ, pregnancy, hyperthyroidism, thrombocytopenia, and ozone allergy [2–4].

Ozone in Dentistry

Fisch used ozonated water in dentistry in 1930 for the first time [1]. Following him, the German surgeon Erwin Payr used ozone in surgery and reported his results at the 59th Congress of the German Surgical Society in Berlin [3].

Ozone has been used in various disciplines of dentistry. Ozone is applied to oral tissues in the following forms: ozonated water, ozonated olive oil, and oxygen/ozone gas. Ozonated water and olive oil have the capacity to trap and then release oxygen/ozone which is an ideal delivery system. These forms of application are used singly or in combination to treat dental diseases [8].

Ozone may temporarily arrest the progression of caries by killing bacteria in active carious lesions. This results in preventing or, at the very least, in delaying the need for tooth restorations [8–11]. Our previous systematic review of the applications of ozone in dentistry showed that ozone can be used to manage primary occlusal and root carious lesions [9]. For example, using a KaVo HealOzone device, Baysan et al. [10] showed that ozone exposure for 10–20 s reduced the total levels of *Streptococcus mutans* and *Streptococcus sobrinus* in the primary root caries lesions (PRCLs) to <1 % of the control values. Holmes [12] assessed the effect of a KaVo HealOzone device on PRCLs followed by a professionally applied remineralizing solution containing xylitol, fluoride, calcium, phosphate, and zinc and found that after 18 months, 100 % of PRCLs had improved. However, the clinical application has yet to achieve a strong level of efficacy and cost-effectiveness [8]. Filippi [12] observed the influence of ozonated water on the epithelial wound healing process in the oral cavity. It was found that ozonated water applied daily can accelerate the healing rate in the oral mucosa. This effect can be seen in the first two postoperative days. A comparison with wounds without treatment showed that daily treatment with ozonated water accelerates the physiological healing rate. Ozone has also been used to treat TMJ dysfunctions and trismus [4].

Effects on Dentin Bonding

Schmidlin et al. [13] showed that, despite a possible retention of surface and subsurface oxide-related substances during high-dose ozone application, shear bond strength was not impaired. Magni et al. [14] indicated that ozone gas did not compromise the mechanical properties of the adhesives. Cadenaro et al. [15] demonstrated that using ozone gas to disinfect the cavity before placing a restoration there had no influence on immediate enamel and dentin bond strength. Cehreli et al. [16] revealed that pre-treatment with ozone improved the marginal sealing ability of the fissure sealants. Bojar et al. [17] showed that ozone therapy improved shear bond strength of two root canal sealers (AH26 and EZ-Fill). Gurgan et al. [18] showed that ozone treatment did not impair the shear bond strength of two self-etch adhesives (Clearfil SE Bond and Clearfil Tri-S Bond) used to coronal and radicular dentin. According to Arslan et al. [19] ozone did not significantly affect the dentin bond strength of a silorane-based resin composite, Filtek Supreme. Garcia et al. [20] revealed that ozone gas and ozonated water had no deleterious effects on bond strengths and interfaces. Bitter et al. [21] showed that adhesion of the self-adhesive resin cement RelyX Unicem was significantly reduced after using gaseous ozone. According to Rodriguez et al. [22] ozone decreased the microtensile bond strength of a dentin-composite resin interface. Dalkilic et al. [23] indicated that ozone reduced the initial microtensile bond strength.

In dental surgery, ozonated water was used to promote hemostasis, enhance local oxygen supply, and inhibit bacterial proliferation [4]. One study was found to evaluate the effect of ozone gas in oral and maxillofacial surgery, where ozone therapy was found to be beneficial for the treatment of refractory osteomyelitis in the head and neck in addition to treatment with antibiotics, surgery, and hyperbaric oxygen [4].

Ozone in Endodontics

Ozone gas in a concentration of ~4 g m^3 (HealOzone; KaVo, Biberach, Germany) is already being used clinically for endodontic treatment. The following summarizes the information available to date (July 2014) of the use of ozone in endodontics [24].

Effect of Ozone on Dentin Hypersensitivity

Dentin hypersensitivity (DH) is characterized by a short, sharp pain arising from exposed dentin in response to stimuli that are typically thermal, evaporative, tactile, osmotic, or chemical and cannot be ascribed to any other form of dental defect or pathology [25]. The application of ozone as a treatment of dentin hypersensitivity was described more than 50 years ago [26]. Dähnhardt et al. [27] assessed the effect of treatment with gaseous ozone on DH. Findings revealed no significant reduction in pain compared to the placebo group. More recently, in an 8-week, three-visit, triple-blinded, randomized controlled clinical trial with two HealOzone machines (ozone/air), Azarpazhooh et al. [28] confirmed the findings of Dähnhardt et al. [27]. Another study investigated the effect of ozone, with or without the use of desensitizing agents, on the patency and occlusion of simulated hypersensitive dentin. Results indicated that the combined use of ozone/fluoride resulted in a significantly higher percentage of tubular occlusion than fluoride desensitizer alone. However, no significant difference was found between oxalate desensitizer and the combined use of ozone/oxalate [29]. It has been demonstrated that ozonated olive oil as a monotherapy was not efficient in reducing postsurgical root dentin hypersensitivity. However, using it in combination with a mineral wash containing calcium sodium phosphosilicate had a positive impact on the reversal of postsurgical root dentin hypersensitivity [30].

Antibacterial Activity

Biofilm is a mode of bacterial growth in which dynamic communities of interacting sessile cells are irreversibly attached to a solid surface, as well as each other, and are embedded in a self-made matrix of extracellular polymeric substances [31]. A microbial biofilm is considered a community when it meets the following criteria: possesses the ability to self-organize (autopoiesis), resists environmental perturbations (homeostasis), is more effective in association than in isolation (synergy), and responds to environmental changes as a unit rather than as single individuals (communality) [31].

A systematic review of the applications of ozone in dentistry showed that there was some evidence that ozone (in both gaseous or aqueous phases) was a potentially effective disinfectant agent for removing the biofilms and related microorganisms such as *Legionella pneumophila*, *Mycobacterium* spp., *Pseudomonas aeruginosa*, and *Candida* spp. from dental unit water systems and was an effective bactericidal agent for removing *S. mutans*, methicillin-resistant *Staphylococcus aureus*, *Candida albicans*, and *E. faecalis* from dentures [32]. In endodontics, so far, four in vitro studies investigated the bactericidal effect of ozone as compared to 2.5 % sodium hypochlorite, the standard irrigation solution in endodontics. The results of this outcome are controversial.

While Nagayoshi et al. [33] found nearly the same antimicrobial activity against *E. faecalis* and *S. mutans* and a lower level of cytotoxicity of ozonated water as compared to 2.5 % NaOCl, in a study by Hems et al. [34] NaOCl was found to be superior to ozonated water in killing *E. faecalis* in broth culture and in biofilms, while gaseous ozone had no effect on the *E. faecalis* biofilms. Muller et al. [35] has also found 5 % NaOCl superior to gaseous ozone in eliminating microorganisms organized in a cariogenic biofilm. Moreover, a recent study has found that irrigating infected human root canals with ozonated water, 2.5 % NaOCl, and 2 % chlorhexidine and the application of gaseous ozone for 20 min were not sufficient to inactivate *E. faecalis* [36]. The antibacterial effectiveness of ozone has been revealed in several other studies [37–45].

Antifungal Activity

Fungi constitute a small part of the oral microbiota. The largest proportion of the fungal microbiota is made up of *Candida* species. *Candida* (*C.*) *albicans* is the fungal species most commonly detected in the oral cavity of both healthy and medically compromised individuals [46]. The incidence of *C. albicans* in the oral cavity has been reported to be 30–45 % in healthy adults [47, 48] and 95 % in patients infected with human immunodeficiency virus [46]. Studies using culturing, molecular genetics, and in situ electron microscopy methods have demonstrated that fungi are not common members of the microbiota associated with primary endodontic infections [46, 49]. However, they seem to be more common in the root canals of root-filled teeth in which the treatment has failed [46, 49]. Cardoso et al. [39] evaluated the effectiveness of ozonated water in the elimination of *C. albicans* from root canals and found that it reduced the number of *C. albicans* cells immediately; however, it showed no residual activity. Huth et al. [41] showed that highly concentrated gaseous and aqueous ozone was dose-, strain-, and time-dependently effective against *C. albicans* in suspension and the biofilm test model.

Ozone and Endotoxin

Gram-negative microorganisms not only have different virulent factors and produce toxic products and subproducts in apical and periapical tissues but also contain endotoxin in their cell walls [38, 50, 51]. Endotoxin, which consists of lipopolysaccharides (LPSs), is liberated during bacterial cell multiplication or death and is responsible for a series of important biological effects [38]. Its action on macrophages initiates the release of a series of inflammatory, bioactive, chemical mediators or cytokines such as tumor necrosis factor and interleukins 1, 6, and 8 [38]. There are very few studies on the effect of ozone on endotoxin. Cardoso et al. [27] showed that ozonated water did not neutralize endotoxin. Furthermore, Noguchi et al. [39] indicated that ozonated water had the ability to improve LPS-induced inflammatory responses and the suppression of odontoblastic properties of KN-3 cells (a rat odontoblastic cell line) through direct inhibition of LPS.

Conclusion

Despite the promising in vitro evidence, the clinical application of ozone in dentistry (so far used in the management of dental and root caries) has not achieved a strong level of efficacy and cost-effectiveness. More well-designed and conducted double-blind randomized clinical trials with adequate sample size, limited or no loss to follow-up, and carefully standardized methods of measurement and analyses are needed to evaluate the possible use of ozone as a treatment modality in dentistry.

References

1. Bocci VA. Scientific and medical aspects of ozone therapy: state of the art. Arch Med Res. 2006;37:425–35.
2. Sunnen GV. Ozone in medicine: overview and future directions. J Adv Med. 1988;1:159–74.
3. Nogales CG, Ferrari PH, Kantorovich EO, Lage-Marques JL. Ozone therapy in medicine and dentistry. J Contemp Dent Pract. 2008;9:75–84.
4. Stubinger S, Sader R, Filippi A. The use of ozone in dentistry and maxillofacial surgery: a review. Quintessence Int. 2006;37:353–9.
5. Schönbein CF. On the production of ozone by chemical means. Philos Mag. 1844;24:466–7.
6. Saini R. Ozone therapy in dentistry: a strategic review. J Nat Sci Biol Med. 2011;2:151–3.
7. Linetskiy SV, Stankova HH, Mazanek SR. Ozone and its usage in general medicine and dentistry: a review article. Prague Med Rep. 2008;109:5–13.
8. Rickard GD, Richardson R, Johnson T, McColl D, Hooper L. Ozone therapy for the treatment of dental caries. Cochrane Database Syst Rev. 2004;(3):CD004153
9. Tondij LD, Ganichev VV, Kozin JO. Osnovni principy ta metody ozonoterapiji v medicine. Charkov. 2001;20:18–20.
10. Baysan A, Whiley RA, Lynch E. Antimicrobial effect of a novel ozone-generating device on micro-organisms associated with primary root carious lesions in vitro. Caries Res. 2000;34:498–501.
11. Holmes J. Clinical reversal of root caries using ozone, double-blind, randomized controlled 18-month trial. Gerodontology. 2003;20:106–14.
12. Filippi A. The influence of ozonized water on the epithelial wound healing process in the oral cavity. Clinic of Oral Surgery, Radiology and Oral Medicine, University of Basel. WWW.OXYPLUS.NET.
13. Schmidlin PR, Zimmermann J, Bindl A. Effect of ozone on enamel and dentin bond strength. J Adhes Dent. 2005;7:29–32.
14. Magni E, Ferrari M, Hickel R, Huth KC, Ilie N. Effect of ozone gas application on the mechanical properties of dental adhesives bonded to dentin. Dent Mater. 2008;24:1428–34.
15. Cadenaro M, Delise C, Antoniollo F, Navarra OC, Di Lenarda R, Breschi L. Enamel and dentin bond strength following gaseous ozone application. J Adhes Dent. 2009;11:287–92.
16. Cehreli SB, Yalcinkaya Z, Guven-Polat G, Cehreli ZC. Effect of ozone pretreatment on the microleakage of pit and fissure sealants. J Clin Pediatr Dent. 2010;35:187–90.
17. Bojar W, Czarnecka B, Pryliński M, Walory J. Shear bond strength of epoxy resin-based endodontic sealers to bovine dentin after ozone application. Acta Bioeng Biomech. 2009;11:41–5.
18. Gurgan S, Firat E, Baysan A, Gutknecht N, Imazato S. Effects of ozone and ND:YAG laser pretreatment on bond strength of self-etch adhesives to coronal and root dentin. Photomed Laser Surg. 2010;28 Suppl 2:S3–9.
19. Arslan S, Yazici AR, Gorucu J, Ertan A, Pala K, Ustun Y, Antonson SA, Antonson DE. Effects of different cavity disinfectants on shear bond strength of a silorane-based resin composite. J Contemp Dent Pract. 2011;12:279–86.
20. Garcia EJ, Serrano AP, Urruchi WI, Deboni MC, Reis A, Grande RH, Loguercio AD. Influence of ozone gas and ozonated water application to dentin and bonded interfaces on resin-dentin bond strength. J Adhes Dent. 2012;14:363–70.
21. Bitter K, Noetzel J, Volk C, Neumann K, Kielbassa AM. Bond strength of fiber posts after the application of erbium:yttrium-aluminum-garnet laser treatment and gaseous ozone to the root canal. J Endod. 2008;34:306–9.
22. Rodrigues PC, Souza JB, Soares CJ, Lopes LG, Estrela C. Effect of ozone application on the resin-dentin microtensile bond strength. Oper Dent. 2011;36:537–44.
23. Dalkilic EE, Arisu HD, Kivanc BH, Uctasli MB, Omurlu H. Effect of different disinfectant methods on the initial microtensile bond strength of a self-etch adhesive to dentin. Lasers Med Sci. 2012;27:819–25.
24. Mohammadi Z, Shalavi S, Soltani MK, Asgary S. A review of the properties and applications of ozone in endodontics: an update. Iran Endod J. 2013;8:40–3.

25. Orchardson R, Gillam DG. Managing dentin hypersensitivity. J Am Dent Assoc. 2006;137:990–8.
26. Ciriello G. Ozone and dentinal sensitivity. Riv Ital Stomatol. 1955;10:159–64.
27. Dähnhardt JE, Gygax M, Martignoni B, Suter P, Lussi A. Treating sensitive cervical areas with ozone. A prospective controlled clinical trial. Am J Dent. 2008;21:74–6.
28. Azarpazhooh A, Limeback H, Lawrence HP, Fillery ED. Evaluating the effect of an ozone delivery system on the reversal of dentin hypersensitivity: a randomized, double-blinded clinical trial. J Endod. 2009;35:1–9.
29. Raafat Abdelaziz R, Mosallam RS, Yousry MM. Tubular occlusion of simulated hypersensitive dentin by the combined use of ozone and desensitizing agents. Acta Odontol Scand. 2011;69:395–400.
30. Patel PV, Patel A, Kumar S, Holmes JC. Evaluation of ozonated olive oil with or without adjunctive application of calcium sodium phosphosilicate on post-surgical root dentin hypersensitivity: a randomized, double-blinded, controlled, clinical trial. Minerva Stomatol. 2013;62:147–61.
31. Mohammadi Z, Palazzi F, Giardino L, Shalavi S. Microbial biofilms in endodontic infections: an update review. Biomed J. 2013;36:59–70.
32. Azarpazhooh A, Limeback H. The application of ozone in dentistry: a systematic review of literature. J Dent. 2008;36:104–16.
33. Nagayoshi M, Fukuizumi T, Kitamura C, Yano J, Terashita M, Nishihara T. Efficacy of ozone on survival and permeability of oral micro-organisms. Oral Microbiol Immunol. 2004;19:240–6.
34. Hems RS, Gulabivala K, Ng YL, Ready D, Spratt DA. An in vitro evaluation of the ability of ozone to kill a strain of Enterococcus faecalis. Int Endod J. 2005;38:22–9.
35. Müller P, Guggenheim B, Schmidlin PR. Efficacy of gasiform ozone and photodynamic therapy on a multispecies oral biofilm in vitro. Eur J Oral Sci. 2007;V115:77–80.
36. Estrela C, Estrela CRA, Decurcio DA, Hollanda ACB, Silva JA. Antimicrobial efficacy of ozonated water, gaseous ozone, sodium hypochlorite and chlorhexidine in infected human root canals. Int Endod J. 2007;40:85–93.
37. Thanomsub B, Anupunpisit V, Chanphetch S, Watcharachaipong T, Poonkhum R, Srisukonth C. Effects of ozone treatment on cell growth and ultrastructural changes in bacteria. J Gen Appl Microbiol. 2002;48:193–9.
38. Polydorou O, Pelz K, Hahn P. Antibacterial effect of an ozone device and its comparison with two dentin-bonding systems. Eur J Oral Sci. 2006;114:349–53.
39. Cardoso MG, de Oliveira LD, Koga-Ito CY, Jorge AO. Effectiveness of ozonated water on Candida albicans, Enterococcus faecalis, and endotoxins in root canals. Oral Surg Oral Med Oral Pathol Oral Radiol Endod. 2008;105:e85–91.
40. Stoll R, Venne L, Jablonski-Momeni A, Mutters R, Stachniss V. The disinfecting effect of ozonized oxygen in an infected root canal: an in vitro study. Quintessence Int. 2008;39:231–6.
41. Huth KC, Jacob FM, Saugel B, Cappello C, Paschos E, Hollweck R, Hickel R, Brand K. Effect of ozone on oral cells compared with established antimicrobials. Eur J Oral Sci. 2006;114:435–40.
42. Kuştarci A, Sümer Z, Altunbaş D, Koşum S. Bactericidal effect of KTP laser irradiation against Enterococcus faecalis compared with gaseous ozone: an ex vivo study. Oral Surg Oral Med Oral Pathol Oral Radiol Endod. 2009;107:e73–9.
43. Case PD, Bird PS, Kahler WA, George R, Walsh LJ. Treatment of root canal biofilms of Enterococcus faecalis with ozone gas and passive ultrasound activation. J Endod. 2012;38:523–6.
44. Eick S, Tigan M, Sculean A. Effect of ozone on periodontopathogenic species–an in vitro study. Clin Oral Investig. 2012;16:537–44.
45. Zan R, Hubbezoglu I, Sümer Z, Tunç T, Tanalp J. Antibacterial effects of two different types of laser and aqueous ozone against Enterococcus faecalis in root canals. Photomed Laser Surg. 2013;31:150–4.
46. Siqueira JF, Sen BH. Fungi in endodontic infections. Oral Surg Oral Med Oral Pathol Oral Radiol Endod. 2004;97:632–41.
47. Lucas VS. Association of psychotropic drugs, prevalence of denture-related stomatitis and oral candidosis. Community Dent Oral Epidemiol. 1993;21:313–6.
48. Arendorf TM, Walker DM. The prevalence and intra-oral distribution of *Candida albicans* in man. Arch Oral Biol. 1980;25:1–10.
49. Waltimo TM, Haapasalo M, Zehnder M, Meyer J. Clinical aspects related to endodontic yeast infections. Endod Topics. 2004;9:66–78.
50. Mohammadi Z. Endotoxin in endodontic infections: a review. J Calif Dent Assoc. 2011;39:152–5.
51. Noguchi F, Kitamura C, Nagayoshi M, Chen KK, Terashita M, Nishihara T. Ozonated water improves lipopolysaccharide-induced responses of an odontoblast-like cell line. J Endod. 2009;35:668–72.

Irrigation of the Root Canal System by Laser Activation (LAI): PIPS Photon-Induced Photoacoustic Streaming

13

David E. Jaramillo

Abstract

Root canal debridement and disinfection control are two of the main steps in root canal therapy. Control of bacterial load from an infected root canal before obturation is necessary to have a more predictable outcome. Bacteria will be present as biofilm colonies and will be responsible to establish disease and infection. Inside the root canal, it will be attached to the canal walls, well within dentinal tubules, fins, lateral canals, and foramina. In a different study, Nair found the presence of bacteria within these areas such as the root canal, fins, webs, isthmuses, etc., even after cleaning, shaping, and filling of the root canal system. When bacteria colonize the root canal system, it becomes very hard to effectively remove it from these inaccessible areas.

During root canal therapy, the endodontist faces all types of complications, one of which is the root canal morphology. There are several studies where several authors have verified the complexity of the root canal system. Root canals can present difficulty with accessibility, and in some areas of the root canal system, accessibility by instrumentation, irrigation, or even intra-canal medication is not possible. Because of this inaccessibility, different irrigation techniques have been proposed in order to obtain better disinfection rates.

Root canal debridement and disinfection control are two of the main steps in root canal therapy [1, 2]. Control of bacterial load from an infected root canal before obturation is necessary to have a more predictable outcome [3]. Bacteria will be present as biofilm colonies and will be responsible to establish disease and infection [4, 5]. Inside the root canal, it will be attached to the canal walls, well within dentinal tubules, fins, lateral canals, and foramina [6]. In a different study, Nair [7] found the presence of bacteria within these areas such as the root canal, fins, webs, isthmuses, etc., even after cleaning, shaping, and

D.E. Jaramillo, DDS
Department of Endodontics,
University of Texas Health Science Center
at Houston, School of Dentistry,
7500 Cambridge St. Suite 6415,
Houston, TX 77054, USA
e-mail: David.E.Janamillo@Uth.tmc.edu

B. Basrani (ed.), *Endodontic Irrigation: Chemical Disinfection of the Root Canal System*,
DOI 10.1007/978-3-319-16456-4_13

filling of the root canal system. When bacteria colonize the root canal system, it becomes very hard to effectively remove it from these inaccessible areas.

During root canal therapy, the endodontist faces all types of complications, one of which is the root canal morphology. There are several studies where several authors Hess [8], Weine [9], Pineda [10], and Vertucci [11, 12] have verified the complexity of the root canal system. Root canals can present difficulty with accessibility, and in some areas of the root canal system, accessibility by instrumentation, irrigation, or even intra-canal medication is not possible. Because of this inaccessibility, different irrigation techniques have been proposed in order to obtain better disinfection rates.

Access to these areas is basically impossible for hand and/or rotary instruments [13], intra-canal medications [14, 15], or through a conventional irrigation technique. Several techniques have been developed for the irrigation of the root canal system. One of the most effective has been the passive ultrasonic irrigation technique described by Weller [16] and van der Sluis [17]. Once the root canal has been shaped, the irrigation solution will flow better inside the root canal and an ultrasonically activated wire can vibrate and produce an acoustic action. Ahmad [18] said the streaming produced will help free canal walls of debris and biofilm from the surfaces. The irrigation solution is used to reach inaccessible areas; however, the streaming might not be strong enough to remove the debris, smear layer, or even biofilm.

Schwalow and Townes following Einstein's theory of simulated emission described the principles of microwave amplification by stimulated emission of radiation. After the development of laser (light amplification by stimulated emission of radiation), it was introduced to dentistry in 1965 by Stern [19]. Today lasers widely used in dentistry include diodes, Nd:YAG, erbium, and even CO2 which produces radiation in both the near and far infrared electromagnet spectrum [20].

Several authors Saks [21], Klein [22], and McGuff [23] had demonstrated a good effect using lasers against microorganisms. In the mid-1980s, some areas of dentistry started to explore the use of the laser, primarily CO2 laser in periodontal therapy, oral surgery, and endodontics. Pini [24] using the excimer laser was successful in removing organic tissue from inside the root canals.

In an effort to accomplish a better seal of the apical constriction, Weichman et al. [25, 26] used a neodymium-yttrium-aluminum-garnet (Nd:YAG) from both inside and outside of the apical foramen unsuccessfully. Dederich [27] found a reduced permeability on the canal walls once it had been irradiated with Nd:YAG lasers due the melting and thermal ablation of the laser beam on the dentin surface. Levy [28] compared the cleaning and shaping of Nd:YAG laser to conventional files. He reported no increased of temperature in the outer surface of the root. The shape (taper) of the canals was equal, and according to his grading, he found smoother and cleaner root canal surface in the laser group. Kantola [29] found higher levels of calcium and phosphorous after applying the CO2 laser which he attributed to the increase in organic content resulting after burning off of the organic component by the laser energy.

Gordon [30], using an in vitro model, found the use of Er,Cr:YSGG (erbium, chromium: yttrium-scandium-gallium-garnet) laser to have a good antimicrobial effect on dentital tubules infected with *E. faecalis*. The FDA has approved this type of laser to clean, shape, and enlarge the root canal as well as for its use in osseous, apical, and periodontal surgery. This laser frequency is highly absorbed by water and as such has a significant impact on the bacterial cell itself. This laser works by penetrating into the dentin surface by several factors. The wavelength of the Er,Cr:YSGG laser (2.78 μm) is absorbed by dentin due to the presence of hydroxide and interstitial water (chromophores of this wavelength). Each laser pulse is composed of 150 μs duration, and each one of these pulses is responsible for the penetration of its energy about 3 μm into the water. The penetration of water and the collapse of water vapor formed can penetrate as deep as 1,000 μm or more into the dentin tubules. This is known as a micropulse-induced sequential absorption. The expansion and collapse of water vapor will produce acoustic waves that will be strong enough to disrupt intratubular bacteria. The author found the largest reductions in bacterial load (CFU) have occurred when the laser was used in the absence of a water spray. An increase in the outer surface of the root temperature of 2.6 °C was documented. The heat generated from these settings creates deleterious effect on the root canal surface, i.e., charring, necrosis, and melting of dentin.

There are many different types of lasers and wavelengths used in dentistry to perform endodontic procedures today. They all function primarily by direct radiation of light energy to tooth surfaces by way of thermal reaction. Low-level laser therapy (LLLT) is a noninvasive and simple technique mainly used for different regenerative medicine procedures. In endodontics, the use of this low-energy laser has been introduced with satisfactory results. Erbium lasers are solid-state lasers whose lasing medium is primarily erbium doped. Er:YAG lasers typically emit light with a wavelength of 2,940 nm, which is infrared light. Unlike Nd:YAG lasers, the output of an Er:YAG laser is strongly absorbed by water. This unique characteristic leads to new applications in root canal therapy such as LAI. Farges [31] found an increase of temperature with Nd:YAG lasers up to 7.2 °C. Folwaczny [32] stated good antibacterial effect of Nd:YAG laser due to radiation energy. But the increased in temperature could be an undesirable effect. A very important fact to be seriously considered in this study was the sampling technique they described in this paper. The NaOCl solution used as irrigation solution was not inactivated after the procedure, which could lead to inaccurate results in the microbiology aspect of this study.

According to Peters [33], 35 % of the root canal wall surface remained untouched by instruments after the cleaning and shaping phase of the root canal therapy. This is important data that has been misinterpreted and misunderstood in a large number of papers and presentations. The results were obtained by mathematical operation, by doing an average of 3 root canals, instead of doing it canal by canal. There is a big difference in between the root canal areas left untouched on buccals and palatal canal. While buccals canals were touched in an average of 85 %, the palatal canal remained untouched 80 %. This would indicate that the root canal cleaning and shaping is totally dependent on the root canal morphology itself.

Kerekes and Tronstad [34] studied the morphology and found it hard to standardized a root canal preparation protocol due to the diversity and differences of root canal morphology. They found that 1 mm from the apex sizes varied from mesio-buccal canal to be as large as a number 40 hand file. The distal-buccal canal was equivalent to a number 60 hand instrument at the 3 mm level, and the palatal canal had even greater differences at the 1 mm level varying from 0.15 to 3.4 mm. The most rounded area found was present at the 1–3 mm level. According to these findings, it is more evident why some canals showed more untouched areas after root canal instrumentation. Wu [35] observed and confirmed oval root canals areas to be left untouched and unfilled depending on the obturation technique used. Tatsuta [36] found the presence of calcospherites (predentin) (Fig. 13.1) in the untouched areas of the root canal. These areas are an excellent niche for necrotic pulp tissue and bacteria to hide away

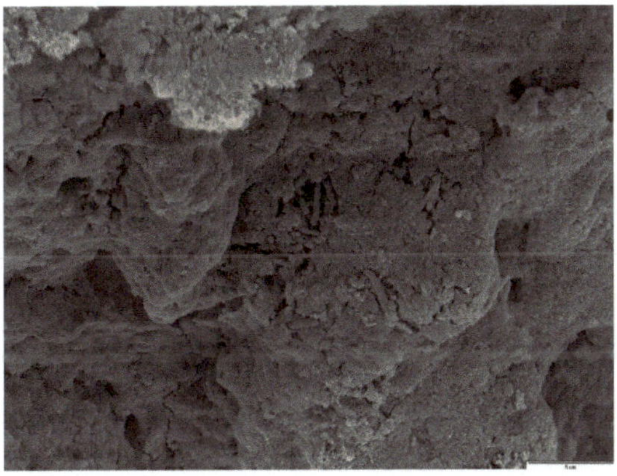

Fig. 13.1 SEM image of predentin area. It is evident the presence of bacteria hiding in these areas that remained untouched and unaltered after the cleaning, shaping, and conventional (needle) irrigation of the root canal system

from instruments, irrigation agents, and intracanal medication.

Due to the lack of predictable ways to completely clean and shape the root canal system, the chemical aspect of the root canal therapy is very important. Sodium hypochlorite (NaOCl) was introduced in endodontics in 1920 [37]. Since its introduction into the root canal therapy, NaOCl is considered to be the best irrigation solution used in root canal therapy. It posses excellent characteristics needed during the endodontic procedure as disinfectant, lubricant, and both vital and necrotic tissue dissolvent [38]. On the other hand, van der Sluis [39] found the frequent replenishment of NaOCl during root canal therapy makes the solution more effective, especially when ultrasonic is added as a final rinse of the irrigation protocol.

The acoustic streaming created by ultrasonic irrigation helps in the removal of pulp and dentin debris, microorganism, as well as the smear layer. By applying an ultrasonic force within the root canal, it will create and generate a turbulence that will enhance and produce a better flushing of this debris. Ahmad [18] mentioned the velocity of the streaming could be influenced by factor such as file size, position, and power setting of the ultrasonic unit. He also noticed that the greater streaming activity was found at the level of the minor radius of the file. The smaller the file and the higher the power setting of the ultrasonic unit, the stronger and greater will the streaming velocities be. Williams [40] showed acoustic streaming caused disruption of biological cells.

Newer Laser Technology

PIPS

Photon-induced photoacoustic streaming is based on the radial firing stripped tip with laser impulses of subablative (to evaporized at very low temperature) energies of 20 mJ at 15 Hz for an average power of 0.3 W at 50 μs impulses. The impulses create an interaction of water molecules with peak powers of 400 W. This creates an expansion and successive shock waves leading to the formation of a very powerful streaming of the fluid located inside the root canal, with no rising of temperature.

PIPS is a form of laser-activated irrigation that works indirectly and without thermal effects by activating irrigants. Its mechanism of action is by creating a strong photoacoustic shockwave that streams irrigants three dimensionally throughout the root canal system (Figs. 13.2 and 13.3). Unlike the other conventional laser applications, the unique tapered and stripped PIPS tip is not required to be placed inside the canal system itself but rather in the pulp chamber only. This reduces the need for using larger files and rotary instruments to create larger canal shapes to open the system so that irrigants used during treatment can effectively get to the delicate apical one-third of the root apex, fins, isthmuses, and lateral canals. This nonthermal pressure wave has been shown to effectively remove both vital and necrotic tissues, kill bacteria, remove biofilm, and even disinfect dentin tubules. Peters [41] compared the disinfection and disruption of biofilm within the root canal in the apical third. PIPS did not completely remove bacteria from infected dentinal tubules but did generate less infection and removed biofilm better than passive ultrasonic irrigation technique group.

Jaramillo et al. [42] found the combinations of 20 s irradiation with Er:YAG laser via this photoacoustic delivery system PIPS, and 6 % sodium hypochlorite was very effective in inhibiting *Enterococcus faecalis* growth. The PIPS technology can be used as an efficient additional tool in the decontamination of infected root canals during

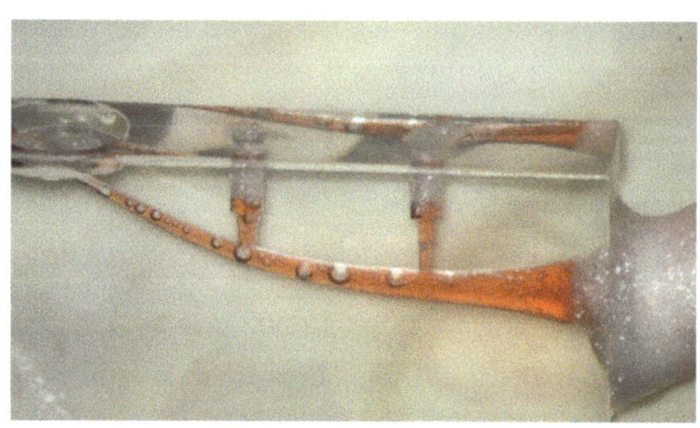

Fig. 13.2 Streaming acoustic produced by the use of PIPS in this simulated plastic root canal

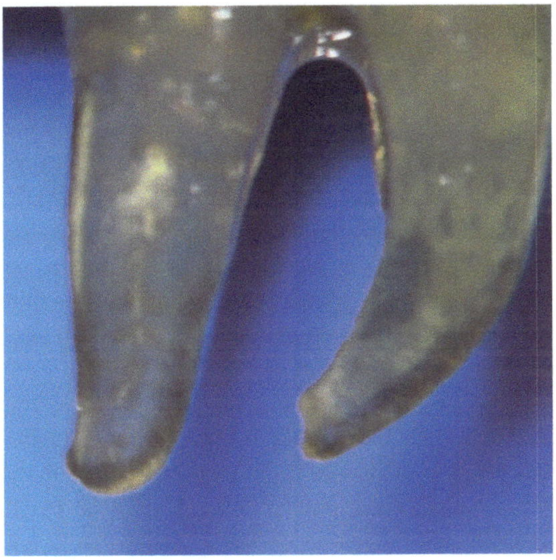

Fig. 13.3 Natural #30 tooth cleared by diaphanization technique showing the steaming acoustic produced by PIPS reaching the apical portion of the distal root canal

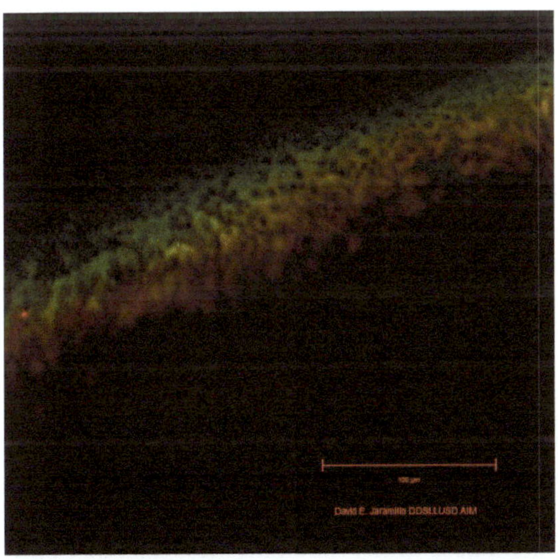

Fig. 13.4 Backlight (live/dead) confocal staining technique. After root canal irrigation with PIPS, the root canal wall and dentinal tubules are free of either live (*green*) or dead (*red*) bacteria

endodontic treatment (Figs. 13.4 and 13.5). Divito et al. [43] studying the removal of smear layer used PIPS at a wavelength of 2,940 nm with a 12 mm, 400 μm quartz tip at 20 mJs, 15 Hz, and 50 μs pulse duration. Placing the tip stationary in the pulp chamber area only revealed higher quantity of open

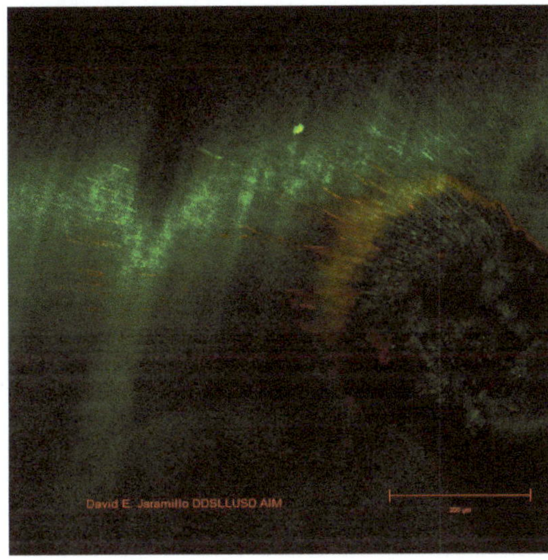

Fig. 13.5 Root canal wall and dentin visualization on the presence of live (*green*) and dead (*red*) bacteria after conventional (needle) irrigation. Baclight technique

dentinal tubules when compared to different timing and solutions to just water. Temperature was checked on the outer root surface and an increase of 1.4 °C after a continuous activation of 40 s was found. Heat generation is a very important aspect of laser usage in dentistry. CO_2 and Nd:YAG lasers are used as photothermal, the hard tissues surrounding the irradiation area will absorb the laser energy and convert it into heat.

According to Saunders [44], an increment of more than 10 °C for more than 1 min may be sufficient to cause bone tissue injury.

Er:YAG lasers are highly absorbed by water. The penetration depth into enamel and dentin is minimal, and the mechanical ablation process is by micro-explosion without the significant rise in temperature. Sonntag [45] showed pulp histological reaction to Er:YAG laser was similar to that generated by a high-speed handpiece. Armengol [46] compared high-speed carbide bur to Er:YAG at 140 mJ pulse repetition of 4 Hz and Nd:YAP at 240 mJ and a pulse repetition of 10 Hz with and without water. As expected Nd:YAP laser created the higher increment in temperature when compared to Er:YAG laser and high-speed handpiece. This two showed the same parameters of rise in temperature when water spray was used.

Because bacteria can be sensitized to light, Wilson [47] tested light-activated disinfection and obtained good results treating localized bacterial-mediated infections. Following this principle, Lim [48] studied the advanced non-Invasive light-activated disinfection (*ANILAD*) that is a more efficient type of light-activated disinfection. According to George [49], in order for the photoactivation to be effective, certain factors need to be in place: the interaction of photosensitizer molecules, the physicochemical environment at the site of application, the half-life of the free radicals generated, and the oxygen availability at the site of application. *ANILAD* improves the penetration into dentinal tubules and the bacterial kill rate. It is also a better oxygen carrier and is less toxic than NaOCl. Unfortunately, the time needed for application is too long and is not clinically convenient at this time. The author found the combination of *ANILAD*, cleaning, and shaping of the root canal had favorable disinfection rates.

Many studies have been conducted in an effort to understand the behavior of the irrigant solution within the root canal system. Boutsioukis [50] looked at the needle design and clinical realistic flow rate values recorded using virtual studies with computational fluid dynamic models with FLUENT 6.2 software. The flow rate, velocity, and turbulence were recorded. According to the experiment findings, a laminar flow was always detected regardless of the pressure applied to the solution. The maximum velocity was detected near the end of the needle suggesting that the needle should be placed 1 mm short of the working length. The same author [51] studied the formation and removal of the vapor lock during the root canal irrigation when a needle was used following the same type of virtual experiments. Their results showed that there is a direct correlation between the size of the root canal preparation and the size of the needle used and the penetration of the needle to disrupt or avoid vapor lock from occurring. Similar findings made by Hsieh et al. [52] found that the diameter of the irrigating needle and the distance from the working length in instrumented canals will prevent the irrigation solution from reaching the apical portion of the root canal during the cleaning and shaping phase. Shen [53] also studied needle designs and penetration depths at 3 and 5 mm from working length. The results showed that the design of the needle tip influences the flow pattern, flow velocity, and the apical wall pressure. The evidence of needle irrigation demonstrated irrigation solution would not reach the target area. After this evidence, researchers looked into a different direction with respect to the root canal irrigation.

Passive ultrasonic irrigation is defined as the agitation of an irrigation solution located inside the root canal system. This is done with the help of an ultrasonic unit equipped with a small smooth wire oscillating freely inside the root canal system to induce a powerful acoustic streaming [54].

Fincham et al. [55] studied the fluid movements generated with PIPS and ultrasonic irrigation by means of microscopic digital velocimetry. The fluid movement was analyzed directly to the activation probe at 3, 5, 10, and 15 mm distances. On spatial structure, PIPS showed a velocity in excess of 1.2 m/s at 3 mm from the tip. The peak velocity at 5, 10, and 15 mm demonstrated the same range of 0.3 m/s. With this, PIPS demonstrated that, after the initial fall-off of energy distal from the probe tip, there was no further attenuation with distance in the velocity field measured in this vial, and vortical structures were also clearly identifiable at 5, 10, and 15 mm. Meanwhile, PUI shows an instantaneous velocity field corresponding to the measurement directly under the ultrasonic tip, which was the initial peak in velocity. The average velocity was 0.036 m/s, which is 20 times less than that measured for the PIPS data, obtained immediately under the probe's tip. In this group at 5 mm from the probe tip, the velocities measured were less than 0.01 m/s.

Ordinola et al. [56] studied the effect of PIPS using a solution of 6 % NaOCl for the removal of an ex vivo biofilm in a novel dentin bovine model. The authors found an improved cleaning of the infected dentin on the PIPS groups when compared to the PUI group. The extraordinary result from this specific experiment was the fact PIPS tip was placed 22 mm away from the target area, while ultrasonic, sonic, and passive irrigation were made at the exact target area.

Jaramillo et al. [57] in an in-vitro model infected single rooted teeth with *E. faecalis* irrigated with three 20 s interval periods replenishing a buffered 0.5 % NaOCl solution and applied PIPS, and compared to conventional needle irrigation. Apical segments were sectioned, and then were immersed in liquid nitrogen and crushed. Serial dilutions were made and then plated. Our results showed an 83 % disinfection of the conventional group after 20 min of continuous irrigation versus 100 % disinfection on PIPS group, with a total of 1 min of irrigation with the same solution.

Alshahrani et al. [58] also found the combination of PIPS+NaOCl 6 % was more effective than water+PIPS or just irrigation with NaOCl 6 %.

According to Ordinola and Alshahrani, a better disinfection rate can be obtained with the combination of PIPS and NaOCl 6 %.

Vera et al. [59] performed root canal treatment in-vivo following standardized protocol for the cleaning and shaping of the root canals, in necrotic cases in one versus two appointments, with placement of intra-canal medication. The general and constant finding was the presence of bacteria (biofilm), infected pulp tissue, inorganic components, etc., inside the root canal lumen, isthmuses, finds, lateral canals, etc. Being aware of the fact that we will always leave all this debris behind after a root canal cleaning, shaping, and irrigation, Lloyd et al. [60] studied by means of high-resolution microcomputed tomography the effect of PIPS in the debris removal from mesial canals of lower molars, including isthmuses, fins, and lateral canals, as well as the volumetric area reached by the irrigation solution used. They compared PIPS to standard needle irrigation. Their findings were a better debris removal when PIPS was used in about 2.6 times greater than SNI group. The effect of the shockwave produced by PIPS is clearly demonstrated in this paper. These Strong Photo-acoustic shockwaves stream irrigants three dimensionally throughout the root canal system. Its also effective debriding the isthmus area where debris tend to be trapped, allowing a better dislodgment of pulp tissue, bacteria, inorganic debris, etc., from these areas.

PIPS Protocol

According to the manufacturer, the following is the current correct protocol that should be followed when using PIPS for the irrigation of the root canal system.

The PIPS tip is placed in the pulp chamber only (not in the root canal) and held stationary throughout the activation process. During the time of laser activation, the dental assistant applies a continuous flow of the solution from the dental irrigating syringe. It is extremely important that the pulp chamber is always kept flooded with enough irrigating solution to keep the PIPS tip submerged. The laser activation period for PIPS is in 30 s cycles. The current protocol is six 30 s cycle of laser activation, with three [3] 30 s off (rest phase) between activation when using NaOCl. Immediately after 3–30 s cycles of laser-activated irrigation with NaOCl, the canals are irrigated for an additional 30 s using PIPS with water only (Fig. 13.6). The pulp chamber is then emptied, and 17 % EDTA is used with PIPS and continuous flow for an additional 30 s. The final step in the PIPS protocol is laser activation with

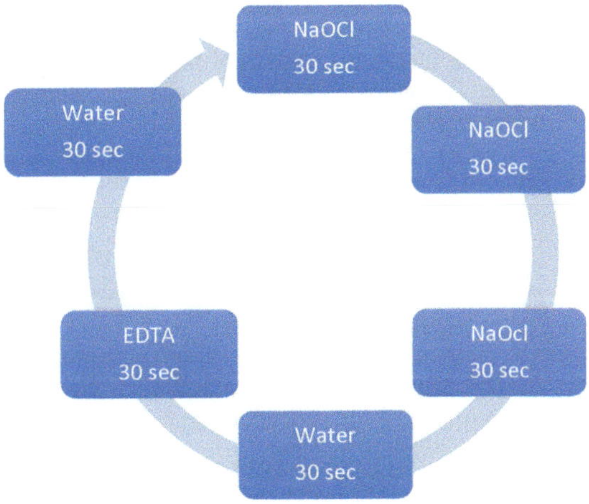

Fig. 13.6 PIPS current correct protocol

an additional 30 s of water only. The canal system is now ready for obturation.

A new era of laser-activated root canal irrigation is now available with excellent results on the smear layer removal and disinfection of the root canal walls, dentinal tubules, isthmuses, lateral canals, fins, etc.

References

1. Schilder H. Cleaning and shaping of the root canal. Dent Clin North Am. 1974;18(2):269–96.
2. Bystrom A, Sundqvist G. Bacteriologic evaluation of the efficacy of mechanical root canal instrumentation in endodontic therapy. Scand J Dent Res. 1981;89(4):321–8.
3. Sjogren U, Hagglund B, Sundqvist G, Wing K. Factors affecting the long-term results of endodontic treatment. J Endod. 1990;16(10):498–504.
4. Costerton W, Veeh R, Shirtliff M, Pasmore M, Post C, Ehrlich G. The application of biofilm science to the study and control of chronic bacterial infections. J Clin Invest. 2003;112(10):1466–77.
5. Chavez de Paz LE. Redefining the persistent infection in root canals: possible role of biofilm communities. J Endod. 2007;33(6):652–62.
6. Nair PN. Pathogenesis of apical periodontitis and the cases of endodontic failures. Crit Rev Oral Biol Med. 2004;15(6):348–81.
7. Nair PNR, Henry S, Cano V, Vera J. Microbial status of the apical root canal system of human mandibular first molars with primary apical periodontitis after one visit endodontic treatment. Oral Surg Oral Med Oral Pathol Oral Radiol Endod. 2005;99:231–52.
8. Hess W. Formation of root canals in human teeth. J Am Den Assoc. 1921;8:704–34.
9. Wine FS, Healey HJ, Gerstein H, Evanson L. Canal configuration in the mesiobuccal root of the maxillary first molar and its endodontic significance. Oral Surg Oral Med Oral Pathol. 1969;28:419–25.
10. Pineda F, Kuttler Y. Mesiodistal and buccolingual roentgenographic investigation of 7,275 root canals. Oral Surg Oral Med Oral Pathol. 1972;33:101–10.
11. Verticcu FJ. Root canal anatomy of the human permanent teeth. Oral Surg Oral Med Oral Pathol. 1984;58:589–99.
12. Vertucci FJ. Root canal morphology and its relationship to endodontic procedures. Endod Topics. 2005;10:3–29.
13. Arnold M, Ricucci D, Siqueira Jr JF. Infection in a complex network of apical ramifications as the cause of persistent apical periodontitis: a case report. J Endod. 2013;39(9):117–84.
14. Sjogren U, Figdor D, Spangberg L, Sundqvist G. The antimicrobial effect of calcium hydroxide as a short-term intracanal dressing. J Endod. 1990;16(12):589–95.
15. Safavi KE, Dowdenn WE, Introcaso JH, Langeland K. A comparison of antimicrobial effects of calcium hydroxide and iodine-potassium iodide. J Endod. 1985;11(10):454–6.
16. Weller RN, Brady JM, Bernier WE. Efficacy of ultrasonic cleaning. J Endod. 1980;6(9):740–3.
17. Van der Sluis LW, Wu MK, Wesselink PR. The efficacy of ultrasonic irrigation to remove artificially placed dentine debris from human root canals prepares using instruments of varying taper. Int Endod J. 2005;38(10):746–8.
18. Ahmad M, Pitt Ford TJ, Crum LA. Ultrasonic debridement of root canals: acoustic streaming and its possible role. J Endod. 1987;13(10):490–9.
19. Stern RH, Sognnaes RF. Laser effect on dental hard tissues. A preliminary report. J South Calif Dent Assoc. 1965;33:17–9.
20. Meral G, Tasar F, Kocagøz S, Sener C. Factors affecting the antibacterial effects of Nd:YAG Laser in vivo. Laser Surg Med. 2003;32(3):197–202.
21. Nm S, Roth CA. Ruby laser as a microsurgical instrument. Science. 1963;141:46–7.
22. Klein E, Fine S, Ambrus J. Interaction of laser irradiation with biological system. III. Studies on biological systems in vitro. Fed Proc. 1965;14:5101–10.
23. McGuff PE, Bell EJ. The effect of laser irradiation on bacteria. Med Biol III. 1966;16:191–3.
24. Pini R, Salimbeni R, Vannini M. Laser dentistry: a new application of excimer laser in root canal therapy. Laser Surg Med. 1989;9:352–7.
25. Weichman JA, Johnson FM. Laser in endodontics. A preliminary investigation. Oral Surg Oral Med Oral Pathol. 1971;31:416–20.
26. Weichman JA, Johnsosn FM, Nitta LK. Laser use in endodontics. Part II. J Oral Surg. 1972;34:828–30.
27. Dederich D, Zachariensen K, Tulip J. Scanning electron microscopic analysis of root canal wall dentin follow Neodymium Yttrium garnet laser irradiation. J Endod. 1984;10:428.
28. Levy G. Cleaning and shaping the root canal with Nd:YAG laser beam: a comparative study. J Endod. 1992;18:123–7.
29. Kantola S. Laser induced effects on the tooth structure. IV. A study of changes in the calcium and phosphorous contents in dentine by electron probe microanalysis. Acta Odontol Scand. 1972;30:463–74.
30. Gordon W, Atabakhsh VA, Meza F, Doms A, Nissan R, Nissan R, Risoiu I, Stevens RH. The antimicrobial efficacy of the erbium, chromium:yttrium-scandium-gallium-garnet laser with emitting tips on the root canal dentin walls infected with Enterococcus faecalis. J Am Dent Assoc. 2007;138(7):992–1002.
31. Farges P, Nahas P, Bonin P. In vitro study of a Nd:YAG laser in endodontic retreatment. J Endod. 1998;24:359–63.
32. Folwaczny M, Mehl A, Jordan C, Hickel R. Antibacterial effects of pulsed Nd:YAG laser

radiation at different energy settings in root canals. J Endod. 2002;28:24–9.
33. Peters OA, Schönenberger K, Laib A. Effects of four Ni-Ti preparation techniques on root canal geometry assessed by micro computed tomography. Int Endod J. 2001;34(3):221–30.
34. Kerekes K, Tronstad L. Morphological observation on the root canals of human molars. J Endod. 1977;3(3):114–8.
35. Wu MKL, Wesselink PR. A primary observation on the preparation and obturation of oval canals. Int Endod J. 2001;34(2):137–41.
36. Tatsuta CT, Morgan LA, Baumgartner JC, Adey JD. Effect of calcium hydroxide and four irrigation regimens on instrumented and uninstrumented canal wall topography. J Endod. 1999;25(2):93–8.
37. Crane AB. A practicable root canal technique. Philadelphia: Lea & Febinger; 1920.
38. Zehnder M, Kosicki D, Luder H, Sener B, Waltimo T. Tissue – dissolving capacity and antibacterial effect of buffered and unbuffered hypochlorite solutions. Oral Surg Oral Med Oral Pathol Oral Radiol Endod. 2002;94(6):756–62.
39. Van der Sluis LW, Vogels MP, Verhaagen B, Macedo R, Wesselink PR. Study on the influence of refreshment/activation cycles and irrigants on mechanical cleaning efficiency during ultrasonic activation of the irrigant. J Endod. 2010;36(4):737–40.
40. Williams AR. Disorganization and disruption of mammalian and amoeboid cells by acoustic microstreaming. J Acoust Soc Am. 1972;52:688–93.
41. Peters OA, Bardsley S, Fong J, Pandher G, Divito E. Disinfection of root canals with photon-initiated photoacoustic streaming. J Endod. 2011;37(7):1008–12.
42. Jaramillo DE, Aprecio R, Angelov N, Divito E, McClammy TV. Efficacy of photon induced photoacoustic streaming (PIPS) on the root canals infected with *Enterococcus faecalis*: a pilot study. Endod Prac. 2012;7(3):28–32.
43. Divito E, Peters OA, Olivi G. Effectiveness of the erbium:YAG laser and new design radial and stripped tips in removing the smear layer after toot canal instrumentation. Laser Med Scue. 2012;27:273–80.
44. Saunders EM. In vivo findings associated with heat generation during thermomechanical compaction of gutta-percha. 1. Temperature levels at the external surface of the root. Int Endod J. 1990;23(5):263–7.
45. Sonntag KD, Kutzman B, Burkes J, Hoke J, Moshonov J. Pulpal response to cavity preparation with the Er:YAG and Mark III free electron lasers. Oral Sug Oral Med Oral Pathol Oral Radiol Endod. 1996;81:695–702.
46. Armengol V, Jean A, Marion D. Temperature rise during Er:YAG and Nd:YAP laser ablation of dentin. J Endod. 2000;26(3):138–41.
47. Wilson M. Lethal photosensitisation of oral bacteria and its potential application in the photodynamic therapy of oral infections. Photochem Photobiol Sci. 2004;3(5):412–8.
48. Lim Z, Cheng JL, Kim TW, Teo EG, Wong J, George S, Kishen A. Light-activated disinfection: an alternative endodontic disinfection strategy. Aust Dent J. 2009;54(2):108–14.
49. George S, Kishen A. Influence of photosensitizer solvent on the mechanisms of photoactivated killing of enterococcus faecalis. Photochem Photobiol. 2008;84(3):734–40.
50. Boutsioukis C, Lambdrianidis T, Kastrinakis E. Irrigant flow within a prepared root canal using various flow rates: a computational fluid dynamic study. Int Endod J. 2009;42(2):144–55.
51. Boutsioukis C, Kastrinakis E, Lambrianidis T, Verhaagen B, Versluis M, van der Sluis LW. Formation and removal of apical vapor lock during syringe irrigation. A combined experimental and computational fluid dynamics approach. Int Endod J. 2014;47(2):191–201.
52. Hsieh YD, Gau CH, Kung Wu SF, Shen EC, Hsu PW, Fu E. Dynamic recording of irrigating fluid distribution in the root canals using thermal image analysis. Int Endod J. 2007;40(1):11–7.
53. Shen Y, Gao Y, Qian W, Ruse ND, Zhou X, Wu H, Haapasalo M. Three-dimensional numeric simulation of root canal irrigant flow with different irrigation needles. J Endod. 2010;36(5):884–9.
54. van der Sluis LW, Versluis M, Wu MK, Wesselink PR. Passive ultrasonic irrigation of the root canal: a review of the literature. Int Endod J. 2007;40(6):415–26.
55. Fincham AM, Jaramillo DE, Divito E, Peters OA. Irrigant flow during Photo Induced Photoacoustic streaming (PIPS) using micro digital particle image velocimetry (μDPIV): a pilot study. IEJ. 2014;47:659–66.
56. Ordinola-Zapata R, Bramante CM, Aprecio RM, Handysides R, Jaramillo DE. Biofilm removal by 6% sodium hypochlorite activated by different irrigation techniques. Int Endod J. 2013. doi:10.1111/iej/12202.
57. Jaramillo DE, Aguilar E, Aprecio RM, Tran K. Dentin disinfection using PIPS and conventional needle irrigation. LLUSD CDR, 2011. Unpublished data.
58. Alsharhrani M, Divito E, Hughes C, Nathanson D, Huang G. Enhanced removal of enterococcus faecalis biofilms in the root canal using sodium hypochlorite plus Photon Induced Photoacoustic Streaming: an in vitro study. Photomed Laser Surg. 2014;32(5):524–30. doi:10.1089/pho2014.3714.
59. Vera J, Siqueira Jr JF, Ricucci D, Loghin S, Fernandes N, Flores B, Cruz AG. One-versus two-visit endodontic treatment of teeth with apical periodontitis: a histobacteriological study. J Endod. 2012;38(8):1040–52.
60. Lloyd A, Uhles J, Clement DJ, Garcia-Godoy F. Elimination of intracanal tissue and debris through a novel laser-activated system assessed using high-resolution micro-computed tomography: a pilot study. Jendod, 2014:40(4):584–7. doi:http://dx.doi.org/10.1016/j.joen.2013.10.040.

Photodynamic Therapy for Root Canal Disinfection

14

Anil Kishen and Annie Shrestha

Abstract

Emergence of antimicrobial-resistant microbial strains, rise of transplants, medically compromised patients, advanced cancer patients, and global spread in infection are few in the major issues related to difficulties of managing infectious diseases. The widespread recognition of microbial biofilm as the contributory factor for human infection warrants the identification of a reliable and effective antimicrobial strategy to combat infectious diseases. On similar lines, treatment of infected root canals presents with a major challenge of bacterial persistence after treatment. Photodynamic therapy (PDT) is considered as one of the potential treatment modalities for the treatment of localized infections irrespective of the causative microorganism, including those that are recalcitrant to conventional antimicrobial therapies/disinfectants. The ongoing research is focused to bring about tissue-specific innovative improvements of antimicrobial PDT by modifying photosensitizer formulation and light delivery system and increasing number of clinical trials and appropriate regulatory approvals for the usage of new photosensitizers. Cumulatively these efforts demonstrate increasing interest in the application of PDT in the coming years.

Introduction

Approximately 60 % of the current human infections have been associated with the presence of bacterial biofilms, which includes both implant-related infections and chronic non-implant-related infections [1]. The conservative management of such infections involving topical or systemic antibiotics has been shown to be ineffective mainly due to multidrug-resistant strains and widespread systemic use of antibiotics and misuse of antibiot-

A. Kishen, PhD, MDS, BDS (✉)
Department of Endodontics, Facility of Dentistry, University of Toronto, Toronto, ON, Canada
e-mail: anil.kishen@utoronto.ca

A. Shrestha, PhD, MSc, BDS
Faculty of Dentistry, Department of Endodontics, University of Toronto, Toronto, ON, Canada

B. Basrani (ed.), *Endodontic Irrigation: Chemical Disinfection of the Root Canal System*,
DOI 10.1007/978-3-319-16456-4_14

ics [2]. Antimicrobial resistance is constantly on rise leading to a major hindrance in the treatment of many infectious diseases [3–5]. Emergence of resistant microbial strains, rise of transplants, medically compromised patients, advanced cancer patients, and spread of infection due to increasing global travel between developed and developing nations are few of the major issues related to difficulties of managing infectious diseases [5, 6]. Photodynamic therapy (PDT) is considered as one of the potential treatment modalities for the treatment of localized infections irrespective of the causative microorganism, including those that are recalcitrant to conventional antimicrobial therapies [7–10].

PDT involves the use of a nontoxic dye or photosensitizer (PS) in combination with visible light, which in the presence of molecular oxygen leads to the production of cytotoxic oxygen radicals such as singlet oxygen. This reactive oxygen species are responsible for the PDT cytotoxic action [11], and its production and activity depend on the PDT dose [12]. PDT was discovered by chance during the early 1900s, when a combination of nontoxic dyes and visible light resulted in the killing of cells. Oscar Raab used acridine dyes and showed that the combination of light and dyes was much more effective to kill a paramecium [13]. Application of PDT as an alternative treatment for tumors has been explored and tested widely. For the last two decades, series of in vitro and in vivo studies have proven the efficacy of PDT in the management of various infectious and noninfectious diseases. The increase in the interest toward PDT is evident as seen by the exponential increase in the number of publications in the recent years (Fig. 14.1). The introduction of photosensitizers for in vivo applications and their approval in certain countries such as Canada, the United States, the European Union, Japan, Australia, and New Zealand show increased surge in using PDT for various systemic and topical pathogenic conditions [14]. The ongoing research is focused to bring about tissue-specific innovative improvements of antimicrobial PDT by modifying photosensitizer formulation and light delivery system and increasing number of clinical trials and appropriate regulatory approvals for the usage of new photosensitizers [15–17]. Cumulatively these efforts demonstrate increasing interest in the application of PDT in the coming years.

Mechanism of Photodynamic Inactivation of Microbial Cells

Antimicrobial photodynamic therapy works as a combination of photosensitizer and light. Photosensitizer is a light-sensitive chemical that

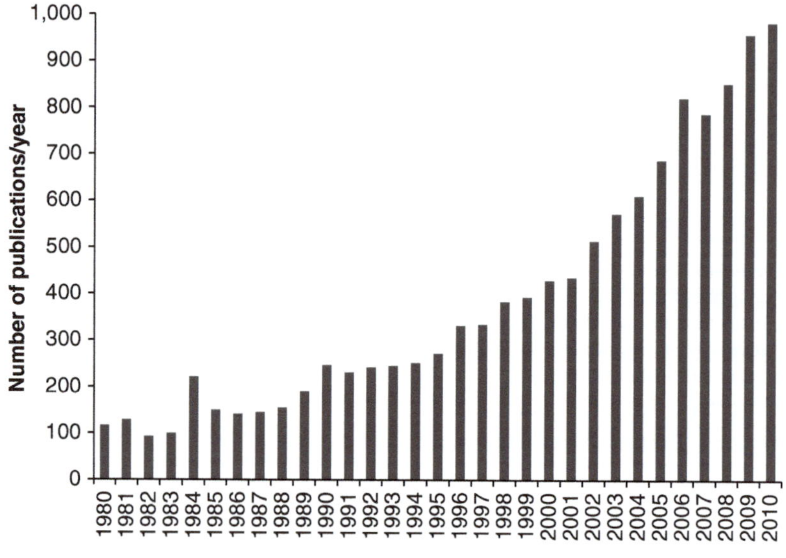

Fig. 14.1 Number of publications (English language) on the PDT since 1980 till 2010 (Source—Pubmed)

possesses low toxicity in the absence of light. Photosensitization of the infected tissue with a photosensitizer allows uptake into the bacterial cells, and irradiation of the photosensitized tissue results in the destruction of bacteria and infected tissue. It is extremely important that the light should be at a specific wavelength, which corresponds to the absorption wavelength of the photosensitizer being used. PDT can be utilized with a suitable photosensitizer and irradiation conditions to treat infections in cases where antibiotic-based therapeutic strategies have failed [8]. Unlike in cancer therapy where the photosensitizer is administered intravenously, for localized infections, the photosensitizer is delivered locally by various methods such as topical application, instillation, and interstitial injection or aerosol delivery. Selectivity of photosensitizer toward microorganisms over mammalian cells and effective removal of the causative microorganisms are the key points in achieving success of PDT to manage localized infections [7].

Photosensitizers are chemicals, when excited, capable of transferring the energy absorbed to other compounds in the vicinity that, in turn, generate very reactive metastable species. The triplet-excited state of the photosensitizer releases energy to come to the ground state via two specific mechanisms: type I or type II pathway [18]. Type I pathway involves production of radical ions of oxygen due to electron transfer from the photosensitizer triplet-excited state to the substrate. Radical ions such as superoxide, hydroxyl, and lipid-derived ions are the cytotoxic species responsible for type I photoreaction [19]. Type II pathway involves production of excited singlet oxygen due to energy transfer from the photosensitizer triplet-excited state to the ground-state molecular oxygen, which is responsible for the oxidation of various cellular constituents [20]. The antimicrobial effect of PDT is mainly due to type II reaction. Singlet oxygen is a strong oxidizing agent and thus highly reactive, with a lifetime of less than 0.04 μs in a biological environment and a radius of action of less than 0.02 μm [21]. The reactions of singlet oxygen with the cellular targets lead to cell death. The above two basic mechanisms account for this lethal damage to the bacterial cell by DNA damage and cytoplasmic membrane damage. Figure 14.2 shows the photodynamic inactivation of bacterial cells in a stepwise manner. It should be noted that the differences in microbial cell wall characteristics and bacterial growth mode should be accounted while determining the duration of photosensitization before light illumination [22, 23]. The photosensitizer with slower uptake could result only in cell wall damage and with longer incubation times; other nuclear effects such as nucleic acid strand breakage might be apparent. The choice of photosensitizer is thus critical in obtaining effective bacterial elimination.

One of the significant advantages of PDT is the targeted antibacterial effect. Choosing a photosensitizer that has high affinity for microbial cells and irradiating the specific area of infection could result in the targeted effect of antimicrobial PDT. As the photosensitizer typically shows a higher affinity toward microbial cells, the host cells could be affected less during PDT. Toxicity of the photosensitizer usually occurs when high concentration/volume of photosensitizer is applied to a tissue to obtain more significant treatment response. The instant antimicrobial activity also offers added advantage as antibiotics take several days to produce comparable efficacy. The broad therapeutic window of PDT because of the high reactivity of ROS could effectively eliminate bacteria as well as the bacterial virulence factors such as endotoxins and proteolytic enzymes. Furthermore, due to the multiple targets of PDT on a bacterial cell, the probability of bacteria developing resistance to this treatment has been considered to be almost impossible [7, 8, 24].

Photosensitizers such as porphyrins, chlorins, and phthalocyanines, for treatment of cancer or other diseases, are chosen based upon their low dark toxicity to mammalian cells and ability to target tumor cells [8]. The photosensitizers for antibacterial PDT are chosen based on their specificity to bacterial cells. Large numbers of photosensitizer potentially useful in LAD are currently in various stages of clinical trials for FDA approval. The commonly used photosensitizers

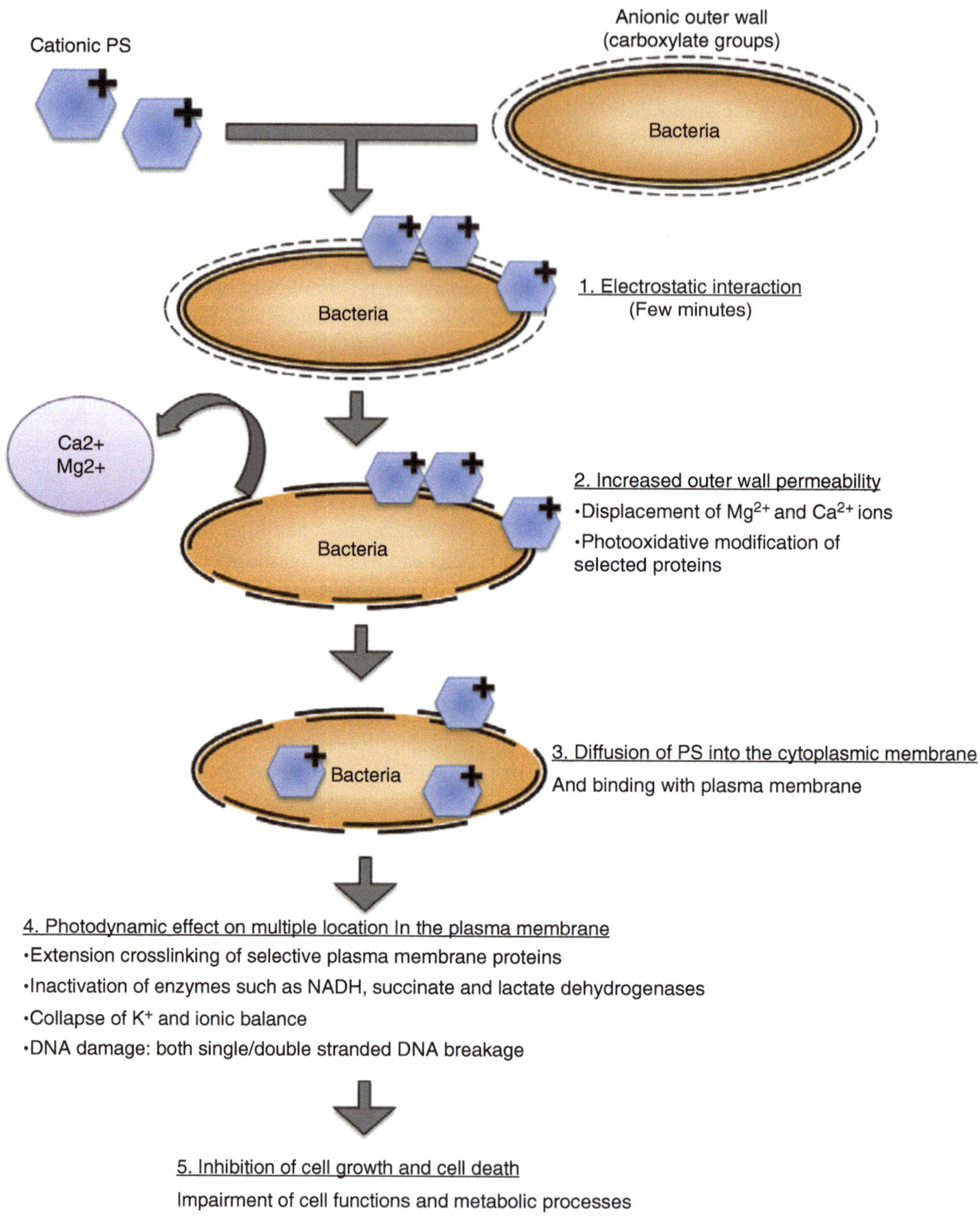

Fig. 14.2 Schematic showing the stepwise mechanism of photodynamic inactivation of microbial cells

for antibacterial purpose are halogenated xanthenes such as rose bengal (RB) [25], phenothiazines such as methylene blue (MB) and toluidine blue (TBO) [9, 22, 26], and perylenequinones such as hypericin [27]. The factors that determine the effectiveness of antibacterial PDT are method/vehicle of topical application, effective time of interaction with the microbes at the site of infection, selectivity of the photosensitizer to microbes, relative non-toxicity toward host tissues at the site of infection, and ability to eliminate the microbes effectively to avoid regrowth of surviving pathogens following treatment [8].

Antimicrobial PDT on gram-positive and gram-negative bacteria induced breaks in both single and double-stranded DNA and the disappearance of the plasmid supercoiled fraction [28, 29]. In addition, the photooxidative effect caused by the phenothiazinium photosensitizer in bacteria led to the damage of multiple targets in bacterial cells such as DNA [28], membrane integrity [30], protease activity, and lipopolysaccharide (LPS) [31]. George and Kishen reported functional impairment of cell wall, extensive damage to chromosomal DNA, and degradation of membrane proteins following methylene blue-mediated APDT of *E. faecalis* [32]. These findings support the hypothesis that antimicrobial PDT is a feasible alternative to antibiotics since the mode of action is markedly different from that typical of most antibiotics and chances of resistance are potentially none.

Antimicrobial PDT in Root Canal Disinfection

The use of PDT in conjunction with conventional root canal disinfection methods resulted in significantly better bacterial elimination as compared to either of these treatments when used alone. Over the years, various efforts were made to optimize different PDT-related parameters for endodontic application. Several in vitro and in vivo studies have shown the effectiveness of PDT in eliminating root canal biofilms [9, 33–42]. Endodontic pathogens such as *E. faecalis*, *P. intermedia*, *F. nucleatum*, *S. intermedius*, and *A. actinomycetemcomitans* have been shown to be killed by using photosensitizers such as methylene blue (MB), toluidine blue (TBO), and rose bengal (RB) [43–46].

Currently PDT is not considered a replacement for the existing root canal disinfection protocols but rather considered as a potential adjunct to improve antibiofilm efficacy following current disinfection protocols during the root canal treatment. Meire et al. [47] and George and Kishen [41, 43] used antimicrobial PDT to enhance the root canal disinfection. They showed that antimicrobial PDT could effectively kill biofilms of *E. faecalis* with photosensitizers such as MB and TBO along with red light. Soukos et al. conducted PDT experiments on a range of endodontic pathogens (methylene blue as photosensitizer) and reported complete elimination of all bacteria except *E. faecalis* (53 %) [34]. In yet another study, significant antibacterial effects on suspensions of *S. intermedius*, *P. micros*, *P. intermedia*, and *F. nucleatum* were reported by Williams et al. following PDT with TBO and red light [44]. Different in vivo studies that examined the efficacy of antimicrobial PDT in root canal disinfection have been summarized in Table 14.1 [26, 36–38]. These studies concluded that a combination of chemomechanical preparation and PDT would bring about maximum reduction in microbial loads.

Singlet oxygen is known to diffuse approximately 50 nm [18]. This emphasizes the close proximity of a photosensitizer molecule to the bacterial cell surface that allows diffusion of singlet oxygen. In a biofilm, only 30 % of the total mass is bacteria and remaining is the self-secreted extracellular polymeric matrix. The ability of the photosensitizer to diffuse and uniformly distribute in the biofilm structure is important for effective killing efficacy [48]. This clearly could be seen in the higher level of energy required to eliminate bacterial biofilms as compared to the planktonic counterparts [22, 46, 48, 49]. Bacteria existing in biofilms are also known to express active efflux pumps that confer their ability to transport amphiphilic chemicals and photosensitizers outside the cell [50]. This is the protective mechanism exerted by the cell to expel potentially toxic compounds. Both prokaryotic and eukaryotic cells possess various membrane proteins termed efflux pumps. Use of efflux pump inhibitors (EPI) such as verapamil would restore the antibacterial activity of a compound that is specific to an efflux mechanism. Both the phenothiazinium dyes such as MB and TBO are amphipathic cations that are potential substrate for multidrug efflux pumps [51]. Use of EPI with

Table 14.1 Table showing clinical studies where PDT was used for root canal disinfection

No	Author/date	Objective and materials	Methodology	Conclusion
1	Bonsor et al. (2006) [36]	Aimed to evaluate the antimicrobial efficacy of root canal disinfection by combining conventional endodontic treatment with PDT Clinical study on 32 root canals from 14 patients	Irrigation with 20 % citric acid and 2.25 % sodium hypochlorite PDT with TBO and diode laser (12.7 mg/L^{-1}, 100 mW, 120 s) Samples collected by filing	Cleaning and shaping resulted in complete bacterial killing in 86.7 % of samples Combination of cleaning and shaping + PDT resulted in complete bacterial killing in 96.7 % of samples
2	Bonsor et al. (2006) [26]	Aimed to compare the effect of a combination of 20 % citric acid and PDT with the use of 20 % citric acid and 2.25 % sodium hypochlorite on bacterial load in prepared root canals 64 patients were used	Procedure similar to previous study	Combination of 20 % citric acid and PDT resulted in complete bacterial killing in 91 % of samples 20 % citric acid and 2.25 % sodium hypochlorite resulted in complete bacterial killing in 82 % of samples
3	Garcez et al. (2008) [38]	This study analyzed the antimicrobial effect of PDT in association with endodontic treatment 20 patients were selected First session of cleaning and shaping + PDT At the end of first session, the root canal was filled with Ca(OH)(2), and after 1 week, a second session of PDT was performed	Irrigation with 2.5 % sodium hypochlorite, 3 % hydrogen peroxide, and 17 % EDTA PDT with polyethylenimine (PEI) chlorin (e6) conjugate (2 min, 9.6 J, 240 s) Paper point sampling	First session produced 98.5 % bacterial reduction (1.83 log reduction) Second session produced 99.9 % bacterial reduction (1.14 log reduction) Second session PDT was observed to be more effective than first session
4	Garcez et al. (2010) [37]	Studied antimicrobial effect of PDT combined with endodontic treatment in patients with necrotic pulp infected with microflora resistant to a previous antibiotic therapy 30 teeth from 21 patients with periapical lesions that had been treated with conventional endodontic treatment and antibiotic therapy were selected	PDT used polyethylenimine chlorin (e6) as a photosensitizer and a diode laser (40 mW, 4 min, 9.6 J)	Endodontic therapy alone produced a significant reduction in numbers of microbial species (only 3 teeth were free of bacteria) The combination of endodontic therapy with PDT eliminated all drug-resistant species and all teeth were bacteria-free

phenothiaziniums resulted in significantly enhanced biofilm elimination at much lower PDT dosage [45, 52, 53]. Since efflux pumps are highly active in bacterial biofilms, use of EPI could potentially enhance the antibiofilm efficacy of PDT inside root canals. Kishen et al. have demonstrated the enhanced ability of EPI in combination with MB photosensitizer to disinfect biofilm bacteria as well biofilm-derived bacteria [45, 52].

In addition to the limitations associated with the interaction/uptake of photosensitizer by intracanal bacterial biofilms, tissue-specific constraining factors in the application of PDT for endodontic disinfection also need special consideration. Some of the tissue-specific constraining factors in the application of PDT for endodontic disinfection are the limited penetration of the light energy into the infected tissue, lack of optimum photosensitizer concentration within the infected tissue, low oxygen tension inside the root canals, and dentin discoloration by the photosensitizer. These issues need to be addressed before establishing PDT as a definitive treatment step in root canal disinfection [33, 41].

In biological tissue, absorption of light is mainly due to the presence of free water molecules, proteins, pigments, and other macromolecules. The absorption coefficient strongly depends on the wavelength of the incoming light/laser irradiation. Scattering of light in tissue has the utmost effect on light intensity and directionality. Scattering, together with refraction, causes a widening of light beam, resulting in the loss of fluence rate (power per unit area) and a change in directionality of the light beam. Tissue-specific approach has been highlighted by George and Kishen, which improved the antimicrobial efficacy of PDT in root canal system. Methylene blue was dissolved in different formulations such as water, 70 % glycerol, 70 % poly ethylene glycol, and a mixture of glycerol-ethanol-water (MIX) in a ratio of 30:20:50 and analyzed for the photophysical, photochemical, and photobiological characteristics [43]. The aggregation of methylene blue molecules was significantly higher in water when compared to other formulations. In addition, the MIX-based methylene blue formulation had effective penetration into dentinal tubules and enhanced singlet oxygen generation, which in turn improved bactericidal action. A significantly higher impairment of bacterial cell wall and extensive damage to chromosomal DNA were observed when methylene blue in a MIX-based formulation was used and when compared to water [32]. The same group also showed that the incorporation of an oxidizer and oxygen carrier with photosensitizer formulation in the form of an emulsion would produce significant photooxidation capabilities, which in turn facilitated comprehensive disruption of matured endodontic biofilm structure [41].

Antimicrobial PDT has the potential to destroy microbial cells as well as mammalian cells. However, the selective killing of microbial cells over host cells is specific to the photosensitization periods and light fluence required for the antimicrobial effects. Soukos et al. compared the effect of PDT using a combination of toluidine blue O (TBO) and red light against *S. sanguis* and human gingival keratinocytes and fibroblasts. They reported no reduction in the human cell viability, whereas the bacteria were effectively killed [54]. Soncin et al. reported the selective killing of *S. aureus* over human fibroblasts and keratinocytes (four to six fold) when subjected to PDT using cationic phthalocyanine and relatively low light fluencies [55]. George and Kishen demonstrated a 97.7 % killing of *Enterococcus faecalis* compared to a 30 % human fibroblast dysfunction following methylene blue-mediated PDT [9]. Even the newer photosensitizer-conjugated chitosan nanoparticles showed favorable cell survival (fibroblasts) as compared to highly effective antibiofilm properties [48, 56]. All these in vitro studies suggested the targeted killing efficacy of antimicrobial PDT.

Conjugating photosensitizer to various agents or chemical moieties can result in improved photosensitizers for PDT. These modified photosensitizers are expected to bind more effectively to the outer membrane of bacteria and upon activation of generated reactive oxygen species, which then diffused into the cells, resulting in cell death. Therefore, photo-generated oxidative species are well confined to the cell wall and its vicinity, which is a highly susceptible domain for photodynamic action. Soukos and coworkers formed a hypothesis that by covalently conjugating a suitable photosensitizer to a *poly-l-lysine* chain, a bacteria-targeted photosensitizer delivery vehicle could be constructed that would efficiently inactivate both gram-positive and gram-negative species [57]. This was demonstrated by preparing a conjugate of chlorin (e6) and a *poly-l-lysine* chain (20 lysine residues), which after 1 min incubation and illumination with red light killed >99 % of the gram-positive *Actinomyces viscosus* and gram-negative *Porphyromonas gingivalis* [58]. Conjugates of polyethylenimine and chlorin (e6) when used as a photosensitizer eliminated all the drug-resistant bacteria during retreatment in failed root canal-treated teeth [37]. This PEI-ce6 conjugate eliminated both gram-positive and gram-negative bacteria in vitro and in vivo as compared to the commonly used photosensitizer TBO [59]. Anionic photosensitizer (rose bengal) conjugated with positively charged chitosan has also been shown to be highly effective in removing biofilms of gram-positive, gram-negative, and multispecies bacteria [48, 60, 61] (Fig. 14.3). Shrestha et al. showed that the rose bengal-conjugated chitosan presented a synergistic effect of the antimicrobial polymer chitosan and singlet oxygen that was generated following photoactivation [48, 56]. The chitosan-conjugated rose bengal nanoparticles (CSRBnp) penetrated deep into the biofilm structure and photoactivation resulted in total elimination of the multispecies biofilms of bacteria associated with endodontic infection [61]. These modified photosensitizers in nano-form were found to envelope the bacterial cells within minutes of the photosensitization period (Fig. 14.4) [48]. Irradiation of these bacteria with closely adhered CSRBnp resulted in total killing with various stages of membrane damage as well as release of cell constituents.

Constituents of the infected root canal such as tissue remnants (pulp tissue), serum products, and dentin matrix compromised the antimicrobial efficacy of not only the common endodontic irrigants [62] but also the antimicrobial efficacy of PDT [63]. Most studies concerning the antimi-

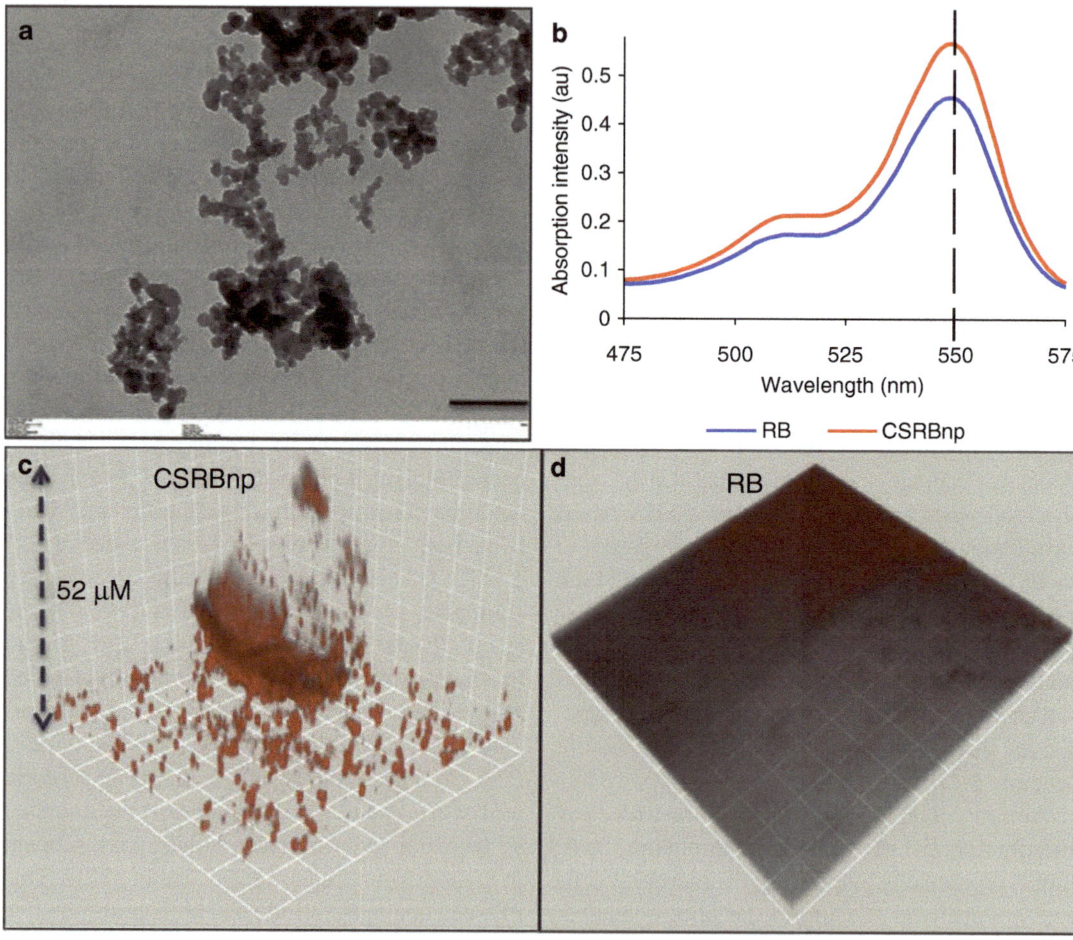

Fig. 14.3 (**a**) Transmission electron microscopic image of CSRBnp (scale bar = 200 nm). The CSRBnps were 60 ± 20 nm in size. (**b**) A typical graph showing the absorption spectrum of RB and CSRBnps. The absorption peak at 550 nm was not affected after conjugation of CSRBnps with RB. (**c**, **d**) The uptake of CSRBnps and RB into the *E. faecalis* biofilms as observed under CLSM. (**e**–**g**) Scanning electron microscopic images of multispecies biofilms on dentin sections. (**e**) The 3-week-old biofilms presented as a uniformly thick matlike structure covering the entire dentin surface. Three specific bacterial morphologies are evident in higher magnification (Denoted by *, + and *block white arrowhead*). The surface showed an abundant polymeric matrix (*open arrowhead*) (magnified area shown by the *open arrow*). (**f**) CSRBnp treatment rendered the dentin surface clean of the biofilm with open dentinal tubules. (**g**) RB treatment showed cleaner areas of dentin along with dense bacterial aggregates (*inset*: magnified area shown by the *white arrow*) (Adapted with permission from Shrestha and Kishen [61])

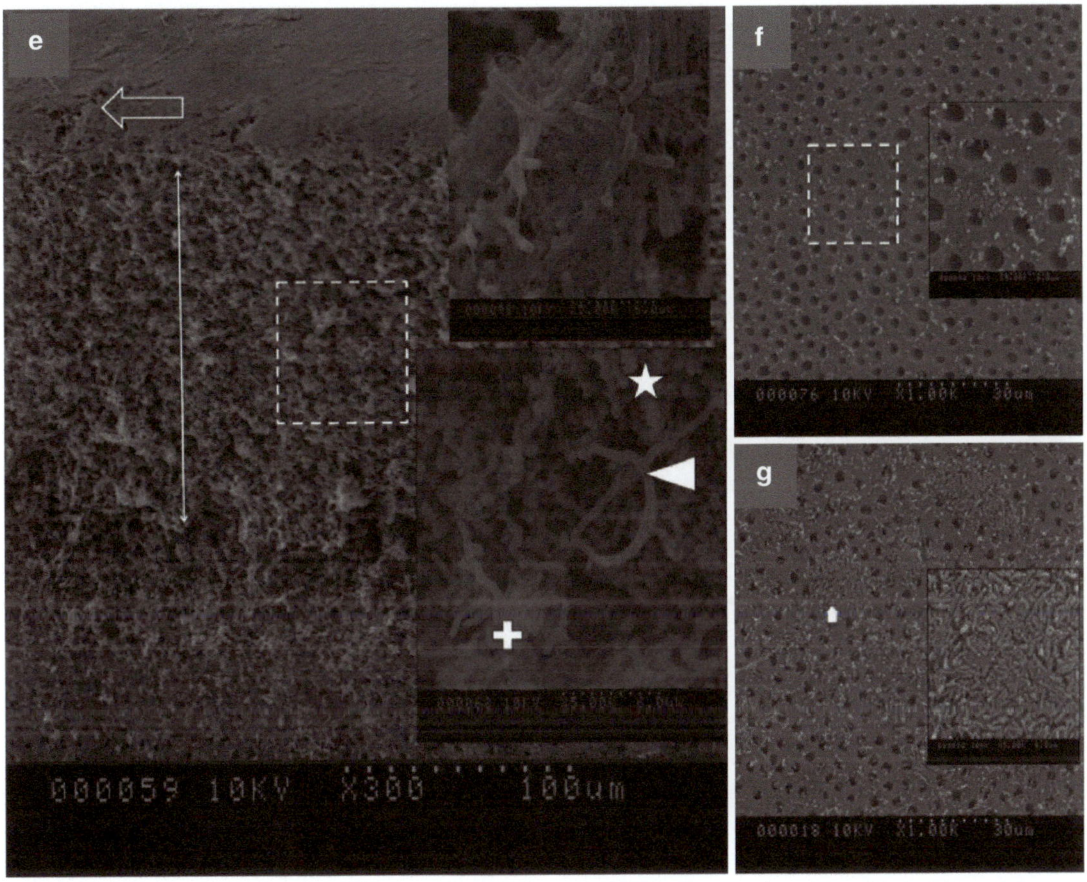

Fig. 14.3 (continued)

crobial PDT of microbial pathogens use deionized water or phosphate-buffered saline to dissolve the photosensitizer. In some studies the photosensitizer was dissolved in brain-heart infusion broth wherein reduced bactericidal effect was reported. This reduction in antibacterial effect was attributed it to the presence of serum proteins in the broth [34, 64]. This effect is either due to cross-linking action or the compromised half-life of singlet oxygen in the presence of proteins.

Both coherent (lasers) and noncoherent (lamps) light sources are used for antimicrobial PDT. The choice of light source is dictated by the location, the required light dose, and the choice of photosensitizer. Laser provides monochromatic, coherent, and collimated light, offering wide range of output power. Laser light can be easily coupled into a fiber-optic cable, which can serve as a delivery system (probe) while irradiating complex anatomy such as a root canal. Nd:YAG, KTP, HeNe, GaAlAs and diode lasers, light-emitting diodes (LEDs), and xenon arc lamps have been employed for APDT. The superiority of one type of light source over the other has not been clearly demonstrated [65]. Recent study evaluated the importance of using optical fiber/diffuser inside the root canal instead of laser tip at the root canal orifice [66] (Fig. 14.5). The rationale for using the optical fiber is mainly to allow better distribution of light energy throughout the infected root canal/root dentin. Notched optical fiber was also used to allow light distribution in 360° [39]. Optical fiber/diffuser allowed uniform light distribution throughout the canal length and enhanced the antimicrobial efficacy of PDT by reducing the bacterial biofilm 2 logs more than the PDT with laser tip at the canal orifice.

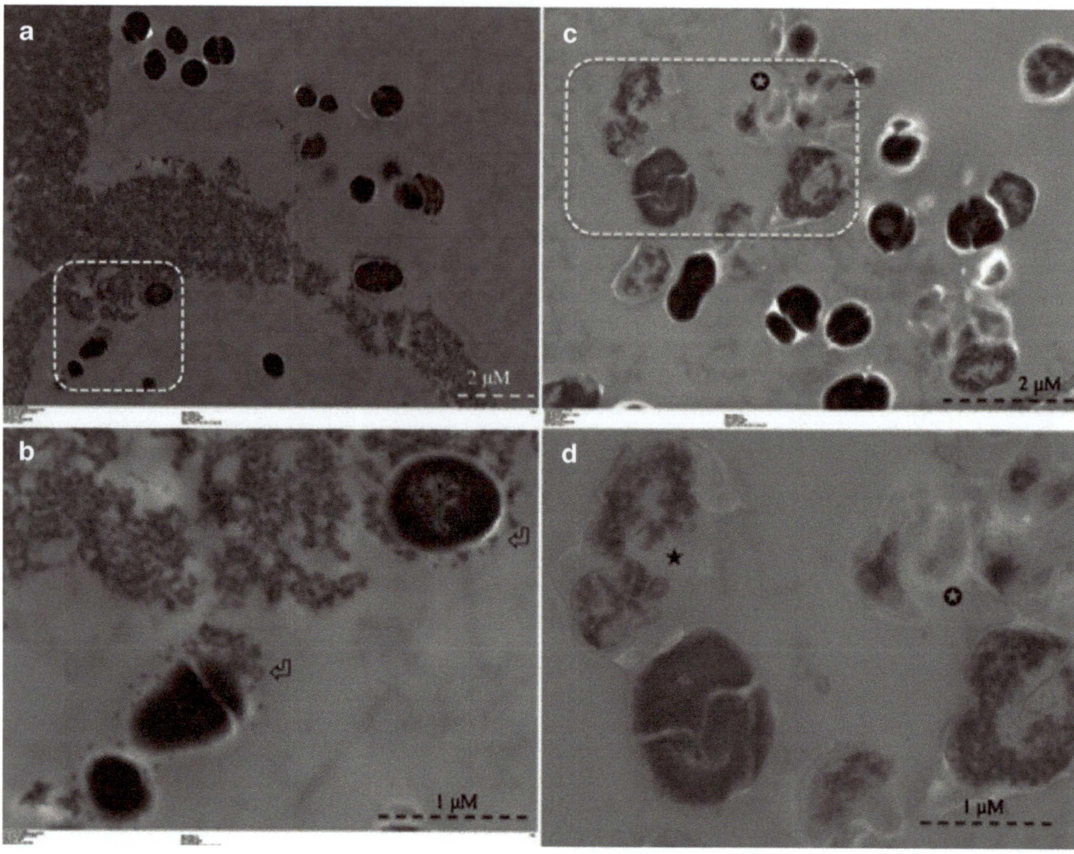

Fig. 14.4 Transmission electron microscopy images for planktonic *E. faecalis* after treatment with CSRBnp for 15 min (**a**, **b**). Aggregates of CSRBnp could be seen surrounding the bacterial cell. Nanoparticles were found attached to the bacterial cell surface and forming an envelope (*open arrows*) (**b**). The cells did not show any disruption of morphology. Following PDT of the sensitized bacteria, various stages of membrane damage as well as release of cell constituents were evident (**c, d**). Most of the bacteria showed some kind of cell membrane disruption (*black star*) and release of cell constituents at higher magnification (**d**) (Adapted with permission from Shrestha et al. [48])

There are a number of commercial PDT systems available for root canal and caries disinfection. Some of the available systems are Savedent, Denfotex PAD, and HELBO photodynamic systems that use TBO and methylene blue as photosensitizers, respectively [67]. These two systems differed in the choice of photosensitizers and their concentration, photosensitization time, fiber-optic probe design, and wavelengths of the lasers used. Although the Denfotex PAD showed significant reduction of planktonic *E. faecalis* [47], both these systems failed to reduce the biofilm bacteria grown on dentin discs. A recent systematic review by Siddiqui et al. [68] reported results of seventeen studies that used various forms of PDT to eliminate *E. faecalis* from infected root canals. The review clearly highlights that the discrepancies in the use of PDT for root canal disinfection are wide, resulting in highly variable findings from each of the studies included in the review (Tables 14.2 and 14.3). Out of the 17 studies included in the review [34, 37, 65, 70–83], 70 % concluded the beneficial effects of PDT in removing *E. faecalis* from root canals as compared to conventional disinfection treatments.

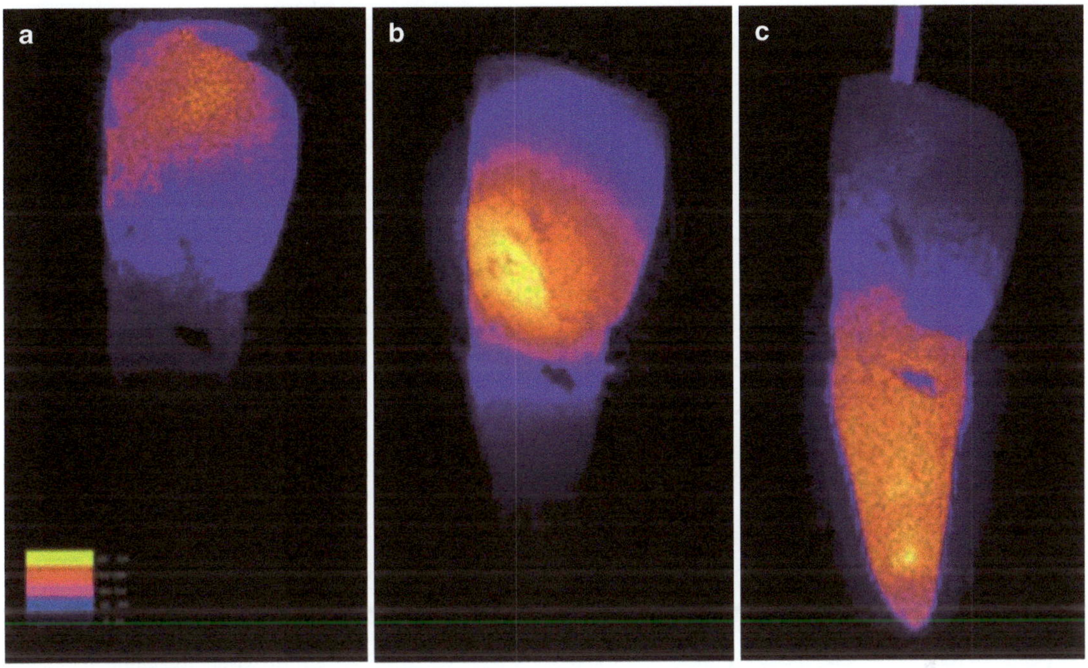

Fig. 14.5 Representative image of the light-scattering intensity of each group. Image J software transforms the black-white image in a false color image according to the light intensity between values minimum of 0 for no light and 256 for maximum light intensity. (**a**) G3, irradiation with the larger laser tip; (**b**) G4, irradiation with the smaller laser tip; and (**c**) G5, irradiation with the laser optical fiber/diffuser (Adapted with permission from Garcez et al. [67])

Conclusion

Elimination of bacterial biofilm from the infected root canal system remains to be the primary focus in the management of endodontic disease. Current research is directed to potentiate the antibiofilm efficacy of PDT by developing newer photosensitizers, by altering the photosensitizer formulation, and by combining the advantages of photodynamic effect with bioactive antimicrobial microparticles [56, 60, 84] and nanoparticles [48, 61, 74]. The key to the successful application of these newer antibacterial strategies for the treatment of root canal biofilms is to address all the tissue-specific issues in entirety rather than focusing only on the antibacterial aspect. Further research is mandatory to improve the antibiofilm efficacy of PDT in the presence of tissue inhibitors, to optimize light delivery within the root canal, and to optimize new photosensitizers and/or formulations for application within the root canal. A standardized protocol for photosensitization and light activation is paramount for endodontic disinfection using PDT.

Table 14.2 Laser parameters of studies showing positive outcomes of photodynamic therapy toward elimination of *Enterococcus faecalis* from infected root canals

Authors et al.	Laser wavelength (nm)	Diameter of fiber in µm	Power output (in mW)	Power density (mW/cm^2)	Energy fluence (in J/cm^2)	Duration of irradiation (in min)	Photosensitizer (concentration in µg/mL)
Bago et al. [70]	660	320	100	–	–	1	(a) Phenothiazine chloride (10^3 µg/mL) (b) TBO (155 µg/mL)
Vaziri et al. [71]	625	–	–	200	12	1	TBO (15 µg/mL)
Foschi et al. [65]	665	500	–	100	60	5	MB (6.25 µg/mL)
Soukos et al. [34]	665	500	1,000	100	30	5	MB (25 µg/mL)
Rios et al. [73]	628	–	–	–	–	0.5	TBO (–)
Pagonis et al. [74]	665	250	1,000	100	60	10	MB (6.25 µg/mL)
Fonseca et al. [75]	660	600	50	–	400	5	TBO (–)
Bergmans et al. [76]	635	300	100	–	–	1.5	TBO (12.5×10^3 µg/mL)
Poggio et al. [77]	628	–	1,000	–	–	0.5 1.5	(a) TBO (100 µg/mL) (b) TBO (100 µg/mL)
Nagayoshi et al. [78]	805	400	5,000	–	–	2	Indocyanine green (12.5×10^3 µg/mL)
Schlafer et al. [79]	628	4×10^3	1,000	–	–	0.5	TBO (100 µg/mL)
Garcez et al. [37]	660	200	40	–	–	4	Conjugate between polyethylenimine and chlorin (~19 µg/mL)

Adapted and modified with permission from Siddiqui et al. [69]
MB methylene blue, *TBO* toluidine blue

Table 14.3 Laser parameters of studies that reported photodynamic therapy to be ineffective toward elimination of *Enterococcus faecalis* from infected root canals

Authors et al.	Laser wavelength (nm)	Diameter of fiber in µm	Power output (in mW)	Power density (mW/cm^2)	Energy fluence (in J/cm^2)	Duration of irradiation (in min)	Photosensitizer (concentration in µg/mL)
Nunes et al. [72]	660	216	90	–	–	5	MB (100 µg/mL)
Hecker et al. [80]	635	–	200	–	–	6	TBO (–)
Souza et al. [81]	660	300	40	–	–	4	(a) MB (–) (b) TBO (–)
Cheng et al. [83]	660	2,000	200	–	–	1	MB (10 µg/ml)

Adapted and modified with permission from Siddiqui et al. [69]
MB methylene blue, *TBO* toluidine blue

References

1. Lewis K. Riddle of biofilm resistance. Antimicrob Agents Chemother. 2001;45:999–1007.
2. Finegold SM. Intestinal microbial changes and disease as a result of antimicrobial use. Pediatr Infect Dis. 1986;5:S88–90.
3. del Pozo JL, Patel R. The challenge of treating biofilm-associated bacterial infections. Clin Pharmacol Ther. 2007;82:204–9.
4. Vakulenko SB, Mobashery S. Versatility of aminoglycosides and prospects for their future. Clin Microbiol Rev. 2003;16:430–50.
5. Cunha BA. Antibiotic resistance. Control strategies. Crit Care Clin. 1998;14:309–27.
6. Smith AW. Biofilms and antibiotic therapy: is there a role for combating bacterial resistance by the use of novel drug delivery systems? Adv Drug Deliv Rev. 2005;57:1539–50.
7. Dai T, Huang YY, Hamblin MR. Photodynamic therapy for localized infections–state of the art. Photodiagnosis Photodyn Ther. 2009;6:170–88.
8. Hamblin MR, Hasan T. Photodynamic therapy: a new antimicrobial approach to infectious disease? Photochem Photobiol Sci. 2004;3:436–50.
9. George S, Kishen A. Advanced noninvasive light-activated disinfection: assessment of cytotoxicity on fibroblast versus antimicrobial activity against Enterococcus faecalis. J Endod. 2007;33:599–602.
10. Jori G, Brown SB. Photosensitized inactivation of microorganisms. Photochem Photobiol Sci. 2004; 3:403–5.
11. Weishaupt KR, Gomer CJ, Dougherty TJ. Identification of singlet oxygen as the cytotoxic agent in photoinactivation of a murine tumor. Cancer Res. 1976;36:2326–9.
12. Niedre MJ, Secord AJ, Patterson MS, Wilson BC. In vitro tests of the validity of singlet oxygen luminescence measurements as a dose metric in photodynamic therapy. Cancer Res. 2003;63:7986–94.
13. Raab O. Ueber die Wirkung fluorescirender Stoffe auf Infusorien. Z Biol. 1900;39:524–46.
14. Hamblin MR, Paweł M. History of PDT: the first hundred years. In: Hamblin MR, Paweł M, editors. Advances in photodynamic therapy- basic, translational, and clinical. Norwood: Artech House; 2007. p. 1–9.
15. Wollensak G, Wilsch M, Spoerl E, Seiler T. Collagen fiber diameter in the rabbit cornea after collagen crosslinking by riboflavin/UVA. Cornea. 2004;23: 503–7.
16. Rafat M, Li F, Fagerholm P, Lagali NS, Watsky MA, Munger R, et al. PEG-stabilized carbodiimide crosslinked collagen-chitosan hydrogels for corneal tissue engineering. Biomaterials. 2008;29:3960–72.
17. Chan BP, Kochevar IE, Redmond RW. Enhancement of porcine skin graft adherence using a light-activated process. J Surg Res. 2002;108:77–84.
18. Ochsner M. Photophysical and photobiological processes in the photodynamic therapy of tumours. J Photochem Photobiol B. 1997;39:1–18.
19. Athar M, Mukhtar H, Bickers DR. Differential role of reactive oxygen intermediates in photofrin-I- and photofrin-II-mediated photoenhancement of lipid peroxidation in epidermal microsomal membranes. J Invest Dermatol. 1988;90:652–7.
20. Redmond RW, Gamlin JN. A compilation of singlet oxygen yields from biologically relevant molecules. Photochem Photobiol. 1999;70:391–475.
21. Moan J, Berg K. The photodegradation of porphyrins in cells can be used to estimate the lifetime of singlet oxygen. Photochem Photobiol. 1991;53:549–53.
22. George S, Hamblin MR, Kishen A. Uptake pathways of anionic and cationic photosensitizers into bacteria. Photochem Photobiol Sci. 2009;8:788–95.
23. Hamblin MR, O'Donnell DA, Murthy N, Rajagopalan K, Michaud N, Sherwood ME, et al. Polycationic photosensitizer conjugates: effects of chain length and Gram classification on the photodynamic inactivation of bacteria. J Antimicrob Chemother. 2002;49:941–51.
24. Wainwright M. Antimicrobial application- photodynamic antimicrobial chemotherapy. In: Wainwright M, editor. Photosensitizers in biomedicine. West Sussex: Wiley-Blackwell; 2009. p. 237–54.
25. Dahl TA, Midden WR, Neckers DC. Comparison of photodynamic action by Rose Bengal in gram-positive and gram-negative bacteria. Photochem Photobiol. 1988;48:607–12.
26. Bonsor SJ, Nichol R, Reid TMS, Pearson GJ. An alternative regimen for root canal disinfection. Br Dent J. 2006;201:101–5.
27. Kubin A, Wierrani F, Jindra RH, Loew HG, Grunberger W, Ebermann R, et al. Antagonistic effects of combination photosensitization by hypericin, meso-tetrahydroxyphenylchlorin (mTHPC) and photofrin II on Staphylococcus aureus. Drugs Exp Clin Res. 1999;25:13–21.
28. Menezes S, Capella MAM, Caldas LR. Photodynamic-action of methylene-blue – repair and mutation in escherichia-coli. J Photochem Photobiol B. 1990; 5:505–17.
29. Bertoloni G, Lauro FM, Cortella G, Merchat M. Photosensitizing activity of hematoporphyrin on Staphylococcus aureus cells. Biochim Biophys Acta. 2000;1475:169–74.
30. Wakayama Y, Takagi M, Yano K. Photosensitized inactivation of E. coli cells in toluidine blue-light system. Photochem Photobiol. 1980;32:601–5.
31. Komerik N, Wilson M, Poole S. The effect of photodynamic action on two virulence factors of gram-negative bacteria. Photochem Photobiol. 2000;72: 676–80.
32. George S, Kishen A. Influence of photosensitizer solvent on the mechanisms of photoactivated killing of Enterococcus faecalis. Photochem Photobiol. 2008; 84:734–40.

33. Lim Z, Cheng JL, Lim TW, Teo EG, Wong J, George S, et al. Light activated disinfection: an alternative endodontic disinfection strategy. Aust Dent J. 2009;54:108–14.
34. Soukos NS, Chen PS, Morris JT, Ruggiero K, Abernethy AD, Som S, et al. Photodynamic therapy for endodontic disinfection. J Endod. 2006;32: 979–84.
35. Soukos NS, Ximenez-Fyvie LA, Hamblin MR, Socransky SS, Hasan T. Targeted antimicrobial photochemotherapy. Antimicrob Agents Chemother. 1998;42:2595–601.
36. Bonsor SJ, Nichol R, Reid TM, Pearson GJ. Microbiological evaluation of photo-activated disinfection in endodontics (an in vivo study). Br Dent J. 2006;200:337–41, discussion 29.
37. Garcez AS, Nunez SC, Hamblim MR, Suzuki H, Ribeiro MS. Photodynamic therapy associated with conventional endodontic treatment in patients with antibiotic-resistant microflora: a preliminary report. J Endod. 2010;36:1463–6.
38. Garcez AS, Nunez SC, Hamblin MR, Ribeiro MS. Antimicrobial effects of photodynamic therapy on patients with necrotic pulps and periapical lesion. J Endod. 2008;34:138–42.
39. Fimple JL, Fontana CR, Foschi F, Ruggiero K, Song X, Pagonis TC, et al. Photodynamic treatment of endodontic polymicrobial infection in vitro. J Endod. 2008;34:728–34.
40. Ng R, Singh F, Papamanou DA, Song X, Patel C, Holewa C, et al. Endodontic photodynamic therapy ex vivo. J Endod. 2011;37:217–22.
41. George S, Kishen A. Augmenting the antibiofilm efficacy of advanced noninvasive light activated disinfection with emulsified oxidizer and oxygen carrier. J Endod. 2008;34:1119–23.
42. Silva LA, Novaes Jr AB, de Oliveira RR, Nelson-Filho P, Santamaria Jr M, Silva RA. Antimicrobial photodynamic therapy for the treatment of teeth with apical periodontitis: a histopathological evaluation. J Endod. 2012;38:360–6.
43. George S, Kishen A. Photophysical, photochemical, and photobiological characterization of methylene blue formulations for light-activated root canal disinfection. J Biomed Opt. 2007;12:034029.
44. Williams JA, Pearson GJ, Colles MJ. Antibacterial action of photoactivated disinfection {PAD} used on endodontic bacteria in planktonic suspension and in artificial and human root canals. J Dent. 2006;34: 363–71.
45. Upadya MH, Kishen A. Influence of bacterial growth modes on the susceptibility to light-activated disinfection. Int Endod J. 2010;43(11):978–87.
46. Kishen A, Upadya M, Tegos GP, Hamblin MR. Efflux pump inhibitor potentiates antimicrobial photodynamic inactivation of Enterococcus faecalis biofilm. Photochem Photobiol. 2010;86:1343–9.
47. Meire MA, De Prijck K, Coenye T, Nelis HJ, De Moor RJG. Effectiveness of different laser systems to kill Enterococcus faecalis in aqueous suspension and in an infected tooth model. Int Endod J. 2009;42:351–9.
48. Shrestha A, Hamblin MR, Kishen A. Photoactivated rose bengal functionalized chitosan nanoparticles produce antibacterial/biofilm activity and stabilize dentin-collagen. Nanomedicine. 2014;10:491–501.
49. Kishen A. Advanced therapeutic options for endodontic biofilms. Endod Topics. 2012;22:99–123.
50. Kvist M, Hancock V, Klemm P. Inactivation of efflux pumps abolishes bacterial biofilm formation. Appl Environ Microbiol. 2008;74:7376–82.
51. Tegos GP, Hamblin MR. Phenothiazinium antimicrobial photosensitizers are substrates of bacterial multidrug resistance pumps. Antimicrob Agents Chemother. 2006;50:196–203.
52. Upadya M, Shrestha A, Kishen A. Role of efflux pump inhibitors on the antibiofilm efficacy of calcium hydroxide, chitosan nanoparticles, and light-activated disinfection. J Endod. 2011;37:1422–6.
53. Tegos GP, Masago K, Aziz F, Higginbotham A, Stermitz FR, Hamblin MR. Inhibitors of bacterial multidrug efflux pumps potentiate antimicrobial photoinactivation. Antimicrob Agents Chemother. 2008; 52:3202–9.
54. Kishen A, Upadya M, Tegos GP, Hamblin MR. Efflux pump inhibitor potentiates antimicrobial photodynamic inactivation of Enterococcus faecalis biofilm. Photochem Photobiol. 2010;86(6):1343–9.
55. Soukos NS, Wilson M, Burns T, Speight PM. Photodynamic effects of toluidine blue on human oral keratinocytes and fibroblasts and Streptococcus sanguis evaluated in vitro. Lasers Surg Med. 1996;18: 253–9.
56. Soncin M, Fabris C, Busetti A, Dei D, Nistri D, Roncucci G, et al. Approaches to selectivity in the Zn(II)-phthalocyanine-photosensitized inactivation of wild-type and antibiotic-resistant Staphylococcus aureus. Photochem Photobiol Sci. 2002;1:815–9.
57. Shrestha A, Hamblin MR, Kishen A. Characterization of a conjugate between Rose Bengal and chitosan for targeted antibiofilm and tissue stabilization effects as a potential treatment of infected dentin. Antimicrob Agents Chemother. 2012;56:4876–84.
58. Gross S, Brandis A, Chen L, Rosenbach-Belkin V, Roehrs S, Scherz A, et al. Protein-A-mediated targeting of Bacteriochlorophyll-IgG to Staphylococcus aureus: a model for enhanced site-specific photocytotoxicity. Photochem Photobiol. 1997;66:872–8.
59. Soukos NS, Hamblin MR, Hasan T. The effect of charge on cellular uptake and phototoxicity of polylysine chlorin(e6) conjugates. Photochem Photobiol. 1997;65:723–9.
60. Demidova TN, Hamblin MR. Effect of cell-photosensitizer binding and cell density on microbial photoinactivation. Antimicrob Agents Chemother. 2005;49: 2329–35.
61. Shrestha A, Kishen A. Polycationic chitosan conjugated photosensitizer for antibacterial photodynamic

therapy(dagger). Photochem Photobiol. 2012;88(3): 577–83.
62. Shrestha A, Kishen A. Antibiofilm efficacy of photosensitizer-functionalized bioactive nanoparticles on multispecies biofilm. J Endod. 2014;40(10):1604–10.
63. Portenier I, Haapasalo H, Orstavik D, Yamauchi M, Haapasalo M. Inactivation of the antibacterial activity of iodine potassium iodide and chlorhexidine digluconate against Enterococcus faecalis by dentin, dentin matrix, type-I collagen, and heat-killed microbial whole cells. J Endod. 2002;28:634–7.
64. Shrestha A, Kishen A. The effect of tissue inhibitors on the antibacterial activity of chitosan nanoparticles and photodynamic therapy. J Endod. 2012;38: 1275–8.
65. Foschi F, Fontana CR, Ruggiero K, Riahi R, Vera A, Doukas AG, et al. Photodynamic inactivation of Enterococcus faecalis in dental root canals in vitro. Lasers Surg Med. 2007;39:782–7.
66. Prasad PN. Introduction to biophotonics. John Wiley & Sons: Hoboken, New Jersey; 2003.
67. Garcez AS, Fregnani ER, Rodriguez HM, Nunez SC, Sabino CP, Suzuki H, et al. The use of optical fiber in endodontic photodynamic therapy. Is it really relevant? Lasers Med Sci. 2013;28:79–85.
68. Meire MA, Coenye T, Nelis HJ, De Moor RJ. Evaluation of Nd:YAG and Er:YAG irradiation, antibacterial photodynamic therapy and sodium hypochlorite treatment on Enterococcus faecalis biofilms. Int Endod J. 2012;45:482–91.
69. Siddiqui SH, Awan KH, Javed F. Bactericidal efficacy of photodynamic therapy against Enterococcus faecalis in infected root canals: a systematic literature review. Photodiagnosis Photodyn Ther. 2013;10: 632–43.
70. Bago I, Plecko V, Gabric Panduric D, Schauperl Z, Baraba A, Anic I. Antimicrobial efficacy of a high-power diode laser, photo-activated disinfection, conventional and sonic activated irrigation during root canal treatment. Int Endod J. 2013;46:339–47.
71. Vaziri S, Kangarlou A, Shahbazi R, Nazari Nasab A, Naseri M. Comparison of the bactericidal efficacy of photodynamic therapy, 2.5% sodium hypochlorite, and 2% chlorhexidine against Enterococcous faecalis in root canals; an in vitro study. Dent Res J (Isfahan). 2012;9:613–8.
72. Nunes MR, Mello I, Franco GC, de Medeiros JM, Dos Santos SS, Habitante SM, et al. Effectiveness of photodynamic therapy against Enterococcus faecalis, with and without the use of an intracanal optical fiber: an in vitro study. Photomed Laser Surg. 2011; 29:803–8.
73. Rios A, He J, Glickman GN, Spears R, Schneiderman ED, Honeyman AL. Evaluation of photodynamic therapy using a light-emitting diode lamp against Enterococcus faecalis in extracted human teeth. J Endod. 2011;37:856–9.
74. Pagonis TC, Chen J, Fontana CR, Devalapally H, Ruggiero K, Song X, et al. Nanoparticle-based endodontic antimicrobial photodynamic therapy. J Endod. 2010;36:322–8.
75. Fonseca MB, Junior PO, Pallota RC, Filho HF, Denardin OV, Rapoport A, et al. Photodynamic therapy for root canals infected with Enterococcus faecalis. Photomed Laser Surg. 2008;26:209–13.
76. Bergmans L, Moisiadis P, Huybrechts B, Van Meerbeek B, Quirynen M, Lambrechts P. Effect of photo-activated disinfection on endodontic pathogens ex vivo. Int Endod J. 2008;41:227–39.
77. Poggio C, Arciola CR, Dagna A, Florindi F, Chiesa M, Saino E, et al. Photoactivated disinfection (PAD) in endodontics: an in vitro microbiological evaluation. Int J Artif Organs. 2011;34:889–97.
78. Nagayoshi M, Nishihara T, Nakashima K, Iwaki S, Chen KK, Terashita M, et al. Bactericidal effects of diode laser irradiation on Enterococcus faecalis using periapical lesion defect model. ISRN Dent. 2011;2011:870364.
79. Schlafer S, Vaeth M, Horsted-Bindslev P, Frandsen EV. Endodontic photoactivated disinfection using a conventional light source: an in vitro and ex vivo study. Oral Surg Oral Med Oral Pathol Oral Radiol Endod. 2010;109:634–41.
80. Hecker S, Hiller KA, Galler KM, Erb S, Mader T, Schmalz G. Establishment of an optimized ex vivo system for artificial root canal infection evaluated by use of sodium hypochlorite and the photodynamic therapy. Int Endod J. 2013;46:449–57.
81. Souza LC, Brito PR, de Oliveira JC, Alves FR, Moreira EJ, Sampaio-Filho HR, et al. Photodynamic therapy with two different photosensitizers as a supplement to instrumentation/irrigation procedures in promoting intracanal reduction of Enterococcus faecalis. J Endod. 2010;36:292–6.
82. Miranda RG, Santos EB, Souto RM, Gusman H, Colombo AP. Ex vivo antimicrobial efficacy of the EndoVac system plus photodynamic therapy associated with calcium hydroxide against intracanal Enterococcus faecalis. Int Endod J. 2013;46:499–505.
83. Cheng X, Guan S, Lu H, Zhao C, Chen X, Li N, et al. Evaluation of the bactericidal effect of Nd:YAG, Er:YAG, Er, Cr:YSGG laser radiation, and antimicrobial photodynamic therapy (aPDT) in experimentally infected root canals. Lasers Surg Med. 2012;44: 824–31.
84. Wainwright M, Giddens RM. Phenothiazinium photosensitisers: choices in synthesis and application. Dyes Pigm. 2003;57:245–57.

15 Local Applications of Antibiotics and Antibiotic-Based Agents in Endodontics

Zahed Mohammadi and Paul V. Abbott

Abstract

Antibiotics are valuable adjunctives for the management of bacterial infections. During endodontic treatment and when managing trauma to the teeth, antibiotics may be applied systemically or locally. Due to the potential risk of adverse effects following systemic application, and the ineffectiveness of systemic antibiotics in necrotic and pulpless teeth (due to the lack of blood supply which is required to distribute the antibiotic to the root canal system), the local application of antibiotics is a more effective mode for delivery during root canal treatment.

Tetracyclines are bacteriostatic antibiotics with substantivity for up to 12 weeks when used as intracanal medicaments. They are typically used in conjunction with corticosteroids, and these combinations have anti-inflammatory, antibacterial, and anti-resorptive properties, all of which help to reduce the periapical inflammatory reaction including clastic-cell-mediated tooth and bone resorption. Tetracycline-based irrigants possess substantivity for up to 4 weeks. Clindamycin and a combination of three antibiotics (metronidazole, ciprofloxacin, and minocycline) have also been reported to be effective at reducing bacterial numbers in the root canal systems of infected teeth.

Introduction

Animal models and clinical studies have clarified the essential role of microorganisms in the development and perpetuation of pulp and periapical diseases [1–3]. Studies have also shown that the outcome of treatment of these diseases is dependent on the elimination of microorganisms from infected root canal systems which is a complicated task. Numerous measures have been

Z. Mohammadi, DMD, MSD
Iranian Center for Endodontic Research (ICER), Research Institute of Dental Sciences, Shahid Beheshti University of Medical Sciences, Tehran, Iran

P.V. Abbott, BDSc, MDS, FRACDS(Endo), FIADT (✉)
Department of Endodontics, School of Dentistry, The University of Western Australia, Nedlands, WA, Australia
e-mail: paul.v.abbott@uwa.edu.au

B. Basrani (ed.), *Endodontic Irrigation: Chemical Disinfection of the Root Canal System*, DOI 10.1007/978-3-319-16456-4_15 described to reduce or eliminate microorganisms from the root canal systems (RCS), such as the use of various instrumentation techniques, irrigation regimens, and intracanal medicaments. There is no evidence in the literature to suggest that mechanical instrumentation alone results in a bacteria-free root canal system. Studies have shown that, at best, instrumentation only reduces the number of microorganisms in the RCS. Considering the complex anatomy of the RCS [4], this is not at all surprising. There are both in vitro and clinical evidences that mechanical instrumentation leaves significant portions of the root canal walls untouched [5] and complete elimination of bacteria from the RCS by instrumentation alone is unlikely [6]. It is assumed, but not proven, that any pulp tissue left in the root canals can serve as bacterial nutrient. Furthermore, tissue remnants also impede the antimicrobial effects of root canal irrigants and medicaments, and they prevent intimate adaptation of the root canal filling to the dentin. Therefore, specific irrigation and disinfection procedures are necessary to remove tissue from the RCS and to kill microorganisms, respectively [7]. The purpose of this chapter is to review these studies regarding the use of common antibiotic-based irrigants and medicaments currently used during root canal treatment and when managing trauma to the teeth.

History

Antibiotics were first discovered in 1928, but they were not routinely used clinically until the early 1940s during the Second World War. Prior to this, most wartime deaths were due to bacterial infections of wounds, rather than from the wounds themselves. The use of antibiotics was popularized as a result of the rapid recovery of wounded military personnel, and this popularity continued after the end of the war [8]. For several decades now, antibiotics have been prescribed in different disciplines of medicine and dentistry [8]. In endodontics and dental traumatology, antibiotics may be applied systemically (orally or parenterally) and/or locally (intradentally). The first reported local use of an antibiotic in endodontics was in 1951 when Grossman [9] used a polyantibiotic paste known as PBSC (a mixture of penicillin, bacitracin, streptomycin, and caprylate sodium suspended in a silicone vehicle) as a root canal medicament. PBSC contained penicillin to target Gram-positive organisms, bacitracin for penicillin-resistant strains, streptomycin for Gram-negative organisms, and caprylate sodium to target yeasts. Later, nystatin replaced the caprylate sodium as an antifungal agent in a similar medicament, known as PBSN [10].

The Rationale for Local Application of Antibiotics

While systemic antibiotics appear to be clinically effective as an adjunct in certain surgical and nonsurgical cases of infection, their administration is not without the potential risk of adverse systemic effects – such as allergic reactions, toxicity, various side effects, and the development of resistant strains of microbes. In addition, the systemic administration of antibiotics relies on patient compliance with the dosing regimens, followed by absorption through the gastrointestinal tract and then distribution via the circulatory system to bring the drug to the infected site at an effective concentration. Hence, the infected area (i.e., the tooth root) requires a normal blood supply which is no longer the case for teeth with a necrotic pulp, a pulpless and infected RCS, or a root-filled tooth that has become infected. Therefore, the local application of antibiotics within the RCS may be a more effective mode for delivering these drugs to the required site of action [11].

Several antibiotic agents have been used in endodontics, and these will be discussed below.

Tetracyclines

Structure and Mechanisms of Action

These drugs are so named for their four ("tetra-") hydrocarbon rings ("-cycl-") derivation ("-ine"). Tetracyclines are collectively known as derivatives of polycyclic naphthacene carboxamide (Fig. 15.1). They are defined as a subclass of

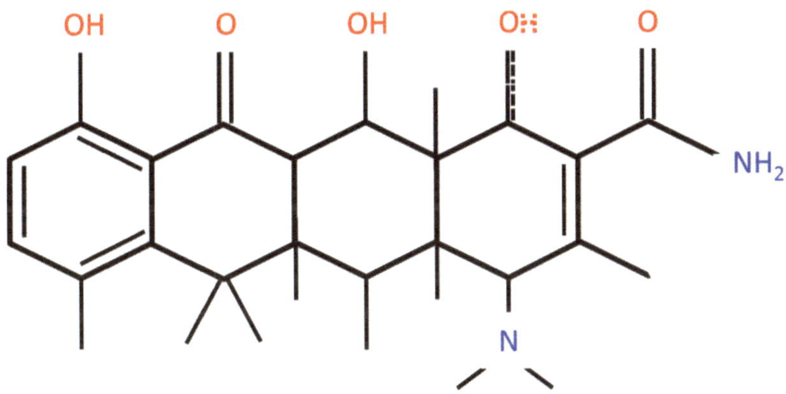

Fig. 15.1 Structure of tetracyclines

polyketides having an octahydrotetracene-2-carboxamide skeleton [12].

Tetracycline antibiotics are protein synthesis inhibitors which inhibit the binding of aminoacyl-tRNA to the mRNA-ribosome complex. They do this mainly by binding to the 30S ribosomal subunit in the mRNA translation complex [13].

Properties

Tetracyclines, including tetracycline HCl, minocycline, demeclocycline, and doxycycline, are a group of broad-spectrum antibiotics that are effective against a wide range of microorganisms [13, 14]. Tetracyclines are bacteriostatic in nature [15]. This property may be advantageous because, in the absence of bacterial cell lysis, antigenic by-products such as endotoxin are not released [16]. Tetracyclines also have many unique properties other than their antimicrobial action, such as the inhibition of mammalian collagenases, which prevent tissue breakdown [17], and the inhibition of clastic cells [17, 18], which results in antiresorptive activity [18]. Inflammatory diseases such as periodontitis include an excess of tissue collagenases which may be blocked by tetracyclines, thus leading to enhanced formation of collagen and bone [16].

Applications in Endodontics

In endodontics, tetracyclines have been used as part of an irrigant to remove the smear layer from instrumented root canal walls [16, 19], for irrigation of retrograde cavities during periapical surgical procedures [20], and as an intracanal medicament [21].

Barkhordar et al. [16] showed that doxycycline HCl eliminated smear layer in a concentration-dependent manner with 100 mg/ml doxycycline being more effective than lower concentrations. In another investigation, Haznedaroğlu and Ersev [19] reported that tetracycline was as effective as citric acid in removing the smear layer. Barkhordar and Russell [20] evaluated the effect of doxycycline on the apical penetration of dye through the margins of retrograde fillings. The teeth with retrograde IRM or amalgam fillings placed following doxycycline irrigation had significantly less dye penetration than those that were not irrigated with doxycycline.

Pinheiro et al. [22] evaluated the antibiotic susceptibility of *Enterococcus faecalis* isolates from canals of root-filled teeth with periapical radiolucencies. The antibiotics were benzylpenicillin, amoxicillin, amoxicillin with clavulanic acid, erythromycin, azithromycin, vancomycin, chloramphenicol, tetracycline, doxycycline, ciprofloxacin, and moxifloxacin. The vast majority (85.7 %) of the isolates were susceptible to tetracycline and doxycycline.

Based on the hypotheses that microorganisms can reach the apical area of recently replanted teeth from the oral cavity (or from contaminated root surfaces during the extra-oral time) and that tetracyclines can potentially inhibit this route of bacterial contamination, Cvek et al. [23] developed a protocol for the topical treatment of exposed roots with doxycycline before replantation of avulsed teeth. Their aim was to eliminate the microorganisms from the root surface via direct local application of the antibiotic in order to decrease the frequency and severity of the inflammatory response. They showed that topical doxycycline significantly increased the chances of successful pulp revascularization and decreased the number of microorganisms that could be isolated from the root canals. They also reported a decreased frequency of ankylosis, external replacement resorption, and external inflammatory resorption. The beneficial effect of soaking a tooth in doxycycline has also been confirmed by Yanpiset and Trope [24].

Using laser Doppler flowmetry (LDF), radiography, and histology, a study investigated the effect of topical antibiotic treatment on pulp revascularization in replanted teeth in a dog model [25]. After extraction, the teeth were kept dry for 5 min and either covered with minocycline, soaked in doxycycline, or soaked in saline, and then they were replanted. Teeth in the positive control group were not extracted. Postoperative radiographs and LDF readings were obtained for 2 months after replantation. After sacrifice of the animals, the jaws were collected and processed for light microscopy. Pre- and post-replantation LDF readings and radiographs and the histological findings were analyzed to assess revascularization. Pulp revascularization occurred in 91 % of the teeth treated with minocycline, 73 % of those soaked in doxycycline, and only 33 % of the teeth soaked in saline [25].

Bryson et al. [26] evaluated the effect of minocycline on the healing of replanted dog teeth after extended dry times of 60 min. Their results indicated that the roots with and without minocycline treatment showed no significant differences in the remaining root mass or the percentage of favorably healed root surfaces. In addition, no benefit was found from the use of topically applied minocycline in the attenuation or prevention of external root resorption. The lack of significant differences is likely to have been a result of the extended dry period before replantation as most of the periodontal ligament cells would have died within this time period and therefore external replacement resorption is the typical result.

Further details and applications of tetracyclines in endodontics and dental traumatology are outlined below in the sections regarding Ledermix paste and triple antibiotic pastes.

Substantivity of Tetracyclines

Tetracyclines readily attach to dentin and are subsequently released without losing their antibacterial activity [15]. This property creates a reservoir of active antibacterial agent, which is then released from the dentin surface in a slow and sustained manner. In an in vivo periodontal study, Stabholz et al. [27] compared the antibacterial substantivity of two concentrations of tetracycline HCl (50 mg/ml, 10 mg/ml) and 0.12 % chlorhexidine. Their findings showed that both concentrations of tetracycline demonstrated residual antibacterial activity and the antibacterial substantivity of the three solutions in descending order was 50 mg/ml tetracycline >10 mg/ml tetracycline >0.12 % CHX.

Abbott et al. [28] demonstrated that tetracyclines form a strong reversible bond with the dental hard tissues and that they exhibit slow release and diffusion through dentin over an extended period of time up to at least 12 weeks. [89] compared the antibacterial substantivity of 2 % CHX, 100 mg/ml doxycycline HCl, and 2.6 % NaOCl in bovine root dentin (Figure 15.2) over five experimental periods of 0, 7, 14, 21, and 28 days in vitro. Their findings indicated that after 7 days, the NaOCl and doxycycline groups showed the lowest and the highest number of colony-forming units (CFUs), respectively. However, after the longer time periods, the CHX group showed the lowest number of CFUs.

Mohammadi et al. [29] evaluated the antibacterial substantivity of three concentrations of doxycycline HCl (100, 50, and 10 mg/ml) in bovine root dentin over five experimental periods of 0, 7, 14, 21, and 28 days. At 7 days, the 100 mg/ml group and the 10 mg/ml group showed the lowest and highest numbers of CFUs, respectively. In each group, the numbers of CFUs increased significantly over time (Table 15.1).

MTAD

BioPure (Dentsply, Tulsa Dental, Tulsa, OK, USA), otherwise known as MTAD, was introduced by Torabinejad et al. [15]. It is composed of 3 % doxycycline, 4.25 % citric acid, and a detergent (0.5 % polysorbate 80) [15].

Antimicrobial Activity

Several studies have evaluated the effectiveness of MTAD for disinfection of root canals. Torabinejad et al. [15] showed that MTAD was able to remove the smear layer and was effective against *E. faecalis* [30–32]. Using a human tooth model, Shabahang et al. [32] showed that the use of MTAD was more effective than 5.25 % NaOCl for disinfecting root canals. Torabinejad et al. [30] also demonstrated that MTAD was significantly more effective than the combination of NaOCl and EDTA against *E. faecalis*. Kho and Baumgartner [33] showed consistent disinfection of infected root canals when a combination of 5.25 % NaOCl/15 % EDTA was used. However, the combination of 1.3 % NaOCl/BioPure MTAD left nearly 50 % of the canals contaminated with *E. faecalis*. Krause et al. [34] compared the antimicrobial effect against *E. faecalis* of MTAD, two of its components (doxycycline and citric acid), and sodium hypochlorite in two in vitro models using two different methods. In the tooth model, NaOCl and doxycycline were more effective than the control in killing *E. faecalis* at shallow bur depths into dentin, but at deeper bur depths, the NaOCl was superior. In the agar diffusion model, NaOCl produced less inhibition of bacteria than MTAD or doxycycline. Ghoddusi et al. [35] indicated that removing the smear layer using MTAD as a final irrigant delayed bacterial penetration of filled root canals. Using the agar diffusion method, Davis et al. [36] determined that MTAD was significantly more effective than 5.25 % NaOCl, 2 % CHX, and Dermacyn against *E. faecalis*. Newberry et al. [37] showed that MTAD inhibited most strains of *E. faecalis* growth when diluted 1:8,192 times and it killed most strains of *E. faecalis* when diluted 1:512 times. Shabahang et al. [38] showed that the addition or substitution of chlorhexidine for doxycycline did not negatively impact the efficacy of MTAD. However, the substitution of this antimicrobial agent for doxycycline significantly reduced the efficacy of the solution. Furthermore, the contents of the root canal system may inhibit or decrease the antibac-

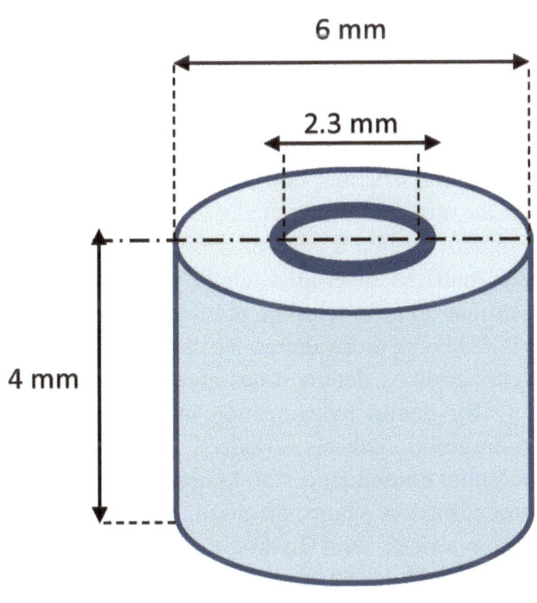

Fig. 15.2 Schematic view of used dentin tubes (Adopted from Mohammadi and Shahriari [40])

Table 15.1 Means of the CFU and the standard deviation of *E. faecalis* in experimental groups (three concentrations of doxycycline) [29]

	Day 0	Day 7	Day 14	Day 21	Day 28
100 mg/ml	0.40±0.69	4.66±2.34	9.70±2.75	20.20±3.22	44.44±5.52
50 mg/ml	0.50±3.97	9.00±3.74	15.40±4.55	37.00±5.33	59.66±5.36
10 mg/ml	4.70±3.68	16.11±8.05	37.40±8.99	61.80±11.11	88.55±5.50

terial activity of MTAD. Portenier et al. [39] investigated the inhibitory effects of dentin and bovine serum albumin (BSA) on the antibacterial activity of MTAD and found that the presence of dentin or BSA caused a marked delay in the killing of bacteria.

Substantivity of MTAD

Tetracyclines (including doxycycline) readily attach to dentin and are subsequently released without losing their antibacterial activity [15]. The presence of doxycycline in MTAD suggests that MTAD may have some substantive antimicrobial action [15]. In an in vitro study using a human tooth model, Mohammadi and Shahriari [40] showed that, during a 4-week period, the substantivity of MTAD was significantly greater than CHX and NaOCl (Table 15.2). In another study, the substantivity of 100 % MTAD was significantly greater than the two other concentrations of MTAD [41]. Tay et al. [42] found that when MTAD was applied to 1.3 % NaOCl-irrigated dentin, its antimicrobial substantivity was reduced. They attributed this phenomenon to the oxidation of MTAD by NaOCl in a manner similar to the peroxidation of tetracycline by reactive oxygen species.

MTAD and Biofilms

Clegg et al. [43] reported that 6 % NaOCl was the only irrigant capable of both rendering bacteria nonviable and physically removing the biofilm. Dunavant et al. [44] showed that MTAD killed 16.08 % of the bacterial cells in *E. faecalis* biofilms, while Giardino et al. [45] showed that MTA was not able to disintegrate and remove bacterial biofilms.

In summary, based on the available literature, MTAD does not appear to be effective against bacterial biofilms.

Smear Layer Removal and Effect on Dentin

Torabinejad et al. [15] showed that MTAD was an effective solution for the removal of the smear layer and that it did not significantly change the structure of the dentinal tubules when root canals were irrigated with NaOCl, followed by a final rinse of MTAD. In another study [30], they showed that although MTAD removed most of the smear layer when used as an intracanal irrigant, some remnants of the organic component of the smear layer remained scattered on the surface of the root canal walls. The effectiveness of MTAD in completely removing the smear layer was enhanced when low concentrations of NaOCl were used as intracanal irrigants before using MTAD as a final rinse. Lotfi et al. [46] showed that MTAD could not remove the smear layer and their regimen did not significantly change the structure of the dentinal tubules [30]. On the other hand, Tay et al. [47] found that both irrigants created a zone of demineralized collagen matrices in eroded dentin and around the dentinal tubules, with the mildly acidic BioPure MTAD being more aggressive than EDTA. These demineralized dentin zones create the opportunity for dentin hybridization by infiltration of hydrophilic adhesives/sealers. However, the potential consequences of compaction of hydrophobic sealers against air-dried, collapsed collagen matrices, and hydrolytic degradation of incompletely infiltrated matrices remain unresolved. In an ultrastructural study, Tay et al. [47] showed that MTAD created a thicker demineralized dentin matrix (5–6 μm) than EDTA

Table 15.2 Means of the CFU and the standard deviation of *E. faecalis* in the experimental groups [40]

	Day 0	Day 7	Day 14	Day 21	Day 28
NaOCl	0.31±0.58	17.16±7.05	34.40±8.79	66.78±10.11	95.25±5.61
CHX	3.56±3.72	10.35±3.77	14.49±4.67	34.35±4.22	51.53±5.35
MTAD	0.70±3.85	4.46±2.24	8.68±2.71	19.25±3.49	40.44±5.42

(1–2 μm). De-Deus et al. [48] found that the demineralization kinetics prompted by MTAD were significantly faster than those prompted by a 17 % EDTA solution.

There is only one study on the effect of MTAD on dentin. Machnick et al. [49] evaluated the effect of MTAD on the flexural strength and modulus of elasticity of dentin. Their findings showed that there was no significant difference in flexural strength and modulus of elasticity between the dentin specimens exposed to saline or MTAD.

MTAD and Dentin Bonding (Anti-collagenolytic Activity)

Machnick et al. [50] compared the effect of MTAD and phosphoric acid on the bond strength to enamel and dentin using a conventional OptiBond Solo Plus dentin adhesive system. They reported that teeth endodontically treated with the MTAD protocol for clinical use (20 min 1.3 % NaOCl/5 min MTAD) might not need any additional dentin conditioning prior to the application of the dental adhesive. Garcia-Godoy et al. [51] evaluated the structure of the hybrid layer formed after the use of EDTA or MTAD solutions when used as a final rinse. Findings showed that the BioPure MTAD hybrid layer was thicker than the 17 % EDTA hybrid layer. Both the BioPure MTAD and EDTA caused collapse of the dentin matrix structure, which impeded sealer infiltration and the formation of high-quality hybrid layer bonding. The hybrid layers created in smear layer-covered dentin exhibited less potential for fluid penetration than the MTAD or EDTA hybrid layer. It was also shown that neither EDTA nor MTAD significantly improved Epiphany-dentin bond strengths when compared with NaOCl used alone [52]. Yurdaguven et al. [53] showed that the bonding of Clearfil SE Bond to coronal dentin was significantly reduced after using MTAD to irrigate the root canal system.

In summary, due to its broad-spectrum MMP-inhibitory effect, MTAD can significantly improve the stability of the resin-dentin bond.

Toxicity of MTAD

There are few studies regarding the toxicity of MTAD. Zhang et al. [54] examined the cytotoxicity of MTAD compared with that of commonly used irrigants and medicaments. L929 fibroblasts were grown on cell culture plates and placed in contact with various concentrations of test irrigants and medicaments. The cytotoxicity of these materials was evaluated 24 h after incubation using MTT assay. Results showed that MTAD was less cytotoxic than eugenol, 3 % H_2O_2, $Ca(OH)_2$ paste, 5.25 % NaOCl, Peridex, and EDTA, while it was more cytotoxic than 2.63, 1.31, and 0.66 % NaOCl. Yasuda et al. [55] evaluated the cytotoxicity of MTAD on MC3T3-E1 and periodontal ligament cells at various concentrations. They reported that it was less cytotoxic and did not affect differentiation into osteoblasts compared with other irrigants such as H_2O_2, NaOCl, EDTA, and chlorhexidine.

Tetraclean

Tetraclean (Ogna Laboratori Farmaceutici, Muggiò (Mi), Italy), like MTAD, is a mixture of an antibiotic, an acid, and a detergent. However, the concentration of the antibiotic, doxycycline (50 mg/ml), and the type of detergent (polypropylene glycol) differ from those of MTAD [56]. Giardino et al. [57] compared the surface tension of 17 % EDTA, Cetrexidin, SmearClear, 5.25 % NaOCl, MTAD, and Tetraclean. The NaOCl and EDTA had the highest surface tensions, whereas Cetrexidin and Tetraclean had the lowest values.

Antibacterial Activity

There are only a few studies on the antibacterial activity of Tetraclean. Giardino et al. [45] compared the antimicrobial efficacy of 5.25 % NaOCl, MTAD, and Tetraclean against an *E. faecalis* biofilm generated on cellulose nitrate membrane filters. Only the NaOCl could disaggregate and remove the biofilm at every time interval tested although treatment with Tetraclean caused a high degree of biofilm disaggregation at each time interval when compared with MTAD [45]. Neglia et al. [58] showed that Tetraclean was very effective against *E. faecalis* in vitro.

Ardizzoni et al. [59] evaluated the effectiveness of Tetraclean against *E. faecalis* using an agar diffusion test and showed that it was 100 % effective against 54 clinical isolates at dilutions up to 1:256. Giardino et al. [60] showed that Tetraclean was more effective than CHX against common endodontic bacteria. Pappen et al. [61] demonstrated that Tetraclean was more effective than MTAD against *E. faecalis* in planktonic culture and in mixed species in an in vitro biofilm. Using the agar diffusion test, Poggio et al. [62] showed that the efficacy of Tetraclean against *Enterococcus faecalis*, *Streptococcus mutans*, and *Staphylococcus aureus* was significantly better than NaOCl, Chloreximid, and hydrogen peroxide. Mohammadi et al. [63] investigated the efficacy of sodium hypochlorite, chlorhexidine, Tetraclean, Hypoclean, and Chlor-XTRA against *Enterococcus faecalis*, *Candida albicans*, *Actinomyces israelii*, *Pseudomonas aeruginosa*, and *Lactobacillus casei* using the agar diffusion method. According to their findings, Hypoclean was the most effective irrigant against *C. albicans*, *P. aeruginosa*, and *L. casei*.

Substantivity of Tetraclean

Mohammadi et al. [64] demonstrated that the substantivity of Tetraclean was significantly higher than MTAD and it was retained in root canal dentin for at least 28 days (Table 15.3). In additional studies, Mohammadi et al. [65] showed that the substantivity of Tetraclean was significantly greater than Hypoclean and 5.25 % NaOCl, and there was a direct relationship between dentin treatment time with Tetraclean and its substantivity [66]. Pretreatment of dentin with NaOCl significantly decreased the substantivity of Tetraclean [67].

Smear Layer Removal Ability

Poggio et al. [68] compared the demineralizing capability on root canal dentin of Tetraclean, Largal Ultra, 17 % ethylenediaminetetraacetic acid and Tubuliclean in vitro. Results indicated that the higher release of Ca^{+2} observed in samples treated with Tetraclean demonstrated its significantly higher demineralizing capability compared to the other irrigants tested.

Ledermix Paste

Ledermix paste is a glucocorticosteroid-antibiotic compound which was developed and was released for sale in Europe by Lederle Pharmaceuticals in 1962 [69]. The sole reason for adding the antibiotic component to Ledermix paste was to compensate for what was perceived to be a possible corticoid-induced reduction in the host immune response. Schroeder and Triadan initially incorporated chloramphenicol in their first trials, but when Lederle Pharmaceuticals became the manufacturer, the antibiotic was changed to demeclocycline HCl. Today, Ledermix paste remains a combination of the same tetracycline antibiotic, demeclocycline HCl (at a concentration of 3.2 %), and a corticosteroid, triamcinolone acetonide (concentration 1 %), in a polyethylene glycol base [69].

The two therapeutic components of Ledermix paste (i.e., triamcinolone and demeclocycline) are capable of diffusing through dentinal tubules and cementum to reach the periodontal and periapical tissues [70]. Abbott et al. [28] showed that dentinal tubules were the major supply route of the active components to the periradicular tissues,

Table 15.3 Mean of the CFU and the standard deviations of *E. faecalis* in the experimental groups [64]

	Day 0	Day 7	Day 14	Day 21	Day 28
Tetraclean	0.00±0.00	0.00±0.00	0.37±0.65	6.68±2.59	15.35±3.21
MTAD	0.71±3.79	4.41±2.21	8.74±2.75	19.20±3.41	39.55±5.43
NaOCl	0.29±0.57	17.13±7.02	33.42±8.72	65.71±10.14	93.22±5.64

while the apical foramen was not as significant as a supply route. Various factors can affect the supply of the active components to the periradicular tissues – these include the presence or absence of the smear layer [71], the presence or absence of cementum [71], and the presence of other materials within the canal, for example, calcium hydroxide [72, 73]. The concentration of demeclocycline within Ledermix paste itself (i.e., as it would be when placed within the root canal) is high enough to be effective against susceptible species of bacteria [74]. However, within the peripheral parts of the dentine and in the periradicular tissues, the concentration achieved through diffusion is insufficient to inactivate bacteria, especially over time [74]. Immediately adjacent to the root canal, inhibitory levels of demeclocycline are achieved for all reported bacteria within the first day of application, but this level drops to about one tenth of the initial level after 1 week in both the mid-root and the apical third levels. Further, away from the root canal toward the cementum, the concentration of demeclocycline after one day is not high enough to inhibit growth of 12 of the 13 strains of commonly reported endodontic bacteria [74].

When investigated in monkeys, Ledermix paste eliminated experimentally induced external inflammatory root resorption in vivo [75]. Furthermore, it has been revealed that Ledermix paste had no damaging effects upon the periodontal membrane and that this paste was an effective medication for the treatment of progressive root resorption in traumatically injured teeth [75]. Taylor et al. [73] showed that Ledermix paste reversibly inhibited mitosis in mouse fibroblasts in concentrations ranging from 10^{-3} to 10^{-6} mg/ml. Furthermore, they showed that Ledermix paste killed *S. mutans* at about the same concentration at which it killed the mammalian cells but required a one thousand-fold greater concentration to kill *L. casei*. Thong et al. [76] found that periodontal ligament inflammation and inflammatory root resorption were markedly inhibited by Ledermix paste relative to untreated controls. Wong and Sae-Lim [77] evaluated the effect of immediately placed intracanal Ledermix paste on root resorption of delayed-replanted monkey teeth. Their findings revealed that the use of Ledermix paste resulted in a significantly higher occurrence of complete healing (35.46 %) compared to the positive control group (16.58 %), but there were no significant differences in external inflammatory and replacement resorption. Bryson et al. [18] evaluated the effect on healing of immediately placing Ledermix paste in the root canals of replanted dog teeth after extended dry times (60 min). Their findings showed that the roots treated with Ledermix paste had statistically significantly more healing and less resorption than the roots treated with $Ca(OH)_2$. Medicating the canals with Ledermix paste also resulted in significantly less loss of root mass due to resorption compared to those roots filled with $Ca(OH)_2$. Chen et al. [78] evaluated the individual influence of triamcinolone and demeclocycline on external root resorption after extended extra-oral dry time (60 min.) and found that there was no statistically significant difference between Ledermix paste group and the triamcinolone group, while the demeclocycline group showed less favorable healing than the Ledermix paste and triamcinolone groups.

Ehrmann et al. [79] found that painful teeth with acute apical periodontitis that had been dressed with Ledermix paste gave rise to less postoperative pain than that experienced by patients who had a dressing of calcium hydroxide or no dressing at all. The authors even commented in the discussion that the rapidity of action of the Ledermix paste medicament was "striking" as patients in that group commenced with greater pain levels prior to treatment and its effect in reducing pain was measurable after just 4 h [79].

Kim et al. [80, 81] demonstrated that after 12 weeks, sunlight exposure had caused dark gray-brown staining of teeth when Ledermix paste had been placed in the canals, but this did not occur when the teeth were kept in the dark. Staining was confined to areas of the tooth where the paste had been placed so in cases where there was no paste in the pulp chamber there was no discoloration of the crown. Furthermore, immature teeth were more severely stained than the mature teeth.

Combination of Ledermix Paste and Calcium Hydroxide

A 50:50 mixture of Ledermix paste and calcium hydroxide has been advocated as an intracanal dressing in cases of infected root canals, pulp necrosis and infection with incomplete root formation (as an initial dressing prior to using calcium hydroxide alone for apexification), perforations, inflammatory root resorption, and inflammatory periapical bone resorption and for treatment of large periapical radiolucent lesions [70, 82]. It has been shown that the 50:50 mixture results in slower release and diffusion of the active components of Ledermix paste which makes the medicament last longer in the canal [72]. This in turn helps to maintain the sterility of the canal for longer and also maintains a higher concentration of all components within the canal [72] without affecting the function of each component of both medicaments [72, 73].

Taylor et al. [73] also showed that for two indicator microorganisms, *Lactobacillus casei* and *Streptococcus mutans*, the 50:50 mixture was marginally more effective than either paste used alone. However, Seow [83] showed that for *Streptococcus sanguis* and *Staphylococcus aureus*, the addition of only 25 % by volume of Calyxl (a calcium hydroxide in saline paste) (Otto and Co., Frankfurt, Germany) to Ledermix paste converted the zone of complete inhibition originally seen with Ledermix paste to one of only partial inhibition.

Triple Antibiotic Paste

Because of the complexity of the root canal infection, it is unlikely that any single antibiotic could result in effective sterilization of the canal. More likely a combination would be needed to address the diverse flora encountered. A combination of antibiotics would also decrease the likelihood of the development of resistant bacterial strains. The combination that appears to be most promising consists of metronidazole, ciprofloxacin, and minocycline [84, 85]. Sato et al. [86] showed that no bacteria were recovered from infected dentin of the root canal wall 24 h after application of a mixture of ciprofloxacin, metronidazole, and minocycline, except in one case in which a few bacteria were recovered. Hoshino et al. [87] investigated the antibacterial effect of a mixture of ciprofloxacin, metronidazole, and minocycline on bacteria taken from infected dentin of root canal walls and found that it was able to consistently sterilize all samples. Takushige et al. [88] evaluated the efficacy of a poly-antibiotic paste consisting of ciprofloxacin, metronidazole, and minocycline, on the clinical outcome of so-called "lesion sterilization and tissue repair (LSTR)" therapy in primary teeth with periradicular radiolucencies. Their results showed that in all cases, clinical symptoms such as gingival swelling, sinus tracts, dull pain, spontaneous pain, and pain on biting disappeared after treatment. However, there were four cases where the clinical signs and symptoms were only finally resolved after further treatment using the same procedures. Windley et al. [32] assessed the efficacy of a triple antibiotic paste in the disinfection of immature dog teeth with apical periodontitis. The canals were sampled before (S1) and after (S2) irrigation with 1.25 % NaOCl and after dressing with a triple antibiotic paste (S3), consisting of metronidazole, ciprofloxacin, and minocycline. At S1, 100 % of the samples cultured positive for bacteria with a mean CFU count of 1.7×10. At S2, 10 % of the samples cultured bacteria-free with a mean CFU count of 1.4×10. At S3, 70 % of the samples cultured bacteria-free with a mean CFU count of only 26. Reductions in mean CFU counts between S1 and S2 as well as between S2 and S3 were statistically significant.

Conclusions

1. The local application of antibiotics within the root canal system may be a more effective mode for delivering such drugs than systemic routes of administration.
2. Tetracyclines have been used to remove the smear layer from instrumented root canal walls, for irrigation of retrograde cavities during periapical surgical procedures, and as intracanal medicaments.
3. Substantivity of tetracyclines has been shown for up to at least 12 weeks.

4. BioPure (MTAD) is effective in removing the smear layer. However, the antimicrobial efficacy against *E. faecalis* of 1.3 % NaOCl/MTAD compared with that of the combined alternate use of 5.25 % NaOCl and 15 % EDTA is still controversial.
5. Substantivity of MTAD has been shown to last for up to 4 weeks. Furthermore, application of MTAD to 1.3 % NaOCl-irrigated dentine may reduce its substantivity.
6. Tetraclean, a mixture of an antibiotic (doxycycline), an acid, and a detergent has a very low surface tension and a high degree of efficacy against bacterial biofilms.
7. Ledermix paste, a glucocorticosteroid-antibiotic compound, has anti-inflammatory, antibacterial, and anti-resorptive properties, all of which help to reduce the periapical inflammatory reaction including clastic-cell-mediated resorption. This material has been shown to significantly lower the incidence of inflammatory and replacement resorption and thus promotes more favorable healing in replanted and luxated teeth.
8. A 50:50 mixture of Ledermix paste and calcium hydroxide has been advocated as an intracanal dressing in cases of pulpless infected root canals, pulp necrosis and infection with incomplete root formation (as an initial dressing prior to apexification), perforations, inflammatory root resorption, and inflammatory periapical bone resorption and for the treatment of large periapical radiolucent lesions.
9. A triple antibiotic paste consisting of metronidazole, ciprofloxacin, and minocycline has been reported to be very effective in the disinfection of the root canal system.

References

1. Kakehashi S, Stanley HR, Fitzgerald RJ. The effects of surgical exposure of dental pulps in germ – free and conventional laboratory rats. Oral Surg Oral Med Oral Pathol. 1965;18:340–8.
2. Möller ÅJ. Microbiological examination of root canals and periapical tissues of human teeth Methodological studies (thesis). Odontol Tidscrift. 1966;74:1–380.
3. Sundqvist G. Ecology of the root canal flora. J Endod. 1992;18:427–30.
4. Hess W. Anatomy of root canals on the teeth of the permanent dentition. Part I. New York: William Wood; 1925. p. 3–49.
5. Peters OA, Laib A, Gohring TN, Barbakow F. Changes in root canal geometry after preparation assessed by high resolution computed tomography. J Endod. 2001;27:1–6.
6. Byström A, Sundqvist G. Bacteriologic evaluation of the efficacy of mechanical root canal instrumentation in endodontic therapy. Scand J Dent Res. 1981;89:321–8.
7. Mohammadi Z, Abbott PV. The properties and applications of chlorhexidine in endodontics. Int Endod J. 2009;42:288–302.
8. Abbott PV. Selective and intelligent use of antibiotics in endodontics. Aust Endod J. 2000;26:30–9.
9. Grossman LI. Polyantibiotic treatment of pulpless teeth. J Am Dent Assoc. 1951;43:265–78.
10. Weine FS. Endodontic therapy. 3rd ed. St. Louis: Mosby; 2003. p. 325.
11. Mohammadi Z, Abbott PV. Antimicrobial substantivity of root canal irrigants and medicaments: a review. Aust Endod J. 2009;35:131–9.
12. Chopra I, Roberts M. Tetracycline antibiotics: mode of action, applications, molecular biology, and epidemiology of bacterial Resistance. Microbiol Mol Biol Rev. 2001;65:232–60.
13. Bahrami F, Morris DL, Pourgholami MH. Tetracyclines: drugs with huge therapeutic potential. Mini Rev Med Chem. 2012;12:44–52.
14. Nelson ML, Levy SB. The history of the tetracyclines. Ann N Y Acad Sci. 2011;1241:17–32.
15. Torabinejad M, Khademi AA, Babagoli J, Cho Y, Johnson WB, Bozhilov K, Kim J, Shabahan S. A new solution for the removal of the smear layer. J Endod. 2003;29:170–5.
16. Barkhordar RA, Watanabe LG, Marshall GW, Hussain MZ. Removal of intracanal smear by doxycycline *in vitro*. Oral Surg Oral Med Oral Pathol Oral Radiol Endod. 1997;84:420–3.
17. Pierce A, Lindskog S. The effect of an antibiotic/corticosteroid paste on inflammatory root resorption *in vivo*. Oral Surg Oral Med Oral Pathol Oral Radiol Endod. 1987;64:216–20.
18. Bryson E, Levin L, Banchs F, Abbott P, Trope M. Effect of immediate intracanal placement of Ledermix paste on healing of replanted dog teeth after extended dry times. Dent Traumatol. 2002;18:316–21.
19. Haznedaroğlu F, Ersev H. Tetracycline HCl solution as a root canal irrigant. J Endod. 2001;27:738–40.
20. Barkhordar RA, Russell T. Effect of doxycycline on the apical seal of the retrograde filling materials. J Calif Dent Assoc. 1998;26:842–5.
21. Molander A, Dahlen G. Evaluation of the antibacterial potential of tetracycline or erythromycin mixed with

calcium hydroxide as intracanal dressing against *E. faecalis in vivo*. Oral Surg Oral Med Oral Pathol Oral Radiol Endod. 2003;96:744–50.
22. Pinheiro ET, Gomes BP, Drucker DB, Zaia AA, Ferraz CC, Souza-Filho FJ. Antimicrobial susceptibility of Enterococcus faecalis isolated from canals of root filled teeth with periapical lesions. Int Endod J. 2004;37:756–63.
23. Cvek M, Cleaton-Jones P, Austin J, Lownie J, Kling M, Fatti P. Effect of topical application of doxycycline on pulp revascularization and periodontal healing in reimplanted monkey incisors. Endod Dent Traumatol. 1990;6:170–6.
24. Yanpiset K, Trope M. Pulp revascularization of replanted immature dog teeth after different treatment methods. Endod Dent Traumatol. 2000;16:211–7.
25. Ritter AL, Ritter AV, Murrah V, Sigurdsson A, Trope M. Pulp revascularization of replanted immature dog teeth after treatment with minocycline and doxycycline assessed by laser Doppler flowmetry, radiography, and histology. Dent Traumatol. 2004;20:75–84.
26. Bryson EC, Levin L, Banchs F, Trope M. Effect of minocycline on healing of replanted dog teeth after extended dry times. Dent Traumatol. 2003;19:90–5.
27. Stabholz A, Kettering J, Aprecio R, Zimmerman G, Baker PJ, Wikesjo UM. Retention of antimicrobial activity by human root surfaces after in situ subgingival irrigation with tetracycline HCl or chlorhexidine. J Periodontol. 1993;64:137–41.
28. Abbott PV, Heithersay GS, Hume WR. Release and diffusion through human tooth roots *in vitro* of corticosteroid and tetracycline trace molecules from Ledermix paste. Endod Dent Traumatol. 1988;4:55–62.
29. Mohammadi Z, Farhad A, Ardakani FE. Antibacterial Substantivity of three concentrations of Doxycycline on bovine root dentin infections: an *in vitro* study. Dent Res J. 2007;4:48–52.
30. Torabinejad M, Shabahang S, Aprecio R, Kettering JD. The antimicrobial effect of MTAD: an *in vitro* investigation. J Endod. 2003;29:400–3.
31. Shabahang S, Torabinejad M. Effect of MTAD on *Enterococcus faecalis*-contaminated root canals of extracted human teeth. J Endod. 2003;29:576–9.
32. Shabahang S, Pouresmail M, Torabinejad M. *In vitro* antibacterial efficacy of MTAD and sodium hypochlorite. J Endod. 2003;29:450–2.
33. Kho P, Baumgartner JC. A comparison of the antimicrobial efficacy of NaOCl/BioPure MTAD versus NaOCl/EDTA against *Enterococcus faecalis*. J Endod. 2006;32:652–5.
34. Krause TA, Liewehr FR, Hahn CL. The antimicrobial effect of MTAD, sodium hypochlorite, doxycycline, and citric acid on *Enterococcus faecalis*. J Endod. 2007;33:28–30.
35. Ghoddusi J, Rohani E, Rashed T, Ghaziani P, Akbari M. An evaluation of microbial leakage after using MTAD as a final irrigation. J Endod. 2007;33:173–6.
36. Davis JM, Maki J, Bahcall JK. An *in vitro* comparison of the antimicrobial effects of various endodontic medicaments on Enterococcus faecalis. J Endod. 2007;33:567–9.
37. Newberry BM, Shabahang S, Johnson N, Aprecio RM, Torabinejad M. The antimicrobial effect of BioPure MTAD on eight strains of *Enterococcus faecalis*: an *in vitro* investigation. J Endod. 2007;33:1352–4.
38. Shabahang S, Aslanyan J, Torabinejad M. The substitution of chlorhexidine for doxycycline in MTAD: the antibacterial efficacy against a strain of *Enterococcus faecalis*. J Endod. 2008;34:288–90.
39. Portenier I, Waltimo T, Ørstavik D, Haapasalo M. Killing of *Enterococcus faecalis* by MTAD and chlorhexidine digluconate with or without cetrimide in the presence or absence of dentin powder or BSA. J Endod. 2006;32:138–41.
40. Mohammadi Z, Shahriari S. Residual antibacterial activity of chlorhexidine and MTAD in human root dentin *in vitro*. J Oral Sci. 2008;50:63–7.
41. Mohammadi Z. Evaluation of residual antibacterial activity of three concentrations of new root canal irrigation solution. N Y State Dent J. 2008;74:31–3.
42. Tay FR, Hiraishi N, Schuster GS, Pashley DH, Loushine RJ, Ounsi HF, Grandini S, Yau JYY, Mazzoni A, Donnelly A, King NM. Reduction in antimicrobial substantivity of MTAD after initial sodium hypochlorite irrigation. J Endod. 2006;32:970–5.
43. Clegg MS, Vertucci FJ, Walker C, Belanger M, Britto LR. The effect of exposure to irrigant solutions on apical dentin biofilms *in vitro*. J Endod. 2006;32:434–7.
44. Dunavant TR, Regan JD, Glickman GN, Solomon ES, Honeyman AL. Comparative evaluation of endodontic irrigants against *Enterococcus faecalis* biofilms. J Endod. 2006;32:527–31.
45. Giardino L, Ambu E, Savoldi E, Rimondini R, Cassanelli C, Debbia EA. Comparative evaluation of antimicrobial efficacy of sodium hypochlorite, MTAD, and Tetraclean against *Enterococcus faecalis* biofilm. J Endod. 2007;33:852–5.
46. Lotfi M, Vosoughhosseini S, Saghiri MA, Vahid Zand V, Bahram Ranjkesh B, Ghasemi N. Effect of MTAD as a final rinse on removal of smear layer in ten-minute preparation time. J Endod. 2012;38:1391–4.
47. Tay FR, Pashley D, Loushine RJ, Doyle MD, Gillespie WT, Weller RN, King NM. Ultrastructure of smear layer-covered intraradicular dentin after irrigation with BioPure MTAD. J Endod. 2006;32:218–21.
48. De-Deus G, Reis C, Fidel S, Fidel R, Paciornik S. Dentin demineralization when subjected to BioPure MTAD: a longitudinal and quantitative assessment. J Endod. 2007;33:1364–8.
49. Machnick TK, Torabinejad M, Munoz CA, Shabahang S, Macknick T. Effect of MTAD on flexural strength and modulus of elasticity of dentin. J Endod. 2003;29:747–50.
50. Machnick TK, Torabinejad M, Munoz CA, Shabahang S. Effect of MTAD on the bond strength to enamel and dentin. J Endod. 2003;29:818–21.
51. Garcia-Godoy F, Loushine RJ, Itthagarun A, et al. Application of biologically-oriented dentin bonding

principles to the use of endodontic irrigants. Am J Dent. 2005;18:281–90.
52. Wachlarowicz AJ, Joyce AP, Roberts S, Pashley DH. Effect of endodontic irrigants on the shear bond strength of epiphany sealer to dentin. J Endod. 2007;33:152–5.
53. Yurdagüven H, Tanalp J, Toydemir B, Mohseni K, Soyman M, Bayirli G. The effect of endodontic irrigants on the microtensile bond strength of dentin adhesives. J Endod. 2009;35:1259–63.
54. Zhang W, Torabinejad M, Li Y. Evaluation of cytotoxicity of MTAD using the MTT-tetrazolium method. J Endod. 2003;29:654–7.
55. Yasuda Y, Tatematsu Y, Fujii S, Maeda H, Akamine A, Mahmoud Torabinejad M, Saito T. Effect of MTAD on the differentiation of osteoblast-like cells. J Endod. 2010;36:260–3.
56. Giardino L, Pecora G, Ambu E, Savoldi E. A new irrigant in the treatment of apical periodontitis: from research to clinic. 12th Biennial congress European Society of endodontology, Dublin; Sept 2005. p. 15–7.
57. Giardino L, Ambu E, Becce C, Rimondini L, Morra M. Surface tension comparison of four common root canal irrigants and two new irrigants containing antibiotic. J Endod. 2006;32:1091–3.
58. Neglia R, Ardizzoni A, Giardino L, Ambu E, Grazi S, Calignano S, Rimoldi C, Righi E, Blasi E. Comparative *in vitro* and *ex vivo* studies on the bactericidal activity of Tetraclean, a new generation endodontic irrigant, and sodium hypochlorite. New Microbiol. 2008;31:57–65.
59. Ardizzoni A, Blasi E, Rimoldi C, Giardino L, Ambo E, Righi E, Neglia R. An *in vitro* and *ex vivo* study on two antibiotic-based endodontic irrigants: a challenge to sodium hypochlorite. New Microbiol. 2009; 32:57–66.
60. Giardino L, Savoldi E, Ambu E, Rimondini R, Palezona A, Debbia EA. Antimicrobial effect of MTAD, Tetraclean, Cloreximid, and sodium hypochlorite on three common endodontic pathogens. Indian J Dent Res. 2009;20:391.
61. Pappen FG, Shen Y, Qian W, Leonardo MR, Giardino L, Haapasalo M. *In vitro* antibacterial action of Tetraclean, MTAD and five experimental irrigation solutions. Int Endod J. 2010;43:528–35.
62. Poggio C, Colombo M, Scribante A, Sforza D, Bianchi S. *In vitro* antibacterial activity of different endodontic irrigants. Dent Traumatol. 2012; 28:205–9.
63. Mohammadi Z, Shalavi S, Giardino L, Palazzi F, Mashouf RY, Soltanian A. Antimicrobial effect of three new and two current root canal irrigation solutions. Gen Dent. 2012;60:534–9.
64. Mohammadi Z, Giardino L, Mombeinipour A. Antibacterial substantivity of a new antibiotic-based endodontic irrigation solution. Aust Endod J. 2012;38:26–30.
65. Mohammadi Z, Mombeinipour A, Giardino L, Shahriari S. Residual antibacterial activity of a new modified sodium hypochlorite-based endodontic irrigation solution. Med Oral Patol Oral Cir Bucal. 2011;16:e588–92.
66. Mohammadi Z, Giardino L, Shahriari S. Effect of dentin treatment time with Tetraclean on its residual antibacterial activity. J Calif Dent Assoc. 2010;38:853–6.
67. Mohammadi Z, Giardino L, Palazzi F, Shahriari S. Effect of initial irrigation with sodium hypochlorite on the residual antibacterial activity of Tetraclean. NY State Dent J. 2013;79(1):32–6.
68. Poggio C, Dagna A, Colombo M, Rizzardi F, Marco Chiesa M, Andrea Scribante A, Alberti G. Decalcifying effect of different ethylenediaminetetraacetic acid irrigating solutions and Tetraclean on root canal dentin. J Endod. 2012;38:1239–43.
69. Athanassiadis B, Abbott PV, Walsh LJ. The use of calcium hydroxide, antibiotics and biocides as antimicrobial medicaments in endodontics. Aust Dent J. 2007;52:S64–82.
70. Abbott PV. Medicaments: aids to success in endodontics. Part 1. A review of literature. Aust Dent J. 1990;35:438–48.
71. Abbott PV, Hume WR, Heithersay GS. Barriers to diffusion of Ledermix paste in radicular dentine. Endod Dent Traumatol. 1989;5:98–104.
72. Abbott PV, Hume WR, Heithersay GS. Effect of combining Ledermix and calcium hydroxide pastes on the diffusion of corticosteroid and tetracycline through human tooth roots *in vitro*. Endod Dent Traumatol. 1989;5:188–92.
73. Taylor MA, Hume WR, Heithersay GS. Some effects of Ledermix paste and Pulpdent paste on mouse fibroblasts and on bacteria *in vitro*. Endod Dent Traumatol. 1989;5:266–73.
74. Abbott PV, Hume WR, Pearman JM. Antibiotics and endodontics. Aust Dent J. 1990;35:50–60.
75. Pierce A, Heithersay G, Lindskog S. Evidence for direct inhibition of dentinoclasts by a corticosteroid/antibiotic endodontic paste. Endod Dent Traumatol. 1988;4:44–5.
76. Thong YL, Messer HH, Siar CH, Saw LH. Periodontal response to two intracanal medicaments in replanted monkey incisors. Dent Traumatol. 2001;17:254–9.
77. Wong KS, Sae-Lim V. The effect of intracanal Ledermix on root resorption of delayed-replanted monkey teeth. Dent Traumatol. 2002;18:309–15.
78. Chen H, Teixeira FB, Ritter AL, Levin L, Trope M. The effect of intracanal anti-inflammatory medicaments on external root resorption of replanted dog teeth after extended extra-oral dry time. Dent Traumatol. 2008;24:74–8.
79. Ehrmann EH, Messer HH, Adams GG. The relationship of intracanal medicaments to postoperative pain in endodontics. Int Endod J. 2003;36:868–75.
80. Kim ST, Abbott PV, McGinley P. The effects of Ledermix paste on discolouration of mature teeth. Int Endod J. 2000;33:227–32.
81. Kim ST, Abbott PV, McGinley P. The effects of Ledermix paste on discolouration of immature teeth. Int Endod J. 2000;33:233–7.

82. Abbott PV. Medicaments: aids to success in endodontics. Part 2. Clinical recommendations. Aust Dent J. 1990;35:491–6.
83. Seow WK. The effects of dyadic combinations of endodontic medicaments on microbial growth inhibition. Pediatr Dent. 1990;12:292–7.
84. Windley 3rd W, Teixeira F, Levin L, Sigurdsson A, Trope M. Disinfection of immature teeth with a triple antibiotic paste. J Endod. 2005;31:439–43.
85. Trope M. Treatment of immature teeth with non-vital pulps and apical periodontitis. Endod Topics. 2006;14:51–9.
86. Sato I, Ando-Kurihara N, Kota K, Iwaku M, Hoshino E. Sterilization of infected root-canal dentine by topical application of a mixture of ciprofloxacin, metronidazole and minocycline in situ. Int Endod J. 1996;29:118–24.
87. Hoshino E, Ando-Kurihara N, Sato I, Uematsu H, Sato M, Kota K, Iwaku M. *In vitro* antibacterial susceptibility of bacteria taken from infected root dentine to a mixture of ciprofloxacin, metronidazole and minocycline. Int Endod J. 1996;29: 125–30.
88. Takushige T, Cruz EV, Asgor Moral A, Hoshino E. Endodontic treatment of primary teeth using a combination of antibacterial drugs. Int Endod J. 2004;37:132–8.
89. Khademi AA, Mohammadi Z, Havaee A. Evaluation of the antibacterial substantivity of several intra-canal agents. Aust Endod J. 2006; 32:112–5.

Intracanal Medication

16

José F. Siqueira Jr. and Isabela N. Rôças

Abstract

Intracanal medication comprises application of a chemical substance into the root canal in order to exert some desired therapeutic effect. The most common indication for intracanal medication is to improve disinfection after chemomechanical preparation. Calcium hydroxide is the most commonly recommended antimicrobial agent to be used as an interappointment dressing. However, it has some limitations and it seems advantageous to combine it with a biologically active vehicle. Other substances, such as chlorhexidine and antibiotics, have also been used as intracanal medicaments. This chapter reviews the rationale for using an intracanal medication, the indications of use, and the mechanisms of action and clinical outcomes of the most commonly used substances.

The Infectious Problem

In a nutshell, clinicians face basically two conditions that require endodontic treatment: uninfected and infected root canals. The former are represented by teeth with vital pulps, which usually need root canal treatment because of irreversible pulpitis. The latter include teeth with necrotic pulps and usually associated with primary apical periodontitis and root canal-treated teeth that require retreatment because of posttreatment apical periodontitis. In teeth with irreversible pulpitis, infection is generally restricted to the area of exposure or the coronal pulp, with the radicular pulp being inflamed or not, but not infected [1, 2]. In these cases, root canal treatment should be completed as soon as possible, with asepsis as the key element to

J.F. Siqueira Jr., DDS, MSc, PhD (✉)
PostGraduate Program in Endodontics,
Faculty of Dentistry, Estácio de Sá University,
Av. Alfredo Baltazar da Silveira, 580/cobertura,
Recreio, Rio de Janeiro, RJ 22790-710, Brazil
e-mail: jf_siqueira@yahoo.com

I.N. Rôças, DDS, MSc, PhD
PostGraduate Program in Endodontics
and Molecular Microbiology Laboratory,
Faculty of Dentistry, Estácio de Sá University,
Av. Alfredo Baltazar da Silveira, 580/cobertura,
Recreio, Rio de Janeiro, RJ 22790-710, Brazil
e-mail: isabela.siqueira@estacio.br

B. Basrani (ed.), *Endodontic Irrigation: Chemical Disinfection of the Root Canal System*,
DOI 10.1007/978-3-319-16456-4_16

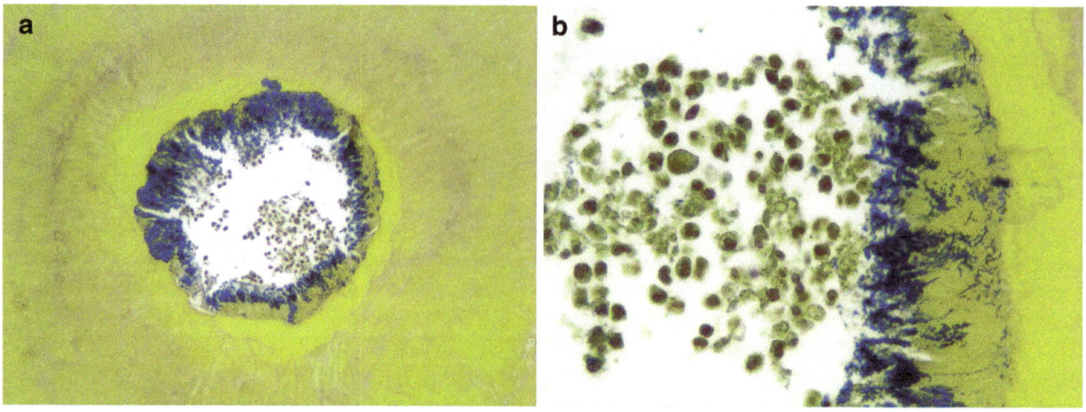

Fig. 16.1 Biofilm is the main form that bacteria are found in endodontic infections. (**a**) Bacterial biofilm covering the entire perimeter of the canal in cross section. (**b**) Higher magnification showing the biofilm attached to the canal walls. An accumulation of polymorphonuclear neutrophils can be seen close to the biofilm. These defense cells are usually ineffective in eliminating the endodontic biofilm (Taylor's modified Brown & Brenn staining, courtesy of Dr. Domenico Ricucci)

influence a successful outcome [3]. It seems consensual that treatment of uninfected teeth should be accomplished in a single visit, provided time, professional skills, and equipment are favorable.

Infected root canals are a completely different problem. Intraradicular infection is the primary cause of both primary and posttreatment apical periodontitis [4–7]. In infected cases, endodontic procedures need to focus not only on asepsis but also on eliminating bacteria from the canal system [8–10]. An optimal outcome of the endodontic treatment will depend on how effective the clinician is in accomplishing these goals.

The success rate of the endodontic treatment of teeth with apical periodontitis is 10–25 % lower than vital teeth or necrotic teeth with no detectable disease [11–17]. Nonetheless, the outcome of treatment of infected teeth filled in the absence of detectable cultivable bacteria (negative culture) is very high and matches that of vital teeth [18]. One can thereby infer that for treatment of infected teeth (necrotic and retreatment cases) to reach a success rate comparable to that of uninfected teeth (vital cases), bacteriologic conditions within the root canals should be similar. This means that maximal bacterial reduction must be achieved in infected teeth before filling.

Bacteria colonizing the infected root canal associated with either primary or posttreatment apical periodontitis are usually organized in biofilm structures attached to the dentinal walls (Fig. 16.1) [6, 7, 19–23]. In addition to the main root canal, bacterial biofilms can be disclosed in anatomical variations including apical ramifications, lateral canals, and isthmuses [2, 24–26]. Biofilms adhered to the apical root surface (extraradicular biofilms) have also been described in some teeth evincing posttreatment apical periodontitis [27–29]. Bacteria that invade and colonize dentinal tubules are a challenge to disinfection procedures and may affect the treatment outcome [20, 30, 31].

The main steps of endodontic treatment involved with infection control are represented by chemomechanical preparation and intracanal medication. Chemomechanical preparation is of paramount importance for root canal disinfection, since instruments and irrigants act primarily in the main canal, which is the most voluminous area of the system and consequently harbors the largest bacterial density. Bacterial elimination from the root canal is carried out by means of the mechanical action of instruments and irrigation as well as the chemical (antibacterial) action of the irrigant solutions. Although substantial amounts of bacteria are eliminated by chemomechanical preparation, studies have demonstrated that 40–60 % of the root canals still present detectable levels of bacteria after instrumentation using either NaOCl or chlorhexidine as the irrigant [18, 32–44]. Because treatment outcome is significantly improved in the absence of detectable bacteria at the time of filling [18, 45–49], some additional step is apparently necessary to optimize disinfection. Several approaches have been proposed to improve disinfection after the instrumentation/irrigation phase [50], including single-visit strategies, but predictably enhanced results have been obtained mostly after an interappointment antimicrobial medication is used.

Intracanal Medication to Supplement Disinfection

Bacteria that escape from the effects of chemomechanical procedures are usually located in areas not reached by instruments and irrigants [7, 24, 26, 51, 52]. These unaffected areas include root canal walls untouched by instruments, dentinal tubules, isthmuses, lateral canals, and apical ramifications [2, 24–26, 31, 53–55].

Irrigants such as NaOCl and chlorhexidine have excellent antimicrobial activities, with pronounced and rapid effects against a large spectrum of species commonly found in endodontic infections. However, these effects are mostly observed when the contact area with the microbial cells is optimal. In the clinical setting, the irrigant should diffuse to reach the areas mentioned above, but the short time they remain in the canal during preparation represents a major limitation. Whereas the irrigant remains in the canal for 10–30 min, which is the usual time taken for preparing most canals, the intracanal medication will remain in the canal for 7 days. This substantial difference in time is the main reason why intracanal medication can enhance disinfection. Because the intracanal medication remains in the canal longer than the irrigation solution, it has more time to diffuse, reach, and eliminate bacteria in areas not affected by chemomechanical procedures.

Numerous substances have been proposed as intracanal medication over the years. The most commonly used substance is calcium hydroxide, so it will be the main focus of this chapter.

Calcium Hydroxide

Calcium hydroxide is possibly the most commonly used intracanal medication. It was introduced in dentistry in 1920 by Bernhard Hermann [56], a German dentist, and since then it has been widely used, especially in endodontics and dental traumatology, for diverse therapeutic purposes [57, 58].

Calcium hydroxide is an inorganic compound, with the formula $Ca(OH)_2$ and molecular weight 74.1 g/mol. The most common presentation is an odorless white powder, obtained by mixing calcium oxide with water:

$$CaO + H_2O \rightarrow Ca(OH)_2$$

Under laboratory conditions, it can also be prepared by mixing aqueous solutions of calcium chloride and sodium hydroxide. Calcium hydroxide is a strong base, with a pH of approximately 12.4. Solubility in water is approximately 1.7 g/L at 20 °C. It is soluble in glycerol and insoluble in alcohol.

In the presence of water, calcium hydroxide dissociates into hydroxyl and calcium ions and most of the biological effects attributed to this substance are related to its alkaline pH (hydroxyl ions) [59]. In the presence of carbon dioxide, calcium carbonate is generated through the following process:

$$Ca(OH)_2 + CO_2 \rightarrow CaCO_3 + H_2O$$

Formation of calcium carbonate negatively affects the activities of calcium hydroxide and should be avoided by preventing contact of this substance with air during storage. Calcium hydroxide should be stored at room temperature.

Vehicles for Calcium Hydroxide

Pure calcium hydroxide is available as a powder. Although some clinicians have developed strategies to apply calcium hydroxide powder in the canal, it is undeniable that mixing this substance with a liquid, gel, or creamy carrier (or vehicle) makes application easier and more predictable. Because calcium hydroxide effects are pH-dependent, the ideal vehicle should

Table 16.1 Classification of the vehicles for calcium hydroxide

Classification according to the consistency and solubility			Classification according to the antimicrobial behavior	
Aqueous	Viscous	Oily	Inert	Biologically active
Distilled water Saline Dental anesthetics Ringer's solution Anionic detergent solution	Glycerin Polyethylene glycol Propylene glycol	CPMC Olive oil Silicone oil	Saline Distilled water Dental anesthetics Glycerin Propylene glycol Polyethylene glycol	CPMC Chlorhexidine Iodine potassium iodide

CPMC camphorated paramonochlorophenol

enable the ionic dissociation of calcium hydroxide. Dissociation will vary according to the type of vehicle used. Because of that, vehicles have been classified according to its consistency and ability to permit calcium hydroxide dissociation as aqueous, viscous, and oily (Table 16.1) [57]. Actually, it is questionable if viscous or oily vehicles are of any value, since they do not permit a high dissociation and consequent release of hydroxyl ions, which is responsible for the main biological effects of calcium hydroxide. Because these effects depend on the magnitude of pH reached in the vicinities where calcium hydroxide was applied, a slow release of calcium hydroxide may not be sufficient to exert the desired effects.

From the standpoint of antimicrobial activity, which is the main property required for an intracanal medicament, vehicles have been classified as inert and biologically active (Table 16.1) [3]. Inert vehicles are for the most part biocompatible but do not significantly influence the antimicrobial properties of calcium hydroxide. These include distilled water, saline, anesthetic solution, glycerin, polyethylene glycol, and propylene glycol. Biologically active vehicles in turn provide additional effects to the calcium hydroxide paste, including improved antimicrobial effects. Examples include camphorated paramonochlorophenol (CPMC), chlorhexidine (CHX), and iodine potassium iodide.

Mechanisms of Antimicrobial Effects

Most bacterial species commonly found in infected root canals are eliminated *in vitro* after a short period of exposure to the high pH of calcium hydroxide [60]. Calcium hydroxide antimicrobial activity depends on the release of hydroxyl (OH^-) ions in an aqueous environment. The hydroxyl ion has a single unpaired electron and is a highly oxidant free radical [61]. The oxidation of organic substrates by hydroxyl ions may occur either by addition of OH^- to an organic molecule or due to removal of a hydrogen atom from it. Hydroxyl ions are short-lived and present high and indiscriminate reactivity. As a consequence, they usually react with biomolecules close to its point of generation [61]. Such reactions usually lead to adverse alterations [62].

Actually, lethal effects of hydroxyl ions on bacterial cells are resultant of the effects on lipids, proteins, and DNA, leading to subsequent damage to the cellular apparatus and drastically altered cellular functions. The effects are as follows: [59]

(a) *Effects on lipids.* Polyunsaturated fatty acids present in membrane phospholipids are particularly sensitive to attack by hydroxyl ions. These free radicals induce lipid peroxidation. A single OH^- can result in peroxidation of many polyunsaturated fatty acids in a cyclic chain reaction. Hydroxyl ions remove hydrogen atoms from polyunsaturated fatty acids, generating a free lipidic radical. This free lipidic radical reacts with oxygen to form a lipidic peroxide radical, which is highly reactive and able to propagate the chain reaction. The peroxide radical removes another hydrogen atom from a second fatty acid, generating another lipidic radical. Therefore, peroxides themselves act as free radicals, initiating an autocatalytic chain reaction and resulting in further loss of polyunsaturated fatty acids, with chain breakage, and extensive membrane damage with increased fluidity and permeability [63, 64].

(b) *Effects on proteins*. The effects of hydroxyl ions on structural proteins or enzymes can cause dramatic effects on the cell and lead to death. Protein damage may be resultant of oxidation induced by hydroxyl ions, either causing oxidative modification of specific amino acids or peptide cleavage. Protein containing the amino acids methionine, cysteine, arginine, and histidine seems to be more prone to oxidation [64]. Hydroxyl ions can also induce the breakdown of ionic bonds that maintain the tertiary structure of proteins. As a consequence, the affected protein maintains its covalent structure but the polypeptide chain is randomly unraveled in variable and irregular spatial conformation. These changes frequently result in loss of biological activity, and if the protein is an enzyme, the cellular metabolism can be disrupted. Structural proteins present in the bacterial cell membranes can also be damaged by hydroxyl ions.

(c) *Effects on DNA*. Hydroxyl ions cause DNA damage through an oxidative attack that results in deoxyribose oxidation, strand breakage, alteration and removal of nucleotides, and DNA-protein cross-links. Hydroxyl ions react with purine and pyrimidine bases and the deoxyribose backbone [65]. The oxidative attack to DNA bases is usually related to addition of OH^- to double bonds; damage to the sugar backbone is mostly related to removal of hydrogen from deoxyribose [65]. Attack to the sugar backbone results in single-strand breaks [61]. The oxidative effects of hydroxyl ions on both DNA and the proteins associated with it may also lead to DNA-protein cross-link formation. DNA-protein cross-links may not be readily repaired and result in cell death under certain circumstances [61].

Antimicrobial Effectiveness in Endodontic Therapy

Laboratory studies have demonstrated that calcium hydroxide is effective against several bacterial species found in endodontic infections [60, 66–68]. Optimum effects were reported when the substance was in direct contact with the test bacteria in solution. In such conditions, concentration of hydroxyl ions is very high, reaching incompatible levels to survival of most bacterial species. However, in the clinical setting, such a direct contact is not always possible to attain.

In fact, clinical studies reveal that the effectiveness of calcium hydroxide in significantly improving disinfection following chemomechanical procedures is somewhat inconsistent [35, 36, 44, 46, 69–71]. This indicates that this substance has its own limitations when it comes to intracanal disinfection. In addition to the difficulties of establishing optimal contact of the medicament with bacteria colonizing the intricacies of the root canal system, other factors may help explain the limitations of calcium hydroxide in promoting predictable root canal disinfection.

Killing of bacteria by calcium hydroxide depends on the availability of hydroxyl ions in solution, which is much higher where the paste is applied (the main root canal). Calcium hydroxide exerts antibacterial effects in the root canal as long as a very high pH is sustained. If this substance needs to diffuse to tissues and the hydroxyl ion concentration is decreased as a result of the action of tissue buffering systems (bicarbonate and phosphate), acids, proteins, and carbon dioxide, its antibacterial effectiveness may be reduced or even impeded [59].

The ability of a medicament to dissolve and diffuse in the root canal system is essential for its successful antimicrobial action. A saturated aqueous suspension of calcium hydroxide possesses a high pH, which has a great toxic potential not only to bacteria but also to host cells. Nevertheless, this highly alkaline substance owes its biocompatibility to its low water solubility and diffusibility [9]. Because of these properties, cytotoxicity is limited to the tissue area in direct contact with calcium hydroxide. On the other

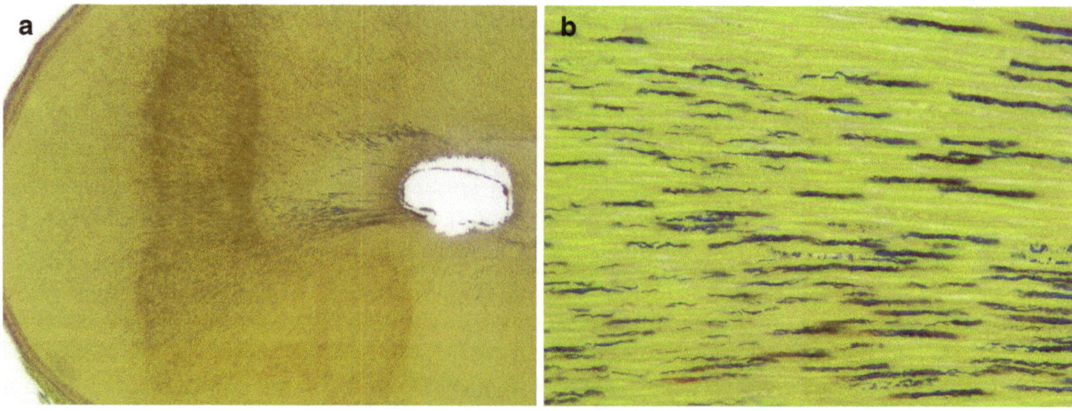

Fig. 16.2 Bacteria colonizing dentinal tubules of the root canal are a challenge for proper disinfection. (**a**) Cross section of the root canal of a tooth with apical periodontitis showing bacterial invasion of dentinal tubules. (**b**) Higher magnification revealing heavy dentinal tubule infection (Taylor's modified Brown & Brenn staining, courtesy of Dr. Domenico Ricucci)

hand, the same properties (low solubility and diffusibility) make it difficult for calcium hydroxide to promote a rapid and significant increase in the pH to eliminate bacteria present in biofilms, dentinal tubules, tissue remnants, and anatomical variations. Likewise, the buffering ability of serum and dentin controls pH changes and thereby reduces calcium hydroxide antimicrobial effectiveness [72–74]. As a consequence of all these factors, calcium hydroxide is a slowly working antimicrobial agent and requires prolonged exposure to allow for saturation of the buffering ability of dentin and tissue remnants. Therefore, long-term use of calcium hydroxide, preferably with exchanges of the medication, is necessary to maximize disinfection of the root canal system.

Bacteria located within dentinal tubules can escape from the effects of chemomechanical preparation. Thus, infected dentinal tubules may serve as a reservoir of bacteria to cause persistent infection and posttreatment apical periodontitis (Fig. 16.2) [7, 75, 76]. Intratubular infection is also the main cause of progressive external inflammatory root resorption [77]. One of the effects expected for intracanal medication is to reach and eliminate bacteria located deep within tubules. Numerous *in vitro* studies demonstrated that calcium hydroxide in inert vehicles has limited effectiveness against intratubular bacteria

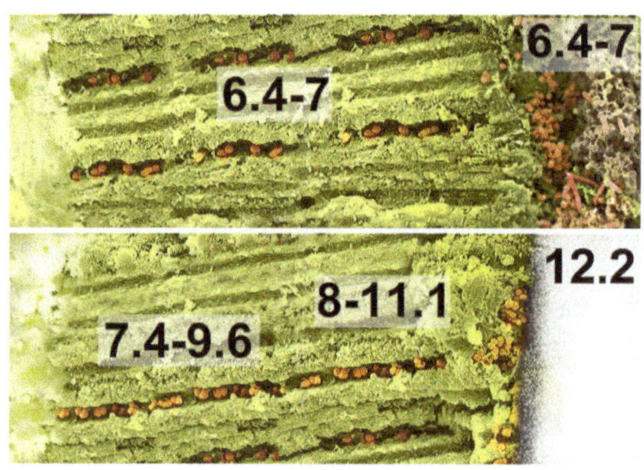

Fig. 16.3 pH changes in different regions of the radicular dentin before and after calcium hydroxide medication (Data according to Tronstad et al. [87])

[78–86]. This is very likely to be resultant of the fact that after a short-term intracanal dressing with calcium hydroxide, the magnitude of pH reached deep in dentin may still be compatible with survival of many microbial species (Fig. 16.3) [87]. Most human bacterial and fungal pathogens grow well within a range of 5–9 pH [88, 89]. Certain bacteria, such as some enterococci, may tolerate even high pH values, varying from 9 to 11.

In fact, resistance to calcium hydroxide has been reported for some microbial species. *Enterococcus faecalis* and some *Candida* species can be highly resistant to the alkaline effects of calcium hydroxide [60, 79, 83, 90, 91]. *E. faecalis* ability to resist high pH values seems to be related to a functioning proton pump, which drives protons into the cell to acidify the cytoplasm [91]. *E. faecalis* and *Candida* species are commonly found in root canal-treated teeth with posttreatment disease [49, 92–97].

Inactivation of Bacterial Virulence Factors

Structural components of the bacterial cell are important virulence factors that stimulate and modulate the inflammatory response and induce indirect damage to host tissues. The main examples are lipopolysaccharides (LPS, a.k.a., endotoxins) and the lipoteichoic acid (LTA), components of the cell wall of gram negative and gram-positive bacteria, respectively.

Lipid A is the portion of LPS that has been regarded as the main responsible factor for the biological effects of this molecule [98, 99]. *In vitro* studies demonstrated that calcium hydroxide can inactivate LPS by acting primarily on the lipid A portion, inducing the alkaline hydrolysis of ester bonds with consequent release of free hydroxy fatty acids with no or reduced toxic and pro-inflammatory effects [100–106]. However, this inactivating effect has been observed *in vitro* under optimal contact between LPS and calcium hydroxide. It is highly unlikely that hydroxyl ions released from calcium hydroxide can reach LPS molecules present in areas distant from the main canal in magnitude sufficient to inactivate these molecules. A clinical study revealed that the levels of LPS were reduced but still relatively high in the canal after chemomechanical preparation, and these levels were virtually unaltered after intracanal medication with calcium hydroxide, CHX, or a combination of both [107].

LTA is a polymer of glycerol phosphate linked to fatty acids. It has been demonstrated that calcium hydroxide can detoxify LTA and attenuate its pro-inflammatory ability [108]. These inactivating effects are supposed to be related to deacylation of LTA induced under high alkaline conditions. Deacylated LTA does not stimulate Toll-like receptor 2, the host molecule responsible for recognition of and response to LTA, and the consequent release of pro-inflammatory cytokines [108]. There are no clinical studies reporting on the effects of calcium hydroxide medication on LTA intracanal levels.

Thus far, it remains to be determined whether these inactivating effects of calcium hydroxide on LPS and LTA can be consistently observed *in vivo* and, if so, what is the actual relevance for the long-term treatment outcome. After all, there is no clear indication that LPS or LTA molecules, in the absence of living bacteria, can induce or maintain periradicular inflammation beyond a certain point in time. Moreover, it is important to point out that virulence factors other than LPS and LTA can also be involved in the pathogenesis of apical periodontitis, usually in a mixture of factors released from multispecies biofilms [109]. This scenario makes the analysis of the effects against specific factors like LPS or LTA somewhat simplistic.

Combination with Biologically Active Vehicles

In an attempt to sidestep the limitations of calcium hydroxide pastes in inert vehicles (*e.g.*, distilled water, saline, glycerin), association of this substance with other antibacterial medicaments, such as CPMC or CHX, has been evaluated [68, 83, 110, 111].

Paste in CPMC

In vitro studies have demonstrated that calcium hydroxide paste in CPMC has a broader antimicrobial spectrum (eliminating microorganisms that are resistant to calcium hydroxide) and a larger radius of antimicrobial action (eliminating microorganisms located in regions more distant from the vicinity where the paste was applied) kills microorganisms faster and is less affected by serum and necrotic tissue than mixtures of calcium hydroxide with inert vehicles [59, 68, 72, 83, 84, 112–119]. The larger radius of action may be a result of the low surface tension of CPMC and/or its high solubility in lipids. Glycerin has been added to the paste to dilute CPMC and facilitate both handling and further removal of the paste from the canal. Although CPMC exhibits high toxicity when used alone, satisfactory biocompatibility results have been observed in animal studies [120, 121]. Clinical studies evaluating the incidence of postoperative pain [122], antibacterial activity [37, 40], and treatment outcome [123] have demonstrated optimal results when using an antibacterial protocol for treatment that includes a 7-day interappointment medication with calcium hydroxide/CPMC/glycerin paste.

Paste in CHX

In vitro studies investigating the antimicrobial effectiveness of the combination calcium hydroxide and CHX have shown conflicting results. Some studies demonstrated that the antimicrobial effects of calcium hydroxide are significantly increased when adding CHX in a paste [110, 124–126], while others have shown no significant increase in activity [112, 127]. However, the antibacterial efficacy of CHX may be significantly reduced after mixing with calcium hydroxide [112, 126, 127].

Although some clinical studies have shown no advantage in using calcium hydroxide combined with CHX [71, 107], others have reported good results for this association [38, 128–130]. Zerella et al. [128] reported that intracanal dressing with a mixture of 2 % CHX and calcium hydroxide was at least as effective as calcium hydroxide in an inert vehicle in the disinfection of root canal-treated teeth with apical periodontitis. In a clinical study evaluating the antibacterial effectiveness of a treatment protocol against primary infections, Siqueira et al. [38] used 0.12 % CHX as the irrigant during chemomechanical preparation and found an incidence of positive cultures of 54 %. Further intracanal medication with calcium hydroxide paste in 0.12 % CHX significantly decreased the number of positive cultures to 8 %. Paiva et al. [129] used several sensitive molecular biology techniques to evaluate the clinical antibacterial effects of chemomechanical preparation using NiTi rotary instrumentation and NaOCl irrigation (S2), a final rinse with CHX (S3), and then 1-week interappointment medication with calcium hydroxide/CHX paste (S4). Treatment procedures promoted a decrease in microbial diversity and significantly reduced the incidence of positive results and the bacterial counts. In general, each subsequent treatment step improved disinfection. In S2, 64 % of samples were still positive for the presence of bacteria, decreasing to 43 % in S3 and then to 14 % in S4. The number of positive results was significantly lower for S4 when compared with S2, and the same was true for bacterial counting analysis. The authors concluded that supplementary steps consisting of a final rinse with CHX followed by calcium hydroxide/CHX interappointment medication promoted further decrease of the bacterial bioburden to levels significantly below those achieved by the chemomechanical procedures alone. Oliveira et al. [130] demonstrated that intracanal medication with calcium hydroxide/CHX paste had significant supplementary effects in eliminating endotoxins from infected canals and/or neutralizing their cytotoxic effects.

CHX remains stable at pH 5–8 and, as the pH increases, ionization decreases. Association of calcium hydroxide with CHX maintains a high pH value, which is similar to calcium hydroxide paste using water as vehicle [110, 128]. CHX antimicrobial activity is influenced by pH conditions, with the optimal range of 5.5–7, and at high pH values, it precipitates and may be unavailable as an antimicrobial agent [128]. Despite the expected high loss of CHX when mixed with calcium hydroxide, the combined resulting antimicrobial effect may still be of clinical significance, as demonstrated by the studies discussed above [38, 128–130]. This combination presents significant antibacterial effects, which may be related to small residues of active CHX still present in the paste, even though the effects of the high pH of the paste cannot be disregarded.

Table 16.2 summarizes several clinical studies investigating the percentage of cases that remained positive for the presence of detectable bacteria after using different treatment protocols.

Table 16.2 Clinical studies evaluating the antimicrobial effects of chemomechanical preparation and intracanal medication

Study	Irrigation	Medication	Time of medication	Microbiological technique	Cases positive for bacteria after medication[a]
Byström et al. (1985) [60]	0.5 or 5 % NaOCl	Calcium hydroxide	30 days	Culture	0/35 (0 %)* 1/35 (3 %)** 2–4 dl
Reit and Dahlén (1988) [156]	0.5 % NaOCl	Calcium hydroxide	14 days	Culture	8/32 (25 %)* 9/32 (28 %)** 7 dl
Orstavik et al. (1991) [157]	Saline	Calcium hydroxide	7 days	Culture	8/22 (36 %)*
Sjögren et al. (1991) [69]	0.5 % NaOCl	Calcium hydroxide	7 days	Culture	0/18 (0 %)* 0/18 (0 %)** 1–5 wl
Yared and Dagher (1994) [158]	1 % NaOCl	Calcium hydroxide	7 days	Culture	19/60 (32 %)*
Shuping et al. (2000) [35]	1.25 % NaOCl	Calcium hydroxide	7–203 days	Culture	3/40 (7.5 %)*
Lana et al. (2001) [159]	2.5 % NaOCl	Calcium hydroxide	7 days	Culture	4/27 (15 %)* 7/27 (26 %)** 7 dl
Peters et al. (2002) [70]	2 % NaOCl	Calcium hydroxide	28 days	Culture	15/21 (71 %)*
Kvist et al. (2004) [160]	0.5 % NaOCl	Calcium hydroxide	7 days	Culture	16/43 (37 %)*
McGurkin-Smith et al. (2005) [33]	5.25 % NaOCl	Calcium hydroxide	7–110 days	Culture	4/24 (17 %)*
Waltimo et al. (2005) [46]	2.5 % NaOCl	Calcium hydroxide	7 days	Culture	6/18 (33 %)*
Zerella et al. (2005) [128][b]	1 % NaOCl	Calcium hydroxide	7–10 days	Culture	10/20 (50 %)*
Zerella et al. (2005) [128][b]	1 % NaOCl	Calcium hydroxide/ 2 % chlorhexidine	7–10 days	Culture	7/20 (35 %)*
Chu et al. (2006) [161]	0.5 % NaOCl	Calcium hydroxide	7 days	Culture	11/35 (31 %)*
Manzur et al. (2007) [71]	1 % NaOCl	Calcium hydroxide	7 days	Culture	2/11 (18 %)*
Manzur et al. (2007) [71]	1 % NaOCl	Calcium hydroxide/ 2 % chlorhexidine	7 days	Culture	3/11 (27 %)*
Manzur et al. (2007) [71]	1 % NaOCl	2 % chlorhexidine (gel)	7 days	Culture	5/11 (45.5 %)*
Paquette et al. (2007) [32]	2.5 % NaOCl	2 % chlorhexidine (liquid)	7–15 days	Culture	15/22 (68 %)*
Vianna et al. (2007) [107]	2 % chlorhexidine (gel)	Calcium hydroxide	7 days	Culture	5/8 (62.5 %)*
Vianna et al. (2007) [107]	2 % chlorhexidine (gel)	2 % chlorhexidine (gel)	7 days	Culture	4/8 (50 %)*
Vianna et al. (2007) [107]	2 % chlorhexidine (gel)	Calcium hydroxide/ 2 % chlorhexidine	7 days	Culture	4/8 (50 %)*
Wang et al. (2007) [162]	2 % chlorhexidine (gel)	Calcium hydroxide/2 % chlorhexidine	14–29 days	Culture	3/36 (8 %)*

(continued)

Table 16.2 (continued)

Study	Irrigation	Medication	Time of medication	Microbiological technique	Cases positive for bacteria after medication[a]
Sakamoto et al. (2007) [163]	2.5 % NaOCl	Calcium hydroxide/ CPMC	7 days	PCR	10/15 (67 %)*
Siqueira et al. (2007) [36]	2.5 % NaOCl	Calcium hydroxide	7 days	Culture	2/11 (18 %)*
Siqueira et al. (2007) [37]	2.5 % NaOCl	Calcium hydroxide/ CPMC	7 days	Culture	1/11 (9 %)*
Siqueira et al. (2007) [38]	0.12 % chlorhexidine	Calcium hydroxide/0.12 % chlorhexidine	7 days	Culture	1/13 (8 %)*
Rôças and Siqueira (2010) [42]	2.5 % NaOCl	Calcium hydroxide/ CPMC	7 days	PCR	10/15 (67 %)*
Rôças and Siqueira (2010) [42]	2.5 % NaOCl	Calcium hydroxide/ CPMC	7 days	RT-PCR	8/15 (53 %)*
Rôças and Siqueira (2010) [42]	2.5 % NaOCl	Calcium hydroxide/ CPMC	7 days	checkerboard	8/15 (53 %)*
Huffaker et al. (2010) [44]	0.5 % NaOCl	Calcium hydroxide	>14 days	Culture	20/74 (27 %)*
Rôças and Siqueira (2011) [40]	2.5 % NaOCl	Calcium hydroxide	7 days	PCR	5/12 (42 %)*
Rôças and Siqueira (2011) [40]	2.5 % NaOCl	Calcium hydroxide/ CPMC	7 days	PCR	4/12 (33 %)*
Beus et al. (2012) [164]	1 % NaOCl	Calcium hydroxide	>7 days	Culture	6/46 (13 %)*
Paiva et al. (2013) [129]	2.5 % NaOCl	Rinsing with 2 % chlorhexidine + calcium hydroxide/ 2 % chlorhexidine	7 days	PCR	2/14 (14 %)*

[a]Number of cases positive for bacteria in posttreatment samples/number of cases positive for bacteria in initial samples
[b]Retreatment cases
*Samples taken at the same visit as medication was removed
**Samples taken some days after the dressing was removed (dl, days later; wl, weeks later)
CPMC camphorated paramonochlorophenol, *PCR* polymerase chain reaction

Chlorhexidine Alone for Intracanal Medication

CHX alone has also been used and evaluated as an intracanal medication. This substance is a topical antiseptic solution that has been used worldwide since 1954 [131]. CHX is a cationic bis-biguanide that is insoluble in water and is formulated with either gluconic or acetic acid to form water-soluble digluconate or diacetate salts. CHX is highly effective against several gram-positive and gram-negative oral bacterial species as well as yeasts [114, 132–137]. In addition to its antimicrobial activity, CHX also presents substantivity in dentin [138–140] and displays low irritation to living tissues [141, 142]. Because of these properties, CHX has emerged as a potential interappointment medication to be used alternatively to calcium hydroxide.

CHX is bacteriostatic at low concentrations and bactericidal at high concentrations [136]. The initial site of CHX action is the cytoplasmic membrane. CHX crosses the cell wall, presumably by passive diffusion, and subsequently attacks the cytoplasmic membrane. CHX binds to the negatively charged bacterial cell membrane and, at low concentrations, can affect its integrity, leading to rupture of the membrane (without lysis of the cell wall) and release of the cell constituents at a very low rate [143]. This effect is usually insufficient to induce cell death. However, at the high concentrations used under antiseptic/disinfectant conditions, CHX enters the cytoplasm via the damaged cytoplasmic membrane and promotes precipitation of cytoplasmic contents, particularly phosphated entities, with resulting cell death [144, 145].

While hydroxyapatite has little or no inhibitory effects on CHX [73], dentin matrix [146], bovine serum albumin [73], and necrotic tissue [72] have been shown to significantly inhibit its activity. CHX solutions may be stored at room temperature and a shelf-life of at least 1 year is expected, provided that packaging is adequate. Prolonged exposure to high temperature or light should be avoided.

Several *in vitro* studies have demonstrated that CHX is more effective than calcium hydroxide in eliminating *E.* faecalis or *C. albicans* from dentinal tubules [112, 127, 147–149]. There are not many clinical studies evaluating the effects of CHX alone as an intracanal medication. One study showed no significant difference in the incidence of postoperative pain in treatment or retreatment cases following chemomechanical preparation and intracanal medication with either CHX or a calcium hydroxide paste [150]. In terms of antimicrobial effectiveness, Vianna et al. [151] evaluated the antibacterial effects of a treatment protocol using chemomechanical preparation with 2 % CHX gel as auxiliary chemical substance followed by 7 days of intracanal dressing with calcium hydroxide, 2 % CHX gel, or calcium hydroxide/2 % CHX gel. The incidence of positive cultures after these medications was 62.5 %, 50 %, and 50 %, respectively, with no significant difference between them. Manzur et al. [71] reported an incidence of positive cultures of 18 % after calcium hydroxide medication, 45.5 % after 2 % CHX, and 27 % after calcium hydroxide/CHX. They concluded that the antibacterial efficacy of the 3 medications was statistically comparable. Paquette et al. [32] evaluated the antibacterial efficacy of intracanal medication with 2 % CHX liquid and reported 68 % positive cultures. Malkhassian et al. [152] assessed the antibacterial efficacy of a final rinse with BioPure MTAD and intracanal medication with 2 % CHX gel and concluded that these approaches did not reduce bacterial counts beyond levels achieved by chemomechanical preparation with NaOCl. Teles et al. [153] observed that a 14-day intracanal medication with calcium hydroxide in inert vehicle performed significantly better than 2 % CHX gel as for reducing bacterial counts in teeth with apical periodontitis.

A study [154] evaluated the 2- to 4-year outcome of treatment using 2 % CHX liquid as the intracanal medication for 7–15 days. Findings revealed that 94 % of the teeth were healed and this finding did not differ significantly from that in a historical control using calcium hydroxide (90 %), suggesting a comparable outcome after medication with these two substances.

Other Intracanal Medicaments

In the past, several toxic substances were used as intracanal medicaments, including aldehydes (formocresol, tricresol formalin, glutaraldehyde) and phenolics (camphorated phenol or paramonochlorophenol, cresatin, eugenol). Most of them are too toxic to host tissues and some of them were ineffective in the clinical setting. Consequently, their use was abolished and no longer recommended.

Other Indications for Intracanal Medication

In addition to be indicated to improve disinfection in routine cases of primary or posttreatment apical periodontitis, an intracanal medication has also been recommended in the following occasional situations:

(a) To serve as a physicochemical barrier to protect against, or at least delay, bacterial contamination of the canal between appointments in uninfected cases where the endodontic treatment could not be completed in a single visit
(b) To act indirectly on inflammation by helping eliminate its primary cause, i.e., residual microorganisms in the apical canal in cases with persistent symptoms or exudation
(c) To help clean and disinfect areas untouched by instruments in teeth with aberrant internal anatomy, as, for instance, because of internal resorption or developmental anomalies. It has been shown that soft tissue pretreated with calcium hydroxide is more rapidly dissolved by NaOCl than when NaOCl is used alone [155]. It is recommended that a calcium hydroxide paste be packed into irregularities and then in the subsequent visit be removed by using endodontic instruments under copious irrigation with NaOCl and/or ultrasonic activation of NaOCl
(d) To help halt external root resorption processes, either by acting on the cause, i.e., bacteria infecting the root canal system, or by directly interfering with the resorptive process
(e) To eliminate infection and create an appropriate environment for apical closure or for regenerative approaches in immature teeth with necrotic pulps and open apexes

References

1. Langeland K. Tissue response to dental caries. Endod Dent Traumatol. 1987;3:149–71.
2. Ricucci D, Siqueira Jr JF. Fate of the tissue in lateral canals and apical ramifications in response to pathologic conditions and treatment procedures. J Endod. 2010;36:1–15.
3. Siqueira Jr JF. Treatment of endodontic infections. London: Quintessence Publishing; 2011.
4. Kakehashi S, Stanley HR, Fitzgerald RJ. The effects of surgical exposures of dental pulps in germ-free and conventional laboratory rats. Oral Surg Oral Med Oral Pathol. 1965;20:340–9.
5. Sundqvist G. Bacteriological studies of necrotic dental pulps [Odontological Dissertation no.7]. Umea: University of Umea; 1976.
6. Ricucci D, Siqueira Jr JF. Biofilms and apical periodontitis: study of prevalence and association with clinical and histopathologic findings. J Endod. 2010; 36:1277–88.
7. Ricucci D, Siqueira Jr JF, Bate AL, Pitt Ford TR. Histologic investigation of root canal-treated teeth with apical periodontitis: a retrospective study from twenty-four patients. J Endod. 2009;35: 493–502.
8. Orstavik D. Root canal disinfection: a review of concepts and recent developments. Aust Endod J. 2003; 29:70–4.
9. Siqueira Jr JF. Strategies to treat infected root canals. J Calif Dent Assoc. 2001;29:825–37.
10. Haapasalo M, Endal U, Zandi H, Coil JM. Eradication of endodontic infection by instrumentation and irrigation solutions. Endod Topics. 2005;10:77–102.
11. Hoskinson SE, Ng YL, Hoskinson AE, Moles DR, Gulabivala K. A retrospective comparison of outcome of root canal treatment using two different protocols. Oral Surg Oral Med Oral Pathol Oral Radiol Endod. 2002;93:705–15.
12. Cheung GS, Liu CS. A retrospective study of endodontic treatment outcome between nickel-titanium rotary and stainless steel hand filing techniques. J Endod. 2009;35:938–43.
13. Chugal NM, Clive JM, Spångberg LS. Endodontic infection: some biologic and treatment factors associated with outcome. Oral Surg Oral Med Oral Pathol Oral Radiol Endod. 2003;96:81–90.
14. Chugal NM, Clive JM, Spångberg LS. A prognostic model for assessment of the outcome of endodontic treatment: effect of biologic and diagnostic variables. Oral Surg Oral Med Oral Pathol Oral Radiol Endod. 2001;91:342–52.
15. de Chevigny C, Dao TT, Basrani BR, Marquis V, Farzaneh M, Abitbol S, Friedman S. Treatment outcome in endodontics: the Toronto study–phase 4: initial treatment. J Endod. 2008;34:258–63.
16. Orstavik D, Qvist V, Stoltze K. A multivariate analysis of the outcome of endodontic treatment. Eur J Oral Sci. 2004;112:224–30.
17. Sjögren U, Hagglund B, Sundqvist G, Wing K. Factors affecting the long-term results of endodontic treatment. J Endod. 1990;16:498–504.
18. Sjögren U, Figdor D, Persson S, Sundqvist G. Influence of infection at the time of root filling on the outcome of endodontic treatment of teeth with apical periodontitis. Int Endod J. 1997;30:297–306.
19. Nair PNR. Light and electron microscopic studies of root canal flora and periapical lesions. J Endod. 1987;13:29–39.
20. Siqueira Jr JF, Rôças IN, Lopes HP. Patterns of microbial colonization in primary root canal infections. Oral Surg Oral Med Oral Pathol Oral Radiol Endod. 2002;93:174–8.
21. Molven O, Olsen I, Kerekes K. Scanning electron microscopy of bacteria in the apical part of root canals in permanent teeth with periapical lesions. Endod Dent Traumatol. 1991;7:226–9.

22. Carr GB, Schwartz RS, Schaudinn C, Gorur A, Costerton JW. Ultrastructural examination of failed molar retreatment with secondary apical periodontitis: an examination of endodontic biofilms in an endodontic retreatment failure. J Endod. 2009;35:1303–9.
23. Schaudinn C, Carr G, Gorur A, Jaramillo D, Costerton JW, Webster P. Imaging of endodontic biofilms by combined microscopy (FISH/cLSM – SEM). J Microsc. 2009;235:124–7.
24. Nair PN, Henry S, Cano V, Vera J. Microbial status of apical root canal system of human mandibular first molars with primary apical periodontitis after "one-visit" endodontic treatment. Oral Surg Oral Med Oral Pathol Oral Radiol Endod. 2005;99:231–52.
25. Ricucci D, Siqueira Jr JF. Apical actinomycosis as a continuum of intraradicular and extraradicular infection: case report and critical review on its involvement with treatment failure. J Endod. 2008;34:1124–9.
26. Vera J, Siqueira Jr JF, Ricucci D, Loghin S, Fernandez N, Flores B, Cruz AG. One- versus two-visit endodontic treatment of teeth with apical periodontitis: a histobacteriologic study. J Endod. 2012;38:1040–52.
27. Tronstad L, Barnett F, Cervone F. Periapical bacterial plaque in teeth refractory to endodontic treatment. Endod Dent Traumatol. 1990;6:73–7.
28. Ferreira FB, Ferreira AL, Gomes BP, Souza-Filho FJ. Resolution of persistent periapical infection by endodontic surgery. Int Endod J. 2004;37:61–9.
29. Ricucci D, Martorano M, Bate AL, Pascon EA. Calculus-like deposit on the apical external root surface of teeth with post-treatment apical periodontitis: report of two cases. Int Endod J. 2005;38:262–71.
30. Peters LB, Wesselink PR, Buijs JF, van Winkelhoff AJ. Viable bacteria in root dentinal tubules of teeth with apical periodontitis. J Endod. 2001;27:76–81.
31. Vieira AR, Siqueira Jr JF, Ricucci D, Lopes WS. Dentinal tubule infection as the cause of recurrent disease and late endodontic treatment failure: a case report. J Endod. 2012;38:250–4.
32. Paquette L, Legner M, Fillery ED, Friedman S. Antibacterial efficacy of chlorhexidine gluconate intracanal medication in vivo. J Endod. 2007;33:788–95.
33. McGurkin-Smith R, Trope M, Caplan D, Sigurdsson A. Reduction of intracanal bacteria using GT rotary instrumentation, 5.25% NaOCl, EDTA, and $Ca(OH)_2$. J Endod. 2005;31:359–63.
34. Byström A, Sundqvist G. The antibacterial action of sodium hypochlorite and EDTA in 60 cases of endodontic therapy. Int Endod J. 1985;18:35–40.
35. Shuping GB, Ørstavik D, Sigurdsson A, Trope M. Reduction of intracanal bacteria using nickel-titanium rotary instrumentation and various medications. J Endod. 2000;26:751–5.
36. Siqueira Jr JF, Guimarães-Pinto T, Rôças IN. Effects of chemomechanical preparation with 2.5% sodium hypochlorite and intracanal medication with calcium hydroxide on cultivable bacteria in infected root canals. J Endod. 2007;33:800–5.
37. Siqueira Jr JF, Magalhães KM, Rôças IN. Bacterial reduction in infected root canals treated with 2.5% NaOCl as an irrigant and calcium hydroxide/camphorated paramonochlorophenol paste as an intracanal dressing. J Endod. 2007;33:667–72.
38. Siqueira Jr JF, Paiva SS, Rôças IN. Reduction in the cultivable bacterial populations in infected root canals by a chlorhexidine-based antimicrobial protocol. J Endod. 2007;33:541–7.
39. Siqueira Jr JF, Rôças IN, Paiva SS, Guimarães-Pinto T, Magalhães KM, Lima KC. Bacteriologic investigation of the effects of sodium hypochlorite and chlorhexidine during the endodontic treatment of teeth with apical periodontitis. Oral Surg Oral Med Oral Pathol Oral Radiol Endod. 2007;104:122–30.
40. Rôças IN, Siqueira Jr JF. In vivo antimicrobial effects of endodontic treatment procedures as assessed by molecular microbiologic techniques. J Endod. 2011;37:304–10.
41. Rôças IN, Siqueira Jr JF. Comparison of the in vivo antimicrobial effectiveness of sodium hypochlorite and chlorhexidine used as root canal irrigants: a molecular microbiology study. J Endod. 2011;37:143–50.
42. Rôças IN, Siqueira Jr JF. Identification of bacteria enduring endodontic treatment procedures by a combined reverse transcriptase-polymerase chain reaction and reverse-capture checkerboard approach. J Endod. 2010;36:45–52.
43. Paiva SS, Siqueira Jr JF, Rôças IN, Carmo FL, Ferreira DC, Curvelo JA, Soares RM, Rosado AS. Supplementing the antimicrobial effects of chemomechanical debridement with either passive ultrasonic irrigation or a final rinse with chlorhexidine: a clinical study. J Endod. 2012;38:1202–6.
44. Huffaker SK, Safavi K, Spångberg LS, Kaufman B. Influence of a passive sonic irrigation system on the elimination of bacteria from root canal systems: a clinical study. J Endod. 2010;36:1315–8.
45. Fabricius L, Dahlén G, Sundqvist G, Happonen RP, Möller AJR. Influence of residual bacteria on periapical tissue healing after chemomechanical treatment and root filling of experimentally infected monkey teeth. Eur J Oral Sci. 2006;114:278–85.
46. Waltimo T, Trope M, Haapasalo M, Ørstavik D. Clinical efficacy of treatment procedures in endodontic infection control and one year follow-up of periapical healing. J Endod. 2005;31:863–6.
47. Heling B, Shapira J. Roentgenologic and clinical evaluation of endodontically treated teeth with or without negative culture. Quintessence Int. 1978;11:79–84.
48. Engström B, Hard AF, Segerstad L, Ramström G, Frostell G. Correlation of positive cultures with the prognosis for root canal treatment. Odontol Revy. 1964;15:257–70.
49. Sundqvist G, Figdor D, Persson S, Sjogren U. Microbiologic analysis of teeth with failed endodontic treatment and the outcome of conservative re-treatment. Oral Surg Oral Med Oral Pathol Oral Radiol Endod. 1998;85:86–93.

50. Siqueira Jr JF, Rôças IN. Optimising single-visit disinfection with supplementary approaches: a quest for predictability. Aust Endod J. 2011;37:92–8.
51. Siqueira Jr JF, Araujo MC, Garcia PF, Fraga RC, Dantas CJ. Histological evaluation of the effectiveness of five instrumentation techniques for cleaning the apical third of root canals. J Endod. 1997;23: 499–502.
52. Walton RE. Histologic evaluation of different methods of enlarging the pulp canal space. J Endod. 1976;2:304–11.
53. Peters OA, Schönenberger K, Laib A. Effects of four Ni-Ti preparation techniques on root canal geometry assessed by micro computed tomography. Int Endod J. 2001;34:221–30.
54. Siqueira Jr JF, Alves FR, Versiani MA, Rôças IN, Almeida BM, Neves MA, Sousa-Neto MD. Correlative bacteriologic and micro-computed tomographic analysis of mandibular molar mesial canals prepared by self-adjusting file, Reciproc, and Twisted File systems. J Endod. 2013;39:1044–50.
55. Paque F, Balmer M, Attin T, Peters OA. Preparation of oval-shaped root canals in mandibular molars using nickel-titanium rotary instruments: a micro-computed tomography study. J Endod. 2010;36: 703–7.
56. Hermann BW. Calciumhydroxyd als mittel zum behandeln und füllen von zahnwurzelkanälen. Würzburg, Med. Diss. 1920. 48p.
57. Fava LR, Saunders WP. Calcium hydroxide pastes: classification and clinical indications. Int Endod J. 1999;32:257–82.
58. Heithersay GS. Calcium hydroxide in the treatment of pulpless teeth with associated pathology. J Brit Endod Soc. 1975;8:74–92.
59. Siqueira Jr JF, Lopes HP. Mechanisms of antimicrobial activity of calcium hydroxide: a critical review. Int Endod J. 1999;32:361–9.
60. Byström A, Claesson R, Sundqvist G. The antibacterial effect of camphorated paramonochlorophenol, camphorated phenol and calcium hydroxide in the treatment of infected root canals. Endod Dent Traumatol. 1985;1:170–5.
61. Sharma P, Jha AB, Dubey RS, Pessarakli M. Reactive oxygen species, oxidative damage, and antioxidative defense mechanism in plants under stressful conditions. J Botany. 2012;Article ID 217037, doi:10.1155/2012.
62. Lobo V, Patil A, Phatak A, Chandra N. Free radicals, antioxidants and functional foods: impact on human health. Pharmacogn Rev. 2010;4:118–26.
63. Kumar V, Abbas AK, Fausto N, Aster JC. Robbins and Cotran pathologic basis of disease. 8th ed. Philadelphia: Saunders/Elsevier; 2010.
64. Freeman BA, Crapo JD. Biology of disease: free radicals and tissue injury. Lab Invest. 1982;47: 412–26.
65. Halliwell B, Gutteridge JMC. Free radicals in biology and medicine. 3rd ed. Oxford, UK: Oxford University Press; 1999.
66. Stuart KG, Miller CH, Brown Jr CE, Newton CW. The comparative antimicrobial effect of calcium hydroxide. Oral Surg Oral Med Oral Pathol. 1991;72:101–4.
67. Georgopoulou M, Kontakiotis E, Nakou M. In vitro evaluation of the effectiveness of calcium hydroxide and paramonochlorophenol on anaerobic bacteria from the root canal. Endod Dent Traumatol. 1993;9: 249–53.
68. Siqueira Jr JF, de Uzeda M. Influence of different vehicles on the antibacterial effects of calcium hydroxide. J Endod. 1998;24:663–5.
69. Sjögren U, Figdor D, Spångberg L, Sundqvist G. The antimicrobial effect of calcium hydroxide as a short-term intracanal dressing. Int Endod J. 1991;24:119–25.
70. Peters LB, van Winkelhoff AJ, Buijs JF, Wesselink PR. Effects of instrumentation, irrigation and dressing with calcium hydroxide on infection in pulpless teeth with periapical bone lesions. Int Endod J. 2002;35:13–21.
71. Manzur A, Gonzalez AM, Pozos A, Silva-Herzog D, Friedman S. Bacterial quantification in teeth with apical periodontitis related to instrumentation and different intracanal medications: a randomized clinical trial. J Endod. 2007;33:114–8.
72. Oliveira JC, Alves FR, Uzeda M, Rocas IN, Siqueira Jr JF. Influence of serum and necrotic soft tissue on the antimicrobial effects of intracanal medicaments. Braz Dent J. 2010;21:295–300.
73. Portenier I, Haapasalo H, Rye A, Waltimo T, Ørstavik D, Haapasalo M. Inactivation of root canal medicaments by dentine, hydroxylapatite and bovine serum albumin. Int Endod J. 2001;34:184–8.
74. Haapasalo M, Qian W, Portenier I, Waltimo T. Effects of dentin on the antimicrobial properties of endodontic medicaments. J Endod. 2007;33: 917–25.
75. Ricucci D, Siqueira Jr JF. Anatomic and microbiologic challenges to achieving success with endodontic treatment: a case report. J Endod. 2008;34:1249–54.
76. Love RM. Invasion of dentinal tubules by root canal bacteria. Endod Topics. 2004;9:52–65.
77. Barnett F. The role of endodontics in the treatment of luxated permanent teeth. Dent Traumatol. 2002;18: 47–56.
78. Estrela C, Pimenta FC, Ito IY, Bammann LL. Antimicrobial evaluation of calcium hydroxide in infected dentinal tubules. J Endod. 1999;25:416–8.
79. Haapasalo M, Ørstavik D. In vitro infection and disinfection of dentinal tubules. J Dent Res. 1987;66: 1375–9.
80. Heling I, Steinberg D, Kenig S, Gavrilovich I, Sela MN, Friedman M. Efficacy of a sustained-release device containing chlorhexidine and Ca(OH)2 in preventing secondary infection of dentinal tubules. Int Endod J. 1992;25:20–4.
81. Orstavik D, Haapasalo M. Disinfection by endodontic irrigants and dressings of experimentally infected dentinal tubules. Endod Dent Traumatol. 1990;6: 142–9.

82. Safavi KE, Spångberg LS, Langeland K. Root canal dentinal tubule disinfection. J Endod. 1990;16:207–10.
83. Siqueira Jr JF, de Uzeda M. Disinfection by calcium hydroxide pastes of dentinal tubules infected with two obligate and one facultative anaerobic bacteria. J Endod. 1996;22:674–6.
84. Sukawat C, Srisuwan T. A comparison of the antimicrobial efficacy of three calcium hydroxide formulations on human dentin infected with *Enterococcus faecalis*. J Endod. 2002;28:102–4.
85. Siqueira JF Jr, Machado de Oliveira JC, Magalhães FAC, Lopes HP. Efeitos do hidróxido de cálcio associado a diferentes veículos sobre dentina contaminada. Revista Brasileira de Odontologia. 2001;58:44–7.
86. Weiger R, de Lucena J, Decker HE, Lost C. Vitality status of microorganisms in infected human root dentine. Int Endod J. 2002;35:166–71.
87. Tronstad L, Andreasen JO, Hasselgren G, Kristerson L, Riis I. pH changes in dental tissues after root canal filling with calcium hydroxide. J Endod. 1981;7:17–21.
88. Padan E, Zilberstein D, Schuldiner S. pH homeostasis in bacteria. Biochim Biophys Acta. 1981;650:151–66.
89. Atlas RM. Principles of microbiology. 2nd ed. Dubuque, USA: WCB Publishers; 1997
90. Waltimo TM, Siren EK, Ørstavik D, Haapasalo MP. Susceptibility of oral *Candida* species to calcium hydroxide in vitro. Int Endod J. 1999;32:94–8.
91. Evans M, Davies JK, Sundqvist G, Figdor D. Mechanisms involved in the resistance of *Enterococcus faecalis* to calcium hydroxide. Int Endod J. 2002;35:221–8.
92. Pinheiro ET, Gomes BP, Ferraz CC, Sousa EL, Teixeira FB, Souza-Filho FJ. Microorganisms from canals of root-filled teeth with periapical lesions. Int Endod J. 2003;36:1–11.
93. Rôças IN, Jung IY, Lee CY, Siqueira Jr JF. Polymerase chain reaction identification of microorganisms in previously root-filled teeth in a South Korean population. J Endod. 2004;30:504–8.
94. Rôças IN, Siqueira Jr JF, Santos KR. Association of *Enterococcus faecalis* with different forms of periradicular diseases. J Endod. 2004;30:315–20.
95. Siqueira Jr JF, Rôças IN. Polymerase chain reaction-based analysis of microorganisms associated with failed endodontic treatment. Oral Surg Oral Med Oral Pathol Oral Radiol Endod. 2004;97:85–94.
96. Rôças IN, Siqueira Jr JF. Characterization of microbiota of root canal-treated teeth with posttreatment disease. J Clin Microbiol. 2012;50:1721–4.
97. Gomes BP, Pinheiro ET, Jacinto RC, Zaia AA, Ferraz CC, Souza-Filho FJ. Microbial analysis of canals of root-filled teeth with periapical lesions using polymerase chain reaction. J Endod. 2008;34:537–40.
98. Rietschel ET, Kirikae T, Schade U, Mamat U, Schmidt G, Loppnow H, Ulmer AJ, Zahringer U, Seydel U, Padova FD, Schreier M, Brade H. Bacterial endotoxin: molecular relationships of structure to activity and function. FASEB J. 1994;8:217–25.
99. Rietschel ET, Brade H. Bacterial endotoxins. Sci Am. 1992;267:26–33.
100. Safavi KE, Nichols FC. Effect of calcium hydroxide on bacterial lipopolysaccharide. J Endod. 1993;19:76–8.
101. Safavi KE, Nichols FC. Alteration of biological properties of bacterial lipopolysaccharide by calcium hydroxide treatment. J Endod. 1994;20:127–9.
102. Nelson-Filho P, Leonardo MR, Silva LA, Assed S. Radiographic evaluation of the effect of endotoxin (LPS) plus calcium hydroxide on apical and periapical tissues of dogs. J Endod. 2002;28:694–6.
103. Silva L, Nelson-Filho P, Leonardo MR, Rossi MA, Pansani CA. Effect of calcium hydroxide on bacterial endotoxin in vivo. J Endod. 2002;28:94–8.
104. Tanomaru JM, Leonardo MR, Tanomaru Filho M, Bonetti Filho I, Silva LA. Effect of different irrigation solutions and calcium hydroxide on bacterial LPS. Int Endod J. 2003;36:733–9.
105. Jiang J, Zuo J, Chen SH, Holliday LS. Calcium hydroxide reduces lipopolysaccharide-stimulated osteoclast formation. Oral Surg Oral Med Oral Pathol Oral Radiol Endod. 2003;95:348–54.
106. Buck RA, Cai J, Eleazer PD, Staat RH, Hurst HE. Detoxification of endotoxin by endodontic irrigants and calcium hydroxide. J Endod. 2001;27:325–7.
107. Vianna ME, Horz HP, Conrads G, Zaia AA, Souza-Filho FJ, Gomes BP. Effect of root canal procedures on endotoxins and endodontic pathogens. Oral Microbiol Immunol. 2007;22:411–8.
108. Baik JE, Kum KY, Yun CH, Lee JK, Lee K, Kim KK, Han SH. Calcium hydroxide inactivates lipoteichoic acid from *Enterococcus faecalis*. J Endod. 2008;34:1355–9.
109. Siqueira Jr JF, Rôças IN. Bacterial pathogenesis and mediators in apical periodontitis. Braz Dent J. 2007;18:267–80.
110. Siren EK, Haapasalo MP, Waltimo TM, Orstavik D. *In vitro* antibacterial effect of calcium hydroxide combined with chlorhexidine or iodine potassium iodide on *Enterococcus faecalis*. Eur J Oral Sci. 2004;112:326–31.
111. Waltimo TM, Ørstavik D, Siren EK, Haapasalo MP. *In vitro* susceptibility of *Candida albicans* to four disinfectants and their combinations. Int Endod J. 1999;32:421–9.
112. Siqueira Jr JF, Rôças IN, Lopes HP, Magalhaes FA, de Uzeda M. Elimination of *Candida albicans* infection of the radicular dentin by intracanal medications. J Endod. 2003;29:501–4.
113. Siqueira Jr JF, Rôças IN, Magalhaes FA, de Uzeda M. Antifungal effects of endodontic medicaments. Aust Endod J. 2001;27:112–4.
114. Siqueira Jr JF, de Uzeda M. Intracanal medicaments: evaluation of the antibacterial effects of chlorhexidine, metronidazole, and calcium hydroxide associated with three vehicles. J Endod. 1997;23:167–9.

115. Gomes BP, Ferraz CC, Garrido FD, Rosalen PL, Zaia AA, Teixeira FB, de Souza-Filho FJ. Microbial susceptibility to calcium hydroxide pastes and their vehicles. J Endod. 2002;28:758–61.
116. Menezes MM, Valera MC, Jorge AO, Koga-Ito CY, Camargo CH, Mancini MN. In vitro evaluation of the effectiveness of irrigants and intracanal medicaments on microorganisms within root canals. Int Endod J. 2004;37:311–9.
117. Siqueira Jr JF, Lopes HP, Uzeda M. Atividade antibacteriana da pasta de hidróxido de cálcio/PMCC/glicerina contendo diferentes proporções de iodofórmio sobre bactérias anaeróbias estritas e facultativas. Rev Paul Odontol. 1997;19:17–21.
118. Siqueira Jr JF, Lopes HP, Uzeda M. Atividade antibacteriana de medicamentos endodônticos sobre bactérias anaeróbias estritas. Rev Assoc Paul Cir Dent. 1996;50:326–32.
119. Siqueira Jr JF, Magalhães FAC, Uzeda M. Avaliação da atividade antibacteriana de medicação intracanal. Três bases fortes e pastas à base de hidróxido de cálcio e paramonoclorofenol canforado. Rev Gaucha Odontol. 1996;44:271–4.
120. Silveira AM, Lopes HP, Siqueira Jr JF, Macedo SB, Consolaro A. Periradicular repair after two-visit endodontic treatment using two different intracanal medications compared to single-visit endodontic treatment. Braz Dent J. 2007;18:299–304.
121. Grecca FS, Leonardo MR, da Silva LA, Tanomaru Filho M, Borges MA. Radiographic evaluation of periradicular repair after endodontic treatment of dog's teeth with induced periradicular periodontitis. J Endod. 2001;27:610–2.
122. Siqueira Jr JF, Rôças IN, Favieri A, Machado AG, Gahyva SM, Oliveira JC, Abad EC. Incidence of postoperative pain after intracanal procedures based on an antimicrobial strategy. J Endod. 2002;28:457–60.
123. Siqueira Jr JF, Rôças IN, Riche FN, Provenzano JC. Clinical outcome of the endodontic treatment of teeth with apical periodontitis using an antimicrobial protocol. Oral Surg Oral Med Oral Pathol Oral Radiol Endod. 2008;106:757–62.
124. Evans MD, Baumgartner JC, Khemaleelakul SU, Xia T. Efficacy of calcium hydroxide: chlorhexidine paste as an intracanal medication in bovine dentin. J Endod. 2003;29:338–9.
125. Podbielski A, Spahr A, Haller B. Additive antimicrobial activity of calcium hydroxide and chlorhexidine on common endodontic bacterial pathogens. J Endod. 2003;29:340–5.
126. Gomes BP, Vianna ME, Sena NT, Zaia AA, Ferraz CC, de Souza Filho FJ. *In vitro* evaluation of the antimicrobial activity of calcium hydroxide combined with chlorhexidine gel used as intracanal medicament. Oral Surg Oral Med Oral Pathol Oral Radiol Endod. 2006;102:544–50.
127. Schafer E, Bossmann K. Antimicrobial efficacy of chlorhexidine and two calcium hydroxide formulations against *Enterococcus faecalis*. J Endod. 2005; 31:53–6.
128. Zerella JA, Fouad AF, Spångberg LS. Effectiveness of a calcium hydroxide and chlorhexidine digluconate mixture as disinfectant during retreatment of failed endodontic cases. Oral Surg Oral Med Oral Pathol Oral Radiol Endod. 2005;100:756–61.
129. Paiva SS, Siqueira Jr JF, Rôças IN, Carmo FL, Leite DC, Ferreira DC, Rachid CT, Rosado AS. Clinical antimicrobial efficacy of NiTi rotary instrumentation with NaOCl irrigation, final rinse with chlorhexidine and interappointment medication: a molecular study. Int Endod J. 2013;46:225–33.
130. de Oliveira LD, Carvalho CA, Carvalho AS, de Souza Alves J, Valera MC, Jorge AO. Efficacy of endodontic treatment for endotoxin reduction in primarily infected root canals and evaluation of cytotoxic effects. J Endod. 2012;38:1053–7.
131. Davies GE, Francis J, Martin AR, Rose FL, Swain G. 1:6-Di-4'-chlorophenyldiguanidohexane (hibitane); laboratory investigation of a new antibacterial agent of high potency. Br J Pharmacol Chemother. 1954;9:192–6.
132. Milstone AM, Passaretti CL, Perl TM. Chlorhexidine: expanding the armamentarium for infection control and prevention. Clin Infect Dis. 2008;46:274–81.
133. Stanley A, Wilson M, Newman HN. The in vitro effects of chlorhexidine on subgingival plaque bacteria. J Clin Periodontol. 1989;16:259–64.
134. Ohara P, Torabinejad M, Kettering JD. Antibacterial effects of various endodontic irrigants on selected anaerobic bacteria. Endod Dent Traumatol. 1993;9:95–100.
135. Theraud M, Bedouin Y, Guiguen C, Gangneux JP. Efficacy of antiseptics and disinfectants on clinical and environmental yeast isolates in planktonic and biofilm conditions. J Med Microbiol. 2004;53: 1013–8.
136. Denton GW. Chlorhexidine. In: Block SS, editor. Disinfection, sterilization, and preservation. 4th ed. Philadelphia: Lea & Febiger; 1991. p. 276–7.
137. Vianna ME, Gomes BP, Berber VB, Zaia AA, Ferraz CC, de Souza-Filho FJ. *In vitro* evaluation of the antimicrobial activity of chlorhexidine and sodium hypochlorite. Oral Surg Oral Med Oral Pathol Oral Radiol Endod. 2004;97:79–84.
138. Rosenthal S, Spangberg L, Safavi K. Chlorhexidine substantivity in root canal dentin. Oral Surg Oral Med Oral Pathol Oral Radiol Endod. 2004;98: 488–92.
139. Komorowski R, Grad H, Wu XY, Friedman S. Antimicrobial substantivity of chlorhexidine-treated bovine root dentin. J Endod. 2000;26:315–7.
140. Basrani B, Santos JM, Tjaderhane L, Grad H, Gorduysus O, Huang J, Lawrence HP, Friedman S. Substantive antimicrobial activity in chlorhexidine-treated human root dentin. Oral Surg Oral Med Oral Pathol Oral Radiol Endod. 2002;94:240–5.
141. Yesilsoy C, Whitaker E, Cleveland D, Phillips E, Trope M. Antimicrobial and toxic effects of established and potential root canal irrigants. J Endod. 1995;21:513–5.

142. Tanomaru Filho M, Leonardo MR, Silva LAB, Anibal FF, Faccioli LH. Inflammatory response to different endodontic irrigating solutions. Int Endod J. 2002;35:735–9.
143. Maris P. Modes of action of disinfectants. Rev Sci Tech. 1995;14:47–55.
144. Hugo WB, Longworth AR. Some aspects of the mode of action of chlorhexidine. J Pharm Pharmacol. 1964;16:655–62.
145. McDonnel G, Russell AD. Antiseptics and disinfectants: activity, action, and resistance. Clin Microbiol Rev. 1999;12:147–79.
146. Portenier I, Haapasalo H, Ørstavik D, Yamauchi M, Haapasalo M. Inactivation of the antibacterial activity of iodine potassium iodide and chlorhexidine digluconate against Enterococcus faecalis by dentin, dentin matrix, type-I collagen, and heat-killed microbial whole cells. J Endod. 2002;28:634–7.
147. Delgado RJ, Gasparoto TH, Sipert CR, Pinheiro CR, de Moraes IG, Garcia RB, Duarte MA, Bramante CM, Torres SA, Garlet GP, Campanelli AP, Bernardineli N. Antimicrobial activity of calcium hydroxide and chlorhexidine on intratubular Candida albicans. Int J Oral Sci. 2013;5:32–6.
148. Delgado RJ, Gasparoto TH, Sipert CR, Pinheiro CR, Moraes IG, Garcia RB, Bramante CM, Campanelli AP, Bernardineli N. Antimicrobial effects of calcium hydroxide and chlorhexidine on Enterococcus faecalis. J Endod. 2010;36:1389–93.
149. Krithikadatta J, Indira R, Dorothykalyani AL. Disinfection of dentinal tubules with 2% chlorhexidine, 2% metronidazole, bioactive glass when compared with calcium hydroxide as intracanal medicaments. J Endod. 2007;33:1473–6.
150. Gama TG, de Oliveira JC, Abad EC, Rocas IN, Siqueira Jr JF. Postoperative pain following the use of two different intracanal medications. Clin Oral Investig. 2008;12:325–30.
151. Vianna ME, Horz HP, Conrads G, Feres M, Gomes BPFA. Comparative analysis of endodontic pathogens using checkerboard hybridization in relation to culture. Oral Microbiol Immunol. 2008;23:282–90.
152. Malkhassian G, Manzur AJ, Legner M, Fillery ED, Manek S, Basrani BR, Friedman S. Antibacterial efficacy of MTAD final rinse and two percent chlorhexidine gel medication in teeth with apical periodontitis: a randomized double-blinded clinical trial. J Endod. 2009;35:1483–90.
153. Teles AM, Manso MC, Loureiro S, Silva R, Madeira IG, Pina C, Cabeda JM. Effectiveness of two intracanal dressings in adult Portuguese patients: a qPCR and anaerobic culture assessment. Int Endod J. 2014; 47:32–40.
154. Tervit C, Paquette L, Torneck CD, Basrani B, Friedman S. Proportion of healed teeth with apical periodontitis medicated with two percent chlorhexidine gluconate liquid: a case-series study. J Endod. 2009;35:1182–5.
155. Hasselgren G, Olsson B, Cvek M. Effects of calcium hydroxide and sodium hypochlorite on the dissolution of necrotic porcine muscle tissue. J Endod. 1988;14:125–7.
156. Reit C, Dahlen G. Decision making analysis of endodontic treatment strategies in teeth with apical periodontitis. Int Endod J. 1988;21:291–9.
157. Orstavik D, Kerekes K, Molven O. Effects of extensive apical reaming and calcium hydroxide dressing on bacterial infection during treatment of apical periodontitis: a pilot study. Int Endod J. 1991; 24:1–7.
158. Yared GM, Dagher FE. Influence of apical enlargement on bacterial infection during treatment of apical periodontitis. J Endod. 1994;20:535–7.
159. Lana MA, Ribeiro-Sobrinho AP, Stehling R, Garcia GD, Silva BK, Hamdan JS, Nicoli JR, Carvalho MA, Farias LM. Microorganisms isolated from root canals presenting necrotic pulp and their drug susceptibility in vitro. Oral Microbiol Immunol. 2001;16:100–5.
160. Kvist T, Molander A, Dahlen G, Reit C. Microbiological evaluation of one- and two-visit endodontic treatment of teeth with apical periodontitis: a randomized, clinical trial. J Endod. 2004;30: 572–6.
161. Chu FC, Leung WK, Tsang PC, Chow TW, Samaranayake LP. Identification of cultivable microorganisms from root canals with apical periodontitis following two-visit endodontic treatment with antibiotics/steroid or calcium hydroxide dressings. J Endod. 2006;32:17–23.
162. Wang CS, Arnold RR, Trope M, Teixeira FB. Clinical efficiency of 2% chlorhexidine gel in reducing intracanal bacteria. J Endod. 2007;33:1283–9.
163. Sakamoto M, Siqueira Jr JF, Rôças IN, Benno Y. Bacterial reduction and persistence after endodontic treatment procedures. Oral Microbiol Immunol. 2007;22:19–23.
164. Beus C, Safavi K, Stratton J, Kaufman B. Comparison of the effect of two endodontic irrigation protocols on the elimination of bacteria from root canal system: a prospective, randomized clinical trial. J Endod. 2012;38:1479–83.

Disinfection in Nonsurgical Retreatment Cases

17

Rodrigo Sanches Cunha and Carlos Eduardo da Silveira Bueno

Abstract

Clinicians should be prepared to retreat the root canal system if endodontic failure occurs, as a tooth with failed root canal treatment need not be deemed unsalvageable. Successful retreatment requires copious irrigation with particular irrigants to achieve disinfection. The effectiveness of the irrigation process and the level of disinfection achieved are heavily dependent on the thorough removal of the obturation material. Obtaining access to the apical foramen while preserving the root canal system's anatomy and avoiding procedural errors is paramount to achieving a favorable outcome in retreatment cases.

Introduction

As defined by the American Association of Endodontists (AAE), retreatment is the removal of root canal filling materials from the tooth, followed by cleaning, shaping, and obturating the canals [1]. The terms "endodontic re-intervention" and "endodontic revision" have also been used in order to eliminate the negative connotation associated with the term "retreatment" [83].

R.S. Cunha, DDS, MSc, PhD, FRCD(C) (✉)
Department Restorative Dentistry, Faculty of Health Sciences, College of Dentistry, University of Manitoba, Winnipeg, MB, Canada
e-mail: rodrigo.cunha@umanitoba.ca

C.E. da Silveira Bueno, DDS, MSc, PhD
Faculty of Dentistry, São Leopoldo Mandic Centre for Dental Research, Campinas, SP, Brazil

Nonsurgical endodontic treatment has a high rate of success [37]; however, if endodontic failure does occur, the clinician should be prepared to first retreat the root canal system prior to performing apical surgery. Despite the additional challenge of post and crown disassembly, and the removal of root-filling materials, retreatment is reported to have a higher long-term success rate when compared to apical surgery [71] (Fig. 17.1).

Why Does Nonsurgical Root Canal Treatment Fail?

It is of paramount importance to understand the main reasons why nonsurgical root canal treatment fails if the clinician wishes to prevent further occurrences of failure and to optimize the

B. Basrani (ed.), *Endodontic Irrigation: Chemical Disinfection of the Root Canal System*,
DOI 10.1007/978-3-319-16456-4_17

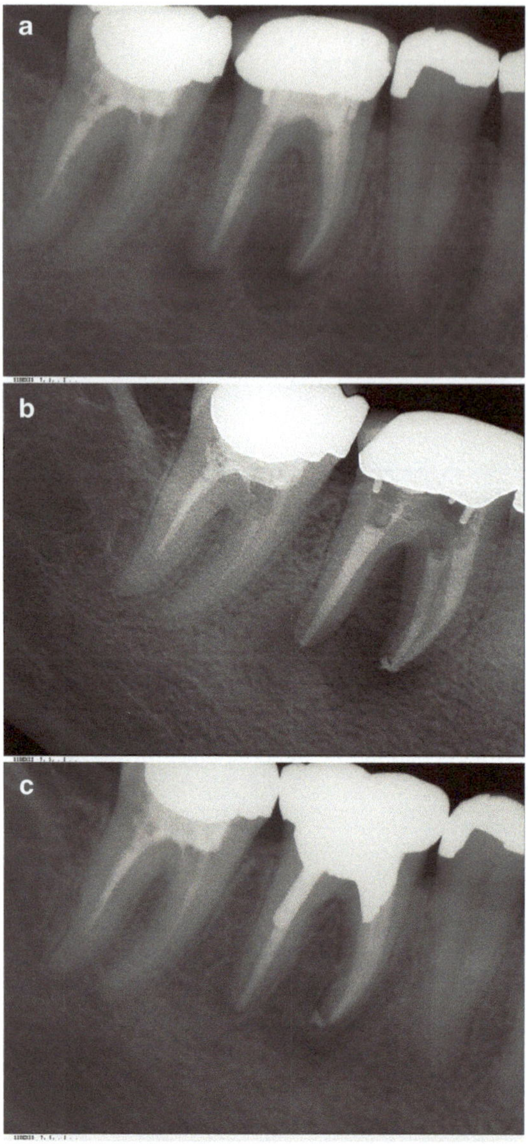

Fig. 17.1 (**a**) Preoperative radiograph of a persistent infection on the first lower mandibular molar. (**b**) Postoperative radiograph after the retreatment. (**c**) A 6-month follow-up radiograph showing signs of healing

likelihood of successful retreatment. The main causes of endodontic therapy failure include: poor technical quality of the previous treatment; the occurrence of procedural errors such as overfilling, underfilling, perforating, missing canals, and breaching the infection control protocol; and inadequate sealing of the root canal system by the permanent restoration (Fig. 17.2).

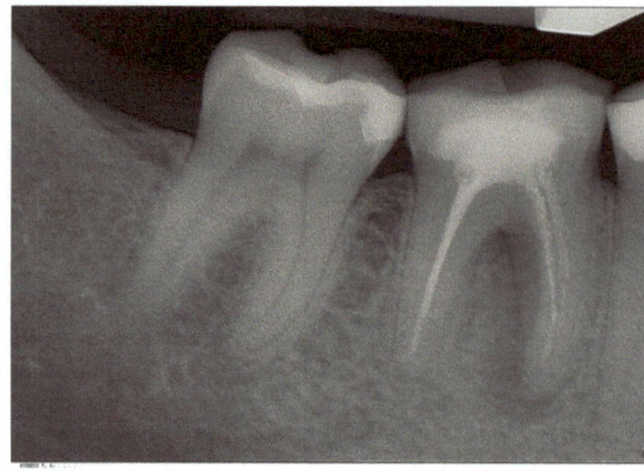

Fig. 17.2 A 36-year-old presented with pain to biting on the mandibular first molar. Nonsurgical root canal treatment and a restoration had been completed 3 years prior to this painful episode. Note the incomplete root canal treatment with a radiolucency surrounding the mesial root

Dugas et al. [20] concluded that the periapical health of root-filled teeth in two Canadian populations was influenced by the quality of both the root filling and the restoration, with the impact of the latter being most critical when the quality of the root filling was adequate. The study also stated that the prevalence of periradicular disease in root-filled teeth did not differ between teeth treated by general dentists and endodontists.

Reports of endodontic failure in cases in which the highest standards of care were followed are prevalent in the literature [42, 63]. Factors beyond the clinician's control, such as a complex root canal system with areas that cannot be cleaned and filled adequately with the instruments and techniques that exist today [25, 35, 45, 46], in combination with the presence of extra-radicular infections [53] are typically the main cause of failure in these cases. Scanning electron microscopic analysis of the apical foramen and external radicular surfaces performed by Signoretti et al. [61] revealed microbial communities embedded in a polysaccharide matrix in a protein-rich environment called a biofilm.

This chapter will briefly focus on three main causes of endodontic failure, as missing canals, vertical root fractures, and infections are the most frequently encountered scenarios.

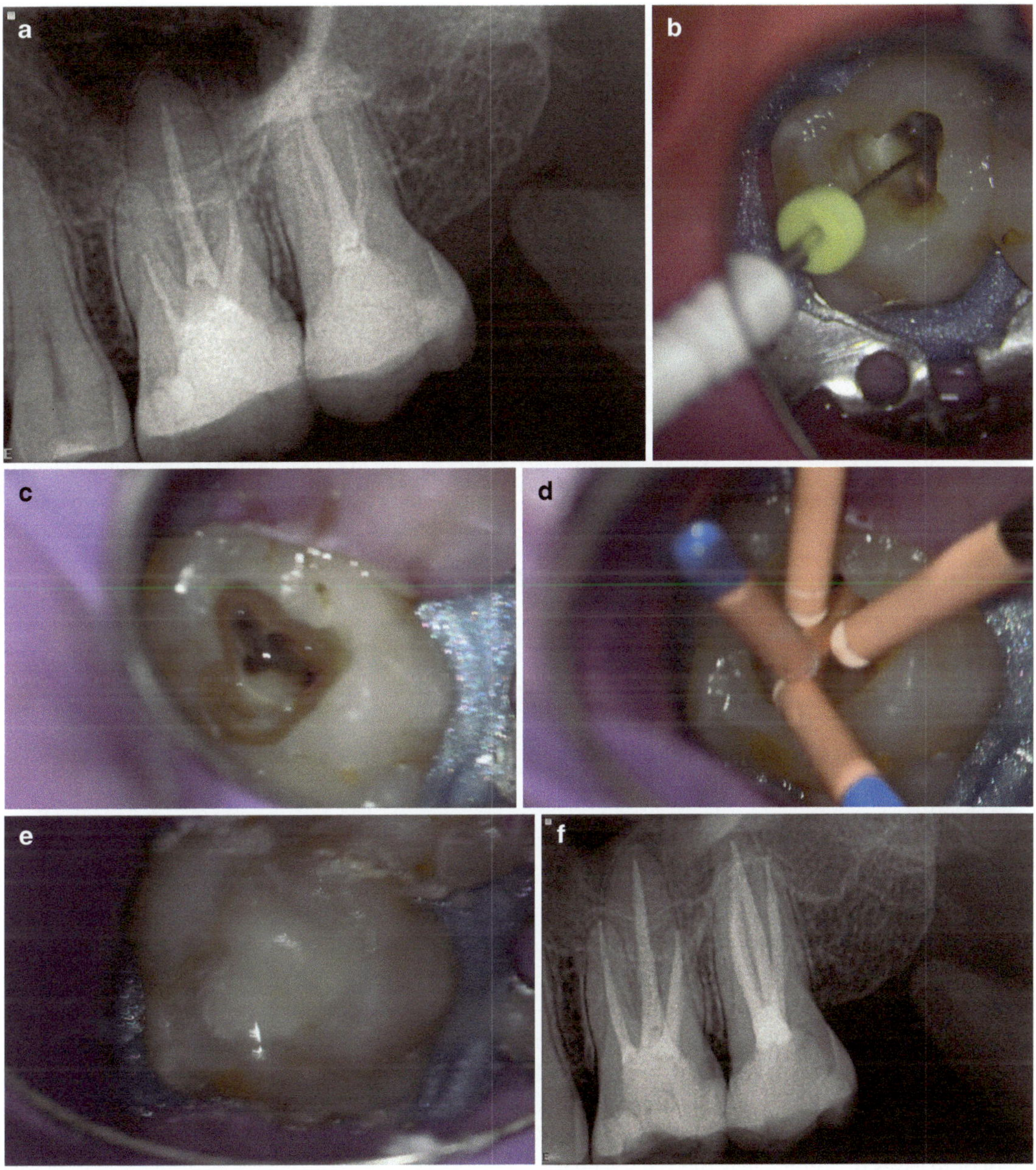

Fig. 17.3 (**a**) Preoperative radiograph showing both first and second maxillary molars with under-filled canals. Patient was percussion sensitive on tooth 27; (**b**, **c**) proper access opening under magnification and illumination allowed negotiation of the second mesial-buccal canal on tooth 27; (**d**) gutta-percha fit; (**e**) Temporary filling with Glass Ionomer; (**f**) postoperative radiograph of the retreatment in both 26 and 27

Missing Canals

Irrigation can play an important role when attempting to locate hidden canal orifices. When used to irrigate the pulp chamber floor, sodium hypochlorite will allow "champagne bubbles" to form in the location of these canals which can then be scouted with a sharp explorer. Magnifying loupes and a dental operating microscope may also increase the likelihood of visualizing the location of canal orifices [31] (Fig. 17.3).

Vertical Root Fracture

Traumatic injuries, restorative procedures, and the excessive removal of tooth structure during endodontic procedures are the main causes for vertical root fracture. Usually, it is diagnosed years after all endodontic and prosthetic treatments have been completed. The diagnostic process for cases of vertical root fracture is often frustrating. It is based on the combination of the patient's subjective complaints and on an objective clinical and radiographic evaluation. Evidence-based data concerning the diagnostic accuracy and clinical efficacy of the objective clinical and radiographic dental evaluation for the diagnosis of vertical root fracture in endodontically treated teeth is lacking [72]. The most common signs and symptoms of vertical root fracture, as described in the literature, are the presence of deep osseous defects especially on the buccal aspect of susceptible teeth and roots and a cervically located sinus tract [69]. Endodontically treated teeth with an expected vertical root fracture typically have a poor prognosis and extraction should be considered (Fig. 17.4).

Infection

A periradicular inflammation may not respond to endodontic treatment due to the persistent nature of the infection. This occurrence is known as persistent disease. It is also possible for a new lesion to appear as a result of the introduction of bacteria into a canal during the treatment process, usually due to either a breach in the infection control protocol or in cases of coronal leakage. This scenario is known as emergent disease. Even after complete healing has occurred, a lesion can reappear after a period of time. This phenomenon is classified as recurrent disease or a late failure [73].

Even though studies have shown that endodontic infections are biofilm-related [10], *Enterococcus faecalis* has been identified as the single most commonly recovered species from teeth with persistent endodontic infections. Yeasts, archaea, and viruses can also be found as part of the microbial diversity of these infections [62].

Success Rate of Nonsurgical Retreatment Cases

Despite the fact that endodontic retreatment has a lower success rate when compared to orthograde treatment [57], according to Salehrabi and Rotstein [58], endodontic retreatment is a procedure with a very good survival rate and patients can be advised that 89 % of these teeth may be retained and functional for at least 5 years after the procedure. The potential for healing is improved if the previous filling material is removed safely and effectively and if patency can be achieved during the retreatment procedure. De Chevigny et al. [15] analyzed the outcome 4–6 years after retreatment was rendered to identify significant outcome predictors that could be determined preoperative such as: root-filling quality, previous perforation, and periradicular radiolucency. In teeth that had an associated radiolucency, the significant outcome predictors included the number of treatment sessions and the previous root-filling quality. The retreatment outcome was seen to be better in teeth with an inadequate previous root filling that did not have a perforation or an associated radiolucency. Gorni and Gagliani [28] differentiated the success rate of retreatment cases into two groups: one in which canal and apical morphology alterations had occurred and the other in which the previous treatment had not lead to adverse alteration of the original morphology. The authors discovered that the success rates differed between the two groups as a higher rate of success resulted when the natural course of the root canals was maintained during the previous endodontic treatment.

Removal of Filling Material

Gutta-percha, in combination with numerous endodontic sealers, is the most widely used material for root canal filling. Effective removal of gutta-percha in endodontic retreatment is necessary in order to obtain access to infected areas of the root canal system. Thorough removal is a significant factor in the successful retreatment of a previously failed procedure as it allows for the

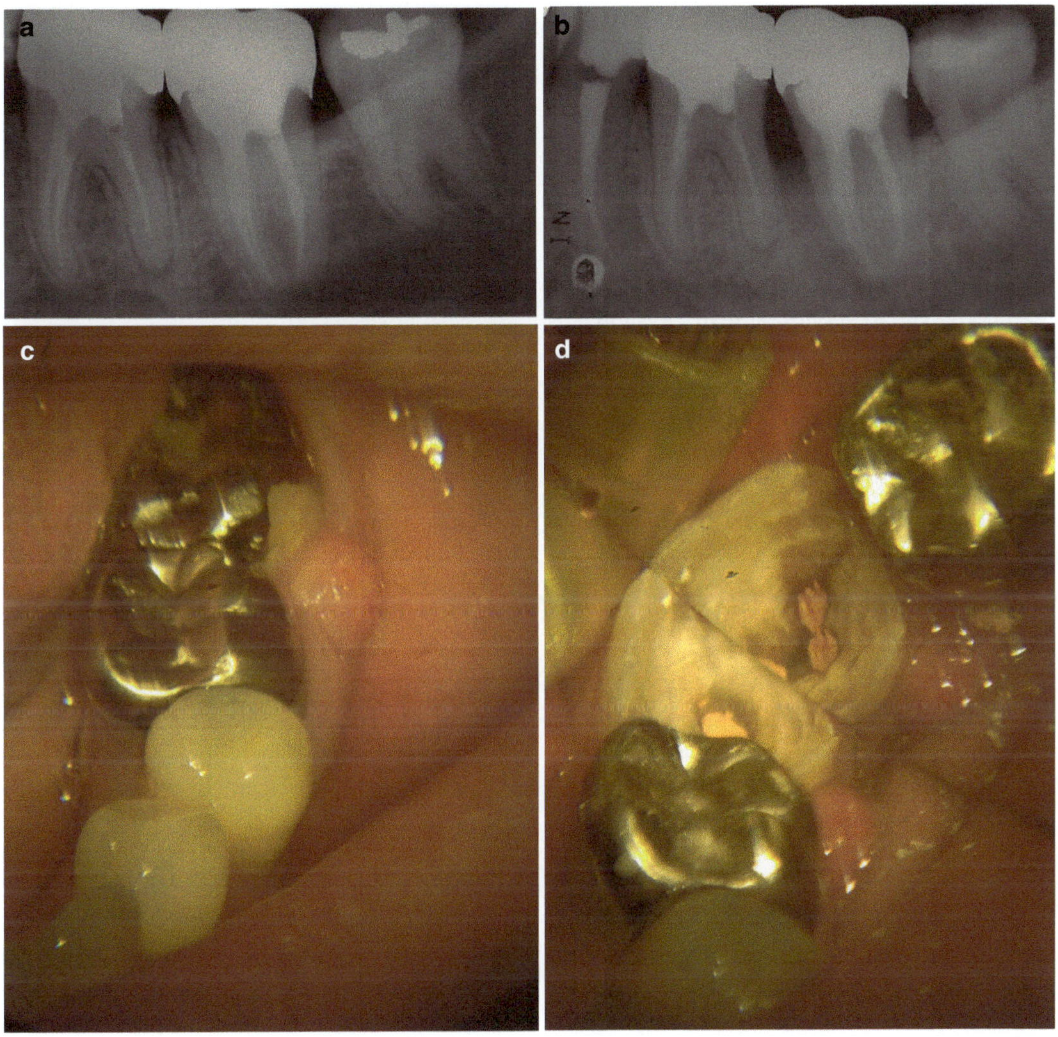

Fig. 17.4 (**a**) A 46-year-old patient had a nonsurgical root canal treatment concluded and a metallic crown was placed immediately after; (**b**) after a little more than 3 years, the patient complained of a throbbing pain and pressure on the left lower jaw. A halo-shaped radiolucency surrounding the mesial root could be seen suggesting the possibility of a vertical root fracture; (**c**) clinically there was a sinus tract close to the gingival margin between the first and second mandibular molars (36 and 37). At this point, a deep narrow pocket was observed in the mesial aspect of the 37; (**d**) once the crown is removed, the fracture is easily visualized

irrigating solution to come in contact with the canal walls and work effectively. Gutta-percha removal can be time consuming and can cause fatigue that may lead to procedural errors that put the success of the retreatment in jeopardy [27]. Oval and long-oval root canals offer an additional challenge to the removal of the previous filling material; there is a tendency to keep the file in the center of the canal, which does not allow adequate preparation in the buccolingual dimension [40, 50, 74, 77]. When previous filling material is not completely removed, it acts as a barrier, preventing the irrigating solution from touching the canal walls. Retention of the filling material also harbors necrotic tissue and microorganisms responsible for endodontic treatment failure.

Cunha et al. [14] assessed the obturation removal in canals filled with Resilon/RealSeal™

(Pentron Clinical Technologies) in comparison to canals filled with gutta-percha/AH Plus in extracted teeth. The obturations were removed from both groups using chloroform, irrigating with 2.5 % NaOCl, and manual re-instrumentation. The teeth were then radiographically analyzed. Specimens without obturation material remnants visible during radiographic examination were selected for analysis under scanning electron microscopy. The Resilon/RealSeal™ system was seen to be removed in greater quantities from the canal walls compared with the gutta-percha cones and the AH Plus™ (Dentsply Maillefer) cement. Scanning electron microscopy revealed material remnants in all portions of the canal. Again, Resilon was seen to be better removed from the canal than the gutta-percha cones and the AH Plus™.

ProTaper Universal™ (Dentsply Tulsa Dental), Mtwo™ (VDW), and D-RaCe™ (FKG Dentaire) are systems that have instruments specifically designed for removing the previous filling material from the root canal. Takahashi et al. [68] evaluated the efficacy of these nickel-titanium rotary instruments used with or without a solvent versus the use of stainless steel hand files for gutta-percha removal in extracted teeth. The results showed that there was no significant difference between the two techniques in regard to the amount of endodontic filling remnants; however, the ProTaper Universal™ rotary retreatment system without chloroform was found to be faster. Numerous studies have continued to evaluate filling material removal using different techniques and file systems. Conventional NiTi rotary files can also be used to remove root-filling material from previously treated root canals with the added advantage of avoiding the removal of excessive tooth structure as frequently occurs when using Gates-Glidden drills (Fig. 17.5). Zuolo et al. [82] compared the efficacy of reciprocating and rotary techniques with that of hand files for removing gutta-percha and sealer from root canals of extracted teeth. The remaining endodontic filling material was observed on the canal walls of all teeth regardless of the technique used. However, hand files combined with Gates-Glidden burs and the use of the reciprocating technique removed more filling material from the canal walls in comparison to the rotary files. Rios et al. [54] assessed the efficacy of 2 reciprocating systems in comparison to a nickel-titanium (NiTi) rotary system in the removal of root canal filling material from canals of extracted teeth. Again, all of the teeth examined had filling remnants within the canal and no significant difference among the file systems was found. Solmonov et al. [65] used a 25.06 ProFile™ (Dentsply Tulsa Dental) instrument followed by the Self-Adjusting File™ (SAF; ReDent Nova) and found this sequence to be less time consuming and more effective at removing the root-filling residue in the canal in comparison to the use of ProTaper Universal™ files for this purpose (Dentsply Tulsa Dental).

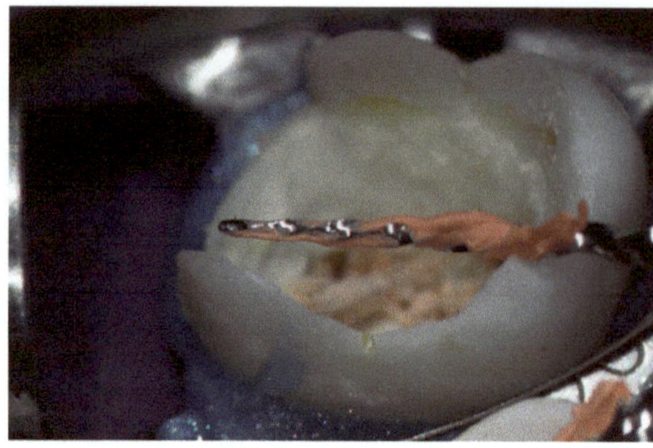

Fig. 17.5 Remnants of gutta-percha threaded in the active portion of a NiTi rotary instrument (ProTaper Universal, Dentsply Tulsa Dental) during the desobturation step

The numerous studies mentioned confirm that it is almost impossible to completely remove the filling material from inside the root canal, and even in cases where this material cannot be seen radiographically, it can be assumed that remnants are still present in areas such as isthmuses, fins, and lateral canals (Figs. 17.6 and 17.7)

In recent years, the predictability of surgical and nonsurgical endodontic procedures has benefited from the combined use of the dental operating microscope (DOM), which allows for improved optics for magnification and illumination, and specially designed ultrasonic tips. Protocols using both devices have been proposed for cases in which nonsurgical retreatment is indicated as they allow for improved precision

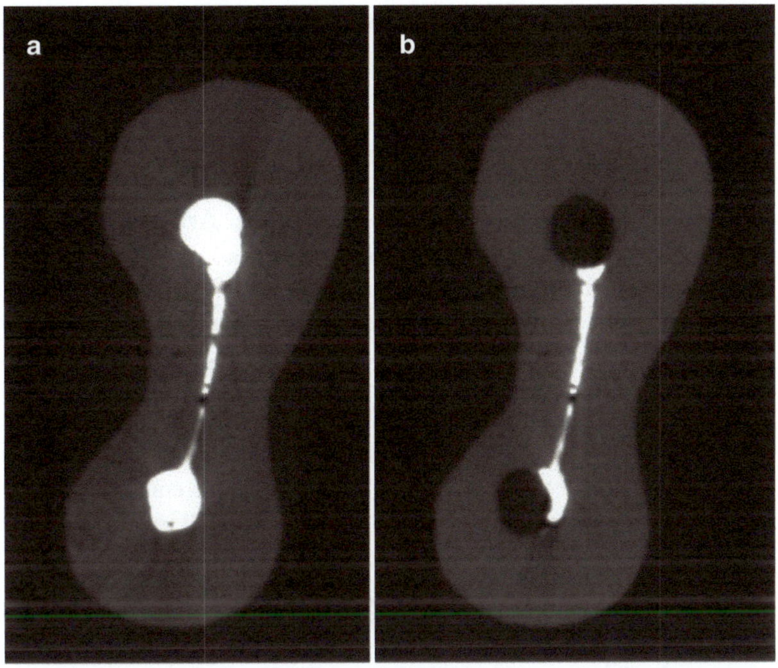

Fig. 17.6 (**a**) A mesial root of a mandibular molar was shaped and filled with gutta-percha and sealer; (**b**) the attempt to completely remove the filling material failed as it was still seen inside the isthmus between both canals at the end of the procedure using a micro-CT scanner

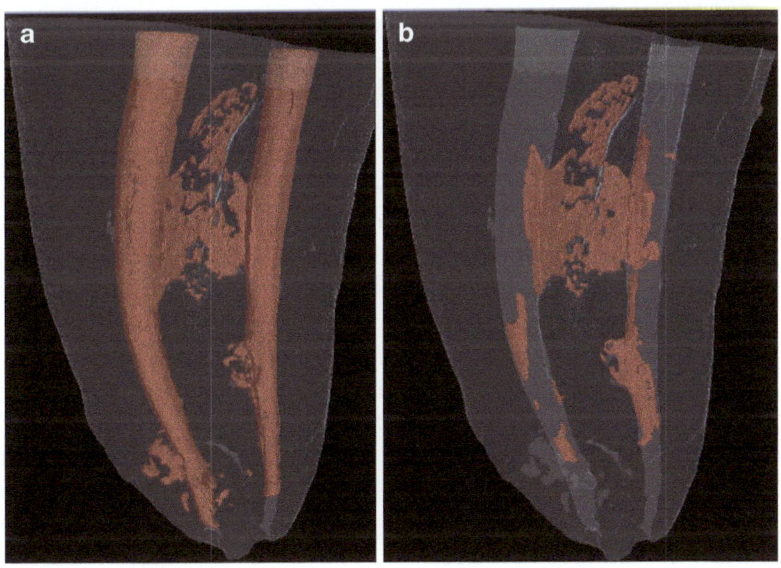

Fig. 17.7 (**a**) A three-dimensional image using a micro-computed tomography scanner of a mandibular molar mesial root showing both MB and ML filled with gutta-percha and sealer; (**b**) after the desobturation procedure, filling material remnants can still be seen on the canal's walls

due to enhanced illumination and magnification. The combination of these devices is especially useful during the removal of filling remnants. De Mello Jr. et al. [17] compared the efficacy of gutta-percha/sealer removal from extracted endodontically treated teeth with and without the aid of a dental operating microscope used in conjunction with ultrasonic instruments. Despite the fact that all teeth had remnants of filling materials at the end of the retreatment, the average amount of remaining gutta-percha/sealer was significantly lower when both devices were used. The remnants of filling materials compacted against the root canal walls after using drills, files, and solvent can easily be removed using ultrasonic instruments due to the cutting efficiency of the piezoelectric oscillation. Grischke et al. [29] compared the efficiency of sonic, ultrasonic, and hydrodynamic devices in the removal of a root canal sealer from the surface and simulated irregularities of root canals. Again, the passive ultrasonic irrigation was seen to be effective in removing sealer from the root canal.

During endodontic therapy, dental instruments may separate within the root canal and impede the renegotiation of the canal path. As such, during radiographic examination in preparation for retreatment, the clinician may unexpectedly encounter one or more retained endodontic instrument fragments. In clinical studies, the incidence of this accident has been reported to range from 0.39 % to 5 % [18, 51].

In a systematic review, Panitvisai et al. [48] assessed the prognosis of teeth after instrument fracture during endodontic therapy and found no statistically significant difference in healing rates between teeth with and without retained instrument fragments. However, the odds of treatment failure are higher when fragments prevent a thorough cleaning and shaping of the entire canal system and when periradicular lesions are present preoperatively [13, 33, 66]. When infection is present, removing or bypassing the fractured instrument is essential to ensure that the irrigation solution reaches the working length in order to obtain disinfection and the associated increased predictability of the outcome. Dental operating microscopes (DOM) and ultrasonic tips have allowed clinicians to obtain access to separated instruments and can assure higher success rates in the removal of instrument fragments, as reported by [43].

Carrier-Based Filling Materials

Carrier-based filling materials provide a straightforward approach to the obturation procedure; however, removal of these materials can be particularly challenging especially when retreating small and curved canals as the plastic core is not soluble in common solvents [4] (Fig. 17.8).

More recently, a 3rd generation of carrier-based obturators named GuttaCore™ (Dentsply Tulsa Dental) was developed and employs cross-linked gutta-percha instead of a plastic carrier. According to a recent research study, this system is easier to remove than those containing plastic carriers [7, 44] (Fig. 17.9).

Solvents: How Effective/Safe Are They?

The use of mechanical techniques and solvents to remove filling materials from previously root canal-treated teeth has been tested throughout the years [9, 11, 68]. The assertion that usage of an organic solvent is necessary for the removal of filling material can be considered inappropriate as several published articles demonstrate both root-filling remnants on the root canal surface and the formation of an artificial smear layer after using these agents [55, 64] (Fig. 17.10). A further disadvantage is the cytotoxic property of organic solvents, which is especially of concern when they are extruded into the periradicular area [5, 60].

Solvents were studied more frequently in the 1980s and 1990s than they are in the present period [30, 70, 76]. Barbosa et al. [5] examined the effects of halothane, turpentine oil, and chloroform solvents on the fibroblastic cells of rats. These authors concluded that the use of solvents should be avoided because all of the agents analyzed were found to be toxic.

In certain cases, the hardening of the sealer is accentuated to such a degree that it is very difficult to remove the gutta-percha in its entirety or even establish a glide path through the gutta-percha, especially in curved canals [30, 70].

A consensus has not yet been reached regarding whether solvents are helpful during the process of gutta-percha removal. Despite this uncertainty, the issue of the cytotoxicity of the solvents used in endodontic retreatment needs to be analyzed more accurately. Although chloroform is generally considered highly effective, the claim that it is cytotoxic has led to the testing of some "alternative" solvents, such as halothane, eucalyptol, orange oil, and xylene [24, 59]. Wilcox [75] and Bueno et al. [9] have reported that chloroform is highly efficient. Recently, a similar study was performed by Sağlam et al. [56] in extracted molars with curved roots. The ProTaper Universal and Self-Adjusting File were used in conjunction with chloroform,

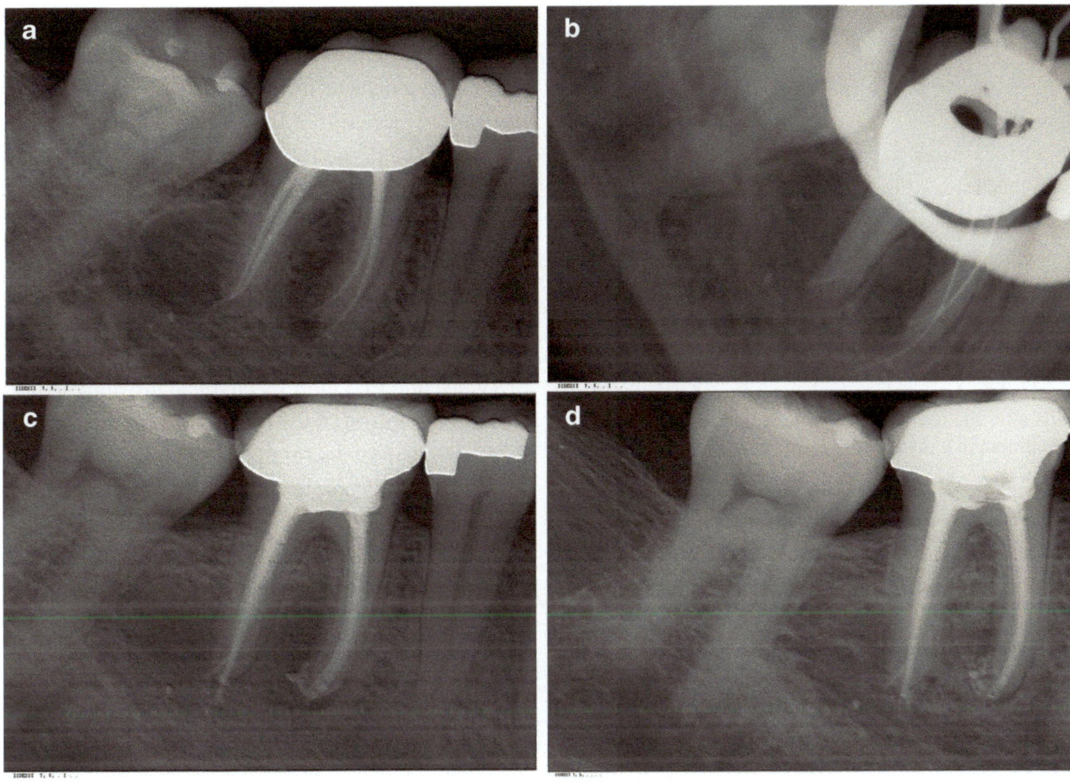

Fig. 17.8 (**a**) A 48-year-old patient had a nonsurgical root canal treatment where the obturation was performed using a carrier-based technique in all four canals. A 7-year follow-up radiograph showed a periradicular lesion in both mesial and distal roots; (**b**) during the attempt to retrieve Thermafil from inside the canals, a ledge and subsequent perforation occurred in the mesial-buccal canal. The carrier inside the distal-lingual canal separated at the apical portion; (**c**) even though a portion of the previous obturation material was kept inside the canals and the perforation inside the mesial-buccal canal perforation, the treatment was concluded and the final restoration was placed; (**d**) a 10-month follow-up showed signs of healing and the patient was asymptomatic. Despite the technical difficulties in this case, the disinfection protocol was essential for a successful outcome

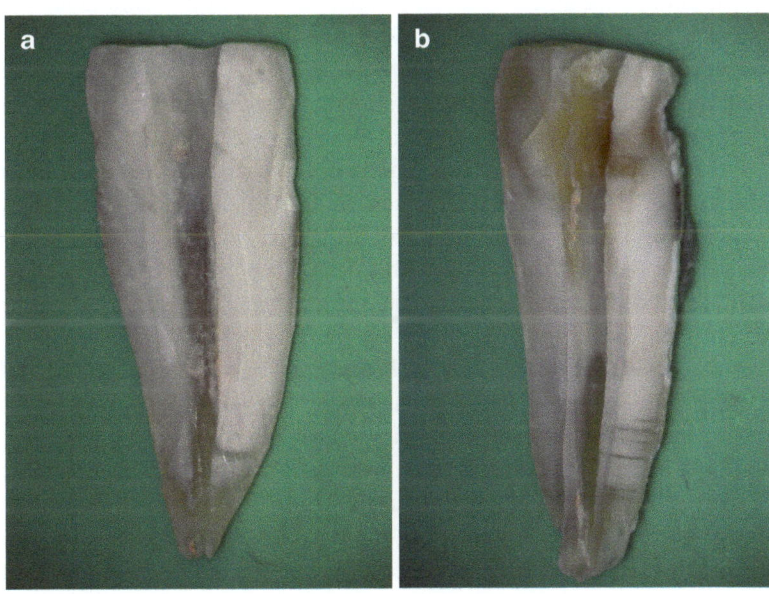

Fig. 17.9 Two specimens representative of root-filling material remnants that remained covering the walls after retreating root canals previously filled with (**a**) GuttaCore and (**b**) Thermafil

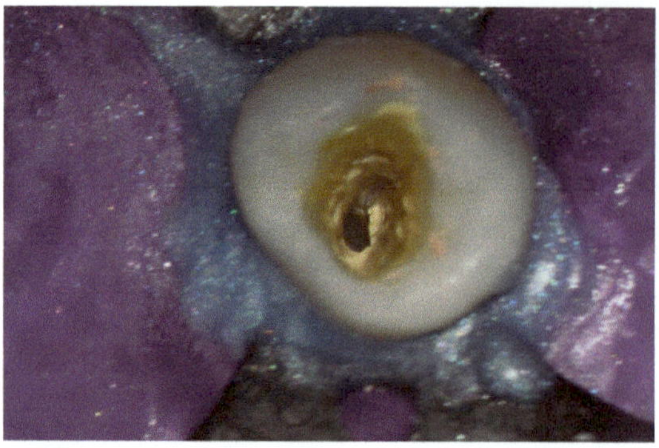

Fig. 17.10 Artificial smear layer adhered to the canal's walls after the usage of chloroform during an endodontic retreatment in a mandibular lower premolar

Endosolv, or no solvent and the residual root-filling material was evaluated using micro-computed tomography (μCT), a noninvasive technology. No significant differences were found between the groups in terms of the percentage volume of residual root canal filling.

Regarding solvent cytotoxicity, McDonald and Vire [39] found that chloroform had no effect on the clinical staff or on the patient who had undergone the treatment involving chloroform. In addition, it was reported that if used under normal conditions, chloroform does not cause any irreversible cytotoxic effects. Chutich et al. [12] analyzed the toxicity of chloroform, halothane, and xylene by quantifying the apically extruded solvent and found that the amount of solvent that was carried through the apical foramen is much lower than the permitted dose. Nevertheless, the US Food and Drug Administration (FDA) specify that chloroform may not be used as an ingredient in drug products or in pharmaceutical compounding.

Fruchi et al. [26] used μCT imaging to evaluate the amount of filling material remaining after instrumentation with reciprocating files and again after passive ultrasonic irrigation (PUI) with xylene. The study concluded that both instruments efficiently, but not completely, removed the filling material from the inside of the curved mesial-buccal canals of extracted maxillary molars. Although the use of xylene with PUI slightly increased the removal of the filling material, this finding was not statically significant. Cavenago et al. [11] evaluated the percentage of remaining filling material in the mesial root canals of mandibular molars after retreatment in which 3 procedures were performed sequentially. The first step involved removal of the filling material, enlargement of the root canals to size 40, and instrumentation with a 0.04 tapered instrument. In the second step, the root canals were irrigated with xylene and an attempt was made to clean the root canals with paper points. In the third step, the PUI technique was performed using 2.5 % sodium hypochlorite. The authors concluded that the filling materials were not completely removed by any of the retreatment procedures alone; however, the use of xylene and PUI after mechanical instrumentation enhanced removal of the materials during endodontic retreatment of anatomically complex teeth.

The antimicrobial effectiveness of chloroform on *Enterococcus faecalis* has also been evaluated. Edgar et al. [21] collected bacterial samples for analysis after gutta-percha had been removed using either chloroform or saline. Negative cultures were obtained in 11 of 17 chloroform samples and 0 of 17 saline samples, demonstrating that the use of chloroform during endodontic retreatment significantly reduced intracanal levels of cultivatable *Enterococcus faecalis*. Martos et al. [38] evaluated the antimicrobial activity of three different solvents solutions (chloroform, eucalyptus oil, and orange oil) alone and in association with various concentration of cetrimide (CTR) against *Enterococcus faecalis* biofilms in dentine. The results obtained in this study suggested that the antimicrobial ability of the solvent agents combined with CTR contributes to the disinfection in endodontic retreatment.

In conclusion, the usage of organic solvents should be avoided in retreatment cases in which the filling material can be easily removed. However, if in the attempt to reach the apical foramen and achieve patency no progress is made, solvents should be used cautiously.

Disinfection Protocol in Nonsurgical Retreatment

In order to obtain an in-depth understanding of the irrigation solutions available for disinfection in endodontic treatment, referral to Chap. 5 is recommended. Briefly, the solutions that, according to our philosophy, have a positive impact during the disinfection phase of nonsurgical retreatment will be discussed.

The disinfection protocol in retreatment cases is similar to that used in conventional endodontic treatment. However, time plays an important role during these cases and should be carefully managed in order to achieve complete disinfection. Multiple visits and intracanal medicaments should be considered in difficult cases [81].

Instrumentation is still considered an important step in the removal of all previous filling materials and necrotic organic tissues from the inside of the canals. This process creates a suitable space for the irrigation solution to make contact with the canal walls. However, the use of irrigation and irrigants has become increasingly relevant as studies are demonstrating that a high percentage of the canal walls are still left untouched after instrumentation [49, 50, 52].

Before beginning retreatment and attempting to regain apical patency, diagnostic radiographs should be carefully examined for evidence of a previous perforation. Extrusion of caustic irrigants such as sodium hypochlorite beyond the apical foramen into the periodontal ligament, alveolar bone, and anatomical structures can cause undue harm and serious accidents. If a perforation is encountered, it is advisable to use a biocompatible solution for irrigation, such as physiologic saline or local anesthetics, until the perforation is sealed.

Numerous factors including delivery of the irrigant closer to the apex, larger irrigation volume, and narrower gauge irrigation needles have shown to improve the efficacy of root canal irrigation [23].

The ideal irrigant should preferably have disinfectant and organic debris dissolving properties. It should also act to remove the smear layer without causing irritation to the periradicular tissues. The irrigation solution should be delivered in copious amounts as close as possible to working length without extruding beyond the foramen. This procedure can be safely and effectively accomplished using a syringe that allows the solution to escape freely into the pulp chamber. It is also important that the irrigant is not delivered with excessive force. The solution may also be agitated while inside the canal using an ultrasonic or sonic system [22]. To date, an ideal irrigating solution that possesses all of these desired properties does not exist; therefore the best protocol to achieve optimal disinfection is a combination of solutions.

Sodium Hypochlorite (NaOCl)

Sodium hypochlorite remains the solution of choice for disinfection throughout the cleaning and shaping procedure, especially in cases where persistent infection is present. NaOCl prepared at a concentration ranging from 2.5 to 6 % is indicated due to the antimicrobial properties, the ability to dissolve necrotic organic tissue, and the price and availability of this solution [80].

Du et al. [19] evaluated the antimicrobial activity of different endodontic disinfecting solutions on *Enterococcus faecalis* biofilms in dentin canals. Sodium hypochlorite at a concentration of 6 % was the most effective antibacterial solution. It has also been proposed that laser activation and passive ultrasonic irrigation of the sodium Hypochlorite solution may enhance the removal of biofilm in infected dentin [45].

Chelants

Ethylenediaminetetraacetic Acid (EDTA)

The advantages of using EDTA to remove the smear layer created by the debridement of the canal are well documented in the literature [2, 3, 78]. A study conducted by Keles et al. [32] indicated that during nonsurgical retreatment, the use of EDTA for removing smear layer assisted in the retreatment process by dissolving calcium hydroxide, polyketone, zinc oxide-eugenol, silicone, and two epoxy resin-based root canal sealers.

It is also noteworthy to state that chelating solutions such as citric acid and EDTA interfere with biofilm cohesion [8]. EDTA should be used after irrigating with NaOCl and before using chlorhexidine in order to avoid the formation of para-chloroaniline (PCA) [6].

Peracetic acid (PAA) in concentrations ranging from 0.5 to 1 % has been proposed as an alternative to the classic decalcifying agents (EDTA and citric acid) due to its capacity to dissolve the smear layer and concomitantly disinfect the root canal system [16, 36, 67].

Chlorhexidine Digluconate (CHX)

Chlorhexidine digluconate (CHX) should be used as the final irrigant. The use of CHX as an auxiliary irrigant in endodontic treatment has been suggested due to its antimicrobial nature and its ability to remain and have a long-lasting effect on the dentin, therefore preventing or delaying recontamination. This long-lasting effect is termed "substantivity." In an in vivo study, Leonardo et al. [34] evaluated the antimicrobial substantivity of 2 % CHX in teeth with pulp necrosis and radiographically visible chronic periradicular lesions. The authors demonstrated that CHX prevented microbial activity in the root canal system with residual effects lasting for up to 48 h after application. When used as a supplemental irrigating solution, CHX has the capacity to reduce the bacterial load inside the root canals [47, 79].

Although CHX is effective against bacterial biofilms, NaOCl is still the only irrigation solution with the capacity of disrupting biofilms [41].

Concluding Remarks

In order to achieve optimal disinfection in retreatment cases, clinicians should be prepared to remove as much of the previous filling material as possible. This removal process may be tiring and time consuming. Solvents may be used if needed; however, caution is advised due to their toxicity. The combined use of the dental operating microscope (DOM) and ultrasonics may enhance the removal of filling material and increase the area of dentin that comes into contact with the disinfecting solutions. A combination of irrigating solutions is important to achieve the objective of ideal disinfection.

References

1. AAE – glossary of endodontic terms. American Association of Endodontics, Chicago, IL, USA. 8th ed. 2012.
2. Ahmetoglu F, Keles A, Yalcin M, Simsek N. Effectiveness of different irrigation systems on smear layer removal: a scanning electron microscopic study. Eur J Dent. 2014;8(1):53–7.
3. Arslan H, Ayrancı LB, Karatas E, Topçuoğlu HS, Yavuz MS, Kesim B. Effect of agitation of EDTA with 808-nanometer diode laser on removal of smear layer. J Endod. 2013;39(12):1589–92.
4. Baratto Filho F, Ferreira EL, Fariniuk LF. Efficiency of the 0.04 taper ProFile during the re-treatment of gutta-percha-filled root canals. Int Endod J. 2002;35:651–4.
5. Barbosa SV, Burkard DH, Spångberg LS. Cytotoxic effects of gutta-percha solvents. J Endod. 1994;20(1):6–8.
6. Basrani BR, Manek S, Sodhi RN, Fillery E, Manzur A. Interaction between sodium hypochlorite and chlorhexidine gluconate. J Endod. 2007;33(8):966–9.
7. Beasley RT, Williamson AE, Justman BC, Qian F. Time required to remove guttacore, thermafil plus, and thermoplasticized gutta-percha from moderately curved root canals with ProTaper files. J Endod. 2013;39:125–8.
8. Brul S, Coote P. Preservative agents in foods. Mode of action and microbial resistance mechanisms. Int J Food Microbiol. 1999;50(1–2):1–17.
9. Bueno CE, Delboni MG, de Araújo RA, Carrara HJ, Cunha RS. Effectiveness of rotary and hand files in gutta-percha and sealer removal using chloroform or chlorhexidine gel. Braz Dent J. 2006;17(2):139–43.
10. Carr GB, Schwartz RS, Schaudinn C, Gorur A, Costerton JW. Ultrastructural examination of failed molar retreatment with secondary apical periodontitis: an examination of endodontic biofilms in an endodontic retreatment failure. J Endod. 2009;35(9):1303–9.
11. Cavenago BC, Ordinola-Zapata R, Duarte MA, del Carpio-Perochena AE, Villas-Bôas MH, Marciano MA, Bramante CM, Moraes IG. Efficacy of xylene and passive ultrasonic irrigation on remaining root filling material during retreatment of anatomically complex teeth. Int Endod J. 2014;47(11):1078–83.
12. Chutich MJ, Kaminski EJ, Miller DA, Lautenschlager EP. Risk assessment of the toxicity of solvents of gutta-percha used in endodontic retreatment. J Endod. 1998;24(4):213–6.
13. Crump MC, Natkin E. Relationship of broken root canal instruments to endodontic case prognosis: a clinical investigation. J Am Dent Assoc. 1970;80:1341–7.
14. Cunha RS, De Martin AS, Barros PP, da Silva FM, Jacinto Rde C, Bueno CE. In vitro evaluation of the cleansing working time and analysis of the amount of gutta-percha or Resilon remnants in the root canal walls after instrumentation for endodontic retreatment. J Endod. 2007;33(12):1426–8.
15. De Chevigny C, Dao TT, Basrani BR, Marquis V, Farzaneh M, Abitbol S, Friedman S. Treatment outcome in endodontics: the Toronto study–phases 3 and 4: orthograde retreatment. J Endod. 2008;34(2):131–7.

16. De-Deus G, Souza EM, Marins JR, Reis C, Paciornik S, Zehnder M. Smear layer dissolution by peracetic acid of low concentration. Int Endod J. 2011;44(6):485–90.
17. De Mello Junior JE, Cunha RS, Bueno CE, Zuolo ML. Retreatment efficacy of gutta-percha removal using a clinical microscope and ultrasonic instruments: part I – an ex vivo study. Oral Surg Oral Med Oral Pathol Oral Radiol Endod. 2009;108(1):e59–62.
18. Di Fiore PM, Genov KA, Komaroff E, Li Y, Lin L. Nickel-titanium rotary instrument fracture: a clinical practice assessment. Int Endod J. 2006;39:700–8.
19. Du T, Wang Z, Shen Y, Ma J, Cao Y, Haapasalo M. Effect of long-term exposure to endodontic disinfecting solutions on young and old Enterococcus faecalis biofilms in dentin canals. J Endod. 2014;40(4):509–14.
20. Dugas NN, Lawrence HP, Teplitsky PE, Pharoah MJ, Friedman S. Periapical health and treatment quality assessment of root-filled teeth in two Canadian populations. Int Endod J. 2003;36(3):181–92.
21. Edgar SW, Marshall JG, Baumgartner JC. The antimicrobial effect of chloroform on Enterococcus faecalis after gutta-percha removal. J Endod. 2006;32(12):1185–7.
22. European Society of Endodontology. Quality guidelines for endodontic treatment: consensus report of the European Society of Endodontology. Int Endod J. 2006;39(12):921–30.
23. Falk KW, Sedgley CM. The influence of preparation size on the mechanical efficacy of root canal irrigation in vitro. J Endod. 2005;31(10):742–5.
24. Faria-Júnior NB, Loiola LE, Guerreiro-Tanomaru JM, Berbert FL, Tanomaru-Filho M. Effectiveness of three solvents and two associations of solvents on gutta-percha and resilon. Braz Dent J. 2011;22(1):41–4.
25. Filipo-Perez C, Bramante CM, Villas-Boas MH, Húngaro Duarte MA, Versiani MA, Ordinola-Zapata R. Micro-computed tomographic analysis of the root canal morphology of the distal root of mandibular first molar. J Endod. 2015;41(2):231–6.
26. Fruchi Lde C, Ordinola-Zapata R, Cavenago BC, Hungaro Duarte MA, Bueno CE, De Martin AS. Efficacy of reciprocating instruments for removing filling material in curved canals obturated with a single-cone technique: a micro-computed tomographic analysis. J Endod. 2014;40(7):1000–4.
27. Gordon MPJ. The removal of gutta-percha and root canal sealers from root canals. N Z Dental J. 2005;101:44–52.
28. Gorni FG, Gagliani MM. The outcome of endodontic retreatment: a 2-yr follow-up. J Endod. 2004;30(1):1–4.
29. Grischke J, Müller-Heine A, Hülsmann M. The effect of four different irrigation systems in the removal of a root canal sealer. Clin Oral Investig. 2014;18(7):1845–51.
30. Hunter KR, Doblecki W, Pelleu Jr GB. Halothane and eucalyptol as alternatives to chloroform for softening gutta-percha. J Endod. 1991;17(7):310–1.
31. Karapinar-Kazandag M, Basrani BR, Friedman S. The operating microscope enhances detection and negotiation of accessory mesial canals in mandibular molars. J Endod. 2010;36(8):1289–94.
32. Keleş A, Köseoğlu M. Dissolution of root canal sealers in EDTA and NaOCl solutions. J Am Dent Assoc. 2009;140(1):74–9.
33. Kerekes K, Tronstad L. Long-term results of endodontic treatment performed with a standardized technique. J Endod. 1979;5:83–90.
34. Leonardo MR, Tanomaru Filho M, Silva LAB, et al. In vivo antimicrobial activity of 2 % chlorhexidine used as a root canal irrigating solution. J Endod. 1999;25:167–71.
35. Leoni GB, Versiani MA, Pécora JD, Damião de Sousa-Neto M. Micro-computed tomographic analysis of the root canal morphology of mandibular incisors. J Endod. 2014;40(5):710–6.
36. Lottanti S, Gautschi H, Sener B, Zehnder M. Effects of ethylenediaminetetraacetic, etidronic and peracetic acid irrigation on human root dentine and the smear layer. Int Endod J. 2009;42(4):335–43.
37. Marquis VL, Dao T, Farzaneh M, Abitbol S, Friedman S. Treatment outcome in endodontics: the Toronto Study. Phase III: initial treatment. J Endod. 2006;32(4):299–306.
38. Martos J, Ferrer Luque CM, González-Rodríguez MP, Arias-Moliz MT, Baca P. Antimicrobial activity of essential oils and chloroform alone and combinated with cetrimide against Enterococcus faecalis biofilm. Eur J Microbiol Immunol (Bp). 2013;3(1):44–8.
39. McDonald MN, Vire DE. Chloroform in the endodontic operatory. J Endod. 1992;118(6):301–3.
40. Metzger Z, Teperovich E, Zary R, Cohen R, Hof R. The self-adjusting file (SAF). Part 1: respecting the root canal anatomy–a new concept of endodontic files and its implementation. J Endod. 2010;36(4):679–90.
41. Mohammadi Z, Abbott PV. The properties and applications of chlorhexidine in endodontics. Int Endod J. 2009;42:288–302.
42. Nair PN. Pathogenesis of apical periodontitis and the causes of endodontic failures. Crit Rev Oral Biol Med. 2004;15(6):348–81.
43. Nevares G, Cunha RS, Zuolo ML, Bueno CE. Success rates for removing or bypassing fractured instruments: a prospective clinical study. J Endod. 2012;38(4):442–4.
44. Nevares G, Albuquerque DS, Zuolo ML, Bueno CES, Cunha RS. Efficacy of retreatment in root canals filled with thermoplasticized techniques. In: 92nd International Association for Dental Research General Session – IADR, 2014, Cape Town. J Dent Res. 93(Special Issue B):1498.
45. Ordinola-Zapata R, Bramante CM, Aprecio RM, Handysides R, Jaramillo DE. Biofilm removal by 6 % sodium hypochlorite activated by different irrigation techniques. Int Endod J. 2014;47(7):659–66.
46. Ordinola-Zapata R, Monteiro Bramante C, Gagliardi Minotti P, Cavalini Cavenago B, Gutmann JL, Moldauer BI, Versiani MA, Hungaro Duarte MA. Micro-CT evaluation of C-shaped mandibular first premolars in a Brazilian subpopulation. Int Endod J. 2014. [Epub ahead of print]

47. Paiva SS, Siqueira Jr JF, Rôças IN, Carmo FL, Ferreira DC, Curvelo JA, Soares RM, Rosado AS. Supplementing the antimicrobial effects of chemomechanical debridement with either passive ultrasonic irrigation or a final rinse with chlorhexidine: a clinical study. J Endod. 2012;38(9):1202–6.
48. Panitvisai P, Parunnit P, Sathorn C, Messer HH. Impact of a retained instrument on treatment outcome: a systematic review and meta-analysis. J Endod. 2010;36:775–80.
49. Paqué F, Ganahl D, Peters OA. Effects of root canal preparation on apical geometry assessed by micro-computed tomography. J Endod. 2009;35(7):1056–9.
50. Paqué F, Peters OA. Micro-computed tomography evaluation of the preparation of long oval root canals in mandibular molars with the self-adjusting file. J Endod. 2011;37(4):517–21.
51. Parashos P, Gordon I, Messer HH. Factors influencing defects of rotary nickel-titanium endodontic instruments after clinical use. J Endod. 2004;30:722–5.
52. Peters OA, Boessler C, Paqué F. Root canal preparation with a novel nickel-titanium instrument evaluated with micro-computed tomography: canal surface preparation over time. J Endod. 2010;36(6):1068–72.
53. Ricucci D, Siqueira Jr JF, Lopes WS, Vieira AR, Rôças IN. Extraradicular infection as the cause of persistent symptoms: a case series. J Endod. 2015;41(2):265–73.
54. Rios Mde A, Villela AM, Cunha RS, Velasco RC, De Martin AS, Kato AS, Bueno CE. Efficacy of 2 reciprocating systems compared with a rotary retreatment system for gutta-percha removal. J Endod. 2014;40(4):543–6.
55. Sae-Lim V, Rajamanickam I, Lim BK, Lee HL. Effectiveness of ProFile.04 taper rotary instruments in endodontic retreatment. J Endod. 2000;26(2):100–4.
56. Sağlam BC, Koçak MM, Türker SA, Koçak S. Efficacy of different solvents in removing gutta-percha from curved root canals: a micro-computed tomography study. Aust Endod J. 2014;40(2):76–80.
57. Salehrabi R, Rotstein I. Endodontic treatment outcomes in a large patient population in the USA: an epidemiological study. J Endod. 2004;30(12):846–50.
58. Salehrabi R, Rotstein I. Epidemiologic evaluation of the outcomes of orthograde endodontic retreatment. J Endod. 2010;36(5):790–2.
59. Scelza MF, Coil JM, Maciel AC, Oliveira LR, Scelza P. Comparative SEM evaluation of three solvents used in endodontic retreatment: an ex vivo study. J Appl Oral Sci. 2008;16(1):24–9.
60. Schirrmeister JF, Meyer KM, Hermanns P, Altenburger MJ, Wrbas KT. Effectiveness of hand and rotary instrumentation for removing a new synthetic polymer-based root canal obturation material (Epiphany) during retreatment. Int Endod J. 2006;39(2):150–6.
61. Signoretti FG, Endo MS, Gomes BP, Montagner F, Tosello FB, Jacinto RC. Persistent extraradicular infection in root-filled asymptomatic human tooth: scanning electron microscopic analysis and microbial investigation after apical microsurgery. J Endod. 2011;37(12):1696–700.
62. Siqueira Jr JF, Rôças IN. Diversity of endodontic microbiota revisited. J Dent Res. 2009;88(11):969–81.
63. Siqueira Jr JF. A etiology of root canal treatment failure: why well-treated teeth can fail. Int Endod J. 2001;34(1):1–10.
64. Só MVR, Saran C, Magro ML, Vier-Pelisser FV, Munhoz M. Efficacy of ProTaper retreatment system in root canals filled with gutta-percha and two endodontic sealers. J Endod Oct. 2008;34(10):1223–5.
65. Solomonov M, Paqué F, Kaya S, Adigüzel O, Kfir A, Yiğit-Özer S. Self-adjusting files in retreatment: a high-resolution micro-computed tomography study. J Endod. 2012;38(9):1283–7.
66. Spili P, Parashos P, Messer HH. The impact of instrument fracture on outcome of endodontic treatment. J Endod. 2005;31:845–50.
67. Subha N, Prabhakar V, Koshy M, Abinaya K, Prabu M, Thangavelu L. Efficacy of peracetic acid in rapid disinfection of Resilon and gutta-percha cones compared with sodium hypochlorite, chlorhexidine, and povidone-iodine. J Endod. 2013;39(10):1261–4.
68. Takahashi CM, Cunha RS, de Martin AS, Fontana CE, Silveira CF, da Silveira Bueno CE. In vitro evaluation of the effectiveness of ProTaper universal rotary retreatment system for gutta-percha removal with or without a solvent. J Endod. 2009;35(11):1580–3.
69. Tamse A, Fuss Z, Lustig J, Kaplavi J. An evaluation of endodontically treated vertically fractured teeth. J Endod. 1999;25:506–8.
70. Tamse A, Unger U, Metzger Z, Rosenberg M. Gutta-percha solvents—a comparative study. J Endod. 1986;12(8):337–9.
71. Torabinejad M, Corr R, Handysides R, Shabahang S. Outcomes of nonsurgical retreatment and endodontic surgery: a systematic review. J Endod. 2009;35(7):930–7.
72. Tsesis I, Rosen E, Tamse A, Taschieri S, Kfir A. Diagnosis of vertical root fractures in endodontically treated teeth based on clinical and radiographic indices: a systematic review. J Endod. 2010;36(9):1455–8.
73. Vieira AR, Siqueira Jr JF, Ricucci D, Lopes WS. Dentinal tubule infection as the cause of recurrent disease and late endodontic treatment failure: a case report. J Endod. 2012;38(2):250–4.
74. Weiger R, ElAyouti A, Löst C. Efficiency of hand and rotary instruments in shaping oval root canals. J Endod. 2002;28(8):580–3.
75. Wilcox LR. Endodontic retreatment with halothane versus chloroform solvent. J Endod. 1995;21(6):305–7.
76. Wourms DJ, Campbel AD, Hicks ML, Pelleu Jr GB. Alternative solvents to chloroform for gutta-percha removal. J Endod. 1990;16(5):224–6.
77. Wu MK, R'oris A, Barkis D, Wesselink PR. Prevalence and extent of long oval canals in the apical third. Oral

Surg Oral Med Oral Pathol Oral Radiol Endod. 2000;89(6):739–43.
78. Yeung W, Raldi DP, Cunha RS, Mello I. Assessment of smear layer removal protocols in curved root canals. Aust Endod J. 2014;40(2):66–71.
79. Zamany A, Safavi K, Spangberg LS. The effect of chlorhexidine as an endodontic disinfectant. Oral Surg Oral Med Oral Pathol Oral Radiol Endod. 2003;96:578–81.
80. Zehnder M. Root canal irrigants. J Endod. 2006; 32(5):389–98.
81. Zehnder M, Paqué F. Disinfection of the root canal system during root canal re-treatment. Endod Topics. 2011;19:58–73.
82. Zuolo AS, Mello Jr JE, Cunha RS, Zuolo ML. Bueno CE Efficacy of reciprocating and rotary techniques for removing filling material during root canal retreatment. Int Endod J. 2013;46(10):947–53.
83. Zuolo ML, Kherlakian D, Mello Jr JE, de Carvalho MC. Fagundes MIRC. Reintervention in Endodontics. São Paulo, Brazil. 1st ed. Quintessence; 2014. p. 314.

18 Irrigation in Regenerative Endodontic Procedures

Anibal R. Diogenes and Nikita B. Ruparel

Abstract

The developing dentition is at risk for pulpal necrosis due to trauma and developmental dental anomalies such as dens evaginatus. Loss of an immature permanent tooth in young patients with mixed dentition can be devastating, leading to loss of function, malocclusion, and inadequate maxillofacial development. These teeth traditionally have been treated with apexification procedures using either long-term calcium hydroxide treatment or immediate placement of a mineral trioxide aggregate (MTA) apical plug. Although these treatments often result in the resolution of signs and symptoms of pathosis, they provide little to no benefit for continued root development. Thus, immature teeth treated with these procedures are considered in a state of "arrested development," and no further root growth, normal pulpal nociception, and immune defense should be expected.

Introduction

The developing dentition is at risk for pulpal necrosis due to trauma and developmental dental anomalies such as dens evaginatus [1–7]. Loss of an immature permanent tooth in young patients with mixed dentition can be devastating, leading to loss of function, malocclusion, and inadequate maxillofacial development. These teeth traditionally have been treated with apexification procedures using either long-term calcium hydroxide treatment [8, 9] or immediate placement of a mineral trioxide aggregate (MTA) apical plug [10]. Although these treatments often result in the resolution of signs and symptoms of pathosis, they provide little to no benefit for continued root development [11]. Thus, immature teeth treated with these procedures are considered in a state of "arrested development," and no further root growth, normal pulpal nociception, and immune defense should be expected.

Regenerative endodontic procedures (REPSs) have emerged as an alternative treatment for these teeth that, in addition to healing of apical periodontitis, aims to promote normal pulpal physiologic functions. These include continued root

A.R. Diogenes, DDS, MS, PhD (✉)
N.B. Ruparel, MS, DDS, PhD
Department of Endodontics, University of Texas Health Center at San Antonio, San Antonio, TX, USA
e-mail: Diogenes@uthscsa.edu

B. Basrani (ed.), *Endodontic Irrigation: Chemical Disinfection of the Root Canal System*,
DOI 10.1007/978-3-319-16456-4_18

development, immunocompetency, and normal nociception, as seen in some published cases [12]. Thus, the ultimate goal of these procedures is to regenerate the components of the pulp-dentin complex. A significant number of case reports and case series have been published since the first reported case in 2001 [12]. These published cases document: 1) commonly observed clinical outcomes such as continued root development and sometimes normal nociceptive responses to vitality testing, 2) commonly found challenges such as technical pitfalls and unwanted adverse reactions such as coronal staining, and 3) great variability in treatment protocols [12]. Despite the lack of randomized clinical trials, these published clinical observations support the hypothesis that patients with otherwise limited treatment options could benefit from these procedures.

In 2011, a study demonstrated that a substantial number of undifferentiated mesenchymal stem cells are delivered into root canal systems following REPS [13]. This finding represented a turning point because treatment protocols previously used in REPS aimed to provide maximum disinfection without consideration for their impact on stem cells. Contemporary regenerative endodontics acknowledges and follows principles of bioengineering regarding the interplay between stem cells, scaffolds, and growth factors [14]. Since stem cells represent one of the pillars of REPS, a series of translational studies evaluating effect of disinfection on stem cell fate have been conducted. These studies have contributed to the foundational framework for the currently American Association of Endodontists (AAE) recommended regenerative endodontic treatment protocol [15]. The present chapter will focus primarily on shedding light on the studies evaluating the role of various irrigants on the survival, differentiation, and other properties of stem cells that are key to an optimal regenerative outcome.

Chemical Debridement in Regenerative Procedures

Clinicians often face the challenge of adequately debriding large infected root canals in REPS. In these procedures, similar to conventional endodontic therapy, microbial control is crucial. These canals with compromised fragile underdeveloped dentinal walls represent a contraindication for mechanical instrumentation; thus, chemical debridement remains the main form of disinfection in REPS. Sodium hypochlorite (NaOCl) is the most widely used agent for chemical debridement in endodontic procedures, including REPS [12]. It has several desirable characteristics including: 1) excellent bactericidal efficacy [16–18], 2) tissue dissolution capacity [19–21], and 3) effective lubrication for endodontic instruments. The first two beneficial properties are crucial for the disinfection of immature teeth in regenerative endodontic procedures, which typically involve minimal to no mechanical preparation. However, what are the effects of NaOCl on stem cells?

A study evaluated the survival of stem cells of apical papilla (SCAP) cultured in an organotype root canal model previously irrigated with various combinations of commonly used chemical agents [22]. It was found that dentin conditioning with 17 % ethylenediaminetetraacetic acid (EDTA) promoted greater survival of SCAP, whereas the use of 6 % NaOCl had a profound detrimental effect on SCAP survival. Importantly, the use of EDTA following 6 % NaOCl attenuated its undesirable effects [22] (Fig. 18.1).

Another *ex vivo* study by Galler et al. [23] evaluated the effects of full-strength (5.25 %) NaOCl compared to 17 % EDTA on dentin surface. Dentin cylinders used as cell carriers were subjected either to 5.25 % NaOCl or 17 % EDTA. Dental pulp stem cells (DPSCs) with biodegradable hydrogel scaffold enhanced with bioactive molecules such as heparin-binding growth factors vascular endothelial growth factor (VEGF), transforming growth factor-beta1 (TGF-β1), and fibroblast growth factor-2 (FGF-2) were loaded into the cylinders which were in turn implanted into immunodeficient mice. The histological results of the study clearly demonstrated that dentin treated with 5.25 % NaOCl leads to resorption and clastic cellular activity along the dentinal walls. On the other hand, dentin conditioned with 17 % EDTA promoted the formation of pulp-like tissue with blood vessels and polarized cells that often extended processes into dentinal tubules and expressed the odontoblastic marker dentin sialoprotein (DSP) (Fig. 18.2). One study evaluated the effects of 5.25 % NaOCl or 17 % EDTA dentin

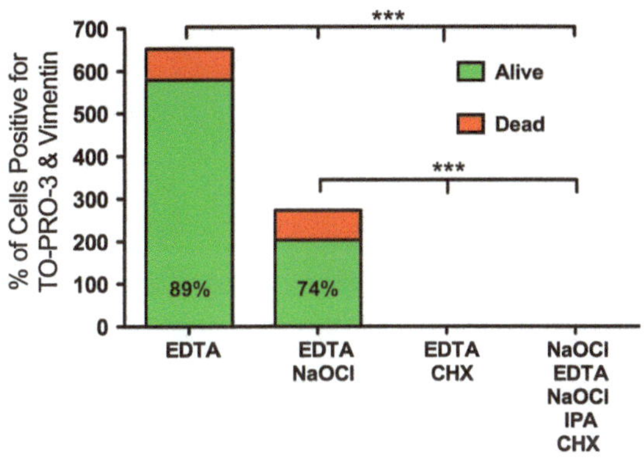

Fig. 18.1 EDTA promotes SCAP survival. Organotype immature teeth root canal models were irrigated with 20 ml of irrigant for 1 min followed by thorough rinsing with Hanks' Balanced Salt Solution for 7 days. SCAPs were then seeded with platelet-rich plasma (PRP) scaffold into the root segments. The percentage of viable cells (vimentin positive) of total cells (TO-PRO-3 positive) were determined by confocal microscopy for each group after 21 days. 17 % EDTA group demonstrated the maximum number of viable cells followed by EDTA/NaOCl. No viable cells were seen for the EDTA/CHX and NaOCl/EDTA/NaOCl/isopropyl alcohol (IPA)/CHX groups (Modified from Trevino et al. [22]). *** P<.001

conditioning on stem cell expression of odontoblastic markers [24]. Dentin disks were treated (conditioned) with 5.25 % NaOCl or 17 % EDTA. The expression of odontoblastic markers such as matrix extracellular phosphoglycoprotein (MEPE), dentin matrix protein-1 (DMP-1), and dentin sialophosphoprotein (DSPP) was evaluated using quantitative reverse-transcription polymerase chain reaction (qRT-PCR). This study demonstrated that tooth slices subjected to 5.25 % NaOCl showed no expression of the abovementioned markers. However, the ones treated with 17 % EDTA showed significant increase in these markers *in vitro* (Fig. 18.3). Moreover, when tooth slices were implanted into the dorsum of immunodeficient mice, similar results were obtained at 14 and 28 days. It is also noteworthy that this prolonged effect of dentin conditioning with NaOCl was detected long after the irrigant had been removed, suggesting that NaOCl has a profound indirect effect on stem cell toxicity [25]. Thus, dentin conditioning with sodium hypochlorite at its maximum used clinical concentration leads to greatly diminished stem cell survival and loss of odontoblast-like cell differentiation.

Another recent study was conducted to evaluate whether other clinically used concentrations of NaOCl were conducive for stem cell (SCAP) survival and differentiation [26]. Standardized root canals were prepared in extracted human teeth. The prepared teeth were then irrigated with NaOCl at the concentrations of 6, 3, and 1.5 %. Approximately half of the samples received a second irrigation with 17 % EDTA, whereas all samples received a copious final flush with saline to remove any residual chemical from the canal space. SCAP in a hyaluronic acid hydrogel were seeded in all canals and cultured for 7 days. The number of viable cells was assessed using a luminescence assay, while the level of DSPP was assessed by real-time RT-PCR. It was found that dentin conditioning with NaOCl decreases both SCAP survival and differentiation in a concentration-dependent manner. However, the concentration of 1.5 % of NaOCl was found to have minimal effects on the survival and differentiation. In addition, it was demonstrated that a final irrigation with 17 % EDTA reverses the deleterious effects of NaOCl (Fig. 18.4). Thus, this study agrees with other studies that dentin conditioning with 6 % NaOCl has a negative effect, while 17 % EDTA has a positive effect on the survival and differentiation of stem cells subsequently cultured in contact with the conditioned dentin [22, 26, 27]. The negative effects of NaOCl do not appear to be directly related to residual NaOCl in the dentinal tubules resulting in direct toxicity since neutralization with sodium thiosulfate (5 %) did not reverse this effect [26]. Thus, NaOCl has a profound effect on dentin resulting in diminished stem cell survival and differentiation. These effects can be minimized by using 1.5 % NaOCl followed by 17 % EDTA [19]. Collectively, all studies mentioned here point to the detrimental effects of full-strength NaOCl and the beneficial effects of 17 % EDTA on dentin.

Irrigants and Dentin Matrix Growth Factors

Important biologically active growth factors are trapped in the dentin matrix during dentinogenesis. Some of these growth factors such as VEGF

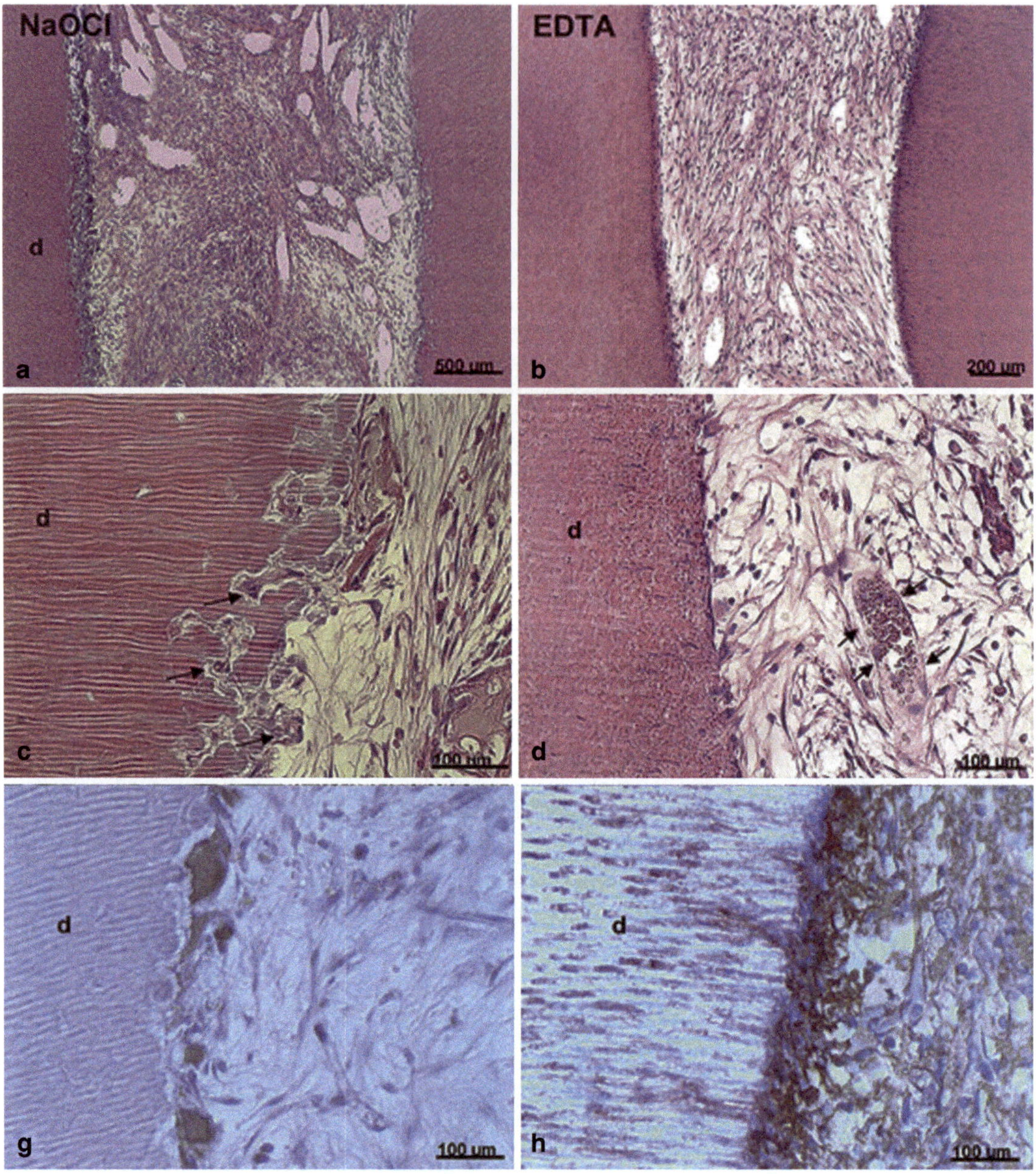

Fig. 18.2 EDTA promotes pulp-like tissue formation and DSP expression. Dentin cylinders were irrigated with 5.25 % NaOCl or 17 % EDTA. DPSCs mixed with hydrogel scaffold were loaded into the cylinders. Dentin cylinders were then implanted into immunodeficient mice. Hematoxylin and eosin staining and tartrate-resistant acid phosphatase (TRAP) done at 6 weeks show the presence of disorganized fibrous connect tissue and presence of large multinucleated giant cells/odontoclasts in the NaOCl group (panels **a**, **c**, **g**) in the NaOCl group. Well-organized vascularized connective tissue with cells at the cell-dentin interface that appear flat and are in close contact with the dentin wall (panels **b**, **d**). Immunohistochemistry for DSP demonstrates that cells adjacent to the dentin surface stain positive for DSP, which indicates that these cells have differentiated into an odontoblast-like phenotype (panel **h**) (Modified from Galler et al. [23])

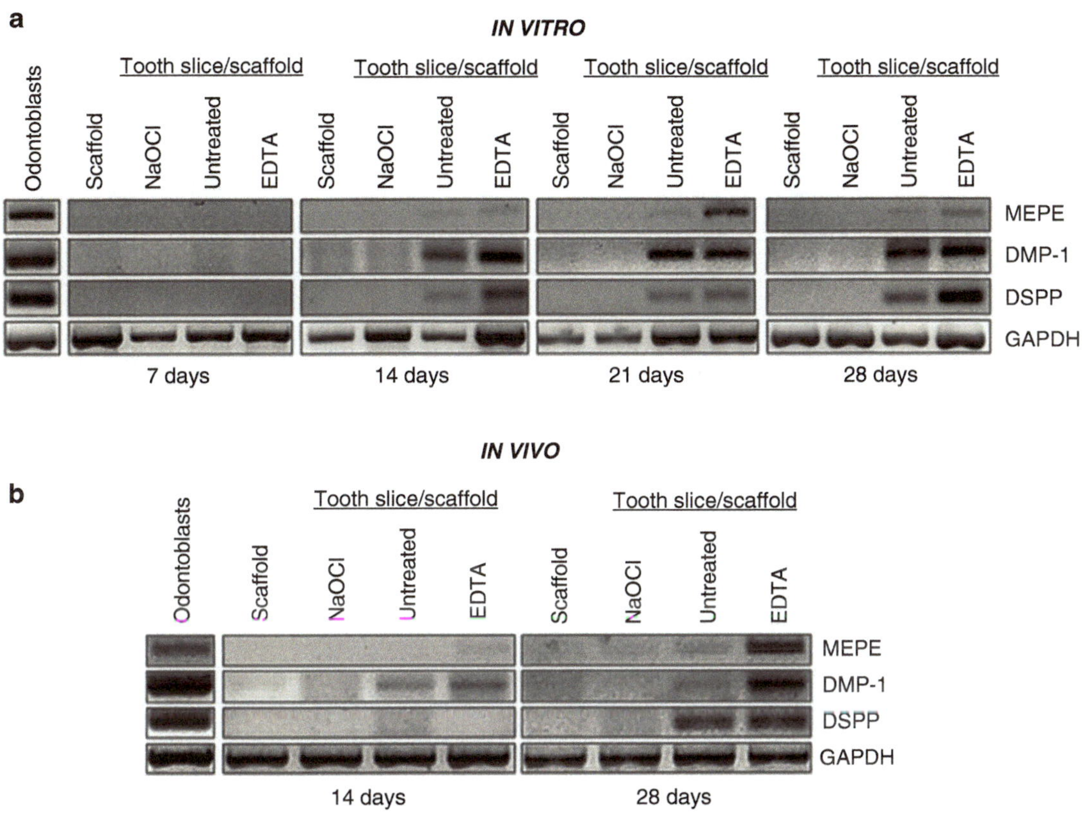

Fig. 18.3 EDTA promotes odontoblastic differentiation of stem cells. Scaffold without tooth slice was used as a negative control. Tooth slices were treated with 5.25 % NaOCl for 5 days (to denature dentin proteins), left untreated, or treated with 17 % EDTA for 1 min (to mobilize dentin proteins). Markers of odontoblastic differentiation, i.e., DSPP, DMP-1, and MEPE, were evaluated by RT-PCR. For in vivo studies, tooth slices were treated with the same irrigation protocol and were then loaded with scaffold and SHED cells. They were then implanted subcutaneously into the dorsum of immunodeficient mice. After 14 or 28 days, markers of odontoblastic differentiation (i.e., DSPP, DMP-1, and MEPE) were evaluated by RT-PCR. Both studies demonstrated increased expression of all markers at in the untreated and 17 % EDTA groups whereas no expression was observed in the scaffold only and 5.25 % NaOCL groups (panels **a**, **b**) (Modified from Casagrande et al. [24])

[28] and TGFB1 [29] are known to have a robust effect on the differentiation and/or proliferation of mesenchymal stem cells. These growth factors appear particularly efficacious in promoting the proliferation of mesenchymal stem cells and directing them toward an odontoblast-like phenotype [30, 31]. Irrigants, especially NaOCl in high concentration, are known to denature these dentin-derived growth factors [32]. In an *in vivo* study, dental pulp stem cells (DPSCs) proliferated at higher rates and expressed higher levels of odontoblastic markers in a tooth slice model compared to DPSCs placed in scaffold only [27]. These findings suggest that morphogens, such as the many growth factors known to be present in dentin, are sufficient to promote the survival, proliferation, and importantly the differentiation of dental stem cells. EDTA is known to solubilize and mobilize these growth factors from dentin, thereby increasing their bioavailability [33, 34].

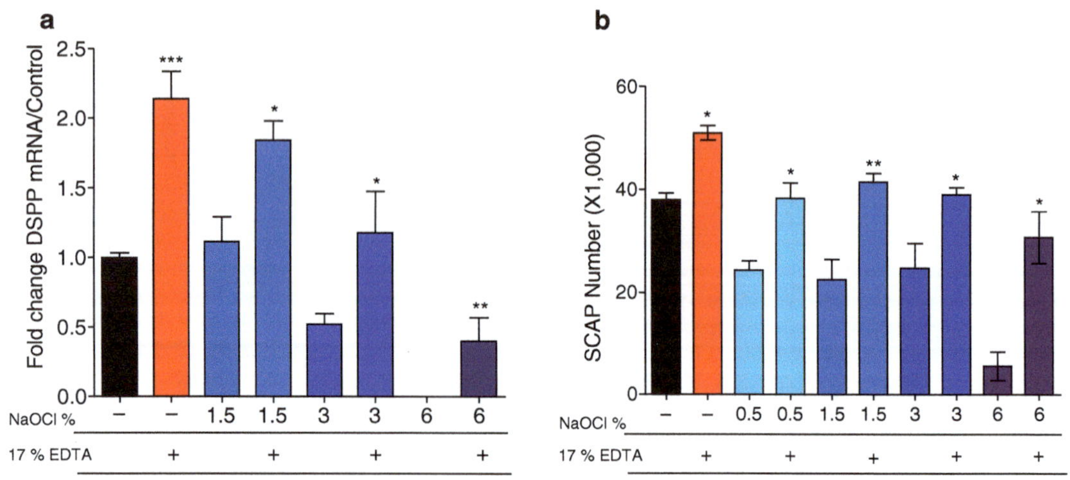

Fig. 18.4 Sodium hypochlorite decreases SCAP survival and differentiation in a concentration-dependent manner. Organotype immature teeth root canal models were irrigated with different concentrations of NaOCl following a standardized protocol that included a final wash of saline or EDTA. SCAPs were seeded into the root segments and cultured in vitro for 7 days. The percentage of viable cells were determined by a luminescence assay. NaOCl concentration-dependent decrease in SCAP survival is partially reversed by a final irrigation with 17 % EDTA (panel **a**). In addition, real-time qRT-PCR was used to determine the expression of the odontoblast-like cell marker dentin sialophosphoprotein (DSPP) mRNA. NaOCl decreases DSPP expression in a concentration-dependent manner with no expression seen in the group treated with 6 %. In addition, EDTA partially reversed the negative effect of NaOCl on DSPP expression (panel **b**). Data are presented by % of maximum observed effect on the EDTA only-treated group (control) (Modified from Martin et al. 2014 [26])

Thus, its use may allow clinicians to harness the inductive properties of dentin-derived morphogens and growth factors normally present in dentin [35]. Therefore, the indirect negative effect of NaOCl and positive effect of EDTA on stem cell proliferation and differentiation appear to be directly related to the denaturing and solubilizing effects of these irrigants, respectively, on dentin matrix proteins. Astute clinicians must use the best available evidence to choose the combinations and concentrations of irrigants to achieve the greatest antimicrobial effect while minimizing stem cells death and loss of differentiation potential.

Stem cell survival, proliferation, and differentiation are also known to be dictated by the surface on which the cells grow [36–38]. Stem cells attach to a specific surface such as a target organ during organogenesis, or repair, via the interaction of specific cell-adhesion molecules such as integrins expressed on the plasma membrane of these cells. The effect of the substrate on stem cell behavior is best illustrated by the effect of the stem cell niche that in addition to growth factors (discussed above) provide attachment signals resulting in cell arrestment in a quiescent state [39, 40]. Cells released from their niche become "activated" and start proliferating and undergoing differentiation. The process of culturing tooth-derived stem cells such as DPSCs or SCAP is a good example of cells leaving their inhibited state in the niche (dental pulp or apical papilla, respectively) and displaying remarkable proliferative and differentiation potentials. This information has strong clinical implications since the dentin matrix composition (stem cell substrate) is altered by chemical treatment during the process of chemical debridement. NaOCl is known to cause changes in dentin matrix composition with decrease in carbon and nitrogen content and demineralization when used at high concentrations [41]. In contrast, the concentration of 1 % NaOCl does not cause any significant changes in dentin composition or mechanical properties. The property of attachment to a substrate has been evaluated using various other irrigants as well [42]. Ten treatment groups with different combinations of irrigants were used to evaluate attachment of stem cells from

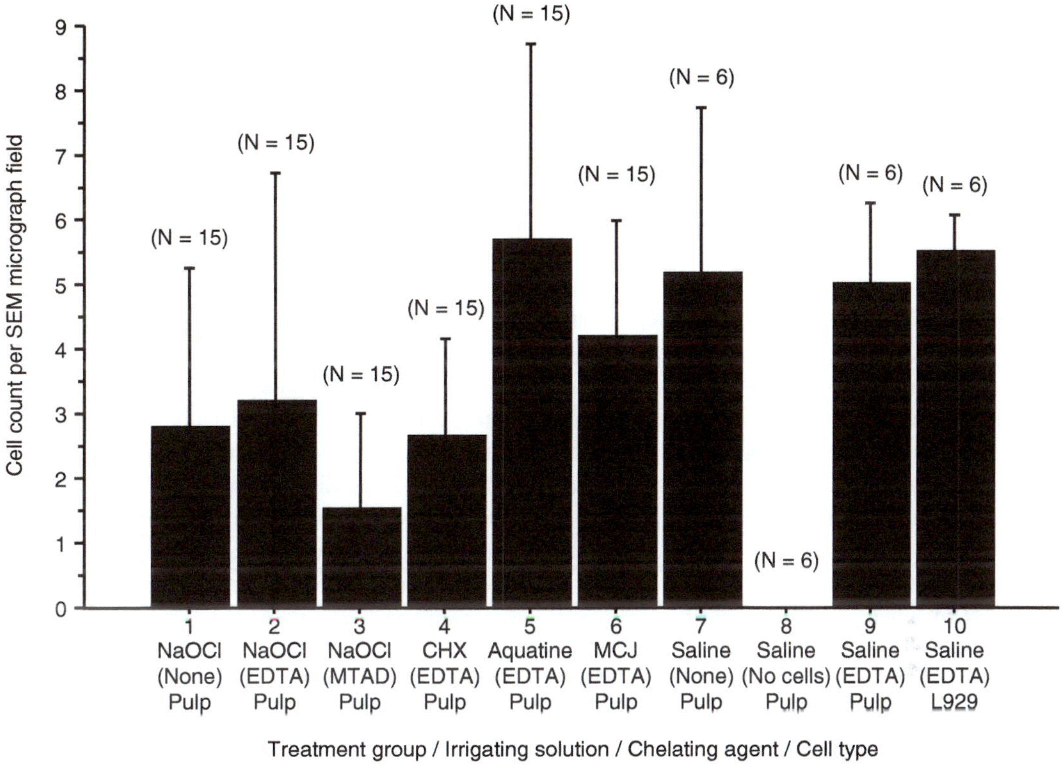

Fig. 18.5 EDTA promotes cell attachment to dentin. Tooth segments were treated with various irrigants during instrumentation followed by the use of a chelating agent and a final rinse with the first irrigant. SHED cells were then loaded into the segments, and after 7 days, the number of cells (L929 and SHED) attached to the root canal walls per SEM micrograph field of view was assessed. Rat fibroblast L929 cells were used as positive control. The rank order of cleaning and shaping treatments from the lowest to the highest mean numbers of attached DPSCs was NaOCl/MTAD, CHX/EDTA, NaOCl, NaOCl/EDTA, MCJ/EDTA, and Aquatine*EC*/EDTA (Modified from Ring et al. [42])

human exfoliated deciduous teeth (SHED) cells to dentin walls. It was found that groups treated with NaOCl and chlorhexidine (CHX) appeared to have the lowest amount of cell attachment compared to the groups that were treated with Aquatine EC and Morinda citrofolia (MCJ) (Fig. 18.5). An interesting finding is that all groups that were treated with EDTA as a chelating agent showed maximum number of cell attachment than groups that were treated with either no chelating agent or MTAD (Fig. 18.5). Thus, changes in dentin's chemical composition could interfere with the ability of stem cells to attach, proliferate, and differentiate on the dentin surface. Thus, NaOCl is likely to affect stem cell fate by altering the dentin's chemical composition, including the denaturation or growth factors and attachment molecules.

Irrigation Techniques

Apart from the choice of chemical irrigant, focus may also be given to the types of techniques used to irrigate these teeth. Apical negative-pressure irrigation has been advocated for its superior disinfection and safety properties [43, 44]. Recent studies comparing bacterial counts in immature dog teeth after use of EndoVac versus conventional positive-pressure irrigation along with triple antibiotic paste (equal mixture of minocycline, metronidazole, and ciprofloxacin (TAP)) failed to demonstrate significant difference in bacterial reduction in the EndoVac group (88.6 %) versus conventional irrigation (78.28 %) [45]. However, the qualitative histological evaluation of the tissues formed following the regenerative/revascularization procedure in both groups suggests that the EndoVac irrigation promoted better formation of connective tissue, blood vessels, and mineralized masses while displaying lesser inflammatory cells in the EndoVac group than in the conventional irrigation group [46]. Moreover, the periapical region showed the presence of osteoclasts and bone resorption. These findings could be due to inadequate disinfection as well as any extrusion of NaOCl that may have impaired pulpal and periapical healing/repair [46]. It is important to emphasize that more studies evaluating the effect of different chemical debridement approaches such as sonic, ultrasonic, and negative pressure on regenerative outcomes are needed. Ideally, these studies should have quantitative outcomes and appropriate sample size to allow for more robust evidence in this important subject. Collectively, additional studies evaluating the effects of other irrigation techniques are warranted to fully optimize the irrigation protocol.

Residual Intracanal Medicaments and Stem Cell Survival

Regenerative procedures are typically performed in multiple visits with placement of an intracanal medicament to maximize disinfection and successful outcomes. Most of the published case reports and case series have utilized either the TAP or calcium hydroxide as inter-appointment medicaments [12]. Although the antimicrobial effect of these agents has been widely appreciated [47–49], their effect on stem cell survival was largely unknown until recently. A study sought to evaluate the direct effect of different medicaments on SCAP survival [50]. It was found that antibiotic paste formulations at the concentration typically used in previously published cases were directly lethal to SCAP. Interestingly, calcium hydroxide had no detrimental effect; instead it promoted survival and proliferation [50]. Another study evaluated the residual effect of calcium hydroxide or TAP on the survival of SCAP [51]. In this study, dentin disks were exposed to TAP or calcium hydroxide for 7 or 28 days, followed by irrigation with 1.5 % NaOCl and 17 % EDTA to remove the medicament. Similar to the direct effect, the TAP at the paste-like consistency had a detrimental residual effect, greatly impacting stem cell survival on the conditioned dentin [51]. Conversely, dentin conditioning with calcium hydroxide promoted survival and proliferation. Therefore, the adequate removal of intracanal medicaments, in particular antibiotic formulations, appears to be a challenging step following irrigation of the root canal system prior to the delivery of stem cells.

A study was conducted to evaluate the effectiveness of different irrigation methods to removal of triple antibiotic medication from the root canal system (canal lumen and dentinal tubules) [52]. Greater than 85 % of the medicament was found remaining within the dentinal walls despite the use of ultrasonic and sonic activation and negative-pressure (EndoVac) and conventional positive-pressure irrigation (Max-i-Probe needle). These findings were surprising and have profound clinical significance. Extensive penetration of TAP was observed as seen by direct visualization of staining often extending to the cementum layer in dentin disks treated with the medication [52]. Although high penetration into dentin appears to be a desirable effect for an antimicrobial agent, its negative effect on stem cell survival must be taken in clinical consideration. Importantly, it has been previously demonstrated that if used at the concentration of 1 mg/ml, it has minimal effect on the survival of stem cells [51]. Thus, the undesirable effects of the triple antibiotic medication can be greatly minimized with the use of a concentration that retains its adequate antimicrobial effect [48] but has minimal residual effect on the survival of stem cells [51]. Nonetheless, irrigation techniques must be optimized to allow better removal of medicaments with possible deleterious effect on stem cell fate and the exposure of attachment molecules and growth factors that maximize the survival, proliferation, and odontoblastic differentiation along the dentinal walls.

Overview of a Regenerative Endodontic Procedure

The following protocol reflects our current personal recommendations for regenerative procedures and is based on the best level of available evidence from clinical or preclinical translational studies. These recommendations are based in part upon the dual requirement of selecting irrigants and medicaments at concentrations that are known to be effective against microorganisms while being least toxic to stem cells. Importantly, it is to recognize that these recommendations are likely to change as the field of regenerative endodontics evolves.

Proposed Regenerative Endodontics Protocol

First treatment visit:

1. Informed consent, including explanation of risks and alternative treatments or no treatment.
2. After ascertaining adequate local anesthesia, rubber dam isolation is obtained.
3. The root canal systems are accessed and working length is determined (radiograph of a file loosely positioned at 1 mm from root end).
4. The root canal systems are slowly irrigated first with 1.5 % NaOCl (20 ml/canal, 5 min) and then irrigated with 17 % EDTA (20 ml/canal, 5 min), with irrigating needle positioned about 1 mm from root end.
5. Canals are dried with paper points.
6. Calcium hydroxide or antibiotic paste at combined concentration no greater than 1 mg/ml is delivered to canal system.
7. Access is temporarily restored.

Final (second) treatment visit:

(The second visit is scheduled 2–4 weeks after the first visit.)

1. A clinical exam is first performed to ensure that there is no moderate to severe sensitivity to palpation and percussion. If such sensitivity is observed, or a sinus tract or swelling is noted, then the treatment provided at the first visit is repeated. At this point the clinician may elect to TAP (at no more than 100 ug of each drug/ml).
2. After ascertaining adequate local anesthesia with 3 % mepivacaine (no epinephrine), rubber dam isolation is obtained.
3. The root canal systems are accessed; the intracanal medicament is removed by irrigating with 17 % EDTA (20 ml/canal, 5 min).
4. The canals are dried with paper points.
5. Bleeding is induced by rotating a pre-curved K-file size #25 at 2 mm past the apical foramen with the goal of having the whole canal filled with blood to the level of the cementoenamel junction.
6. Once a blood clot is formed, a premeasured piece of CollaPlug™ (Zimmer Dental Inc, Warsaw, IN) is carefully placed on top of the blood clot to serve as an internal matrix for the placement of approximately 3 mm of white MTA (Dentsply, Tulsa, OK). To avoid staining of the crown, the chamber may be etched, primed, and bonded prior to placement of MTA.
7. A (3–4 mm) layer of glass ionomer layer (e.g., Fuji IX ™, GC America, Alsip, IL; or other) is flowed gently over the MTA and light cured for 40 s.
8. A bonded reinforced composite resin restoration (e.g., Z-100™, 3 M, St Paul, MN; or other) is placed over the glass ionomer.
9. The case needs to be followed up at 3 months, 6 months, and yearly after that for a total of 4 years.

Concluding Remarks

Clinicians and researchers have focused for more than 100 years in adequately addressing disinfection to prevent and treat apical periodontitis. Regenerative endodontics also has this primordial focus but also acknowledges principles of bioengineering to promote continued tooth development and normal physiology. Although regenerative endodontic procedures have been highly successful in controlling infection, promoting radiographic root development and nociception [12], recent histological reports of teeth previously treated with regenerative endodontic procedures highlight the lack of control over stem cell fate [53, 54]. Mineralized deposits along the dentinal walls resemble cementum or osteodentin. In addition, islands of mineralized tissue that resembles bone were found embedded in the loose connective tissue. These findings are in agreement with histological studies in animal models of regenerative endodontics [46, 55, 56] that do not employ tissue engineering principles. It is fair to say that clinical success does not appear to match the histological success (full regeneration resembling a "naive" undamaged pulp). At this time, the significance of these histological findings to the clinical practice of regenerative endodontics is not clear. Nonetheless, these findings suggest that the regenerated tissue is not fully recapitulating the native pulp-dentin complex. Significantly more translational research must be done for all the mechanistic aspects of regenerative endodontic procedures to reach both clinical and histological success.

The balance between disinfection and the creation of an intracanal microenvironment conducive for the proliferation of stem cells requires further investigation. Choices of irrigants and medicaments must be made based on their antimicrobial efficacy *and* with the least harm to stem cells and growth factors present in the microenvironment. Therefore, astute clinicians must make evidence-based decisions on the various chemical and mechanical interventions on stem cells, scaffolds, and growth factors while maintaining the basic principles of disinfection. To date, this requires interpretation of preclinical studies and this level of evidence should be increased by randomized controlled clinical studies. Additional translational studies and clinical trials evaluating the different aspects of this procedure are required to understand the complexity of interrelated aspects that could result in better and more predictable outcomes.

References

1. Sobhi MB, Rana MJ, Ibrahim M, Chaudary A, Manzoor MA, Tasleem ul H. Frequency of dens evaginatus of permanent anterior teeth. J Coll Physicians Surg Pak JCPSP. 2004;14(2):88–90.
2. McCulloch KJ, Mills CM, Greenfeld RS, Coil JM. Dens evaginatus: review of the literature and report of several clinical cases. J Can Dent Assoc. 1998;64(2):104–6.
3. Yip WK. The prevalence of dens evaginatus. Oral Surg Oral Med Oral Pathol. 1974;38(1):80–7.
4. Kling M, Cvek M, Mejare I. Rate and predictability of pulp revascularization in therapeutically reimplanted permanent incisors. Endod Dent Traumatol. 1986;2(3): 83–9.
5. Andreasen JO, Ravn JJ. Epidemiology of traumatic dental injuries to primary and permanent teeth in a Danish population sample. Int J Oral Surg. 1972;1(5): 235–9.
6. Soriano EP, Caldas Ade Jr F, Diniz De Carvalho MV, Amorim Filho Hde A. Prevalence and risk factors related to traumatic dental injuries in Brazilian schoolchildren. Dent Traumatol Off Publ Int Assoc Dent Traumatol. 2007;23(4):232–40.
7. Andreasen JO, Borum MK, Jacobsen HL, Andreasen FM. Replantation of 400 avulsed permanent incisors. 2. Factors related to pulpal healing. Endod Dent Traumatol. 1995;11(2):59–68.
8. Cvek M. Treatment of non-vital permanent incisors with calcium hydroxide. IV. Periodontal healing and closure of the root canal in the coronal fragment of teeth with intra-alveolar fracture and vital apical fragment. A follow-up. Odontol Revy. 1974;25(3): 239–46.
9. Cvek M. Prognosis of luxated non-vital maxillary incisors treated with calcium hydroxide and filled with gutta-percha. A retrospective clinical study. Endod Dent Traumatol. 1992;8(2):45–55.
10. Witherspoon DE, Small JC, Regan JD, Nunn M. Retrospective analysis of open apex teeth obturated with mineral trioxide aggregate. J Endod. 2008;34(10):1171–6.
11. Bose R, Nummikoski P, Hargreaves K. A retrospective evaluation of radiographic outcomes in immature teeth with necrotic root canal systems treated with regenerative endodontic procedures. J Endod. 2009; 35(10):1343–9.
12. Diogenes A, Henry MA, Teixeira FB, Hargreaves KM. An update on clinical regenerative endodontics. Endod Topics. 2013;28(1):2–23.
13. Lovelace TW, Henry MA, Hargreaves KM, Diogenes A. Evaluation of the delivery of mesenchymal stem cells into the root canal space of necrotic immature teeth after clinical regenerative endodontic procedure. J Endod. 2011;37(2):133–8.
14. Langer R, Vacanti JP. Tissue engineering. Science. 1993;260(5110):920–6.
15. Law AS. Considerations for regeneration procedures. J Endod. 2013;39(3 Suppl):S44–56.
16. Harrison JW, Wagner GW, Henry CA. Comparison of the antimicrobial effectiveness of regular and fresh scent Clorox. J Endod. 1990;16(7):328–30.
17. Vianna ME, Horz HP, Gomes BP, Conrads G. In vivo evaluation of microbial reduction after chemo-mechanical preparation of human root canals containing necrotic pulp tissue. Int Endod J. 2006;39(6): 484–92.
18. Martinho FC, Gomes BP. Quantification of endotoxins and cultivable bacteria in root canal infection before and after chemomechanical preparation with 2.5 % sodium hypochlorite. J Endod. 2008;34(3):268–72.
19. Hand RE, Smith ML, Harrison JW. Analysis of the effect of dilution on the necrotic tissue dissolution

property of sodium hypochlorite. J Endod. 1978;4(2): 60–4.
20. Harrison JW, Hand RE. The effect of dilution and organic matter on the anti-bacterial property of 5.25 % sodium hypochlorite. J Endod. 1981;7(3): 128–32.
21. Yang SF, Rivera EM, Baumgardner KR, Walton RE, Stanford C. Anaerobic tissue-dissolving abilities of calcium hydroxide and sodium hypochlorite. J Endod. 1995;21(12):613–6.
22. Trevino EG, Patwardhan AN, Henry MA, Perry G, Dybdal-Hargreaves N, Hargreaves KM, et al. Effect of irrigants on the survival of human stem cells of the apical papilla in a platelet-rich plasma scaffold in human root tips. J Endod. 2011;37(8):1109–15.
23. Galler KM, D'Souza RN, Federlin M, Cavender AC, Hartgerink JD, Hecker S, et al. Dentin conditioning codetermines cell fate in regenerative endodontics. J Endod. 2011;37(11):1536–41.
24. Casagrande L, Demarco FF, Zhang Z, Araujo FB, Shi S, Nor JE. Dentin-derived BMP-2 and odontoblast differentiation. J Dent Res. 2010;89(6):603–8.
25. Essner MD, Javed A, Eleazer PD. Effect of sodium hypochlorite on human pulp cells: an in vitro study. Oral Surg Oral Med Oral Pathol Oral Radiol Endod. 2011;112(5):662–6.
26. Martin DE, Henry MA, Almeida JFA, Teixeira FB, Hargreaves KM, Diogenes AR. Effect of sodium hypochlorite on the odontoblastic phenotype differentiation of SCAP in cultured organotype human roots. J Endod. 2012;38(3):e26.
27. Demarco FF, Casagrande L, Zhang Z, Dong Z, Tarquinio SB, Zeitlin BD, et al. Effects of morphogen and scaffold porogen on the differentiation of dental pulp stem cells. J Endod. 2010;36(11):1805–11.
28. Roberts-Clark DJ, Smith AJ. Angiogenic growth factors in human dentine matrix. Arch Oral Biol. 2000;45(11):1013–6.
29. Cassidy N, Fahey M, Prime SS, Smith AJ. Comparative analysis of transforming growth factor-beta isoforms 1–3 in human and rabbit dentine matrices. Arch Oral Biol. 1997;42(3):219–23.
30. Smith AJ, Tobias RS, Plant CG, Browne RM, Lesot H, Ruch JV. Morphogenetic proteins from dentine extracellular matrix and cell-matrix interactions. Biochem Soc Trans. 1991;19(2):187S.
31. Smith AJ, Matthews JB, Hall RC. Transforming growth factor-beta1 (TGF-beta1) in dentine matrix. Ligand activation and receptor expression. Eur J Oral Sci. 1998;106 Suppl 1:179–84.
32. Zhao S, Sloan AJ, Murray PE, Lumley PJ, Smith AJ. Ultrastructural localisation of TGF-beta exposure in dentine by chemical treatment. Histochem J. 2000; 32(8):489–94.
33. Caplan AI. Adult mesenchymal stem cells and the NO Pathways. Proc Natl Acad Sci U S A. 2013 110(8): 2695–96.
34. Lin P, Lin Y, Lennon DP, Correa D, Schluchter M, Caplan AI. Efficient lentiviral transduction of human mesenchymal stem cells that preserves proliferation and differentiation capabilities. Stem Cells Transl Med. 2012;1(12):886–97.
35. Smith AJ, Smith JG, Shelton RM, Cooper PR. Harnessing the natural regenerative potential of the dental pulp. Dent Clin N Am. 2012;56(3): 589–601.
36. Walcott S, Sun SX. A mechanical model of actin stress fiber formation and substrate elasticity sensing in adherent cells. Proc Natl Acad Sci U S A. 2010; 107(17):7757–62.
37. Vincent LG, Choi YS, Alonso-Latorre B, del Alamo JC, Engler AJ. Mesenchymal stem cell durotaxis depends on substrate stiffness gradient strength. Biotechnol J. 2013;8(4):472–84.
38. Trappmann B, Gautrot JE, Connelly JT, Strange DG, Li Y, Oyen ML, et al. Extracellular-matrix tethering regulates stem-cell fate. Nat Mater. 2012;11(7): 642–9.
39. Hirao A, Arai F, Suda T. Regulation of cell cycle in hematopoietic stem cells by the niche. Cell Cycle. 2004;3(12):1481–3.
40. Ema H, Suda T. Two anatomically distinct niches regulate stem cell activity. Blood. 2012;120(11): 2174–81.
41. Marending M, Luder HU, Brunner TJ, Knecht S, Stark WJ, Zehnder M. Effect of sodium hypochlorite on human root dentine–mechanical, chemical and structural evaluation. Int Endod J. 2007;40(10): 786–93.
42. Ring KC, Murray PE, Namerow KN, Kuttler S, Garcia-Godoy F. The comparison of the effect of endodontic irrigation on cell adherence to root canal dentin. J Endod. 2008;34(12):1474–9.
43. Desai P, Himel V. Comparative safety of various intracanal irrigation systems. J Endod. 2009;35(4):545–9.
44. Hockett JL, Dommisch JK, Johnson JD, Cohenca N. Antimicrobial efficacy of two irrigation techniques in tapered and nontapered canal preparations: an in vitro study. J Endod. 2008;34(11):1374–7.
45. Cohenca N, Heilborn C, Johnson JD, Flores DS, Ito IY, da Silva LA. Apical negative pressure irrigation versus conventional irrigation plus triantibiotic intracanal dressing on root canal disinfection in dog teeth. Oral Surg Oral Med Oral Pathol Oral Radiol Endod. 2010;109(1):e42–6.
46. da Silva LA, Nelson-Filho P, da Silva RA, Flores DS, Heilborn C, Johnson JD, et al. Revascularization and periapical repair after endodontic treatment using apical negative pressure irrigation versus conventional irrigation plus triantibiotic intracanal dressing in dogs' teeth with apical periodontitis. Oral Surg Oral Med Oral Pathol Oral Radiol Endod. 2010;109(5):779–87.
47. Takushige T, Cruz EV, Asgor Moral A, Hoshino E. Endodontic treatment of primary teeth using a combination of antibacterial drugs. Int Endod J. 2004;37(2):132–8.
48. Sato T, Hoshino E, Uematsu H, Noda T. In vitro antimicrobial susceptibility to combinations of drugs on bacteria from carious and endodontic lesions of

human deciduous teeth. Oral Microbiol Immunol. 1993;8(3):172–6.
49. Shuping GB, Orstavik D, Sigurdsson A, Trope M. Reduction of intracanal bacteria using nickel-titanium rotary instrumentation and various medications. J Endod. 2000;26(12):751–5.
50. Ruparel NB, Teixeira FB, Ferraz CC, Diogenes A. Direct effect of intracanal medicaments on survival of stem cells of the apical papilla. J Endod. 2012; 38(10):1372–5.
51. Althumairy R, Teixeira FB, Henry MA, Diogenes A. The effect of dentin conditioning with intracanal medicaments on the survival of stem cells of apical papilla. J Endod. 2014;40(4):521–5.
52. Berkhoff JA, Chen PB, Teixeira FB, Diogenes A. Evaluation of triple antibiotic paste removal by different irrigation procedures. J Endod. 2014;40(8): 1172–7.
53. Martin G, Ricucci D, Gibbs JL, Lin LM. Histological findings of revascularized/revitalized immature permanent molar with apical periodontitis using platelet-rich plasma. J Endod. 2013;39(1):138–44.
54. Shimizu E, Ricucci D, Albert J, Alobaid AS, Gibbs JL, Huang GT, et al. Clinical, radiographic, and histological observation of a human immature permanent tooth with chronic apical abscess after revitalization treatment. J Endod. 2013;39(8):1078–83.
55. Wang X, Thibodeau B, Trope M, Lin LM, Huang GT. Histologic characterization of regenerated tissues in canal space after the revitalization/revascularization procedure of immature dog teeth with apical periodontitis. J Endod. 2010;36(1):56–63.
56. Yamauchi N, Yamauchi S, Nagaoka H, Duggan D, Zhong S, Lee SM, et al. Tissue engineering strategies for immature teeth with apical periodontitis. J Endod. 2011;37(3):390–7.

Conclusion and Final Remarks 19

Bettina Basrani

Abstract
This final chapter is intended to summarize the main ideas of this irrigation book and give a perpective into the future of root canal disinfection.

Treatment must have a goal and the path to that goal must be based upon the best scientific evidence available. What then are the goals of root canal treatment? The principle goal is the control of infection, be it the elimination of microorganisms from an infected root canal system or the prevention of root canal infection in a tooth that has been successfully treated. The prospects for maintaining the health of the tissues surrounding a treated tooth are also influenced by the nature and quality of the procedures used in restoring the tooth to function. The challenges facing the clinician in achieving these goals however are often hampered by the form (biofilm) and pervasive nature of root canal infection, the complex anatomy in which it exists, and the limitations of the technology currently available to the clinician who routinely addresses these issues. Mainstream endodontic treatment is still based upon the use of metal instruments to clean and shape the principle canals of the root canal system and the disinfecting agents used to address infection that is left behind in the main canal and present in areas unreachable by the cleaning and shaping instruments.

The effectiveness of root canal cleaning and shaping has been improved over the years through the introduction of different instrument shapes and the use of more versatile metals and alloys that were not available in the past. It has been an exciting time in endodontics as new instruments, new alloys, and new modalities of instrumentation came on market to allow preparation of canals that at one time were considered untreatable because of their anatomy. Unfortunately, while the selection of teeth for treatment broadened, the prognosis for success subsequent to their treatment remained the same. Studies have repeatedly shown that even when using state-of-the-art instruments, motors, and devices, biofilm still remains on the walls of the main areas of the root canal and in the irregularities and complex pathways of its anatomy. It is as obvious today as it was many years ago that means other than the mechanical preparation of the root canal system are necessary to reduce and hopefully eliminate a microbial presence or, as stated in terms of our treatment goals, to eliminate the presence of microorganisms.

B. Basrani, DDS, MSc, RCDC (F), PhD
Associate Professor, Director M.Sc. Endodontics Program, Faculty of Dentistry, University of Toronto, 348C-124 Edward Street, Toronto, ON M5G1G6, Canada
e-mail: Bettina.Basrani@dentistry.utoronto.ca

B. Basrani (ed.), *Endodontic Irrigation: Chemical Disinfection of the Root Canal System*,
DOI 10.1007/978-3-319-16456-4_19

Over the years various agents and combination of agents have been used to augment disinfection of the root canal. Interestingly, sodium hypochlorite first introduced over a half century ago has remained the most effective and consequently the most widely used. Despite its effectiveness however, microorganisms still remain, be they in significantly reduced concentrations after use. This is not to say that other agents have not been introduced to augment mechanical preparation of the root canal and it is not surprising that some are currently in use. Chlorhexidine, MTAD, and other proprietary solutions, for example, have been used and are still being used as an adjunct in treatment. The same might be said for interappointment dressings. None however have proven themselves to be more effective or yield a more favorable treatment outcome to than sodium hypochlorite when used alone. The fact that microorganisms continue to persist in the root canal after treatment indicates that while we have been able to successfully treat many more types of teeth, we have not been successful in achieving the intended treatment goal of routine and predictable root canal sterility.

This has not remained unaddressed. As this textbook goes to press, new and exciting methods of root canal irrigation and disinfection are being developed for use in endodontic treatment. These vary from new methods in the delivery of NaOCl, and new methods of NaOCl activation, to improve its anti-biofilm activity and to extend its antimicrobial action to otherwise unreachable areas of the root canal. Innovative researches using lasers and photoactivated nanoparticles for root canal disinfection are also being tried and have also shown some measure of promise. So what does the future hold for the next generation of endodontic clinicians? Will these new methods be simply a variation of the current approach to root canal irrigation with NaOCl, or will they be a vastly different technology that does not rely on NaOCl. Will the treatment outcome be the same, or will it show significant improvement? Only time will tell. Another question remains as to whether these new technologies can be readily incorporated into endodontic practice with the same ease and expense as are the methods of root canal irrigation being used today. As an optimist, I have every expectation that something better than what we currently use will become available and that, with its or their introduction, our ability to eliminate microorganisms from the root canal will improve. Ultimately we will move closer to achieving our goal and ultimately we will witness a rise in treatment outcome.

Dr. Shimon Friedman, in a lecture delivered at the 2014 American Association of Endodontists' annual meeting, said that when new technologies come on the market, they fall into 2 categories: (1) those that claim to facilitate treatment (with no impact on outcome) and (2) those that claim to improve the outcome of treatment for the patients. The 1st category includes the use of apex locators, microscopes, motor-driven endodontic instruments, etc. These improvements make our work as endodontists easier and more predictable. The 2nd category includes the use of MTA for sealing of perforations or in inducing apexification, where clinical evidence has shown that the prognosis of treatment has improved. All these devices, instruments, and materials that either improve our comfort as practitioners or improve the outcome for patients can be incorporated to the clinical practice without delay.

But what about the enhanced irrigation devices described in this chapter? Which category do they fall into? Unfortunately, there is not enough clinical evidence to currently support their use with a better outcome. Perhaps our current ways of measuring the outcome are not sensitive enough to measure the changes that may occur. Maybe the sample size is too small for the type of interventional research that is needed to show a difference, or maybe none of the irrigation enhanced modality is significantly better than sodium hypochlorite in a handheld syringe. Logic suggests that if these irrigation devices are making our irrigation procedure easier without causing harm to the patient, there is nothing wrong with incorporating into practice now. But if we are looking for an improvement in the outcome of treatment of apical periodontitis, we will have to wait for evidence derived from blinded and controlled from clinical studies.

Acknowledgement I would like to thank Dr. Calvin Torneck for his feedback in writing this chapter.

Index

B. Basrani (ed.), *Endodontic Irrigation: Chemical Disinfection of the Root Canal System*,
DOI 10.1007/978-3-319-16456-4

FSC
www.fsc.org
MIX
Papier | Fördert gute Waldnutzung
FSC® C083411

Kolibri 360 GmbH
Ferdinand-Jühlke-Straße 7
99095 Erfurt, Deutschland
produktsicherheit@kolibri360.de